Comprehensive School Physical Activity Programs

Putting Research Into Evidence-Based Practice

Russell L. Carson, PhD

PlayCore
University of Northern Colorado, Professor Emeritus

Collin A. Webster, PhD

University of South Carolina

Editors

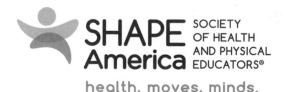

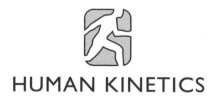

Library of Congress Cataloging-in-Publication Data

Names: Carson, Russell L., 1975- editor. | Webster, Collin A., 1976- editor.
Title: Comprehensive school physical activity programs : putting research into evidence-based
  practice / Russell L. Carson, PhD, University of Northern
  Colorado, Collin A. Webster, PhD, University of South Carolina, Editors.
Description: Reston, VA : Shape America, [2020] | Includes bibliographical
  references and index.
Identifiers: LCCN 2018056298 (print) | LCCN 2018058973 (ebook) | ISBN
  9781492591184 (epub) | ISBN 9781492559726 (PDF) | ISBN 9781492559719
  (print)
Subjects: LCSH: Physical education and training--Research. | Physical
  education and training--Study and teaching.
Classification: LCC GV361 (ebook) | LCC GV361 .C636 2020 (print) | DDC
  613.7--dc23
LC record available at https://lccn.loc.gov/2018056298

ISBN: 978-1-4925-5971-9 (print)

The web addresses cited in this text were current as of January 2019, unless otherwise noted.

Acquisitions Editor: Ray Vallese; **SHAPE America Editor:** Thomas Lawson; **Developmental Editor:** Melissa J. Zavala; **Copyeditor:** Erin Cler; **Proofreader:** Anne Rumery; **Indexer:** Andrea J. Hepner; **Permissions Manager:** Dalene Reeder; **Graphic Designer:** Joe Buck; **Cover Designer:** Keri Evans; **Cover Design Associate:** Susan Rothermel Allen; **Photographs (interior):** ©Human Kinetics, unless otherwise noted; **Photo Production Manager:** Jason Allen; **Senior Art Manager:** Kelly Hendren; **Illustrations:** ©Human Kinetics, unless otherwise noted; **Printer:** Sheridan Books

SHAPE America – Society of Health and Physical Educators

1900 Association Drive
Reston, VA 20191
800-213-7193
www.shapeamerica.org

Printed in the United States of America

10 9 8 7 6 5 4 3 2 1

The paper in this book is certified under a sustainable forestry program.

Human Kinetics
P.O. Box 5076
Champaign, IL 61825-5076
Website: www.HumanKinetics.com

In the United States, email info@hkusa.com or call 800-747-4457.

In Canada, email info@hkcanada.com.

In the United Kingdom/Europe, email hk@hkeurope.com.

For information about Human Kinetics' coverage in other areas of the world,

please visit our website: **www.HumanKinetics.com**

E7201

CONTENTS

Preface   viii

Part IV Contextual Considerations   171

PREFACE

Youth physical inactivity—particularly its correlation with preventable chronic diseases, premature death, and poorer performance in school—is a topic of widespread scientific inquiry and vast media attention. Worldwide, a growing number of developed nations face the same dilemma:

- While it is known that physical activity (PA) is critically important for children's physical, cognitive, social, and emotional health, many children engage in too little PA.
- When placed in positions of influence, many adults do too little to promote active lifestyles in children.

These trends trace to myriad origins, span wide swaths of the societal landscape, and carry implications for multiple scientific disciplines and professional communities. Adopting behavioral patterns, learning competencies, and formulating dispositions that support the recommended accumulation of 60 minutes of PA each day are crucial steps to establishing adaptive and long-term PA habits that continue into adulthood.

As researchers and practitioner advocates so commonly note, the school setting presents a wealth of opportunity for systemic PA infusion into youth behaviors, values, and goals. Virtually all children and adolescents attend school, and existing resources, such as teachers, space, and professional learning initiatives, provide an impressive infrastructure for fostering daily PA promotion. Yet schools generally are ill prepared for making a significant impact on daily youth PA levels, are highly resistant to organizational change efforts, and require strong leadership and coordination across all dimensions of their infrastructure to institutionalize educational innovations. The complex challenges of targeting schools and school professionals as change agents for public health initiatives have stimulated us to collate and share the vast possibilities of promoting youth PA by bridging research and practice in one place.

The primary reason for publishing this book is to provide a scholarly and informative resource on what has become the sine qua non conceptualization for the promotion of PA through schools, affectionately termed a *comprehensive school physical activity program*, or CSPAP. Rooted in an earlier and broader conceptualization for the promotion of school health, known as a *coordinated school health program*, the CSPAP model was initially outlined as a position statement of the National Association for Sport and Physical Education (NASPE) in 2008. In one decade, the model has rapidly spread by way of national task forces; campaigns; resource guides; funding opportunities; trainings; dedicated special issues in journals; academic symposia at national meetings; an updated CSPAP position statement; a web page with its namesake; a CSPAP research special interest group; and, most impressively, a national collaborative of over 90 supporting organizations, known as Active Schools. These initiatives have mobilized a CSPAP field of study and practice into what is now considered a national framework for physical activity and physical education (Centers for Disease Control and Prevention, 2015, 2017).

One of the most important goals in creating this book was to bring together a set of chapters, written by pioneers and recognized practitioners in the CSPAP field, on the most prominent conceptual perspectives, issues, and developments in the field. Because a complete summary of the cumulative work in this growing field does not yet exist, this book is designed to accommodate the growing needs of academic researchers, school practitioners, district coordinators, educators, advocates, organizations, university faculty, and students who want to learn more about CSPAP or undertake ways to increase daily PA opportunities in and around schools. Stakeholder groups likely to benefit from this text include

- *K-12 teachers* (physical education and classroom teachers), who can use this text to plan and implement CSPAP initiatives;
- *K-12 school staff* (administrators and support staff), who can use this text to support, evaluate, and get involved in school-wide PA programming;
- *policy makers* (district coordinators, district councils, and parents), who can use this text to promote and sustain PA initiatives for youth in and around schools;

- *higher education faculty and students* (teacher educators, scientific researchers, and graduate students), who can use this text for courses and research programs in physical education teacher education, PA and public health, and community health education and promotion; and

- *community members and groups* (nonprofit and for-profit organizations, health agencies, and professional membership organizations), who can use this text as a professional reference for partnering with schools to advance PA opportunities for youth.

We are hopeful this book will facilitate new research, accelerated learning, and innovative solutions for diverse audiences about the utility and reality of CSPAPs.

The 22 chapters are organized into six sections. Part I, Foundations and Contemporary Perspectives, includes two chapters, which provide the historical and foundational perspectives and policy landscapes of the CSPAP approach, respectively. Part II, Conceptual Models for CSPAP Implementation, encompasses three chapters, the purpose of which is to outline, in tandem, internal (within-school), external (beyond the school), and psychological (within-individual) factors that should be considered in program design, implementation, and sustainability. In Part III, Research on Program Effectiveness, six chapters are devoted to examining and interpreting the existing research concentrated on the effectiveness of established programs and previous interventions. The first five chapters in the section focus on specific components of the CSPAP model, and the sixth chapter examines the effectiveness of multicomponent approaches to PA promotion through schools. Part IV, Contextual Considerations, includes four chapters. The first two chapters in the section illuminate special considerations for effective programming within urban and rural settings, respectively. The third chapter reviews current and ongoing international CSPAP initiatives, and the fourth chapter considers the application of the CSPAP model to alternative contexts beyond the K-12 school setting. In Part V, Developing, Measuring, and Promoting CSPAPs, issues pertaining to the critical aspects of advancing and promoting sustainable CSPAP

implementation are divided into four chapters, which focus first on using assessments to determine the PA promotion needs of a school community; then on instrumentation and procedures for measuring school-wide PA programming; and finally, on processes for both evaluating and advocating for CSPAPs. Part VI, Looking to the Future, closes the text with three chapters. The first chapter in this section examines current reform efforts, aligned with CSPAP preparation, within preprofessional programs in teacher education and other fields. In the penultimate chapter, the varied tools and future potential for utilizing technology to deliver and assess CSPAP efforts are reviewed. The final chapter summarizes and synthesizes the book's content to gauge promising directions for the disciplines of study that inform the CSPAP knowledge base as well as to recommend strategies to advance and further coalesce the fields of practice where CSPAPs intersect, take root, and blossom.

Chapter content is structured using six subheadings, beginning with a *review of research*. The subsequent sections provide readers with bulleted *knowledge claims* from the research (what we know), *knowledge gaps and directions for future research* (what we need to know), and *evidence-based recommendations and applications* (what we need to do) geared toward at least two practitioner groups: school staff (e.g., teachers, administrators, and support personnel) and community partners (e.g., universities, local policy makers, district offices, parents, and youth organizations). Either real-world or fictitious *case examples* are then presented near the end of the chapters to help demonstrate the practical recommendations and applications presented. To facilitate thought and dialogue around chapter content, each chapter ends with *questions to consider* for discussion. In keeping with this chapter-closing strategy, we have posed six questions to guide the reader's reflection as we embark together on a journey into the pages of this book, navigate the impressive trove of knowledge they hold, and preview the inexorable expansion of CSPAP research and practice. Each question will be revisited in the concluding chapter as a means to advance the science and professional work devoted to CSPAPs. We are hopeful the consistent organizational structure in each chapter allows readers to immerse themselves in the content and its translation and practical relevance. Overall, each chapter section is intended to capture the interest of a broad readership and provide stakeholder groups with information they find most useful for their purposes.

The spirit behind the development of this book is that the CSPAP approach is worth examining. Through the application of CSPAP research to practice, it may be possible to gain unique perspectives about how to generate and sustain successful initiatives in educational settings to increase youth PA and promote long-term engagement in active behavior. The rapid growth of the field and the increasing number of diverse and exceptional scholars (many of whom are contributors to this book) are indications of the need for this resource. We envision that the corpus of work compiled herein will help to espouse continued efforts in both research and practice to generate programs that maximize the potential of educational settings to uniquely serve the PA needs of every child and adolescent. Now, with the publication of this book, those who want to pursue CSPAP research and practice have a comprehensive resource with which to do so, one that offers access to the leading thoughts, invaluable tools, and challenging questions that help propel the CSPAP field to its next level of depth and clarity.

QUESTIONS TO CONSIDER THROUGHOUT THE BOOK

Part I

How does the policy landscape reflect the evolving values and traditions of the CSPAP model?

Part II

What conceptual and theoretical approaches could guide CSPAP practice and collaboration?

Part III

What does the latest evidence say about the effectiveness of each CSPAP component and multicomponent approaches in promoting PA?

Part IV

How does context factor into best practices for CSPAPs?

Part V

What are some promising strategies for planning, researching, evaluating, and promoting CSPAPs?

Part VI

What are the potential contributions of preservice education and technology integration in CSPAP research and practice?

PART I

Foundations and Contemporary Perspectives

CHAPTER 1

CSPAPs: History, Foundations, Possibilities, and Barriers

Hans van der Mars, PhD
Arizona State University

Kent A. Lorenz, PhD
San Francisco State University

This chapter serves as the introduction to this edited text, which focuses on trends and developments around the comprehensive school physical activity program (CSPAP) framework. In it, we provide a brief overview of what constitutes a CSPAP, which also includes possible misconceptions of and resistance to CSPAP development and preparation of professionals who are to deliver CSPAPs. This overview is followed by a description of the factors that led to the development of the CSPAP framework,

CSPAP's link with national physical activity (PA) recommendations for children and youth, and CSPAP's theoretical roots. The final sections will focus on why CSPAPs constitute a critical opportunity for school physical education and will identify the various barriers to full-fledged CSPAP implementation. Subsequent chapters will show that much has happened around the CSPAP framework relative to its promotion and implementation and the empirical study of its multiple aspects.

Emergence of CSPAPs

As of 2017 in the United States, a national framework and guidelines exist for the development and implementation of a CSPAP, which serves as a proposed model for physical education and PA within all schools (Centers for Disease Control and Prevention [CDC], 2013, 2015). CSPAPs are supported by a national collaborative of public and private sector organizations (e.g., CDC), institutes of science and medicine (e.g., Institute of Medicine), and health and physical educators (e.g., SHAPE America). These organizations outline the need for increased access and opportunity for all children to engage in PA before, during, and after the school day. Moreover, CSPAPs create layers of influence and engage families, school staff, and the surrounding community to be physically active role models.

The CSPAP movement has gained momentum in recent years, starting with the guiding model of former First Lady Michelle Obama's *Let's Move!* Active Schools initiative (figure 1.1) and moving to the publication of more peer-reviewed research papers examining the effects of CSPAPs, the creation of a special interest group and web page within the national organization SHAPE America, and an increased emphasis within physical educa-

tion teacher education (PETE) programs across the United States (Kulinna et al., 2017). Since 2013, the CSPAP model has reached over 23,000 schools; 33,000 educators; and 12,000,000 students (Active Schools, 2018).

This chapter serves as an introduction to the history and emergence of the CSPAP framework within the United States and investigates its roots within public health and the national recommendations for increased PA for children and youth. We will explore the theoretical models that provide the conceptual scaffolding for CSPAPs as well as provide a brief discussion regarding the barriers to and prospects of implementation of CSPAPs in schools, which outlines the rest of the book and provides a foundation for the reader.

History and Emergence of CSPAPs

CSPAPs emerged as part of public health efforts to address a shifting culture of increased sedentary time and the rising prevalence of hypokinetic chronic diseases, such as obesity, heart disease, and diabetes (Biddle et al., 2004). The rise in the percentage of overweight and obese children and youth (Ogden et al., 2016) prompted extensive

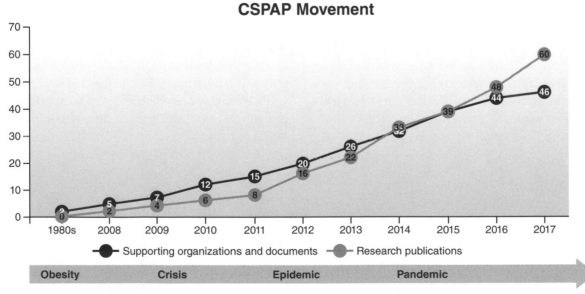

Figure 1.1   Growth of CSPAP-related resources and research since 2008.

© Russell Carson

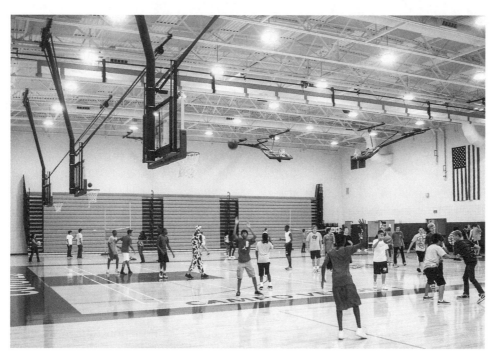

Open access for play opportunities, with appropriate equipment and supervision, is one way to help students meet daily PA recommendations.

© Hans van der Mars

programmatic and research efforts in school settings starting in the early 1980s and the subsequent publication of numerous documents with PA recommendations, policies, and guidelines by government, professional and research societies, and private foundations. The U.S. Department of Health and Human Services (HHS, 1990, 2000, 2010) published its Healthy People objectives, which included objectives specific to increasing PA levels. It also included objectives specific to school physical education. Effectively delivered school physical education is one of only a few interventions for which there is sufficient evidence that it positively affects children and youth (e.g., CDC, 2001; Heath et al., 2012; Pate et al., 2006). In 2008, the first-ever national PA guidelines for all Americans were published along with a midterm follow-up report in 2012, and a second edition released in 2018 (HHS, 2008, 2012, 2018). And finally, the National Physical Activity Plan (National Physical Activity Plan Alliance [NPAPA], 2010, 2016b) reflects a multipronged approach to promoting PA across all age groups. This plan brings together 10 societal sectors, including education. The education sector offers general strategies and specific tactics aimed at increasing PA levels, including

for children and youth (Siedentop, 2009). The NPAPA (2014, 2016a, 2018) also spearheads a recurring U.S. Report Card on Physical Activity for Children and Youth, with schools regularly receiving a nearly failing grade (D-minus). Therefore, despite national efforts to promote PA for youth in schools, it appears that only between 21 and 40 percent of youth are experiencing benefits from increased PA programming within the education sector (NPAPA, 2016b).

A precursor for the NPAP (NPAPA, 2010, 2016b) was the *Guidelines for School and Community Programs to Promote Lifelong Physical Activity Among Young People* (CDC, 1997). These guidelines outlined objectives related to increasing PA participation of school-aged youth. In addition to PA targets, the NPAP also includes recommendations for schools and community programs that span a range of stakeholders. These recommendations include policy and environmental changes, effective physical and health education, extracurricular activities, school and community personnel training, and parental and community involvement. The astute reader will recognize these recommendations to be similar to the five core components of a CSPAP: effective physical education programming, opportunity for PA before and after school, PA during school, staff involvement, and family and community engagement (CDC, 2013).

The first document that specifically references CSPAPs was published in 2008 as a position statement. It included a central recommendation for all schools to implement a CSPAP to assist in meeting newly passed federal legislation (National Association for Sport and Physical Education [NASPE], 2008; SHAPE America, 2013). This legislation (Public Law 108-265) outlined requirements of the Child Nutrition and WIC Reauthorization Act of 2004, which mandated that schools with federally funded meal programs develop wellness policies that addressed the nutrition education, food service, and PA needs of students (NASPE, 2008). The goal of these policies was to engage a range of stakeholders to increase the emphasis on healthy eating, PA, and overall wellness of students in schools. Since then, there has been an explosion of resources specific to promoting and supporting CSPAPs in the form of literature, presentations, professional papers, research publications, position statements, and guidelines (see figure 1.1).

CSPAP's Roots Within Public Health and National Physical Activity Recommendations

In 1991, Sallis and McKenzie wrote a pivotal article suggesting that physical education programs and teachers can play a vital role in public health through the promotion of lifelong PA participation. Twenty years later, a reflection on the progress toward the alignment of physical education with public health revealed some positive developments (Sallis et al., 2012). There is an increased awareness of the physical, emotional, and academic benefits of PA and how physical education and school-based opportunities can help children and youth accumulate the necessary PA (Sallis et al., 2012). However, the authors also noted that there are still opportunities for improvement. Most relevant here is the reflection that education has not fully adopted public health ideals for physical education or school-based PA (Sallis et al., 2012). This is where the CSPAP framework can serve as a benchmark. The ultimate aim of a CSPAP is

to increase the amount of PA all students get in a typical school day that is in direct concordance with public health recommendations (CDC, 2013; HHS, 2008, NASPE, 2008).

The current national PA recommendations in the United States are for every American youth, aged 6 to 17, to accumulate a minimum of 60 minutes of PA per day (HHS, 2018). This includes moderate-to-vigorous PA (MVPA), muscle strengthening activities, and bone strengthening activities to engage youth in developmentally appropriate and enjoyable PA (HHS, 2018). Despite these recommendations, there is surveillance data indicating that PA participation declines as children move through their school years (Katzmarzyk et al., 2017; Pate et al., 2002). By the time the typical student reaches middle school (12-14 years old), less than two-thirds of boys and about half of girls meet PA recommendations, with a further decline to about one-third of boys and one-fourth of girls meeting guidelines during high school (16-18 years old; Katzmarzyk et al., 2017). In combination, this data contributes to consistently poor NPAP U.S. Report Card results for overall PA for children: D minus in both 2014 and 2016 (NPAPA, 2014, 2016a).

Because 97 percent of youth spend time in schools (National Center for Education Statistics, 2016; Sallis & McKenzie, 1991), schools are a logical place for interventions to increase PA and reduce time spent in sedentary behaviors. HHS (1990, 2000, 2010) published its Healthy People objectives, which included objectives specific to increasing PA levels. Objectives specific to school physical education were also included. In 2008, the first-ever national PA guidelines for all Americans were published along with a midterm follow-up report in 2012 and second edition in 2018 (HHS, 2008, 2012, 2018). Moreover, Bassett and colleagues (2013) published a review of school-based PA interventions and noted that a combination of policy and environmental modifications can increase the amount of daily PA in schools consistent with ecological models of healthy behaviors.

CSPAP's Theoretical Roots

The study and implementation of CSPAPs has its roots in various ecological model theories of behavior (e.g., Cohen et al., 2000; Hovell et al.,

2002; Lohrmann, 2010; Sallis et al., 2008). The social-ecological framework (Stokols, 1992) has been a frequently used basis for much of the research aimed at building the evidence base on PA and the improvement thereof. More recently, Carson, Castelli, Beighle, et al. (2014) proposed a CSPAP conceptual framework for the promotion of school-based PA.

The environment is a powerful determinant of PA (Sallis et al., 2012), and Bauer and colleagues (2014) noted that improving our understanding of the role the environment plays is central to developing key PA promotion and intervention strategies. This understanding of the role the environment plays aligns well with Hovell and colleagues' (2002) behavioral ecological model (see figure 1.2). The behavioral ecological model has been the basis for an expansive evidence base supporting changes in other health behaviors as well, such as encouraging child car seat use (i.e., injury prevention), smoking cessation, and condom use.

In the behavioral ecological model, improvements in health behavior (such as PA) can be better achieved through the effective arrangement of environmental and social contingencies along with reinforcement; these contingencies function at a range of levels (from the individual to society). For example, beyond effective physical education, schools that have expansive PA venues, provide easily accessible equipment and adult supervision, and actively promote PA behavior are more likely to have a greater number of students engaging in PA during discretionary times (i.e., before, during, and after school; e.g., Lorenz et al., 2017; Mahar et al., 2011; McKenzie et al., 2000; Stylianou, Hodges-Kulinna, et al., 2016; Stylianou, van der Mars, et al., 2016).

In addition, relative to the during-the-school-day component of CSPAPs, classroom teachers' use of PA recesses to break up academic instruction has been shown to be an effective strategy to improve students' on-task behavior, focus, concentration, academic performance, and PA accumulation (e.g., Erwin et al., 2012; Goh et al., 2014; Mahar, 2011; Mahar et al., 2006). These improvements in students are reinforcing to teachers in that they can focus more on academic instruction and less on managing students' behavior. Moreover, recess on playgrounds with supervision, added equipment, and improved playground markings provides another important PA opportunity for elementary aged students to

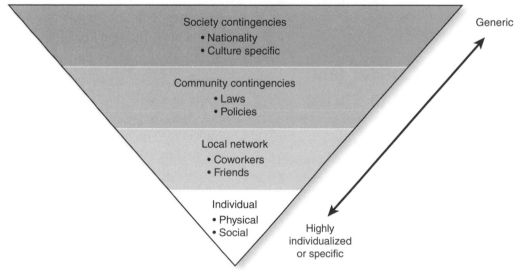

Figure 1.2 Schematic of the behavioral ecological model (Hovell et al., 2002), which outlines how different levels of contingencies influence and reinforce behaviors.

Reprinted by permission from M. F. Howell, D.R.F. Wahlgren, and C.A. Gehrman, Behavioral Ecological Model: Integrating Public Health and Behavioral Science, in *Emerging Theories in Health Promotion Practice and Research: Strategies for Improving Public Health,* edited by R.J. Diclemente, R.A. Crosby, and M.C. Kegler (San Francisco, CA: Jossey-Bass, 2002), 363.

break up the school day (e.g., Ridgers et al., 2007; Stratton & Mullan, 2005; Willenberg et al., 2010).

Similarly, publicly funded school campuses are also environments that can support the health and wellness of teachers and administrative and support staff as well as the health of families and members of the surrounding community. Connecting schools and school campuses to local health and wellness programming would create a stronger and broader PA-supportive culture. Many high school campuses have weight rooms for their athletic teams, which are seldom used during evening and weekend hours. School districts (and individual schools) can be encouraged to employ shared-use agreements (Spengler, 2012), thereby making campus-based PA venues more accessible to individuals and outside organizations, such as sport clubs, during evening and weekend hours. Despite the potential, as of 2014, only 4 out of 10 municipalities had shared-use agreements with their school districts (Omura et al., 2017).

Thus, through the shaping of physical-, social-, and policy-specific contingencies, PA levels can be increased not just at the individual level but also at the cultural level (e.g., school campus). This, in turn, contributes to the reduction in the health risks (and health-care costs) associated with physical inactivity. Schools are one of many social institutions that can directly support or suppress PA of children and youth (others being sport clubs, park and recreation programs, and Boys and Girls Clubs).

Why CSPAPs: A Critical (and Final?) Opportunity to Thrive

For many years, physical education has sought to be viewed as an important and relevant school subject. The previously described emergence of CSPAPs placed schools as a central site among other larger national initiatives aimed at increasing PA levels. Just as school physical education alone did not cause the problems of overweight and obesity, it alone cannot solve these problems. School physical education is only one of several key players that focus on promoting PA and, thus, improving the health status of our nation's children and youth (e.g., Institute of Medicine, 2013; NPAPA, 2018; Pate et al., 2006). Fortunately, the

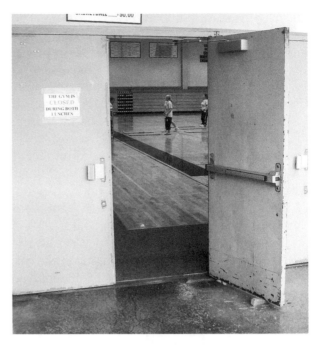

Visual prompts, such as this sign indicating that the gym is closed, suppress PA during school lunch.

© Hans van der Mars

field of physical education is one of many societal sectors, along with other health agencies, professions, nonprofits, and institutions, that share an interest in promoting PA among children and youth (e.g., CDC, 2013; NPAPA, 2016b, 2018).

Core Characteristics Needed Within Physical Education for a Thriving CSPAP Culture

- Increasing *all* students' PA levels within physical education and beyond is a legitimate and credible goal.

- Physical education alone is not enough as an intervention to support and promote health-enhancing PA in schools. Physical educators are uniquely qualified and positioned to be leaders who can push campus communities toward a culture of PA.

- Full-fledged implementation of all five components of the CSPAP framework is the gold standard. However, there is considerable variability in individual school contexts (e.g., administrative leadership, funding, facilities, location [rural vs. suburban], and community resources). This variability will likely produce a wide variety of hybrid CSPAP versions. The key is for *all* schools to provide access and opportunity for PA for *all* students in physical education and throughout the school day to the maximum extent possible.

- Skill learning and PA are *not* mutually exclusive outcomes. Continuing to view them as such will hamper effective delivery of school physical education (e.g., Blankenship, 2013; Harvey et al., 2016; Kretchmar, 2006).

- Strong state-level policies in support of school physical education and school-based PA create the necessary conditions for CSPAPs to become more prevalent.

Importantly, many outside organizations have recognized the significant contributions that school physical education can make to promoting PA among K-12 students. Such recognition has created an opportunity for physical education to be a partner institution. Yet, in many ways, physical education has created its own barriers, which likely will impede progress toward full CSPAP implementation (e.g., Sallis, 2017). As a field, we need to be mindful of the consequences of not embracing the CSPAP framework that is health focused. That is, school physical education likely will continue to be marginalized and lose its place as a contributor to successfully promoting PA among school-aged youth, and we risk not being invited back. There are many other organizations, corporations, and individuals that are part of this broad effort who will gladly take the place of physical education. It is not hard to see how that situation will only widen the existing PA access and opportunity disparity. Thus, the question to consider is this: Why would anyone (i.e., teaching professionals, school administrators, PETE professors, and graduate students) affiliated with school physical education who has a genuine interest in promoting students' engagement in physical activities for a lifetime decline this opportunity to contribute? The health and well-being of children and youth form the foundation for their overall development. Given today's health status of children (notably those who are economically disadvantaged; Annie E. Casey Foundation, 2017), the CSPAP framework is unifying for the field, which is inclusive of all possible philosophical and curricular persuasions.

Possibilities of CSPAPs

Full implementation of CSPAPs in schools would be the ultimate goal. However, the reality for many schools is that their context (e.g., geographic, financial, and social) will affect whether CSPAPs in their community will include only one or all four components beyond effective physical education. However, schools and those in PA leadership positions can choose from a host of CSPAP implementation options (see figure 1.3).

Physical education professionals with assistance and support from others (including other school staff, parents, professionals in the community, and partner organizations with similar goals) can choose from a menu of options (see figure 1.3) aimed at increasing PA of students, school staff, and community members. The school campus can become a central hub in the neighborhood or larger community with increasing health-enhancing PA as the prime target, thereby maximizing the school's "caloric footprint." As outlined by the CSPAP guide for schools (CDC, 2013), school-based PA programs reflect the needs of the students and their families and the surrounding community and create supportive environments for everyone to engage in health-enhancing PA. This places physical education professionals in a prime position to coordinate and facilitate PA opportunities that are relevant within the school and community environment and connect personnel to stakeholders in the area surrounding the school (CDC, 2013).

Barriers to Overcome

Along with the excitement about the available CSPAP options, it is important to be cognizant of both external and internal forces at play that can inhibit or even push back at the development of a CSPAP. To be sure, despite its continuing marginalization, school physical education continues to evolve (e.g., professional resources, research base, standards, better fitness assessments, and a shift from developing fitness to promoting PA). However, there are numerous multidimensional barriers that will make full CSPAP implementation more complex. Recognizing and understanding

Great Ideas-Let's Get Moving

Before and after school

- Early-bird PA program with local YMCA
- After-school sports clubs
- FITT Zone-before school PA program open to all
- Targeted fitness clubs: zumba, yoga, pilates
- Activity clubs with rotating focus
- Xbox Kinect clubs (NIKE fitness trainer)
- Running clubs before and after school
- PA clubs: tag, sport, ultimate frisbee, etc.
- Teach a weekly flash-mob dance in bus room
- Wake-up and walk for 15-20 min/day
- Incorporate technology: relate it to use at home
- Community school activity-based programs on campus
- Monday-Sunday

Physical education

- Require students to take physical education daily
- Improve the quality of physical education to provide increased MVPA and time on task
- Be open to collaborations with other content classes
- Infuse a fitness component in every lesson
- Develop a spiraling, comprehensive, standards-based curriculum for grades P-12
- Provide enough equipment for every student to increase time on task and practice
- Implement teaching strategies and protocols that increase activity time
- Assess student learning and adjust instruction accordingly
- Incorporate technology use to enhance goal-setting

Family and community engagement

- Safe routes to school
- Bike-and-walk-to-school programs
- Community-sponsored physical activity programs
- Adopt an active school: commit time, money, equipment, and volunteers
- Fit City Initiative
- We Can program
- Family fitness nights
- Family Run-4-fun day
- Parents run-walk program
- Partnership with city sports and activity programs
- Invite parents and community partners to participate in before-school activity programs, recess, after-school programs, and help them feel that they are an integral part of the program and needed
- School-sponsored and promoted family time at local activity venues: bowling, swimming, kayaking, fishing

Activities for staff involvement

- Create a school wellness committee: encourage buy-in
- School Health Advisory Councils (SHAC)
- 10K day for staff and students
- Create staff wellness competition
- Develop an employee-wellness program
- Teach eye dominance and cognitive-motor link to use with students
- Add physical activity incentives to benefit program
- Conduct school fundraisers that incorporate physical activity
- Provide teacher training on how to conduct physical activity breaks
- Provide training on how to integrate movement into teaching
- Collaborate with staff to develop pedometer challenges
- Establish a Golden Sneaker Award for active classrooms or supportive principals
- Provide physical activity plans for advisory classes to use

During school

- Establish a 30-min rule, requiring classroom teachers to get students up and moving every 30 min
- Flash-Mob Fridays for middle school and high school
- Holiday celebration days incorporate physical activity segments as part of the activities
- Jog-a-thon as a school fundraiser
- Fitness breaks incorporated during school
- School public service announcements (PSAs) with a physical activity theme; students move with the message!
- Activity rewards for students who complete class work

- Active homeroom environments: fitness corner, yoga mat, exercise tubing, posted quiet body-weight exercise breaks
- Open gym-fitness center and exer-gaming area
- Homeroom competitions and challenges
- Fitness or wellness weeks at school
- Birthday celebrations
- Pull bars located in hallways and doorways
- Physical activity treasure chests with PA equipment located adjacent to play areas

Figure 1.3 Possible CSPAP implementation strategies.

Reprinted by permission from SHAPE America, *PAL Training Manual.*

these barriers will aid in employing strategies to overcome them. In this section, we will outline those barriers that we view as the most critical by highlighting the mostly external barriers and discussing those barriers that are more internal to the profession.

Governance and Funding of Education

Shifts in the composition of federal- and state-level legislatures directly affect priorities in education funding and regulations. For example, as can be seen in recent developments, the initial excitement around the prospects of physical education's benefiting from the 2015 passage of the *Every Student Succeeds Act* (ESSA) has waned in the wake of recent national elections. The planned Title II and IV funding that figured prominently for physical education in terms of creating significant professional development opportunities is in jeopardy.

Moreover, other recent developments since the 2016 election, such as the appointment of the new Secretary of Education, have increased the push for more funding for school vouchers and charter schools, to the detriment of traditional public schools. Charter schools (which are publicly funded) are being built at an unprecedented rate in many states (e.g., Arizona, Florida, and Texas) based on the claims that (1) they will perform better than traditional public schools and (2) competition between different schools will lift up all schools. Apart from the fact that charter schools can inflate their reported student performance by not accepting certain students who likely will not score well (i.e., students with special needs), more importantly, there is little evidence that students in charter schools consistently do better academically (their prime focus) or graduate students at a higher rate than their public school counterparts (Berliner et al., 2014).

Specific to physical education, charter schools are not required to hire certified physical education teachers, if they even offer physical education. And while CSPAP preparation in preservice PETE programs remains sporadic (e.g., Kwon et al., 2017), it is unlikely that noncertified personnel put in charge of physical education have the needed skills and knowledge to be a CSPAP campus leader.

Fluctuations in education funding are largely dependent on the makeup of the state legislatures as well as cycles in the national and state economies. With physical education (along with other offerings and services deemed "less central") continuing to be an easy target for cutbacks in school districts, it is unlikely that more funding for subjects such as physical education in public schools will be forthcoming. However, the field of physical education may find support for CSPAP implementation by teaming up with the health-care industry and private foundations that may be interested in taking more preventive approaches to managing the health of children and youth.

Weak Physical Education Policy Profiles at the State Level

Despite the wide recognition of the importance of physical education and PA, there is wide variability in state-level policy profiles (SHAPE America, 2016). In too many states, strong state-level policies on such issues as number of minutes of physical education and recess, class size, graduation requirements, waivers and substitutions, and state-level assessments are absent. Without these policies in place, such decisions are left to policy makers in individual districts and schools. Coupled with the obsession for improving students' academic performance, this makes the condition for improving the quality and quantity of physical education as well as other expanded PA opportunities more difficult. While stronger policy profiles alone are not the magic elixir, they do create the prerequisite conditions.

On the positive side in physical education, there now appears to be a clear recognition of the important role played by strong policies and the need for proactive advocacy. That advocacy is playing a larger role is evidenced by the improved presence of advocacy resources on SHAPE America's website as well as on the websites of some of the state-level physical education associations. Furthermore, there is evidence of positive impact as a consequence of well-crafted and strong state-level policies on the delivery of physical education, recess, and related student PA levels (e.g., Barroso et al., 2009; Cawley et al., 2007; Evenson et al., 2009; Kahan & McKenzie, 2015; Kelder et al., 2009; Lounsbery et al., 2013; Slater et al., 2012).

What remains unknown is how broad based state-level advocacy efforts are and to what extent the available evidence is translated effectively for policy makers.

Those devoted to making CSPAPs a reality in most schools (along with every other professional and scholar in physical education) will need to become active players in proactive advocacy on a sustained basis. This is an aspect of our work that is still uncharted waters for many, but as van der Mars (2018) noted, without effective proactive advocacy, school physical education will remain marginalized and full CSPAP implementation may remain out of reach. Increased and sustained advocacy efforts will help develop the kind of policy profiles at the state level that support delivery of effective physical education, ensure recess for all students in elementary schools, and create access to all PA venues on school campuses for all students, regardless of the time of day or day of the week.

Labor Relations in Education

Given today's labor relations climate in education, it is hard to see how most physical educators would commit to building a CSPAP without either additional pay or release time from regular day-to-day duties. One possible way of accomplishing this goal would be for teachers to negotiate such arrangements when teachers' contracts are renegotiated during collective bargaining.

State statutes requiring or providing the option of collective bargaining between public school teachers and their district employers gained popularity in the 1950s, thereby strengthening the role of teacher unions. This continued through the mid-1980s, resulting in 35 states having such statutes. Conversely, collective bargaining by state employees is prohibited in seven states (Arizona, Georgia, Mississippi, North Carolina, South Carolina, Texas, and Virginia; Lovenheim & Willén, 2016). In addition, teachers' strikes are illegal in 37 states, though few specify penalties for striking (Katula, 2012). Thus, in states with a "duty to bargain" (in public sector labor relations, this is also referred to as "meet and confer" or "consult" [Malin et al., 2012]) or at least where it is allowed, physical educators have leverage through their local teacher union to strive for labor conditions that would support efforts to develop CSPAPs.

An important positive example thereof is the Seattle public school district in 2015. After contract negotiations broke down, a five-day strike ensued. A new three-year collective bargaining agreement was reached that included mandatory daily recess at all Seattle public elementary schools. For states with collective bargaining options and requirements for public employees, physical educators who belong to their union can collective voice their wishes as part of contract negotiations. This constitutes a potentially effective strategy that can bring about increased support for building CSPAP-supportive school environments.

The next few barriers are more internal or proximal to the field of physical education. These barriers are discussed in the next sections.

Reality of Teaching Position Assignments

With the emergence of CSPAPs, the changing role of physical education professionals has been a focus. As part of efforts to provide professional development around developing and implementing CSPAPs, SHAPE America has developed workshops aimed at introducing teachers to the what, why, and how of CSPAPs as well as to the role that physical educators play in their successful implementation (Carson, Castelli, et al., 2014). After workshop completion, participants gain Physical Activity Leader (PAL) status, and this training appears to increase the number of PA opportunities within a school (Carson, Castelli, et al., 2014).

What remains unclear are the actual time and positional demands for physical educators who commit to implementing CSPAPs beyond the teaching of the regular physical education classes. Metzler (2015, see table 2) reported that, as a group, the six participating physical educators spent a combined total of 20 hours per week on planning and implementing CSPAP components beyond teaching their regular classes. It is unknown whether such a time commitment differs between secondary schools (often made up of several teachers as part of a department) and elementary schools (typically solo or traveling teacher) and how this translates into the willingness of teachers to create additional work for themselves during the school day. Moreover, many physical educators also commit to sport coaching during after-school hours, and many sports have become year-round endeavors, increasing time commitments, and making CSPAP implementation more difficult.

Without fundamental changes to how the typical position description for physical educators is structured, it is difficult to see how a single teacher at an elementary school could not only plan and implement but also sustain a full CSPAP. The obvious solution for full CSPAP implementation would be to provide physical educators release time from teaching a number of physical education lessons per week to function effectively as the campus PA leader. This would require school districts to hire additional physical education teachers to cover those class periods. Other strategies might be to recruit qualified professionals who can assist with planning and implementing expanded PA programming (e.g., community members). Another solution would be for school districts to partner with departments of public health, which could provide funding to hire additional support personnel.

Messaging in Presenting and Promoting CSPAPs

The CSPAP framework has been promoted vigorously in recent years. And, as with any other initiative, there are risks of misconceptions (and fears) emerging about what CSPAPs are and what they seek to accomplish. In addition, misconceptions about CSPAPs may also emerge as a consequence of a lack of accurate knowledge and understanding thereof (Carson, Pulling, et al., 2014).

In efforts to spread the good word about the why, what, and how of CSPAPs, the importance of effective messaging may have been overlooked as well as Luntz's (2007) notion of *it is not what someone says, but rather what is heard.* For example, despite including references to a physical education program being the "centerpiece" CSPAP component (see figure 1.1), the listeners may have only heard about the other four components and come away thinking *They want me to teach PE and all that other stuff? They can't be serious!* That is, an (over)emphasis on the other components may have led physical educators to believe that CSPAP advocates view the physical education program as less critical.

A related misconception is that the planning, implementing, and assessing of CSPAPs falls on the shoulders of just the physical educator. Another misconception may have emerged as a consequence of the introduction of the new titles "physical activity director" and, more recently, "physical activity leader." The names by themselves are perfectly appropriate. However, their introduction contributed to perhaps the most worrisome reactions to and claims about CSPAPs: that the profession has forsaken its historic focus on skill, social, and emotional development and favors just "getting kids active" and that skill development and promotion of PA are incompatible. That is, the profession has capitulated and opted to devalue school physical education as we know it and we are playing into the hands of those who just let kids play (i.e., roll out the ball). This may lead school districts to believe that they do not need licensed professionals to teach and they can simply hire minimum-wage supervisors without any educative expectations because then physical education is only about getting children and youth active and nothing else. The central focus of a CSPAP is effective physical education, which includes meaningful content, developmentally appropriate opportunities for learning, effective assessment practices, and appropriate instruction that facilitates PA (CDC, 2013). Physical activity is part of physical education and vice versa; ignoring one to spite the other is a disservice to our students (Blankenship, 2013).

Continuing Lack of Awareness or Knowledge About CSPAPs

Research on PA levels of children and youth emerged in the 1980s and became a dominant line of inquiry. This research formed the basis for the landmark paper by Sallis and McKenzie (1991). The mid-2000s brought about a plethora of applied and professional publications. Some examples include (1) what constitutes a CSPAP and how to implement it (including resources; e.g., CDC, 2013; Rink et al., 2010); (2) the changing role of physical educators (e.g., Castelli & Beighle, 2007); (3) the skills and knowledge needed for successful implementation (e.g., Metzler et al., 2013a, 2013b); and (4) how to prepare future physical education professionals to plan, implement, and assess a CSPAP (see Kulinna et al., 2017). Moreover, in the past few years, there have been numerous presentations at professional conferences (across national, regional, and state levels). And, in the late 2000s, NASPE (2008) published the first CSPAP-focused publication, a position statement pointing to the need for school physical education to reconceptualize its role in schools. Yet, despite this proliferation of CSPAP-specific information, there is some evidence that, specific to the preparation of future physical educators, only one in four PETE programs has CSPAP-related learning experiences (Kwon et al., 2017). What remains less clear is why, almost a decade later, CSPAP has not gained the desired traction in schools. Though speculative, likely reasons for this lack of awareness and implementation may well include lack of membership in either state- or national-level SHAPE America and lack of engagement in professional development among K-12 and PETE professionals.

Perceived Fear of Job Loss

One outgrowth of the CSPAP messaging and lack of in-depth knowledge is the perceived fear that because of the narrow emphasis on promoting PA, districts may perceive that there is less need to hire certified physical educators. There is no evidence that school and district administrators have used this argument as a reason to reduce the physical education teaching force. Rather, when the physical education teaching force was reduced, it was more likely a consequence of economic factors. Yet perceptions can easily become entrenched and may create outright resistance to CSPAP development. Continued efforts in providing well-designed professional development are needed to bend these perceptions toward more positive outlooks to CSPAP itself and the critical role that physical educators play.

Skill Development Versus PA: An Artificial Split in Perspectives

The "skill versus PA" conundrum is a largely self-inflicted barrier. It has created an artificial wedge between those who view motor skill development as physical education's main function and those who view promotion of PA as a primary mission. The belief that the two outcomes are mutually

exclusive is inherently flawed in that one cannot be achieved without the other. That is, developing competence in fundamental motor skills cannot be achieved without engaging in PA. Conversely, regular engagement in PA (e.g., rock climbing, tennis, golf, or swimming) is unlikely to occur without a sufficient level of competence in fundamental motor skills (e.g., Stodden et al., 2008).

Thus, as Blankenship (2013) noted, motor skill competence (along with related knowledge) and PA are two sides of the same coin. The key is how teachers are able to design learning tasks that maximize opportunities for appropriate practice and PA in combination. A good example of combining motor skill competence and PA is the recent research in the area of games-based approaches to teaching and learning sport games (e.g., Teaching Games for Understanding [TGfU] and Play Practice). There is evidence that well-delivered games-based approaches that combine a focus on technical and tactical development through deliberate game design can produce improved gameplay performance and afford MVPA levels at or above recommended levels (e.g., Harvey et al., 2016; Miller et al., 2016).

Overemphasis on Interscholastic Sport Programs

Interscholastic sport programs have been a dominant institution in secondary schools for decades. In recent years, many school districts have opted to eliminate between-school competition in middle schools and, instead, have instituted pay-to-play fees to offset budget cuts at the district level. And at the high school level, parent booster programs have become a major source of revenue to support the after-school sport programs (e.g., Siedentop & van der Mars, 2012). Successful sport programs become a major source of pride for players, coaches, and school administrators, especially in more rural communities. As pressure builds for programs (especially in football and boys' basketball) to maintain their success level, time for and access to practice and strength conditioning is increased throughout the school day, which results in fewer physical education sections with sport and other content offerings (i.e., less access) that are accessible to students who are not on their school's sport teams (van der Mars, 2017).

Decrease in PETE Program Enrollment

Until about a decade ago, strong enrollment levels in PETE programs was virtually guaranteed. Since then, enrollment in the United States has declined significantly (e.g., Bulger et al., 2015). Coupled with the emergence of a corporate culture within state universities (where enrollment growth has become an increasingly important funding source through tuition), several well-known programs have been closed down. Potential reasons for this decline include a combination of the recent economic depression, low salaries for teachers, teachers' being blamed for poor student performance, portrayal of teachers in the media and entertainment industry, the expense of university education (e.g., increases in tuition and fees), and a general devaluation of public education in the country.

Attention has recently increased in seeking effective strategies to reverse this enrollment decline through national presentations (e.g., Ward et al., 2017) and community discussions. Examples of recruitment strategies include stronger marketing efforts; outreach to high school students; stronger connections between four-year institutions and the surrounding community colleges through articulations; scholarship incentives for high school students who choose to enter a teacher education program; improved partnering of teacher education programs with the offices of admission services, academic advising, and marketing; and the hiring of college-level recruiters. In addition, PETE faculty are asked to engage in various recruitment efforts, such as speaking to junior- and senior-level high school students to showcase a career in teaching physical education. The return on investment in these and other strategies remains unclear as yet. However, for the foreseeable future, failure to engage in aggressive and proactive student recruitment will continue to suppress PETE program enrollment levels. Without appreciable increases in enrollment, additional PETE programs will face the same verdict, add to the already sizable teacher shortage in general, and limit the number of physical educators who potentially could be prepared to plan and facilitate CSPAPs.

CSPAP Preparation in PETE Programs

Future physical educators will need to be prepared in ways that include the development of skills; knowledge; *and* the dispositions associated with planning, implementing, and assessing CSPAPs. These criteria lay well beyond those associated with the more traditional job of teaching physical education. Those charged with preparing physical educators will need to work within the constraints of university credit limits, accreditation requirements set forth by the Council for the Accreditation of Educator Preparation, and teacher education course requirements set by the state departments of education. They are the ones who shape the content and structure of their PETE programs so that CSPAP preparation is assured (for examples, see Kulinna et al., 2017).

The recently revised standards for beginning physical education teachers now include the first reference to "expanded physical activity programming" at the school level in the professionalism standard (number 6, element 3), but PETE candidates are expected to have only the knowledge related to CSPAPs (SHAPE America, 2017). Without expectations for actual hands-on CSPAP experiences being built into PETE programs, it is unlikely that many PETE programs will include them. The next PETE standards revision will constitute a new opportunity to strengthen CSPAP preparation expectations for PETE programs. However, this next revision will not occur until 2024.

In addition, the incoming conceptions of what teaching physical education is like of those entering PETE programs may also be a barrier in that they may not have experienced anything that resembles a CSPAP modeled by their K-12 physical education teachers. The approaches taken within their PETE program to socialize PETE majors into building CSPAPs will be key to whether they will take that initial CSPAP background and build it into their own K-12 programs once they have graduated. However, whether and to what extent those PETE majors who were introduced to CSPAP development in their program transfer that into their own teaching remains unknown. A recent review on physical education teachers' socialization did not yet include reference to this either (Richards & Gaudreault, 2017).

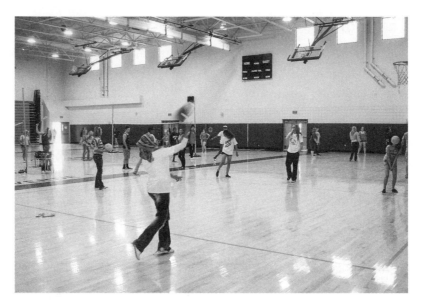

High schools may increase opportunities for free recreational play at lunchtime by using teacher candidates from a local university PETE program to provide necessary equipment and supervision.

© Hans van der Mars

Lack of a Strong and Replication-Based CSPAP Evidence Base

As is evident in other parts of this text, there is a small but growing body of evidence surrounding CSPAPs, and the need for more sustained inquiry remains. Currently, however, the available evidence for CSPAPs represents a "good news–bad news" situation. The good news is that there is now a small evidence base that supports the efficacy of individual CSPAP components targeting students' PA (e.g., Carson, Castelli, Beighle, et al., 2014; Russ et al., 2015). First, effective physical education programs do result in students' PA levels at or above recommended levels (e.g., Harvey et al., 2016; Luepker et al., 1996; McKenzie et al., 1996; Sallis et al., 1997; Young et al., 2006). Beyond physical education, for the during-school component, the aforementioned classroom PA breaks and lunchtime PA programming have a promising evidence base (e.g., Lorenz et al., 2017; Ward, 2011). For the before-school component, there is supportive evidence for strategies such as before-school PA programs (e.g., walking and running clubs; Mahar et al., 2011; Stylianou, Hodges-Kulinna, et al., 2016; Stylianou, van der Mars, et al., 2016). In addition, the aforementioned evidence on recess (through improved equipment and playground markings) is also promising.

The bad news is that, to date, the research has targeted only individual CSPAP components. There continues to be a dearth of evidence supporting full-fledged CSPAP implementation and school staff, parent, and community involvement and a lack of effort in conducting systematic replications. The sidebar includes a brief summary of a two-year case study that constitutes the lone completed research project on full CSPAP implementation (Metzler, 2015).

Another limitation is that the bulk of CSPAP-focused research to date has targeted student-focused CSPAP components. There is only scant published evidence on efforts to engage school staff in additional PA during the school day (Erwin et al., 2013; Russ et al., 2015). Nor is there substantial evidence for the outcome of CSPAP efforts targeting families and surrounding communities specifically related to observable changes in PA (Erwin et al., 2013; Russ et al., 2015).

Finally, the lack of systematic replications mirrors the concerns raised about most of educational research. Makel and Plucker (2014) reported that less than 0.2 percent of all published educational research constituted a replication of previous research. Lack of replication of previous research continues to hamper any effort to affect education practice and policy. To be sure, replication of research that focuses on just one or two non–

Full CSPAP Implementation

Metzler (2015) and colleagues conducted a two-year pilot study of full CSPAP implementation at one ethnically and racially diverse middle school with over a third of the student population qualifying for free or reduced-cost school meals. The CSPAP approach was based on the Health Optimizing Physical Education (HOPE) curriculum design and principles (Metzler et al., 2013a, 2013b). Some of the results were promising across various outcome measures (e.g., FitnessGram measures, attendance at an after-school PA program for students, and attendance at health fair events targeting parents). In addition, relative to students' MVPA accumulation, physical education classes specifically aimed at maximizing PA coupled with PA accrued during the after-school program produced recommended MVPA daily totals.

Concerns raised included the feasibility and sustainability of the program as implemented given the prohibitive monetary, human, and temporal costs associated with implementing it. No doubt, as more experience is gained in doing full CSPAPs, those implementing them will develop a level of expertise we have not yet seen. But more importantly, more in-depth study is needed of what it takes to develop and implement full CSPAPs along with outcomes.

physical education CSPAP components (e.g., before-school programming, classroom PA breaks, and lunchtime programming) certainly should continue. Following are just a few examples of replications that would also help support efforts to make CSPAPs more commonplace. First, research in high school settings is sorely needed. Much of the published literature has been conducted in elementary schools. With the rolled-back graduation requirements for physical education and the established drop in overall PA levels, high school–aged youth may well be the population in greatest need of PA opportunities. Second, we know very little about whether, how, and to what extent even "CSPAP light" (i.e., physical education plus one or two added components) is possible and sustainable in rural schools. Third, evidence is needed on effective strategies to capture participation by students with disabilities. Much like training of school staff to prompt and promote PA among typically developing peers during recess and lunch periods, paraprofessionals who assist students with special needs can be trained in the same way.

Finally, there is the need for "traditional" sport pedagogy research. By that, we mean research that focuses on events in the physical education lessons. For various reasons, the rise of research on PA within and beyond physical education has shifted attention away from the study of pedagogical processes within physical education, which was so prominent in the first three decades of North American sport pedagogy research. For example, what is the evidence for if or how much physical educators actively promote out-of-school PA? SHAPE America's third content standard targets students' out-of-school PA, which represents the importance of students' seeking out independent PA during discretionary out-of-school time. There is evidence that physical educators rarely direct or encourage their students to seek out PA beyond the class or campus (e.g., Kelder et al., 2003; McKenzie et al., 2006; Weaver et al., 2016). More in-depth study around this topic across school levels and settings is needed to determine the efficacy of interventions aimed at increasing students' out-of-class and out-of-school PA levels through explicit teacher promotion thereof as well as its impact on that behavior.

Building greater capacity to conduct CSPAP-focused research could be accomplished through effective programming in doctoral PETE programs where the study of CSPAPs is a central and sustained theme of the research. Moreover, globally there is considerable interest in whole-of-school approaches to promoting PA, similar to CSPAP in purpose. Countries such as Australia, Belgium, Canada, Finland, Ireland, Poland, and Scotland have had initiatives in place aimed at increasing PA levels of school-aged youth (e.g., Cordon & De Bourdeaudhuij, 2002; McMullen, et al., 2015; Naylora et al., 2006; Reid, 2009; Sutherland et al., 2016). Combining efforts with international colleagues who have similar scholarly interests can have important benefits as well.

SUMMARY

We hope that this chapter serves as an appropriate springboard for the next chapters in this text and that it prompts further applications of and research on CSPAPs. Making CSPAPs more prevalent in most schools is a daunting task. Yet there is reason for optimism. For example, while the future of the ESSA is less certain because of the current turbulence within the federal government, related funding is supposed to flow to the states that school districts can use to expand existing programs; create new programs; and, most importantly, provide increased funding for continuing professional development. In addition, there are outside organizations with goals similar to those of CSPAPs (e.g., Active Schools, Alliance for a Healthier Generation, and the NPAPA) and a growing evidence base that supports effective interventions.

Moreover, this chapter's lead author was a witness to the emergence of sport pedagogy research in the United States during the 1970s and 1980s. The focus, enthusiasm, and passion were palpable. We now have been asked to play in a different way, alongside other parties with similar interests. When sport pedagogy and PA researchers respond to this challenge in the same way as the prior generation of scholars and conduct high-quality research on CSPAP planning, implementation, and assessment, we can be optimistic and witnesses to more large-scale implementation thereof.

QUESTIONS TO CONSIDER

1. How do CSPAPs represent a fundamental shift for the field of physical education?
2. How does the behavioral ecological framework reflect the basis for what CSPAPs represent?
3. Explain how CSPAPs are an approach for increasing PA levels of school-aged youth, regardless of the widely varying contexts in which physical education teachers work (e.g., urban or suburban schools vs. rural schools).
4. Describe how full-fledged CSPAPs would affect the day-to-day work of physical education professionals.
5. How does the presence of policies (or lack thereof) affect CSPAP implementation?
6. What are the external barriers that would affect the degree to which CSPAP implementation is feasible?
7. What are internal and proximal barriers that would affect the degree to which CSPAP implementation is feasible?

CHAPTER 2

Emerging Policy Landscape Surrounding CSPAPs

Justin B. Moore, PhD, MS, FACSM
Wake Forest School of Medicine

Abigail Gamble, PhD
University of Mississippi Medical Center

David Gardner, DA
North Carolina Division of Public Health

Alexandra Peluso, BS
University of Texas at Austin

Danny Perry, MAEd, MSA
Bertie County Schools

Policies are formal declarations of action that should be undertaken by entities and individuals. In the context of a CSPAP, policies exist across multiple levels with varying degrees of formality, implementation, evaluation, and enforcement. For example, CSPAP policies can be developed and adopted at the state or local education agency (LEA; i.e., district) level. In some circumstances, policies can be adopted at the school level. A policy can target anticipated outcomes of a CSPAP (i.e., time for PA) or a number of CSPAP components (e.g., physical education or staff involvement) and requires varying levels of accountability and evaluation. Adoption, implementation, and enforcement will vary as functions of the clarity and specificity of a policy. As such, the impact of a CSPAP policy can be difficult to measure and quantify depending on the target and focus of the policy being examined. For example, while the ultimate goal of a CSPAP is to increase PA behaviors in students attending the participating schools, it can be exceptionally challenging to determine if a state-level policy focused on the quality of physical education actually influences students' PA. Similarly, it would be difficult to connect a district policy that forbids using PA as punishment to changes in PA among the students.

Importantly, there is no existing research that formally addresses the implementation of an intact CSPAP policy (i.e., to include all five components). However, there is a body of literature that examines the impact of policies specific to individual components of CSPAPs, and it is clear from this literature that CSPAP policies have utility to increase the PA of youth if they are properly implemented at the local level with fidelity to the ideals envisioned by the writers of the policy (Kim, 2012). This complex systems of schools can provide multiple areas for breakdown between policy and practice. In this chapter, the following will be presented: (1) a review of the research addressing the various levels and settings where CSPAP policy is applied, (2) knowledge claims based on this research, (3) knowledge gaps and recommendations for future research on CSPAP policy, (4) practical implications from the existing research for policy makers and school officials, and (5) a case example of a successful policy implementation initiative.

Review of Research

There is currently a paucity of research available to support the role of policy, especially at the highest levels of organizations, to effect child-level behavior change outcomes (Robertson-Wilson et al., 2012). This is primarily related to the costs associated with large-scale, systematic evaluations of state-level policy adoption and implementation and the impact on opportunities for youth PA or PA itself. For example, if a state were to legally mandate 150 minutes of weekly physical education, someone seeking to determine the effect would need to establish the extent to which all LEAs in the state had adopted this standard, changed staffing to accommodate increased resource needs for staff (i.e., certified physical education teachers), procured equipment, changed class schedules, and delivered the physical education classes. Finally, that person would need to be able to assess the amount of PA children in the schools engaged in before and after adoption and implementation. Understandably, no studies have captured all components of such a large undertaking, and only a few (discussed later) have focused on certain aspects of the equation, such as the quality of the state policies, adoption of the policies by the LEA, or impact of policy

adoption (i.e., increased physical education time) on overall PA levels of youth. The result is that the web of evidence available to support state-, LEA-, and school-level policies is riddled with gaps that weaken the support for policy development and adoption. Taken as a whole, the evidence supports the concept that policies should be strongly and specifically worded and inclusive of the entire school ecosystem. For example, a policy that requires 150 minutes of weekly physical education delivered by a certified physical education teacher who is working from a standardized curriculum in a fully equipped facility and administering annual fitness testing is likely to have a greater impact on students' PA than one that simply recommends 150 minutes of weekly physical education. This is especially true where funding is provided to hire and retain the physical education teacher.

National-Level Policy

At the national level, two prominent laws have been enacted with bearing on state and LEA CSPAP policies. These laws are the Child Nutrition and WIC Reauthorization Act of 2004 (Public Law 108-265) and the Healthy, Hunger-Free Kids Act of 2010 (Public Law 111-296). The former requires that schools participating in the child nutrition programs must have a local school wellness policy, and the latter requires stronger language and transparency for the wellness policy. While one study suggested that compliance with federal policies was related to the presence of policies at the LEA level (Metos & Nanney, 2007), no research to date has been conducted to link compliance with these laws to youth PA.

LEA Policy

LEA policy research is difficult to differentiate from the school-level intervention research, which will be the focus of other chapters of this book, because many cluster randomized trials focus on one or more schools within a district (Cradock et al., 2014). However, these studies test the impact of trained interventionists or other change agents to implement strategies or policies, not the impact of the policies themselves (Webber et al., 2008). As such, the research reviewed in this section is limited to the effects of written LEA policies on school policies and practices and youth behaviors.

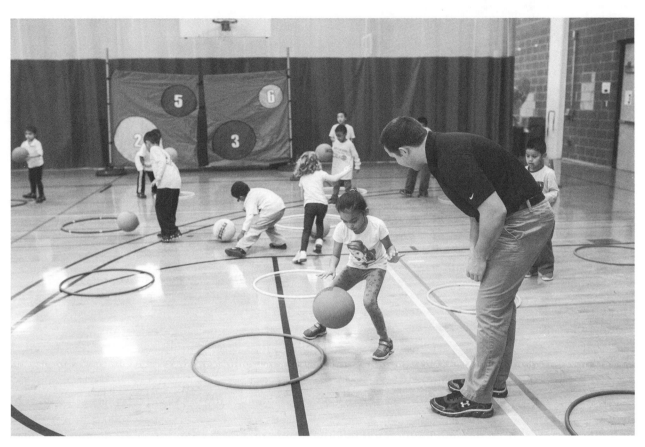

Schools with designated time, teachers, and facilities for physical education support quality instruction, learning, and PA opportunities. Here, a physical education teacher helps elementary students learn to dribble.

Using this definition, few studies qualify for inclusion. However, those that have been conducted focus on LEA policies and opportunities for PA, LEA policies and markers of obesity, and LEA policies and PA behaviors (Larson et al., 2016).

LEA Policies and Opportunities for PA

Few studies have examined the association of district policies and opportunities for PA in youth. One study found no association between the proportion of schools offering intramural or interscholastic athletic programs and the strength of district policies addressing them (Larson et al., 2016). In the same study, the authors found a counterintuitive, inverse relationship between district policy strength and shared-use agreements, where schools with weak policy language were more likely to have shared-use agreements in place (Larson et al., 2016).

LEA Policies and Markers of Obesity

As with state policies, there is little evidence that LEA or school policies are associated with changes in obesity prevalence or indicators of obesity in youth (Williams et al., 2013). Williams and colleagues (2013) conducted a systematic review and meta-analysis examining the impact of school PA policies on markers of obesity and adiposity in youth and concluded that school PA policies are unrelated to obesity status in youth, but as others have stated (Kim, 2012), the available data is insufficient to draw definitive conclusions.

LEA Policies and PA Levels

While few studies have examined the impact of LEA policies on youth PA levels, there is some evidence that individuals working at the LEA or school level can have a positive impact on youth health behaviors. O'Brien and colleagues (2010) found that schools in Maine that employed a part-time or more than part-time school health coordinator demonstrated more positive health behaviors in the observed youth, including lower levels of physical inactivity. In a separate study, Carson and associates (2014) showed that physical education teachers trained to implement CSPAP components were successful in blunting declines in MVPA over the school year relative to youth in comparison schools. Unfortunately, few rigorous studies have examined the impact of policies, other than individual training or staffing efforts, on PA in attending students. This lack of evidence likely stems from the logistical challenge of collecting data across a large number of schools or school districts and the inability to randomize schools or districts to adopt a specific policy.

State-Level Policy

State-level policy has been referred to as "big P" policy to differentiate it from organizational policies (e.g., specific to a school site), or "little P" policy (Brownson et al., 2009). "Big P" policies are those crafted by state legislatures with the input of advocacy groups and topical experts. These policies must often balance between scientific evidence or expert opinion and practical concerns related to constituent desires or budgetary constraints. For example, PA may be considered important by a policy maker, but a local constituent (e.g., a parent or a teachers union) may be concerned about time potentially being taken from more traditional academic subjects. As such, state-level policies often represent a compromise between the desires of PA proponents and proponents of other school activities (e.g., art and music). Thus, not all states have enacted policies, and some of those that have enacted policies have enacted policies that are short of the ideals set forth by CSPAP proponents (Eyler et al., 2010; Taber et al., 2012). Research at the state level has historically focused on examining the quality of state-level policy; the extent state-level policy translates to the LEA or school level; or the association between state-level policies and prevalence of obesity in youth, although a recent study attempted to equate state policy to the quantity of PA time in physical education classes (Chriqui et al., 2013).

Quality of State PA Policy

Few investigations of the quality of state policy have been conducted. In a study by Eyler and colleagues (2010), the investigators conducted a content analysis of bills introduced at the state level to determine how many of the recommendations were evidence based and how many were eventually adopted. The investigators examined 781 proposed bills, of which 162 were enacted, and their findings suggested that the bills enacted were less likely to have evidence-based elements because only 42 of 272 bills that contained at least one evidence-based element were enacted (Eyler et al., 2010). In a separate study, Carlson and colleagues (2013) graded the strength of wording in existing state PA policies. The authors classified policies as weak if they contained vague, aspirational, or unenforceable language (i.e., "can provide up to 30 minutes of physical activity" versus "will provide 30 minutes of moderate-to-vigorous physical activity"). Only 19 state policies were identified, with none rated as "strong." Five of the policies were rated as "moderate," with the remainder considered to have "weak" wording (Carlson et al., 2013). In a third study (Metos & Nanney, 2007), investigators examined the potential impact of federal legislation on the content and quality of policies in Utah school districts that were written after enactment of the federal law. Although the results of the study were promising, with 75 percent of school policies meeting inclusion criteria, few PA-specific policies were included in the school policy documents.

Translation of State Policies to Local Policies

Although limited, the existing research on the translation of state to local policies is promising. One study examined the effect of the North Carolina Healthy Active Children Policy, which required all K-8 children to engage in 30 minutes or more of PA daily (Evenson et al., 2009). Using survey data from school district officials, Evenson et al. (2009) reported increases in PA participation, time on task, and staff involvement. Another study found that physical education classes in elementary schools were more likely to be taught by teachers trained in physical education following state policy adoption and that PA was less often used as punishment (Phillips et al., 2010).

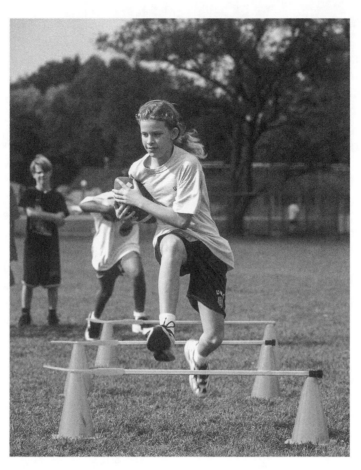

In the United States, national guidelines specify that 50% of physical education class time be spent in moderate to vigorous PA. Here, some students are active while others wait their turn. Teachers should create opportunities to maximize each student's participation in PA and learning.

However, a separate study examining a similar state-level policy found no changes in time for physical education classes or recess (Belansky et al., 2009). These results suggest that it may be important to codify state-level policy changes into local written policies so adoption, implementation, and enforcement guidance is consistent across policy strata.

State-Level Policies and Prevalence of Obesity

Overall, there is little evidence that state PA policies are associated with prevalence of obesity in youth. This is intuitive because obesity is a complex disease with a multifactorial etiology, in which schools play a meaningful but small role (Weinsier et al., 1998). In examining the association between PA policies and obesity, Nanney and

colleagues (2010) found no association between PA and education policies and obesity using 2006 School Health Policies and Practices Study data. Similarly, a study examining five physical education domains of state policy effects on self-reported body mass index found no negative associations (i.e., lower obesity with stricter policies) and three positive associations with obesity, suggesting that states with stronger policies had children with higher rates of obesity (Riis et al., 2012). However, the latter results may be attributable to more aggressive efforts to reduce obesity rates in states with a higher obesity burden.

State-Level Policies and Prevalence of PA

Few studies have attempted to examine the association between state policies and PA of youth. Chriqui et al. (2013) conducted a thorough examination of state and district physical education policies and their impact on reported levels of physical education scheduling and PA time in physical education classes. The authors reported that state and district policies were associated with more time for physical education but not with the proportion of physical education classes dedicated to PA (versus instruction or other activities). Interestingly, the authors found that the state policies were more likely to focus on time allotted for PA, whereas the district policies were more likely to focus on PA time within the physical education class (Chriqui et al., 2013). In a separate study, state legislation that required children to participate in a total of 135 minutes of PA per week was found to be associated with meeting these goals and the proportion of children meeting benchmarks for PA in physical education classes (Kelder et al., 2009).

Knowledge Claims

Based on the available research reviewed in the previous section of this chapter, the following evidence-based claims can be made about policies surrounding CSPAPs.

- State policies vary in clarity, specificity, strength, and consistency with optimal standards.
- The specificity of state policies is associated with the clarity and enforceability of LEA policies.
- State policies are associated with greater physical education time and more time spent being active during physical education classes.
- Neither state nor local PA or physical education policies are associated with prevalence or markers of obesity.

Knowledge Gaps and Directions for Future Research

Given the large differences in the amount and quality of evidence available, the effectiveness of policies to change institutional practices or youth behaviors is one of the most understudied areas in the CSPAP literature. Of the evidence available, the largest body relates to the effectiveness of inter-

ventions targeting the quality of physical education instruction (Russ et al., 2015). Currently, the greatest gap in the scientific knowledge is between the adoption of policies and the implementation of those policies by teachers, staff, and administrators who must serve as the agents of change in the school setting (Robinson et al., 2014). This is especially true for state-level policies, where data collection at the LEA and school levels is especially expensive and time consuming. There is also a lack of evidence to support the contention that implementation of certain policies will result in changes in youth PA. For example, there is currently no evidence that activities to increase staff wellness lead to increased PA in students (Russ et al., 2015).

Currently, little evidence is available to support the relationship between state-level policy and implementation at the LEA or school level. For example, Taber and colleagues (2012) found that improvements in the strength of state-level physical education policies were associated with increases in the strength of district-level physical education policies in a nationally representative sample. However, district scores for PA policies were independent of state policy strength (Taber et al., 2012). This research is further complicated by the fact that few states have policies that specify minutes of PA or the percentage of time to be spent in PA during physical education, making it difficult for LEAs to model best practices in policy development when following state models (Carlson et al., 2013). However, the national physical education standards recommend that a minimum of 50 percent physical education class time be spent in moderate-to-vigorous PA (MVPA; SHAPE America, 2015). Therefore, one can assume that LEAs might best be served by following national standards that have stronger language, rather than modeling state policies that often lack specific guidance.

Evidence-Based Recommendations and Applications

While there is much to learn regarding the impact of state-, local-, and school-level policies on the behaviors of those targeted by the policies, the existing evidence does lead to a series of best

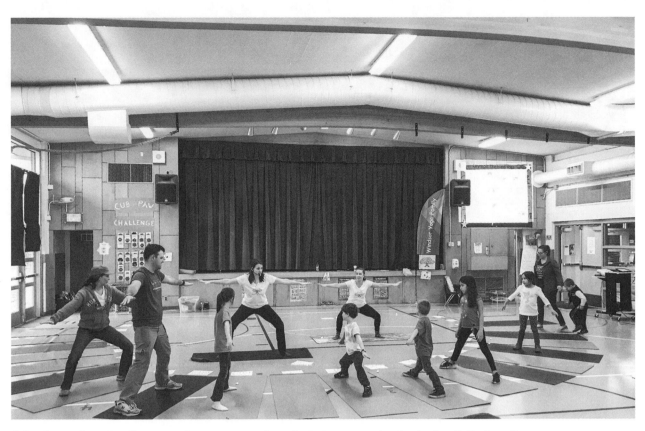

Schools can host family events for parents and students to engage in physical activity together.

Photo courtesy of Veronica Adams.

practices. These best practices can be adopted by community partners and school staff working in coordination to achieve the desired behavioral outcomes. However, it is important to remember that the evidence base is limited at this time and will benefit from additional practice-based research.

For Community Partners

Community partners, especially those working in the policy arena, can greatly assist their colleagues working in schools by supporting the adoption and implementation of a comprehensive state CSPAP policy. An example of a comprehensive state policy based on the recommendations of SHAPE America can be found in table 2.1. While the level of evidence available for these practice recommendations is limited, enough evidence is available to suggest that these recommendations will not adversely affect child health or learning and may benefit one or both. Ideally, these recommendations would be adopted and implemented at

the state level with incentives and accountability measures to ensure implementation at the LEA level, but this may not be realistic for those working at the LEA or school level in states lacking the political capital or desire to stipulate regulations at the local level. All states should strive to require LEAs to address PA and physical education through formal policies. For example, the state of Florida specifies the following:

> Each district school board shall adopt a written physical education policy that details the school district's physical education program, the expected program outcomes, the benefits of physical education, and the availability of one-on-one counseling concerning the benefits of physical education. (Florida Title XLVIII, 1003 § 455, 2010)

Regardless of mandates at the state level, all LEAs should clearly articulate general PA and physical education requirements (separately) in local policy statements. Specifically, LEAs should

TABLE 2.1 Exemplary Policies Enacted by States for Select CSPAP-Related Components

CSPAP component	Content area	Optimal policy	
Physical education	Amount, frequency, and intensity: elementary	All students shall be provided daily physical education or the equivalent of at least 150 minutes per week for the entire school year. At least 50% of physical education class time should be spent in MVPA.	
	Class size	Physical education classes shall have a pupil-to-teacher ratio comparable to the ratio in the classroom context.	
	Curriculum	Each school district shall adopt a curriculum that aligns with state or National Standards for Physical Education for grades K-12, with grade-level benchmarks. The curriculum shall be reviewed every two years. Annual training in the curriculum shall be provided to staff.	
	Student assessment	Student achievement shall be assessed based on physical education standards, and a written physical education grade shall be reported for students according to the district's grading schedule. Data from assessment of student achievement shall be used to improve the physical education program. Fitness assessment shall be performed, using a valid and reliable tool, and used to set student goals and track progress toward those goals. Results of the fitness assessment shall be reported to parents.	
	Teacher certification	Require all physical education teachers to be certified, licensed, and endorsed to teach physical education, and provide funding to school districts to assure their physical education teachers receive adequate professional development specific to their field on an annual basis, especially school districts serving at-risk students and minority populations. Integrate public health into professional development, educating members of the profession on their role within the public health model. Require teachers to keep current on emerging technologies, model programs, and improved teaching methods.	
	Waivers, exemptions, and substitutions	Waivers, exemptions, substitutions, and pass–fail options for physical education are prohibited. Accommodations will be made for those with medical, cultural, or religious considerations.	
PA during school	Opportunities for PA throughout the day	Supplement physical education time with other PA opportunities to facilitate school-aged children accumulating at least 60 minutes of total PA before, during, and after school and avoiding prolonged periods of inactivity.	
	Safe facilities and equipment	Indoor and outdoor facilities shall be available so that PA is not dependent on the weather. Equipment shall be age appropriate, inviting, and available in sufficient quantities for all students to be active. Equipment shall be inspected regularly (at least weekly) for safety and replaced as needed. The ratio of supervisors to students shall not exceed 1:90. For students with special needs, the ratio shall not exceed 1:16.	

Florida Statute 1003.455:

"On any day during which physical education instruction is conducted there are at least 30 consecutive minutes per day."

Texas Admin. 28.002:

"On a weekly basis, at least 50 percent of the physical education class be used for actual student PA and that the activity be, to the extent practicable, at a moderate or vigorous level."

South Carolina Admin. Code 59-10-10, per South Carolina Section 59-10-20:

"Beginning with the 2008-09 school year, the student to certified physical education teacher ratio in the elementary schools for the State must be 500 to 1."

Alabama course of study for physical education

The course of study specifies K-12 content standards for physical education based on the National Standards for Physical Education. Related, administrative Code 290-2-3 (1997) requires that textbooks be purchased from a list of approved textbooks adopted by the Alabama State Board of Education.

California Education Code 60800 Sections (b) and (d):

"Upon request of the department, a school district shall submit to the department, at least once every two years, the results of its physical performance testing," and "pupils shall be provided with their individual results after completing the physical performance testing."

Iowa Admin. Code 282-13.28(14)

Grades 5-12:

"Completion of 24 semester hours in physical education to include coursework in human anatomy, kinesiology, human physiology, human growth and development related to maturational and motor learning, adaptive physical education, curriculum and administration of physical education, personal wellness, and first aid and emergency care. A current certificate of CPR training is required in addition to the coursework requirements."

Arkansas Admin. Code 6-16-132 (c): "The local board shall encourage a student granted a waiver...to take, as an alternative to physical education, appropriate instruction in health education or other instruction in lifestyle modification if an exemption is granted pursuant to this section."

Connecticut Substitute House Bill No. 6525, Public Act No. 13-173: "Each local and regional board of education shall require each school under its jurisdiction to . . . include in the regular school day for each student enrolled in [grades kindergarten to five, inclusive] elementary school time devoted to physical exercise of not less than twenty minutes in total."

South Carolina Code of Laws 59-10-60:

"Each district shall make every effort to ensure that the schools in its district have age appropriate equipment and facilities to implement the physical education curriculum standards."

require schools to provide 150 minutes of physical education to all students weekly throughout the school year at the elementary level and 225 minutes weekly at the secondary level. Physical education should be provided without substitution for participating in athletics or other enrichment activities (e.g., marching band and ROTC). Schools should also require 30 minutes of daily opportunities for PA while at school, which can be provided through activity breaks, recess, or kinesthetic learning opportunities. Related, PA time should not be used or withheld as punishment nor withheld for remediation or other purposes (SHAPE America, 2015). LEAs should utilize a formal curriculum for physical education that specifically aligns to state or National Standards for Physical Education. LEAs should also specify that physical education classes be taught by certified or licensed physical education teachers utilizing the same teacher-to-staff ratio as employed for academic classes. Similarly, physical education classes should be assessed annually for teacher and curriculum effectiveness. LEAs should employ shared-use agreements so youth and community members can access school facilities for PA outside of school hours. Related, these agreements can be used to allow for school use of community facilities for PA programming when similar facilities are not available on school properties. Increasingly, parent organizations (e.g., parent–teacher associations) and health-care and public health advocates are recognizing and supporting increased time for PA and quality physical education. These groups recognize the health and academic success connection and are advocating at local and state levels for policy adoption and change and can be helpful partners when attempting to adopt and implement PA policies. Finally, funding should be provided to schools to support their efforts in all of these areas (Boles et al., 2011).

For School Staff

At the school level, school scheduling policy should accommodate opportunities for PA. Specifically, recess at the elementary level should be scheduled for a minimum of 20 minutes daily, ideally before lunch. Classroom teachers should incorporate kinesthetic learning or activity breaks twice daily to provide opportunities for PA (Bartholomew et al., 2018) and increase time on task (Mahar et al., 2006). Where appropriate, schools should work with partner agencies to develop opportunities to actively commute to school. School-level policy

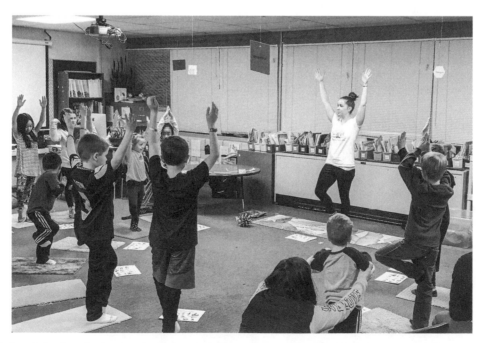

Teacher-led activity breaks in the classroom help increase physical activity levels in students.
Photo courtesy of Veronica Adams.

and practice may hold the greatest potential for affecting PA levels of students. At the school level, the principal is accountable for implementing, monitoring, enforcing, and documenting state and local policies. The principal can establish "little P" policies and practices for her or his school that align with state and local policies and ensure compliance. Such school-level policies and practices become elements of the school culture and environment and, thus, more likely to be understood, embraced, and followed by teachers and staff (Gamble et al., 2017).

Principals should consider the benefits of establishing a CSPAP committee led by a designated PA leader (PAL). The CSPAP committee should include teachers, administrators, and other school-level staff (e.g., school nurses); parents; community members and professionals; and students who will ensure that state-, local-, and school-level PA policies are implemented with fidelity (see chapter 3). The PAL should be a teacher or staff member who understands and is committed to the benefits of PA, possesses leadership skills, and is respected by her or his coworkers. In many schools, a physical educator serves as the PAL, owing to his or her expertise in physical education and PA. However, schools may benefit from designating a classroom teacher, administrator, school nurse, or other staff member as the PAL to broaden the scope of PA in the school environment beyond physical education. Chapter 3 presents further PAL research and discussion.

To affect student behavior and health, state-, LEA-, and school-level policies must be applied and activated at points of contact with students. These points of contact may be in a classroom or gymnasium, on a playground, in hallways, on sidewalks, or in any school setting where students can be active. Principals, PALs, CSPAP committee members, and other school staff should continuously work to establish, implement, and follow policies and practices that ensure students experience the recommended PA during the school day. For example, school leaders should consider the benefits of including increased opportunities for PA when they write the school improvement plan, which can be helpful in providing a level of accountability. Additionally, principals can include the implementation of classroom PA and active recess in teacher observations and evaluations.

SUMMARY

While the evidence base confirming the impact of CSPAP policy adoption on the physical activity of youth is still emerging, preliminary evidence suggests a beneficial effect on student behaviors that warrants further research on this topic. While an optimal CSPAP policy approach has not been empirically developed and tested, a number of states provide exemplary components of a comprehensive policy that can serve as a foundation for future work in this area. It is imperative that future investigations seek to identify the most effective and impactful CSPAP policies at the various levels and settings where these policies are applied. More importantly, effective dissemination and implementation strategies will need to be developed to ensure that effective policies impact all children equally, regardless of their age, race, gender, geography, or socioeconomic status. Only through concerted efforts from the research and practice communities can these goals be accomplished, but their result will be physical activity supportive environments for youth everywhere, which is a truly worthy cause.

QUESTIONS TO CONSIDER

1. What is the optimal state-level policy to promote CSPAPs from the standpoint of acceptability, feasibility, and effectiveness?
2. What are the minimum components of an optimal state-level policy?
3. What is the most effective way to encourage schools to formally adopt and implement state-level CSPAP policies?

4. What resources do schools need to implement the optimal CSPAP policies currently recommended by leading organizations (e.g., 50 percent of physical education time spent in MVPA and 30 minutes of MVPA during school)?

5. Does codifying CSPAPs at the LEA level ensure sustainability of practices?

CASE EXAMPLE

Danny Perry, MAEd, MSA
Director of Safety and Security, Health and Physical Education and Support Services
Bertie County Schools, North Carolina

In November 2014, I assumed the position of school health liaison, which was created to support the nutrition and PA program in Bertie County schools. One of the initial goals of the program was to develop a plan to meet the requirements of the Healthy Active Children Policy in grades K-8, which states in part that "for schools in which Physical Education is not currently offered daily to all K-8 students, a minimum of 30 minutes, daily, of moderate to vigorous physical activity shall be provided by schools for all K-8 students."

The process of meeting the goal of 30 minutes of daily MVPA began with the identification of a school wellness champion at each school. The school wellness champion serves as the point person in the school who recruits and leads the school wellness team. After the wellness team was in place, the school wellness champion and wellness team worked with me as the school health liaison to develop and implement activities to meet the nutrition and PA goals identified in the school action plan.

The school physical education program was in place at all schools prior to the development and implementation of the PA action plan. On average, students were scheduled to participate in physical education class two times per week for 50 minutes during each class. The wellness team at each school was tasked with developing a plan to incorporate PA into the daily schedule to provide all students with at least 30 minutes of MVPA per school day.

The first such PA was the implementation of energizers in the classroom. As stated in the action plan, "By May 31, 2018, 80% of teachers will use grade appropriate energizers and for the duration of 3-5 minutes per energizer activity in the classroom at least 3 times per week." The classroom teachers were provided with online links to resources necessary to incorporate the energizers into their lesson plans. The classroom energizer plan was discussed at monthly staff meetings to encourage participation. As the school health liaison, I visited classes, video recorded the energizer activities, and provided feedback to the classroom teacher.

The school schedule included recess for the students each day for 15 minutes. The recess period was very traditional; the students went to the playground and played on various pieces of equipment. To help meet the goal of 30 minutes of MVPA per day, the wellness team encouraged the classroom teachers to participate in the 100-mile walking club with the goal of each student in every classroom walking 100 miles by the end of the school year. A marked walking trail was designed and constructed at each school. The classroom teachers were encouraged to lead their class on a mile walk on the outside walking trail as part of the recess program. The walking trail at each school was also available for public use after school hours and on weekends.

These small PA additions to the daily school schedule have been both popular and effective. Teachers have reported fewer discipline issues in the classroom when students were offered the opportunity to get out of their seat and move. Students have received more opportunities to participate in MVPA each school day.

The CSPAP in Bertie County schools has created an environment where PA is a valued and planned part of the school curriculum. Teachers and students now realize the importance of PA when considering the whole-child model. The grant that provided the financial support for the PA action plans at the schools ended in May 2018. However, we plan to continue to incorporate the annual PA action plan into the school improvement plan, owing to the success of the program the past four years.

PART II

Conceptual Models for CSPAP Implementation

Internal Capacity Building: The Role of the CSPAP Champion and Other School Professionals

Russell L. Carson, PhD
University of Northern Colorado

Catherine P. Abel-Berei, PhD
Southern Connecticut State University

Laura Russ, PhD
Augusta University

Jessica Shawley
Moscow Middle School

Tanya Peal
Soaring Heights PK-8

Cyrus Weinberger
Soaring Heights PK-8

For a CSPAP to meet its full potential and transform schools into sustainable cultures of integrated PA and healthy living, the creation and re-creation of school-based change agents continues to be recognized as a promising internal (i.e., within-school) approach for capacity building. Carson, Castelli, Beighle, et al. (2014) proposed a tripartite personnel structure, known as the triad of CSPAP leadership, as a guideline for schools to follow when building the internal capacity for a successful and sustainable CSPAP (see figure 3.1). The triad of CSPAP leadership comprises a PA champion (preferably, a physical education teacher), who spearheads efforts; a supportive school administrator; and a CSPAP committee (e.g., the PA champion, administrator, and other influential leaders in and around the school—classroom teacher, parent, or nurse), which advises and assists with CSPAP coordination and implementation (Carson, Castelli, Beighle, et al., 2014).

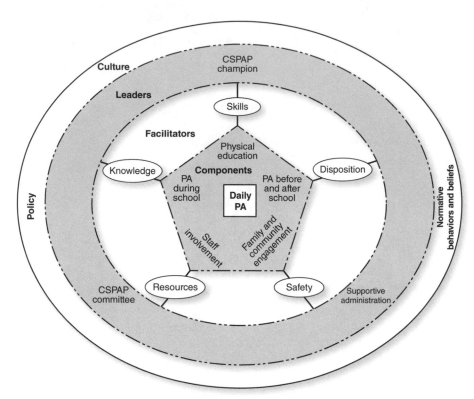

Figure 3.1 A conceptual framework for CSPAP research and practice based on a social-ecological perspective. Dotted lines represent the bidirectional influences of levels. Facilitator-level resources related to personnel, finances, politics, time, space, access, built environment, and transportation support and safety relate to physical, social, and emotional well-being.

Reprinted with permission from R.L. Carson et al., "School-Based Physical Activity Promotion: A Conceptual Framework for Research and Practice," *Childhood Obesity* 10, no. 2 (2014): 100-106.

In this chapter, we review the research and offer existing knowledge claims from the growing evidence for each unit of CSPAP leadership—PA champion, supportive administrator, and CSPAP committee; identify knowledge gaps and provide directions for future research around building internal capacity for CSPAPs; propose evidence-based recommendations and practical applications for building and supporting a synergetic CSPAP leadership triad; and conclude with three nationally recognized case examples of the triad operating in unison to create a thriving CSPAP community where reaching the recommended amounts of daily PA is the norm and students and staff are still learning and smiling.

Review of Research

Research for each unit of the CSPAP leadership triad is reviewed in order, organized within each unit by the central tenets produced from the scholarship to date.

PA Champion

A PA champion is the school-level leader, coordinator, or director of CSPAP initiatives (Carson, 2012). The presence of quality leadership has been identified as the foundation for CSPAP success (Doolittle & Rukavina, 2014; Jones et al., 2014; Kulinna et al., 2012). This section gives an overview of what is currently known about a PA champion based on the available literature.

What a Champion Does

The leadership responsibilities of a PA champion typically include setting school-wide PA goals and priorities, identifying and sharing PA resources, ensuring and maintaining clean and safe PA environments, and coordinating community-engaged health and wellness activities (Carson, 2012; CDC, 2013). In addition, the PA champion must be a transformational leader who strives to influence and enhance major changes within a school setting toward a shared vision (Illg, 2014).

Who Are the Champions?

Because teachers are familiar with the unique school environment, policies, procedures, staff, and students, they are ideal candidates to lead during school daily PA opportunities (Kulinna et al., 2012). The most appropriate teacher with the PA expertise, extensive wellness and PA engagement knowledge, professional training (i.e., physical education teacher education [PETE] programs), and understanding of developmentally appropriate PA opportunities is the physical education teacher (Carson, 2012; Castelli & Beighle, 2007). A physical educator helps children achieve the recommended 60 minutes of daily PA so that children live a healthy, active lifestyle (CDC, 2013), yet this daily recommendation cannot be attained in quality physical education classes alone (SHAPE America, 2016). The CSPAP model provides a guide for the school-wide PA opportunities in addition to quality physical education (CDC, 2017). According to current physical educators, they coordinate and implement CSPAPs because (1) they feel more time for PA is needed to achieve recommended amounts of daily PA and to provide opportunities for students to learn and practice skills related to personal and social responsibility; (2) they have personal reasons (i.e., enjoyment and feelings of doing good for children); (3) they believe it is part of their job description; and (4) they want to promote a positive image of physical education and the physical education teacher (Berei, 2015; Carson, Pulling, et al., 2014; Centeio, Erwin, et al., 2014). In addition, stakeholders in school environments, such as principals and classroom teachers, view the physical educator as the essential change agent for CSPAP implementation (Deslatte & Carson, 2014; Doolittle & Rukavina, 2014).

While the physical educator may be well suited to be a PA champion, it may not always be realistic for a physical educator to fill this role. In these situations, leadership can come from school administrators, classroom teachers, school staff, or any capable and willing parent or community member (Berei, 2015; Jones et al., 2014). Ideally, any potential PA champion participates on a school-level CSPAP committee or team to facilitate CSPAP change (Carson, Castelli, Beighle, et al., 2014). Kulinna and colleagues (2012) found that classroom teachers are willing and able to be part of school-based PA programming but they need assistance from a knowledgeable and skilled leader to provide training and encouragement. In many cases, classroom teacher training programs do not address how to establish healthy and active school environments; therefore, it may be necessary to educate faculty and staff on how to teach and practice healthy behaviors (Beighle et al., 2009; Castelli et al., 2017).

What a Champion Needs

First and foremost, the PA champion must have adequate CSPAP content knowledge (Carson, 2012; Illg, 2014; McMullen et al., 2014), including a deep understanding of how the five CSPAP components interact within the organizational structures of a community and school setting (Centeio, Erwin, et al., 2014; Illg, 2014). The CSPAP champion must be willing and able to go beyond his or her traditional role as the physical educator and provide PA opportunities outside of physical education classes in innovative and creative ways (Carson, 2012; Doolittle & Rukavina, 2014). An effective CSPAP cannot be implemented by the PA champion alone; therefore, effective leadership and advocacy skills are necessary (Centeio, Erwin, et al., 2014; Doolittle & Rukavina, 2014; Illg, 2014; Jones et al., 2014; McMullen et al., 2014). One strategy to ensure PA champions have the knowledge and skills they need to effectively fulfill their role is through CSPAP professional development.

Knowledge for Successful PA Champions

- Adequate foundational CSPAP content knowledge (Carson, 2012; Illg, 2014; McMullen et al., 2014)
- Theoretical orientations to leadership systems and organizational structures (Illg, 2014):
  - Understand the structure of a school and community system
  - Understand factors that affect decision making in school settings
- Thinking beyond the role of the traditional physical educator in innovative ways (Carson, 2012; Doolittle & Rukavina, 2014)

Skills for Successful PA Champions

- Implementing an extensive CSPAP needs assessment (Illg, 2014; Jones et al., 2014)
- Organization, management, and leadership skills:

- Develop and plan short- and long-term CSPAP objectives
- Demonstrate strong communication skills
- Find and organize resources
- Prepare, recruit, educate, and train others to lead and provide PA opportunities
- Utilize effective strategies to implement and promote PA beyond the physical education classroom, such as during the school day (work with classroom teachers and increase PA at recess) and before and after school
- Strategic policy development
- Understand when and how to delegate responsibilities (Doolittle & Rukavina, 2014; Illg, 2014; Jones et al., 2014)
- Advocacy skills:
  - Find support and collaborate and network with colleagues, administrators, and other community partners and stakeholders
  - Build community and share visions
  - Effectively market programs
  - How to relate to and with and motivate others (Centeio, Erwin, et al., 2014; Doolittle & Rukavina, 2014; Illg, 2014; McMullen et al., 2014)

Training Opportunities for Champions

Physical educators are familiar with offering PA programs and components of a CSPAP as a natural expectation or duty of their job (Berei, 2015; Carson, Castelli, Pulling Kuhn, et al., 2014; Centeio, Erwin, et al., 2014). Physical educators want to learn more specifically about CSPAPs (Berei, 2015), and in response, a wide range of CSPAP training opportunities have become more prevalent and diverse (see the sidebar titled "Types of CSPAP Professional Development Opportunities"). Most notable are the 12-month Physical Activity Leader (PAL) Learning System, which builds leadership skills, learning communities, and resources for implementing CSPAPs (SHAPE America, 2017) and PETE programs, which are now integrating CSPAP-specific content and learning experiences (Carson et al., 2017). Collectively, these PA champion training opportunities have the potential to increase awareness and knowledge of CSPAPs, provide implementation strategies, modify the physical educator's role in addressing the sedentary nature of schools, and provide ideas to overcome CSPAP implementation barriers (Deslatte & Carson, 2014; Doolittle & Rukavina, 2014; Jones et al., 2014).

There is some evidence related to the influence of CSPAP training on the PA opportunities and behaviors in school settings. Carson, Castelli, Pulling Kuhn, and colleagues (2014) found PA opportunities during school and for staff were reportedly more frequent with a trained PAL as opposed to no PAL in place. Centeio, Erwin, and colleague (2014) found that PAL-trained physical educators exhibited increased awareness of CSPAPs and a greater ability to overcome barriers and establish the necessary support systems for successful CSPAP implementation. Teachers implement a wide range of CSPAP initiatives after PAL training, and the long-term effects (eight months later) from these CSPAP initiatives on the

Types of CSPAP Professional Development Opportunities

- Physical Activity Leader (PAL) Learning System, available at the SHAPE America website
- University PETE programs (see Kulinna et al., 2017)
- Emerging online coursework and an online master's degree (see Dauenhauer et al., 2018 and Dauenhauer et al., 2017)
- State, regional, national, and international health and physical education workshops and conventions
- Additional popular modes of communication information
  - Informational newsletters, brochures, or emails sent from professional organizations, state departments of education, or district health and physical education coordinators
  - Social media

time students spend in moderate-to-vigorous PA at school ranged from 2.2 minutes per day for boys to 3.4 minutes per day for girls (Carson, Castelli, Pulling Kuhn, et al., 2014).

Barriers for Champions

Every physical educator is encouraged to be the PA champion, yet research has identified two prominent barriers to filling this role: workload demands and role conflict (Berei, 2015; Carson, Pulling, et al., 2014; Deslatte & Carson, 2014; Jones et al., 2014; Patton, 2012). Workload demands are mostly the perceived time constraints from the additional responsibilities or schedule constraints to successfully coordinate a CSPAP (Berei, 2015; Carson, Pulling, et al., 2014; Deslatte & Carson, 2014; Jones et al., 2014; Patton, 2012). In a study investigating the perspectives of teachers attempting to implement a school-wide daily PA program, the teachers reported very little to no time allocated for planning and insufficient time to conduct the program (Patton, 2012). Carson, Pulling, and colleagues (2014) also found increased workload was a perceived inhibitor for CSPAP implementation by trained physical educators. Many teachers, especially physical educators who also coach, already have full schedules; thus, the time and energy dedicated to the additional responsibilities of a PA champion can contribute to teacher burnout or amotivation (Berei, 2015; Deslatte & Carson, 2014; Jones et al., 2014). Furthermore, very little to no additional compensation; lack of infrastructure in facilities, equipment, and supervision (Berei, 2015; Carson, Pulling, et al., 2014; Dwyer et al., 2003); and lack of teacher competence and confidence (Larsen et al., 2012) can hinder PA implementation. As a result, teachers who assume a PA champion role often offer PA opportunities beyond their "normal" teaching duties in a sporadic fashion, initiated by personal initiative, planning, and investment without extra pay or full-time equivalency (Berei, 2015; Jones et al., 2014).

The second barrier, role conflict, relates to the professional expectation that a physical educator's duties are to teach physical education and be the PA champion. Some physical educators feel their role in the school setting is to teach physical education, and others feel that it is their role to offer PA opportunities in most or all of the five CSPAP areas (Berei, 2015; Carson, Pulling, et al., 2014; Centeio, Erwin, et al., 2014). A physical educator's beliefs and perceptions surrounding the place for PA promotion as a physical educator can be the determining factor for whether a physical educator assumes the PA champion role (Carson, Pulling, et al., 2014; Centeio, Erwin, et al., 2014; McMullen et al., 2014). CSPAP training can change physical educators' beliefs and perceptions about their PA expertise from teaching physical education classes solely to coordinating or implementing daily PA opportunities across CSPAP components. McMullen and colleagues (2014) found that a cultural change toward physical education teachers' becoming the PA champion begins by incorporating successful CSPAP experiences in PETE programs. In addition, one year posttraining, physical education teachers reported being more committed to their PAL role, and more experienced teachers (over 20 years of experience) reported being more invigorated in their school setting when compared to untrained, experienced teachers (Pulling Kuhn et al., 2015).

Supportive Administrator

A natural starting place for building leadership is to focus on the school administrator, the leader of the school. It is commonly believed that a supportive administrator is a mediating variable and critical to the success of a CSPAP (Carson, 2012; Carson, Castelli, Beighle, et al., 2014; Deslatte & Carson, 2014; Erwin et al., 2014; Patton, 2012).

The First Step: Gaining Support From Administrators

In a study on characteristics of trained physical education teachers during CSPAP implementation, researchers identified having a supportive administration as a key theme for successful implementation (Centeio, Erwin, et al., 2014). Teachers in training to become CSPAP champions reported gaining administrator endorsement as the first step taken when introducing CSPAPs (Carson, Castelli, Beighle, et al., 2014). Similarly, teachers identify lack of school leadership support as a barrier to PA in schools (Hills et al., 2015); therefore, teachers are encouraged to seek buy-in from administrators early (Heidorn & Centeio, 2012) and build a quality physical education program in order to gain support from their administration (Deslatte & Carson, 2014).

The Role of the Administrator: An Active CSPAP Supporter

There is an absence of research examining the role of a supportive administrator; thus, we know very little about what he or she should know and be able to do related to effective CSPAP efforts. Jones and colleagues (2014) asserted that a supportive administrator can influence all of the transformational change factors (i.e., leadership, environment, and PA access and opportunities), which underpins the claim that successful CSPAP implementation requires the support of an administrator (Centeio, McCaughtry, et al., 2014). Although administrators claim that barriers hindering their ability to facilitate student PA at school exist (Carson, Castelli, Beighle, et al., 2014), they do view healthier school communities as important and believe that quality physical education is linked to successful schools (Deslatte & Carson, 2014). Moreover, the belief exists that supportive administrators, in combination with teachers who implement PA programs, are more likely to make wide-scale changes (Erwin et al., 2014). An overarching recommendation for an administrator to be considered supportive is to develop leadership and build internal capacity (Jones et al., 2014). Specific strategies for achieving this goal are to include administrators in contributing to the overall vision (Elliot et al., 2013), establishing a wellness committee or specific CSPAP committee (Carson, 2012; Castelli et al., 2014; Heidorn et al., 2010; Jones et al., 2014), participating on the wellness or CSPAP committee, or filling the role of the PA champion themselves (Heidorn et al., 2010; Jones et al., 2014).

Effective Strategies for Administrator Support

Teachers believe administrator support is key to the creation, implementation, and sustainability of programs promoting PA in schools (Carson, 2012; Carson, Castelli, Beighle, et al., 2014; Deslatte & Carson, 2014; Patton, 2012). One study that included detailed observations of supportive administrators is a case study of an existing physical education, sport, and PA program in an urban setting (Doolittle & Rukavina, 2014). Administrators not only supported growth of the program but also encouraged it by giving permission to teachers to try new ideas, allocating school funding (i.e., principal discretionary funds and fund-raising to pay for teachers as coaches), pursuing devoted physical education teachers as staff, and valuing and contributing to the greater community (Doolittle & Rukavina, 2014). A second study examined the support of school administration during the implementation of a daily PA program (Patton, 2012). Teachers implementing the PA program reported their administrators valued the program but did not check back on program progress, leading to a lack of accountability and sporadic implementation at the classroom level (Patton, 2012).

While little evidence exists about what a supportive administrator looks like and the impact one has on CSPAP implementation and success, a review of literature yields an abundance of suggestions and recommendations for administrators to be supportive (see the sidebar titled "Characteristics of a Supportive Administrator"). Current CSPAP researchers recommend that administrators provide training opportunities to classroom teachers (Carson, 2012; Castelli et al., 2014; Heidorn et al., 2010), appoint a PAL (Heidorn et al., 2010), provide and lead PA opportunities (Castelli et al., 2014; Elliot et al., 2013), demonstrate that they value and prioritize PA by following up on PA program implementation (Patton, 2012), formally schedule a PA program into the daily school schedule (Patton, 2012), and give teachers autonomy and creativity on how to include PA in their classrooms (Castelli et al., 2014; Centeio, Erwin, et al., 2014; Doolittle & Rukavina, 2014). In addition, administrators can be supportive by providing resources needed for teachers to attend CSPAP trainings, enhancing program marketing (Carson, 2012; Carson, Castelli, Beighle, et al., 2014), allocating funds for physical education programming (Deslatte & Carson, 2014), and recruiting staffing help (Metzler et al., 2013) to assist in the development of PALs and quality physical education programming. While this information illuminates what physical education teachers believe a supportive administrator should do, it does not examine the effectiveness of these characteristics on CSPAP outcomes. The next section defines and discusses the importance and role of the CSPAP committee.

Characteristics of a Supportive Administrator

- Values and prioritizes PA:
  - Has knowledge and appreciation that can enhance and increase participation in and enjoyment of PA (i.e., advocacy)
  - Contributes to the overall vision related to providing PA opportunities
  - Understands PA and its contribution to the greater community
  - Believes before- and after-school PA events are important
  - Follows up on PA program implementation
  - Formally schedules a PA program into the daily school schedule (Doolittle & Rukavina, 2014; Elliot et al., 2013; Metzler et al., 2013; Patton, 2012)
- Serves as a role model and assists or leads district- or school-wide PA programming through the following:
  - Establishing a wellness or CSPAP committee
  - Actively participating on the committee
  - Appointing a PA champion or fulfilling the PA champion role themselves
  - Providing or leading PA opportunities
  - Devoting personal time to help organize or participate in events (Carson, 2012; Castelli et al., 2014; Centeio, Erwin, et al., 2014; Elliot et al., 2013; Heidorn & Centeio, 2012; Heidorn et al., 2010; Hills et al., 2015; Jones et al., 2014)
- Assists or leads in the development of PALs or quality physical education programming through the following:
  - Providing resources needed for teachers to attend CSPAP trainings
  - Enhancing program marketing
  - Allocating funds for physical education programming
  - Recruiting staffing help (Carson, 2012; Carson, Castelli, Beighle, et al., 2014; Deslatte & Carson, 2014; Metzler et al., 2013)
- Assists or leads teachers in the school through the following:
  - Providing permission for teacher autonomy and creativity on how to include PA in their classrooms
  - Allowing teachers to try new ideas when implementing PA opportunities
  - Pursuing devoted physical education teachers as staff
  - Providing training opportunities to classroom teachers
  - Sanctioning attendance at PA professional development opportunities
  - Incentivizing employee wellness programs
  - Influencing the likelihood of teachers to integrate PA and provide extra opportunities for PA
  - Acknowledging efforts of all teachers and students involved (Carson, 2012; Castelli et al., 2014; Centeio, Erwin, et al., 2014; Doolittle & Rukavina, 2014; Erwin et al., 2013; Heidorn et al., 2010)
- Builds community connections to promote PA through the following:
  - Employing shared-use agreements
  - Sponsoring guest speaker programs
  - Viewing the school as a vehicle to help get the community active through understanding and acknowledging the bidirectional influence between the school and the community (Jones et al., 2014)

CSPAP Committee

The necessity and utility of school teams to guide the planning and implementation of health policies, practices, and programs dates back to school wellness legislation for systematically addressing poor nutrition and physical inactivity among students. The Child Nutrition and WIC Reauthorization Act of 2004 (Public Law 108-265) required schools participating in child nutrition programs (e.g., school breakfast and lunch services) to adopt a local school wellness policy that included input from stakeholders, including parents, students, school health professionals, school administrators, the school board, and the public. District officials were encouraged to form a committee to gather this input, but they had the option of meeting this requirement in other ways.

The Healthy, Hunger-Free Kids Act of 2010 (Public Law 111-296) added new provisions related to the implementation, evaluation, and transparency of local school wellness policies with a compliance guideline that includes the participation of the same stakeholders. District officials were recommended to establish a committee to meet the requirements of both laws, led by one designated person at each school authorized to ensure school compliance of the final rule by the end of the 2017 school year. The research to date on CSPAP committees grew from these laws. Next, the scant research on CSPAP committees specifically is reviewed before turning to the broader subject of the earlier research on school-based team approaches, which might inform CSPAP committee research and evidence-based practice moving forward.

CSPAP Committee Research

A CSPAP committee is considered a smaller team of individuals with vested interests in the programming success of school physical education and school-wide PA (Carson, Castelli, Beighle, et al., 2014). CSPAP committees should comprise a diverse set of education and health professions from the school, school district, and local community, pulling from members on preexisting school health teams or district-level school health advisory councils (SHACs; CDC, 2013; Rink et al., 2010). The main function of the committee is to serve as an adviser and decision maker for the establishment, implementation, and evaluation of CSPAP initiatives (CDC, 2013). For instance, the committee might help build awareness and support for physical education and PA at the school and district levels, facilitate a needs assessment process, identify and organize implementation strategies, monitor and evaluate program activities, and secure and manage sustainable resources and community partnerships for the program (Carson, Castelli, Beighle, et al., 2014; CDC, 2013). The recommendation is for CSPAP committees and the work they perform to be led by the CSPAP champion (Carson, Castelli, Beighle, et al., 2014).

CSPAP committee research has been relatively sparse when compared to research on broader school-based health teams. Across many school sites, school-level committees have emerged as a central internal capacity feature for effective CSPAP implementation (Jones et al., 2014). Deslatte and Carson (2014) conducted a mixed methods collective case study of three existing CSPAPs in Louisiana and found that a common element for successful implementation was a supportive network within the school. McMullen and colleagues (2015) presented the CSPAP approaches adopted as a national program in four countries and found that the overarching aims of two programs (Active School Flag in Ireland and Physical Education with Class in Poland) were orchestrated by school-level teams. The CSPAP committee typically includes a physical education teacher; principal; and classroom teacher, whose role can vary from providing an informal support system to being responsible for specific tasks (e.g., managing social media, monitoring evaluation, and coordinating community engagement functions; Deslatte & Carson, 2014; Jones et al., 2014; McMullen et al., 2015). Important community or parent perspectives missing from committee membership can be identified and added through asset mapping of the expertise available in the community (Allar et al., 2017). Above all, the key is that the committee chair (often the physical education teacher as a PA champion) perceives the committee to be readily available to aid with the CSPAP implementation as needed. To no surprise, the first step in establishing a CSPAP nationally and internationally is the formation of a committee (CDC, 2013; McMullen et al., 2015).

School-Based Team Approach

Related published literature that can guide CSPAP committee research and practice is rooted in the comparable school-based team approach adopted in broader comprehensive health frameworks or policies. Both the Coordinated School Health program and the expanded Whole School, Whole Community, Whole Child model depend on an organizational support structure at both the school and district levels, whereby district advisory councils, district coordinators, school health teams, and district policies act in concert to build sustainable school health-promoting practices (Association for Supervision and Curriculum Development & CDC, 2014). Two-year training programs can facilitate the development of a district and school team support infrastructure (Stoltz et al., 2009) and, when prevalent, successfully engage personnel and noticeably improve students' PA levels (Ward et al., 2006), the number of school-wide PA offerings (O'Brien et al., 2010), and the strength of local wellness policy related to PA (Chriqui & Chaloupka, 2011).

The provisions of the Child Nutrition and WIC Reauthorization Act and Healthy, Hunger-Free Kids Act also include district- and school-level representation and participation in wellness policy development and implementation. Compliance with these federal guidelines ranges from 78 to 97 percent, which is commonly met by structures or requirements already in place at the district rather than creating new ones (e.g., a new position or school committee; Buns & Thomas, 2015; Metos & Nanney, 2007). Further complementary school-based team research is subsequently reviewed, which is organized by categories of similar content. The goal is that a review of the broader school-based health team research might help substantiate and supplement the knowledge about CSPAP committees.

Team Composition

Despite laws requiring school wellness policy input from specific stakeholders, the few studies that have examined the makeup and associated outcomes of school health teams have been at the district level. Buns and Thomas (2015) conducted a study in Iowa that examined the composition of individuals involved in the school wellness policy

process and whether the presence of school-based health experts influenced the policies created. Among the 241 districts responding, the majority (97 percent) formed a district committee that typically consisted of 15 members and met for an average of four times during the policy planning process. Committee membership in only 39 percent of the districts included the wide range of school, district, and community representation required by law: food service director (97 percent), school administrator (96 percent), parent (91 percent), school board member (73 percent), student (66 percent), and member of the public (60 percent). Although not a federal mandate, participation from school-based health experts, such as physical education teacher (76 percent), classroom teacher (74 percent), school nurse (72 percent), and health teacher (64 percent), was common and produced slightly stronger policy content and goals, as determined by an objective numeric rating. Policy points improved when policy monitoring and evaluation plans were included, but the institutionalization of such plans can be hindered by excluding school health expertise in the process (Videto & Hodges, 2009). Similarly, barriers to implementing coordinated school health activities often relate to lack of input (and a general lack of set meeting times for this input) from school professionals dedicated to health and wellness (e.g., school nurses; Ward et al., 2006). Taken together, the wide range of stakeholder input at the district level is sensible for school-level teams and should include school health expertise.

Team Function

The main responsibility of school-based health teams documented to date has been to facilitate the school-level implementation of school wellness policy and programming (CDC, 2013). Specific duties have ranged from determining the specific school health activities and necessary changes to undertake (Benjamins & Whitman, 2010), to leading the assessment process using CDC's School Health Index (Videto & Hodges, 2009), to forging partnerships between the school health activities and targeted stakeholders in and around the school (Carson, Castelli, Beighle, et al., 2014). The benefits of school health teams show promise. An intervention study conducted in 12 high schools by Ward and colleagues (2006) reported that the active participation of highly engaged and administration-supportive school-level teams was among the top school environment features found to increase the PA levels of high school girls.

District-Level Coordinator

Stronger evidence exists for the importance of dedicated district-level support for the promotion and protection of wellness initiatives across school campuses. District-level support might be a sole individual, often titled a district wellness coordinator or school health coordinator, or an appointed group of district or school individuals, often referred to as a SHAC, who represent the stakeholder participation required by law: district or school administrators, food service directors, parents, students, and community members. Both forms of district support have functions similar to those of the central body for driving wellness policy development, implementation, and monitoring and evaluation: provide school-level guidance and assistance with logistics, advocate for the importance of school health within the community, recruit community organizations to be involved, act as a liaison with state agencies and partners from various levels of school or district administration, support district-level fiscal planning, and secure additional funding (Chriqui & Chaloupka, 2011; Jain & Langwith, 2013; O'Brien et al., 2010). Most U.S. school boards presume that their district levels have the capacity to provide these supports, but the districts often do not feel equipped to monitor and evaluate wellness policy implementation (Agron et al., 2010).

The potential school health outcomes from district-level support personnel are encouraging. In a qualitative study with 19 key district- and school-level informants from six school districts funded to implement school-based health interventions, Jain and Langwith (2013) found that a district wellness coordinator was the cornerstone to implementation success. Schools reported having little capacity to address school health without the help of a designated district wellness coordinator. This individual reported to the district superintendent and worked primarily with a school champion (mostly a school nurse or physical education teacher) to initiate the intervention, secure funding, assist with logistics, promote and share successes district wide (which also fostered motivation), and encourage partnerships across school campuses (which helped reduce feelings of isolation). The wellness coordinators emphasized greater implementation success when a school-level champion assumed ownership of an intervention that was also aligned with school and district partners' priorities.

A similar district-led change agent was adopted in Maine with equally positive results. There, district superintendents assigned a school health coordinator to work at least 20 hours per week in one to three schools to convene SHACs, coordinate implementation of action plans and fund-raising activities, write grants, make educational presentations to school boards, and organize school-level leadership teams (i.e., CSPAP committees). Maine schools that employed this individual ($n = 123$), compared to schools without a coordinator ($n = 205$), were more likely to offer after-school PA programs (i.e., intramurals and clubs) and provide health education curricula that emphasized PA and fitness benefits, and they had significantly fewer (22 percent) students who reported watching two or more hours of TV per day (O'Brien et al., 2010).

A SHAC as a required element of school wellness policy, along with ongoing communication among building administrators and school boards, can facilitate wellness policy passage by school boards and related school environment changes for more PA breaks, healthier vending machine options, and tobacco-free campuses (Gollub et al., 2014). Unfortunately, the requirements for SHACs are not ubiquitous. Chriqui and Chaloupka (2011) found that policies that required SHACs had significantly stronger wellness policies overall, although they were more prevalent in majority White districts (vs. majority Hispanic districts) and in large districts (vs. small- and medium-sized districts).

Knowledge Claims

The internal capacity recommended for successful CSPAP programming includes a triad composed of the PA champion, a supportive administrator, and a CSPAP committee (Carson, Castelli, Beighle, et al., 2014). The existing literature related to the PA champion is growing, whereas the research on supportive administrators and CSPAP committees is scarce. Based on the research evidence that does exist, the following claims can be made by triad unit:

PA Champion

- The physical educator is the best option to fill the PA champion role.
- CSPAP knowledge and quality leadership skills are essential for effective and sustainable CSPAP implementation.
- Workload and role conflict are two prominent barriers that exist for the PA champion.

Supportive Administrator

- The first step in establishing a CSPAP is to intentionally solicit support from administrators.
- A supportive administrator is an active contributor on the CSPAP committee.
- Strategies and recommendations for administrator support include valuing and prioritizing PA, serving as a role model, assisting or leading the development of PA programming in various areas (district wide, school wide, the PA champion, quality physical education, and teachers), and building community connections to promote PA.

CSPAP Committee

- An early step in building a CSPAP is to establish a CSPAP committee, which serves in an advisory and decision-making capacity.
- At the very least, a CSPAP committee is composed of three members—a CSPAP champion, who likely serves as chair; a building principal; and a classroom teacher.
- Membership may extend to preexisting district-level SHACs or teams to ensure a similar range of input required in school wellness legislation (Public Laws 108-265 and 111-296) is represented: school board member, school health professional, parent, student, and the public.
- The function and impact of CSPAP committees on school PA opportunities may improve

by having a designated district-level support (wellness coordinator) to assist with fundraising, building district- and communitywide partnerships, and monitoring evaluation.

Knowledge Gaps and Directions for Future Research

Despite little research on the triad of CSPAP leadership, knowledge claims and an abundance of suggestions and recommendations exist. However, in the absence of research, there are several areas from which to create new knowledge for future research in all three triad units. The former (National Association for Sport and Physical Education, 2008) and most recent (CDC, 2017) inceptions of CSPAPs as a national framework to promote school PA and provide opportunities for children to achieve 60 minutes of daily PA warrant the need for research to examine the overall effectiveness and influence of CSPAPs on the PA levels of K-12 students. Expanding the research base of each unit within the triad of CSPAP leadership, both separately and collectively, will assist in determining the success of CSPAPs as a PA framework for schools.

It is recommended that the physical educator fill PA champion roles (Deslatte & Carson, 2014; Doolittle & Rukavina, 2014), yet this notion has not been researched extensively. Little is known regarding strategies to recruit and retain current physical educators and their willingness and attitudes in relation to fulfilling PA champion roles (Berei, 2015; Carson, Castelli, Pulling Kuhn, et al., 2014; Pulling Kuhn et al., 2015). Gathering further evidence related to physical educators' prolonged engagement in CSPAP implementation and CSPAP fidelity (Berei, 2015; Centeio, Erwin, et al., 2014; Doolittle & Rukavina, 2014) will support this claim and encourage physical educators to take on this role.

Similarly, it is unclear what kind or amount of support is beneficial for the promotion of school PA (Carson, Castelli, Beighle, et al., 2014), including the influence of the triad of CSPAP leadership on CSPAP-related outcomes (Berei, 2015). Research investigating the role of the physical educator (Berei, 2015) and the types and frequencies of effective administrator support is necessary (Carson, Castelli, Beighle, et al., 2014). For example, there is an ongoing effort by Idaho researchers to examine the perspectives and roles of Idaho school administrators to gather further evidence on effective administrator support for CSPAPs (Goc Karp et al., 2017). Additional research is also warranted pertaining to the impact of a supportive administrator on CSPAP outcomes.

Several recommendations include a call for CSPAP professional development (PD) opportunities that increase CSPAP knowledge and leadership skills for the PA champion, administrators, and CSPAP committee members. While researchers have begun to examine this area in further depth, very little is known about CSPAP PD (Chen & Gu, 2018; Russ et al., 2015), and future research should examine the frequencies and types of effective CSPAP PD. University students in PETE programs are the future of the physical education profession and have the potential to influence the use of the CSPAP framework. Similar to PD, PETE programs have the potential to increase CSPAP knowledge and leadership skills for future PA champions and CSPAP committee members. Research gaps related to this type of PD exist; therefore, it is important to learn how PETE programs prepare physical educators to fill PA champion roles and the effects of CSPAP PD on their knowledge, leadership skills, awareness, beliefs, ability to overcome barriers, and program implementation (Berei, 2015; Centeio, Erwin, et al., 2014; Illg, 2014; McMullen et al., 2014). Interested readers are directed to a two-part special issue of the *Journal of Physical Education, Recreation & Dance*, which details the CSPAP coursework and learning experiences integrated in 12 PETE programs—spanning undergraduate and graduate programs—around the country (Carson et al., 2017).

It is clear from research that the barriers related to CSPAP implementation exist for all areas of the triad of CSPAP leadership as well as on many levels within each unit. To assist in overcoming implementation barriers, future research should examine the strengths and barriers within school systems (Jones et al., 2014) for

effective CSPAP implementation. Although each school environment is unique, it is important to determine the overlapping factors necessary to sustain CSPAPs over time and effective strategies for overcoming barriers in school environments (Berei, 2015; Centeio, Erwin, et al., 2014; Doolittle & Rukavina, 2014). It is also necessary to examine what is known about the way policies influence an administrator's level of support (Carson, Castelli, Beighle, et al., 2014) and the work of the CSPAP committee as a whole (Chriqui & Chaloupka, 2011). This examination includes studying the actions of administrators and how those actions interact with ("decompose") potential effects of policy (Centeio, Castelli, et al., 2014) or how PA policies predominately come from districts rather than from states or even the federal government (Story et al., 2009). Another avenue may be to examine the impact of education (i.e., importance of CSPAPs and how to implement and maximize PA) on CSPAP committees and administrators (Erwin et al., 2013).

Lastly, it is important that CSPAP researchers remember that a CSPAP cannot be effective without the support and collaboration of parents, teachers, administrators, and other professionals and organizations in the local community (Metzler et al., 2013). That is, the leadership triad must operate interdependently and utilize the multilevel support system that exists both within and outside the school setting. Community-based participatory research is an effective approach for forming community partnerships and integrating local opinions (Israel et al., 1998) to develop, implement, and evaluate CSPAP initiatives (Kong et al., 2012) and policies (Hogan et al., 2014). Beyond including input from parents and community partners to build a sustainable CSPAP that improves children's physical behaviors (King & Ling, 2015), researchers may consider how school PA interventions can be facilitated by regular communication and coordination (via technical assistance and regular site visits) from local university personnel (Ward et al., 2006; Webster et al., 2015; see chapter 5). Above all, allowing student voice and perspective to be represented in school wellness discussions and planning is a recommended practice that needs further investigation (Hughes et al., 2015).

Evidence-Based Recommendations and Applications

Informed by the knowledge claims, table 3.1 depicts the evidence-based research and practical applications for each of the three influential units of CSPAP leadership—PA champion, supportive administrator, and CSPAP committee.

For School Staff

Supportive school staff members should consider becoming a PA champion or joining a CSPAP committee and utilizing the associated recommendations in table 3.1. If neither are reasonable options, school staff should utilize strategies to garner support from administrators, such as advocating for a quality physical education program and other CSPAP initiatives, or follow administrator recommendations in table 3.1 pertaining to valuing PA, serving as a role model, and offering a variety of assistance with the development of school-wide PA programming.

For Community Partners

Community members are critical elements to building the internal capacity for a CSPAP and all three units of the CSPAP leadership triad. To aid a CSPAP champion, it is recommended that community members reach out to schools and school PA champions to offer or connect the PA opportunities that are available in close proximity to the school and reaffirm the importance of physical education and school-wide PA programming to the local community and be willing to participate in shared-use agreements. To aid a supportive administrator, community members may consider providing resources and services to market and implement school-wide PA programming or entice participation (student or family incentives) and expand community connections. To aid a CSPAP committee, community members should willingly get involved in the committee work or, better yet, join the committee when asked. Many of these recommendations are embedded and further detailed throughout table 3.1.

SUMMARY

In conclusion, this chapter presented the research and practical evidence supporting the recommended approach to internal capacity building for CSPAP success—for every school to be equipped with a CSPAP leadership triad consisting of a designated PA champion, a supportive school administrator, and a dedicated CSPAP committee (Carson, Castelli, Beighle, et al., 2014). Successful strategies for developing and utilizing each unit of the CSPAP leadership triad are grounded in literature and achievable in practice.

QUESTIONS TO CONSIDER

1. In addition to those presented in this chapter, what other knowledge, skills, and characteristics do you think are necessary for an effective PA champion to possess, and how should the PA champion acquire them?

2. Brainstorm potential barriers to CSPAP implementation and the strategies that could be utilized to help overcome those barriers.

3. How can the PA champion and CSPAP committee solicit support for school-wide PA from administrators? Brainstorm and discuss advocacy strategies that have the potential to result in administrator support for incorporating PA throughout the school and community.

4. It is recommended the CSPAP committee include a variety of personnel. If you were the PA champion and took the role to create a CSPAP committee, who would you include on your committee? Support your answer with an explanation of their role and expected contribution to the committee and the CSPAP.

TABLE 3.1   Evidence-Based Recommendations and Applications Based on Knowledge Claims

Knowledge claims	Evidence-based recommendations and applications
PA CHAMPION	
The physical educator is the best option to fill PA champion role.	• Utilizes his or her movement-related knowledge and PA expertise to promote and advocate CSPAPs. • Leads or is an active member of the CSPAP committee. • Plays an active role in providing PA opportunities to various populations beyond quality physical education.
CSPAP knowledge and quality leadership skills are essential for effective and sustainable CSPAP implementation.	• The PA champion attends and participates in CSPAP-related PD opportunities (PAL, in-person trainings at conferences, webinars, active in professional organizations, informational emails). • PETE programs integrate opportunities for prospective teachers to develop knowledge and skills (see table 1) surrounding the role of a PA champion. (Refer to chapter 20 for further information on CSPAP and PETE programs.)
Workload and role conflict are two prominent barriers that exist for the PA champion.	• Lead a CSPAP committee to delegate responsibilities and workload for CSPAP implementation. • Implement a CSPAP needs assessment during the beginning phases of establishing a CSPAP to determine areas of strength and improvement within the individual school and community setting and decrease redundancy within the program (step 2 of the guide [CDC, 2013]). • Identify barriers for CSPAP implementation in unique school and community environments. • Collaborate with school and community personnel (CSPAP team, wellness committee, administrators, school faculty and staff, and parents) to examine strategies and implement a feasible plan to overcome CSPAP barriers. • Collaborate with school personnel, such as administrators and athletic directors, to negotiate funding and facility shared-use possibilities and opportunities for CSPAPs. • Utilize resources and grants to increase access to PA resources, equipment, and funding for CSPAPs. • Examine and address teacher beliefs regarding the role in physical education and school-wide PA promotion.
SUPPORTIVE ADMINISTRATOR	
The first step in establishing a CSPAP is to intentionally solicit support from administrators.	• Develop and implement a quality physical education program prior to implementing other CSPAP components. • Advocate for the quality physical education program to gain administrator support. • Seek buy-in from administrators early in the CSPAP implementation process.
A supportive administrator is an active contributor on the CSPAP committee.	• Establish and actively participate on a wellness or CSPAP committee. • Appoint a PA champion or fulfill the PA champion role. • Serve as a role model by providing, leading, and participating in PA opportunities. • Devote personal time to help organize or participate in events.
Strategies and recommendations for administrator support include valuing PA, serving as a role model, assisting the development of PA programming in various ways (district wide, school wide, the PA champion, quality physical education, and teachers), and building community connections to promote PA.	• Value the overall contribution of PA for its benefits in relation to the overall school and community vision. • Prioritize PA by formally scheduling a PA program into the daily school schedule. • Hold teachers accountable for implementing a PA program by regularly following up with teachers. • Seek knowledge and gain an appreciation of PA that can enhance and increase participation in and enjoyment of PA (i.e., advocacy). • Assist in the development of PALs and quality physical education programming through providing resources needed for teachers to attend CSPAP trainings, enhancing program marketing, allocating funds for physical education programming, and recruiting staffing help. • Provide CSPAP-specific PD for all teachers, or allow attendance at PD opportunities. • Allow teacher autonomy and creativity on how to include and integrate PA in the classroom, and provide extra opportunities for PA. • Acknowledge the efforts and accomplishments of all teachers and students involved in CSPAP-related opportunities. • Incentivize employee wellness programs. • Build community connections to promote PA, such as using shared-use agreements and guest programs, that service and influence school and community populations.
CSPAP COMMITTEE	
An early step in building a CSPAP is to establish a CSPAP committee, which serves in an advisory and decision-making capacity.	• Pull committee members from preexisting school or district-level wellness teams.
A CSPAP committee is composed of three members: a CSPAP champion, who serves as chair; a building principal; and a classroom teacher. Expand membership to include a wide range of representation and reach: school board member, school health professional, parent, student, and the public.	• Apply the same broad categories of public involvement required from the 2004 and 2010 public laws when creating a CSPAP committee. Select a parent; a student; at least one school physical education or PA expert; a school board member; a school administrator; and a person from the public, which could be a community member with authority in physical education and PA.
The function and impact of CSPAP committees on school PA opportunities may improve by having a designated district-level support person (wellness coordinator) to assist with fund-raising, promotion district and community wide, partnership building, and monitoring evaluation.	Build a case for district support with data and policy mandates. Consider involving nearby university faculty and students (via service learning courses). They can facilitate the collection and interpretation of needs assessment data, the identification of feasible action plans, and implementation of evidence-based CSPAP initiatives. The close proximity will allow for in-person working meetings, sharing written reports, and in-service presentations.

5. Explain and discuss how a school-based team approach for CSPAPs is similar to other comprehensive health frameworks or policies and why the team approach is necessary for effective CSPAP implementation.

CASE EXAMPLES

There are three nationally recognized case examples in this section that illustrate how units of the triad may operate in unison to create a thriving CSPAP community where reaching the recommended amounts of daily PA is the norm. The first two examples are from current physical education teachers as PA champions who share their passion, rationale, and successful implementation strategies for CSPAPs at their school. The third example is from a supportive administrator who describes how and why as a principal he is supportive of school-wide movement opportunities.

PA Champion

Jessica Shawley
Moscow Middle School
Moscow, Idaho

As a physical education teacher, I am proud that our profession has officially recognized the importance of reaching beyond our classroom walls to help our school communities become the active, healthy places students need and deserve. What better way to demonstrate the impact of my physical education program than through the CSPAP approach. As the lead PA champion in my school for several years now, I know the benefits of a CSPAP far outweigh the barriers. Participating in the Fuel Up to Play 60 program provided by my state's United Dairymen association, along with SHAPE America's PA leader training, has been the major catalyst for implementing a CSPAP in my school. This combination of support gave me the knowledge, skills, and confidence to lead efforts in educating administrators and colleagues on the importance of PA before, during, and after the school day.

Being a PAL has led to a plethora of accomplishments at my school, including activity break training and materials, lunchtime intramurals and recess equipment, before- and after-school activity clubs, cross-curricular projects where health-related messaging is infused in technology education, and improvements in our cafeteria culture. Our school culture embraces student and staff wellness. My colleagues are more mindful that students have a need to move. It brings me joy to have conversations with them on how they are incorporating movement into the classroom. We also provide staff wellness initiatives and communicate with parents about community opportunities.

This has all been possible through a purposeful progression of CSPAP implementation in small, achievable steps, of which many are outlined in this chapter. Some of the most important steps deal with leadership and building capacity through a team. The movement may start with the physical education teacher as the primary PA champion, but it should not end there. Others are interested and will support the CSPAP approach. The lead PA champion just needs to initiate the movement so momentum can begin. As you follow the steps to implementing and maintaining a CSPAP in your school, more PA champions will develop, and the workload can be shared, thus reducing barriers and producing a sustainable model for success. I encourage all physical education teachers to become their school's PA champion and to start an official CSPAP initiative so a culture of wellness can thrive.

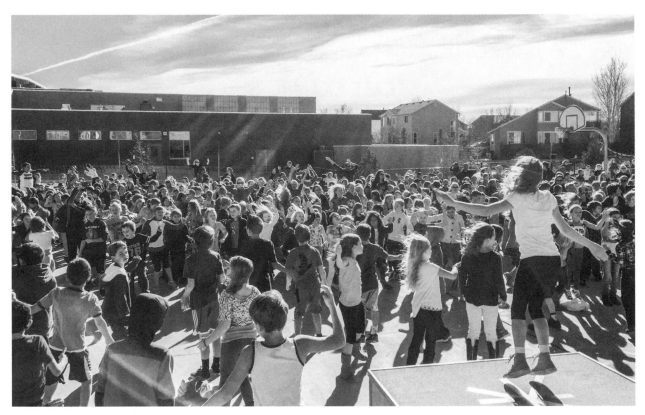

Red Hawk Elementary School's all-school movement program being led by one lucky student.

© Cyrus Weinberger

PA Champion

Tanya Peal
Soaring Heights PK-8
Erie, Colorado

The opening of Red Hawk Elementary in the fall of 2011 was an amazing opportunity for me as the physical educator. Our goal was to get students active every day for 40 minutes in addition to the activity time in recess and physical education. We had this movement concept but did not quite know how to make it happen. As the physical educator, I suspected that both teachers and students might get bored or lose interest in moving if they were stuck in their classrooms and that teachers might burn through their PA materials very quickly because I know that classroom teachers have so much on their plates. The last thing they had time for was to research ways to get their students moving.

I took it upon myself to find ways to keep movement fresh and easy for teachers. I started thinking outside of the box and really looked at the space we had available, both inside and outside of the school, thinking about how to best get students moving during our 20-minute block of morning movement time. I developed a colored day movement schedule, which is still followed today, six years and an additional 400 students later. The colored day movement schedule dictates three days where three grade levels are moving in their classrooms during the morning movement block and three days where they are moving outside their classrooms in a variety of activities. The outside-of-the-classroom activities take place on the playground, in an open field, and through hallways inside the building. Every Friday morning, the entire school population comes together for all-school movement, for which different classes and students are chosen to lead. While building our movement program, we learned as we went and tweaked things as we progressed to make them work for our school.

Six years later, our movement program follows the same colored day schedule, even though our school has doubled in size! I believe the program's success can be attributed to collaboration among our administrative team; school staff, including our custodian; and teachers, whose buy-in is critical to the program's success. Every day, we all work together because we believe that PA enhances student learning. I believe that it is the physical education teacher's role to lead this collaboration because this educator not only knows the importance of movement but also has the knowledge and skills to organize activities and ensure the students are moving. The physical educator is in a unique position because s/he works with all grade levels and, therefore, knows all students, teachers and school dynamics. A physical educator taking on this role adds much more responsibility to his or her job, but the rewards are indescribable. To see and hear of students who have improved focus and better behavior and have gained more self-confidence in themselves is so amazing.

Reflecting back, I see that all of my teaching experiences and training have helped me in the role of being a PAL for Red Hawk Elementary. Teaching a wide range of abilities and ages throughout the years, attending numerous trainings and workshops, and reading the latest research on the effects of PA on the brain have helped me immeasurably in this role. Based on my experiences and training, I had the confidence to take risks when developing a movement program.

Supportive Administrator

Cyrus Weinberger
Soaring Heights PK-8
Erie, Colorado

There has never been a more difficult time to be an educator. The challenges of today can seem overwhelming or impossible to overcome. Students living in poverty, the obesity epidemic, budget cuts and antiquated funding levels, high stakes testing, new data and technologies to examine and learn, and the list goes on. Yet PA truly changes the structure of the school day and alters school culture in such an invigorating way that students, teachers, and parents are able to learn in new ways. They are able to let go of what they have always done.

My interest was "sparked"—which reminds me of *Spark*, the title of the seminal book by Dr. Ratey, one of the chief researchers on the impact of exercise on the brain. The more I delved into the research and the astounding success of school systems such as Naperville, Illinois, which made daily aerobic exercise an essential part of its school day, I was determined, as the principal of a new elementary school, to make a school-wide exercise program a valued part of our curriculum. The frosting on the cake for me was how the introduction of the all-school movement program at Red Hawk not only shifted the culture of the school and raised the satisfaction level of parents, students, and teachers but also how it has become a catalyst for change in our middle and high schools and the creation of an online course through the University of Northern Colorado, which is accessible to 300 teachers in 10 school districts across the state.

As a teacher, I would allow students to stand up at their desks during independent work times and take small activity breaks, and I started a running club on Friday afternoons. I would intuitively bring movement into my classroom, but I had no in-depth pedagogical idea why PA helped my classroom run more smoothly. I always felt like I was going to be caught wasting valuable class time. The prevailing notion that more time in seats would lead to better performance made bringing movement into classrooms a waste of instructional time. The idea of changing the master schedule, training teachers, and talking to parents about the importance of exercise seemed absurd to many—despite the research from *Spark*.

When the opportunity to open a new school, Red Hawk Elementary, came about, it afforded me the opportunity to develop and plan a school from scratch, work with the community members about what they most wanted in a public school, hire all the teachers, and build a school community from the ground up. It turned out that what people wanted most in their public school was quite simple: a rigorous academic environment and happy healthy kids who looked forward to going to school and learning.

From the beginning, we integrated movement into the fabric and culture of our school by bringing 35 to 40 minutes of PA into the school day in addition to recess and physical education. We built movement into the master schedule and created a turnkey program for teachers so that it was not just something extra on their plate but rather a fun and invigorating part of everyone's day.

Despite these perfect conditions, we were met with resistance. It took all of our efforts, especially those of the physical education teacher, Tanya Peal, to educate parents and teachers about why PA is so important to learning, that it is not just about getting the wiggles out but rather creating an optimal learning environment.

By making movement part of the school day for *all* children, we required teachers and students to change their behavior; once this happened, it did not take long for people to embrace the idea. The impact our all-school movement program has had on our students and community is nothing less than amazing—from strong growth rates and high test scores to tremendous student climate surveys and few discipline referrals.

The Red Hawk story is compelling because it is a story of how one school has had a tremendous impact on a large swath of students and schools and even districts. During this time, St. Vrain Valley School District received a $1.4 million grant to bring running clubs, training, and materials to all elementary schools in the district. Other schools began their own all-school movement programs. Even some middle and high schools began to integrate PA into their days. It is important to realize that despite our success in grant funding to support the spread of the Red Hawk movement program, the components of the program itself in terms of how it is implemented have stayed the same since its inception—there is little to no cost to bringing this program to a school. It is more a matter of political will. If we want to create real and lasting cultural changes in our schools, PA has the greatest promise for truly changing people's behavior and in many ways is the least threatening.

Movement is not a panacea, but it certainly touches on the critical elements for how to improve educational outcomes for all our students. It provides a mechanism to enhance existing academic environments and supports health and wellness.

Capitalizing on Internal–External Partnerships to Maximize Program Sustainability

Collin A. Webster, PhD
University of South Carolina

Cate A. Egan, PhD
University of Idaho

Kevin Brabham
Jesse Boyd Elementary School

The issue of sustainability is often left unattended in the development, implementation, and evaluation of public health programs, including those applied within the K-12 school setting (Johnson et al., 2004; Scheirer & Dearing, 2011; Shediac-Rizkallah & Bone, 1998). Empirically based insights into effective strategies for program sustainability are therefore lacking (Schell et al., 2013). Already, the amassing literature on CSPAP recommendations and research mirrors this void. Most people seem to be more interested in how to get a CSPAP up and running than in how to make it last. For example, in the 70-page, step-by-step CSPAP guide for schools developed by the Centers for Disease Control (CDC, 2013) in collaboration with SHAPE America, only half of one page is devoted to developing CSPAP sustainability strategies. Furthermore, the strategies listed (establish and adopt policies; secure internal and external funding and other resources; and provide annual professional development for administrators, teachers, and other school staff) are limited in depth and scope and do not reflect recent advances in thinking about the sustainability of CSPAPs.

The purpose of this chapter is to foreground the issue of CSPAP sustainability. The first section of the chapter is a review of research related to the sustainability of public health programs. Key concepts are defined, and emphasis is placed on school-based health programs, including the developing CSPAP research in this area. Next, knowledge gaps from the existing evidence base are examined. Recommendations for and applications of the current knowledge base for program planning, implementation, and monitoring are then proposed. Finally, a case example is presented that illustrates the translation of the evidence base to professional practice.

Review of Research

Public health researchers have taken different, though often overlapping, views of program sustainability. The term "sustainability" has been defined in numerous ways in the literature on public health programs and is either used interchangeably with or treated as distinct from other terms such as "routinization," "institutionalization," and "continuation." An important consideration in defining sustainability is the extent to which a program is meant to be rigidly or flexibly maintained (Scheirer & Dearing, 2011). Shediac-Rizkallah and Bone (1998) stated the following:

> Sustainability does not imply a static program, in contrast to the notions of institutionalization and routinization which imply something that is repetitive but fixed. A dictionary definition of the word "sustain" is "to supply with sustenance: nourish," suggesting a living entity with the power to respond and change, just as a program must adjust to new needs and circumstances if it is to continue. (pp. 92-93)

This perspective emphasizes the evolutionary quality of sustainable programming: A program is sustained through its capacity to be adapted in ways that are consistent with the dynamic nature of the community it serves.

Defining sustainability also hinges on the targeted outcomes of a given program (Scheirer & Dearing, 2011; Shediac-Rizkallah & Bone, 1998). Programs may be viewed as successful if the intended health benefits are sustained, the program activities persist, or continued capacity building is evident within the recipient community or organization (Shediac-Rizkallah & Bone, 1998). Scheirer and Dearing (2011) identified additional sustainability outcomes, including the extent to which attention to the issue or problem continues and the program is replicated or diffused. Arguably, all of these outcomes are interdependent and should be addressed with equal attention when planning for sustainability as well as when evaluating and monitoring program success. It is possible, for instance, that a program designed to increase children's PA outside of school could be effective in the first but not the second year of implementation because of changes in children's interests. Thus, while program activities may continue from the first to the second year, the intended health benefits of the program may diminish. Using any single sustainability outcome to define program success will limit an evaluator's ability to fully understand program sustainability and predict its future and plan for its continuance.

Aside from the numerous outcomes that can be used to examine sustainability, there is a lack of clear direction in the literature with respect to what constitutes a sustainable program. For example, Scheirer and Dearing (2011) posed such questions as how much modification to the program activities at the organizational or community levels would be considered too much to still identify the program as the "same" program, and what dosage of the original program must be maintained to determine that the program has been sustained. Until such questions can be addressed to provide guidance for the field, it may be most suitable for program developers to specify program-specific indicators of sustainability (e.g., what part of a program or how much of the program is to be sustained, how the program should be sustained, how long the program should be sustained, and who will be responsible for sustaining the program; Shediac-Rizkallah & Bone, 1998).

Schell and colleagues (2013) identified nine core domains that affect a program's capacity for reaching the previously mentioned sustainability outcomes (e.g., sustained health benefits, sustained program activities, and continued capacity building). Each domain showed good face validity and is empirically supported. The domains, which are influenced by factors both internal and external to the program, include

- political support (internal and external political environment that influences program funding, initiatives, and acceptance);
- funding stability (making long-term plans based on stable funding environment);
- partnerships (the connection between program and community);
- organizational capacity (the resources needed to effectively manage the program and its activities);
- program evaluation (monitoring and evaluating process and outcome data associated with program activities);
- program adaptation (the ability to adapt and improve to ensure effectiveness);
- communications (the strategic dissemination of program outcomes and activities with stakeholders, decision makers, and the public);
- public health impacts (the program's effect on the health attitudes, perceptions, and behaviors in the area it serves); and
- strategic planning (the process that defines program direction, goals, and strategies).

Additionally, St. Leger (2001) reviewed the evidence on good practices in school health education and promotion and identified several themes among programs that achieved desired outcomes. Successful programs occurred over several years, provided significant professional development for teachers, and were adequately resourced, holistic (i.e., used whole-school approaches), and designed in light of both opportunities and limitations of schools in effecting meaningful health improvements. These findings suggested that successful, long-term health program implementation in schools is connected to the use of multicomponent approaches that are sensitive to contextual variables and provide substantial support for school professionals.

Specific to CSPAP research, Dowda and colleagues (2005) evaluated the sustainability of the Sports, Play, and Active Recreation for Kids (SPARK) program in schools that had adopted the program one to four years earlier. SPARK originally was a physical education curriculum program developed for elementary and middle school students that focused on fitness, motor skills, and enjoyment (see www.sparkpe.org for details about the current SPARK programming). Earlier research showed that SPARK resulted in sustained positive effects on desired outcomes 18 months following the initial intervention (McKenzie et al., 1997). Subsequent steps taken to diffuse the program included offering the program to schools across the United States on a contractual basis (contracts ranged from 6 to 12 hours of experiential, professional development training for school staff), using certified trainers to lead the trainings, using trained on-site facilitators in schools without physical education specialists, and providing technical assistance for schools via telephone and email communication when needed (Dowda et al., 2005). Program sustainability was assessed using a survey developed for the study to measure current use of SPARK and identify factors that might influence the continued use of the program. Surveys from 111 schools were returned, indicating 81 percent of schools reported still using SPARK. Schools that had continued to use the program reported more principal support, having more adequate equipment, and not using standardized physical education curricula prior to receiving SPARK training. Survey respondents (teachers) who reported currently using SPARK also reported higher participation in PA compared to respondents who reported not using the program. The majority of SPARK users indicated they had program-specific materials (99 percent), could easily adapt predesigned SPARK lessons when needed (99 percent), were given a regular schedule for using needed equipment and facilities (79 percent), and received ongoing training and support for program implementation (54 percent) and their principal or another teacher initiated the program at their school (58 percent; Dowda et al., 2005).

McKenzie and colleagues (2009) provided further information about the procedures used to ensure the sustainability of SPARK. From its inception, the program was designed to be implemented by teachers (physical education and classroom) and was informed by the professional background of the program developers, which included experience in physical education and health teaching, school administration, curriculum development, and teacher education. The investigators understood that school context mattered in the adoption, implementation, and maintenance of any new program. Therefore, the contractual agreements with schools interested in using SPARK begins with a consultation and needs assessment, which allows the trainers to tailor professional development appropriately for each school. Schools are provided with curriculum materials, which include a checklist that those who attend professional development sessions (teachers, principals, and other administrators) are trained to use to assess or evaluate the implementation of SPARK lessons. Other sustainability strategies described include giving schools and teachers certificates of recognition and sending schools a quarterly newsletter and benchmark documents as well as providing online support materials.

Another CSPAP-related program that was tested for its sustainability is the Child and Adolescent Trial for Cardiovascular Health (CATCH). CATCH was a multicomponent program for elementary students that included a food service intervention, a physical education program, classroom curricula, and a home and family component (details about the current iteration of CATCH [Coordinated Approach to Child Health] can be found at http://catchinfo.org). Physical education and classroom teachers received program-specific training and on-site consultations. Teachers also were encouraged to design their own activities to meet the program objectives. The program was tested for two and a half years with students from 96 schools (56 intervention and 40 control) starting in third grade and finishing in fifth grade. McKenzie and colleagues (1996) found that students in the intervention schools engaged in more moderate-to-vigorous PA (MVPA) and expended more energy during physical education lessons than children in the intervention schools. Data from students' fifth-grade year showed the intervention schools scored higher than the control schools on several observed characteristics, including

- teacher encouragement for students to be physically active,
- at least half the class being engaged in MVPA for 40 percent or more of the class time,
- having an adequate child-to-equipment ratio, and

- a warm-up and a cool-down.

Subsequently, Nader and colleagues (1999) found that three years following the end of the original intervention, children in the intervention group (then in eighth grade) reported higher MVPA, dietary knowledge, and dietary intentions compared to children in the control group.

Owen and colleagues (2006) noted an important aspect common to the sustainability approaches used in designing and implementing both the SPARK and CATCH programs. In each case, program development, dissemination, adoption, and diffusion were guided by key principles of the diffusion of innovations theory (Rogers, 1995). Specifically, program attributes known to increase the rate of adoption and facilitate diffusion were highlighted. These attributes include the relative advantage of the innovation compared to what is currently being used, the compatibility of the program with potential adopters' skills and beliefs, the simplicity with which the innovation can be implemented, the "trial-ability" of the innovation (the extent to which it can be implemented on a trial basis), and the observability of the innovation (the extent to which its positive results are observable).

More recently, Goh and colleagues (2017) examined factors related to 15 classroom teachers' continuance in using a classroom movement integration program (TAKE10) five months after the conclusion of an eight-week intervention. TAKE10 is a prepackaged set of classroom-based activities that link PA with academic lessons (see the TAKE10 website at http://take10.net for further information and examples). The teachers, who were from two elementary schools, participated in a one-hour training, which included information about the benefits of movement integration and direct participation in TAKE10 activities. During the intervention period, a member of the research team was on-site at both schools daily to provide additional assistance to the teachers. This assistance ceased after the intervention. Individual interviews and an open-ended questionnaire were used to collect data on program continuance. The findings showed that several of the teachers continued to use TAKE10 activities, although only three teachers used the activities two or more times per week. Factors related to continuance were (1) scheduling movement integration into weekly routines, (2) children's requests for the activities, and (3) collaboration with other teachers.

To the authors' knowledge, Egan and colleagues (2018) have conducted the only study to date that investigates the sustainability of a full, five-component CSPAP. The researchers examined the extent to which a grant-funded CSPAP, which was implemented with the support of a university research team across a two-year period at a charter middle school, continued to be implemented one and a half years after funding for the program ended (for further information about the program and its implementation, please refer to Hunt & Metzler, 2017; Metzler, 2016; and Metzler et al., 2015). The program was based on the Health Optimizing Physical Education (HOPE) curriculum model and included eight components (Metzler et al., 2013):

- Before-, during-, and after-school extended PA programming
- Sports, games, dance, and other movement forms
- Family and home education
- Community-based PA programming
- Health-related fitness
- Diet and nutrition for PA
- PA literacy (consumerism, technology, and advocacy) Integration of HOPE across all school subjects

Physical education teachers at the school received a training specific to the program. Similar to the interventions reviewed previously in this chapter, the goal was for the teachers and others at their school to implement the program as opposed to the university research team taking on this responsibility. During the training, the teachers were provided with information about the HOPE model and asked to decide how best to implement the various program components. The teachers were encouraged to identify ways in which they could integrate the program into existing aspects and areas of the school's current programming. A member of the university research team was assigned to each component to provide support during the implementation.

The study done by Egan and colleagues (2018) found that despite the presence of an extensive support structure during implementation (e.g., seven physical education teachers, the university research team, good school facilities and ample space for PA, support from the school principal, and external funding), most aspects of the program were not sustained when the funding ended and the university research team was unable to provide ongoing support. The reasons for the lack of sustainability included the loss of external funding, not sufficiently planning for sustainability, not initially conducting a needs assessment, and reduced communication between the university research team and the school after the two-year implementation. On balance, the findings make it clear that sustaining a full-scale CSPAP requires considerable resources that even the most well-equipped schools may struggle to provide on a long-term basis.

Knowledge Claims

Based on the available research reviewed in the previous section of this chapter, the following evidence-based claims can be made about CSPAP sustainability:

- Multiple outcomes can be used to conceptualize sustainability.
- CSPAP sustainability requires planning, which should take place prior to program implementation and include decisions about how to define, measure, monitor, and ensure program continuance.
- Resources beyond what the school can provide are needed to sustain CSPAPs in many cases.
- Integrating CSPAPs into routine parts of school life may help to foster program sustainability.
- The diffusion of innovations theory variables (e.g., perceived attributes of the innovation) may provide useful lenses when planning for CSPAP sustainability.
- Tailoring CSPAPs to fit different school contexts may increase the chances that these programs will be sustainable.
- Allowing teachers to take ownership of the CSPAP design, development, and implementation may increase program sustainability, although it is likely that the transfer of responsibility from trained interventionists and researchers to teachers should be gradual, and external support (provided by interventionists and researchers) may need to be extensive initially and continue for a number of years.

- Opportunities for teachers to collaborate and plan together are important to CSPAP sustainability.

Knowledge Gaps and Directions for Future Research

The most important question that needs to be answered is whether CSPAPs can be sustained. In particular, research is needed to examine the life span of comprehensive programs that show progress toward accomplishing both the educational and behavioral goals of CSPAPs, which are to foster lifelong engagement in PA and provide sufficient opportunities to participate in at least 60 minutes of PA each day during one's school years. When such programs are implemented, how long do they last? Is it typical for these programs to continue for more than a period of months, a year, several years? Several studies have tracked students' PA and other health-related outcomes following the intervention (Burns et al., 2017; Carson, Castelli, Pulling Kuhn, et al., 2014; Centeio, McCaughtry, et al., 2014), but investigation into educational outcomes (i.e., student performance in relation to K-12 physical education standards) is also needed to understand whether the comprehensive goals of CSPAPs can be realized.

The characteristics of programs that have lasted for relatively short durations also must be brought to light. In-depth case studies are needed to identify implementation approaches that have led to more and less sustainable CSPAPs in specific school contexts. Information about program history will prove to be invaluable in understanding the factors that have played a role in its sustainability. Who implemented different program components at different points in the program's existence? What enablers or challengers did implementers encounter along the way, what changes were made to facilitate implementation, and what resources were needed to enact these changes? Among variables in the program's life span, were there any constants (e.g., a supportive administrator, a motivated physical education teacher, or a strong policy to provide school-based PA opportunities)? Such research will build upon work that began to explore some of these issues (Carson, Castelli, Beighle, et al., 2014; Carson, Castelli, Pulling Kuhn, et al., 2014).

Concurrently, research must be undertaken to explore a wide variety of alternative CSPAP implementation approaches in terms of both the effectiveness and sustainability of such approaches. Many of the recommendations for implementing CSPAPs focus on physical education teachers as the natural or obvious choice among individuals in their school communities to take on the role of a PA director, CSPAP champion, or other designated expert for leading program implementation (Beighle et al., 2009; Carson, 2012; Carson, Castelli, Beighle, et al., 2014; Castelli & Beighle, 2007; Heidorn & Centeio, 2012). However, little evidence currently exists to demonstrate that most physical education teachers have the requisite training for and are capable of performing this role. In a national survey study with physical education teacher education faculty in the United States (Webster et al., 2016), respondents indicated their programs did little to prepare teacher candidates for CSPAP roles beyond teaching physical education. There is also little research on physical education teachers' perceptions of CSPAPs and willingness to assume new professional responsibilities (beyond teaching physical education lessons, coaching sports, and performing other assigned duties) without extra incentives (e.g., reduction in teaching loads, salary increases, or bonuses). In two U.S.-based studies, only 10 of 50 and 60 of 129 physical education teachers, respectively, who participated in an initial CSPAP-related training chose to continue with the training (Carson, Castelli, Pulling Kuhn, et al., 2014; Centeio, Erwin, et al., 2014). While it is possible that teachers discontinued the training because they felt the initial training was sufficient, this is not likely given there is a lack of focus on CSPAPs in the standards for beginning physical education teachers (used for accreditation; SHAPE America, 2017) and until recently, virtually no continuing education initiatives specific to CSPAPs for physical education teachers. According to a systematic review, the recommended knowledge and skills needed to implement CSPAPs are extensive (Webster, Webster, et al., 2015). Even if in cases where members of a school community (teachers, principals, students, and parents) want to implement a CSPAP and even succeed in doing so, there is still the question of whether a school can independently sustain the program without support from outside organizations and the extra resources they can provide.

Evidence-Based Recommendations and Applications

Although there has been limited research on the sustainability of CSPAPs, an evidence base is emerging to support the conceptual framework for effective and sustainable CSPAPs (see figure 4.1) developed by Webster, Beet, et al. (2015). The model is designed as a moving wheel to signify the potential for program continuance. The wheel's

three spokes represent the bridging of external and internal resources through each partnership to overcome possible barriers faced by the internal support system and achieve an effective and sustainable CSPAP.

The model is built on the assumption that maximizing the effectiveness and sustainability of CSPAPs requires the support of community partners, such as university faculty, service providers, and professional networks. This assumption is based on several perspectives. First, as previously mentioned, many school professionals, including physical education teachers, may not have the competency base to successfully implement, let alone sustain, a CSPAP. In their systematic review, Webster, Webster, and colleagues (2015)

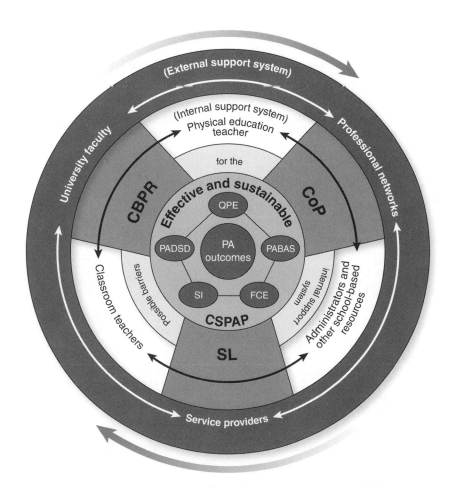

Figure 4.1 Conceptual model for achieving an effective and sustainable CSPAP through internal–external partnerships, including communities of practice (CoPs), community-based participatory research (CBPR), and service learning (SL). (Note: QPE = quality physical education; PABAS = physical activity before and after school; FCE = family and community engagement; SI = staff involvement; and PADSD = physical activity during the school day.)

identified 47 distinct recommendations in the literature related to preparing preservice physical education teachers for CSPAP implementation. Also, as previously mentioned, preservice preparation for such roles appears to be limited (Webster et al., 2016). This may partly be a function of the lack of formal accountability for CSPAP implementation (Carlson et al., 2013; Cradock et al., 2013; McCullick et al., 2012). The current national standards for beginning physical education teachers (SHAPE America, 2017) outline only one CSPAP-related expectation (beyond physical education) for teacher candidates, which is to be able to describe strategies for the promotion and advocacy of expanded PA opportunities. Candidates are not expected to be able to perform any of the skills that would be needed to implement or sustain CSPAPs.

Second, there is a dearth of research to demonstrate whether CSPAP-related professional training, at either the preservice or in-service level, can make a significant impact on program implementation, outcomes, and sustainability. Carson, Castelli, Pulling Kuhn, and colleagues (2014) examined differences in self-reported CSPAP implementation and program outcomes across one year between physical education teachers who received CSPAP training and support and those who did not. Teachers who were trained participated in a six-hour summer workshop where they received information about CSPAPs, practiced skills related to implementing each CSPAP component, and developed an action plan to implement a new PA opportunity at their school. During the academic year, the trained teachers had access to additional resources, including online learning modules as well as technical assistance and support from an assigned mentor. Results showed that trained teachers reported more PA offerings than untrained teachers but that students actually spent decreasingly less time in MVPA and increasingly more time being sedentary during school, with effects blunted in schools with trained teachers. At this time, more research is needed to address questions about the extent and nature of the training needed to increase teachers' rate of CSPAP implementation, students' PA, and program sustainability.

A third consideration is the possible reluctance of many physical education teachers or other school professionals to take on the additional responsibilities tied to implementing and sustaining CSPAPs. Changing teachers' beliefs and professional practices can be challenging (Curtner-Smith, 1999; Evans et al., 1996; Fullan & Pomfret, 1977; Laws & Aldridge, 1995; McLaughlin, 1987). The expansion of PA throughout the school day requires the support and involvement of classroom teachers, who are called upon to provide PA opportunities during regularly scheduled classroom time (Webster, Russ, et al., 2015). However, classroom teachers have expressed numerous concerns about integrating movement into their classroom lessons and routines, such as feeling overloaded with too many other assigned duties to also devote time and energy to PA promotion (see chapter 9 of this book for further information regarding this issue).

Perspectives From the Literature on Organizational Change and Capacity Building

The possible limitations of the school's internal support system (physical education teachers, classroom teachers, administrators, and other school-based resources) for CSPAP implementation and sustainability bring attention to challenges specific to organizational change and capacity building. Multiple models exist to explain organizational change (Heward et al., 2007). Heward and colleagues (2007) posited that two of these models, one proposed by Lewin (1951) and the other proposed by Pettigrew and colleagues (1992), provide particularly useful frameworks. In Lewin's (1951) model, organizational change is viewed as "a process shaped by the balance or equilibrium of the driving and restraining forces for change" (Heward et al., 2007, p. 173). Driving forces catalyze and sustain the change process, whereas restraining forces resist change efforts. Although increasing the driving forces may seem like an effective way to overcome the restraining forces, Heward and colleagues (2007) suggested that this approach will only result in the restraining forces increasing to match the pressure of the driving forces. To evoke change, Iles and Sutherland (2001) and Siler-Wells (1987) recommended (1) developing a state of readiness for change; (2) focusing on decreasing the restraining forces; and (3) attending to the organizational culture, politics, and group norms as important resisting forces.

Pettigrew and colleagues (1992) emphasized the role of historical, cultural, and political contexts in organizational change efforts. The authors distinguished between inner context (elements within the organization that influence the change process) and outer context (elements outside the organization that influence the change process) and suggested that both inner and outer contexts warrant analysis when attempting to initiate and understand organizational change. Another key aspect of the model by Petigrew et al. (1992) is the focus on the interconnectedness between context, content (the targeted area of transformation), and process (the actions, reactions, and interactions of stakeholders). These factors must be considered in relation to one another and viewed as continuously in flux. From this perspective, characterizing the change process, in context and over time, becomes the central aim of inquiry into organizational change. Pettigrew and colleagues (1992) asserted that a common limitation of studies of organizational change is they are "often preoccupied with the intricacies of narrow *changes* rather than the holistic and dynamic analysis of *changing*" (p. 6).

According to Crisp and colleagues (2000), "capacity building" is a term that "can be applied to interventions which have changed an organization's or community's ability to address health issues by creating new structures, approaches and/or values . . . without the need for future funding" (p. 100). Like organizational change, capacity should be viewed as dynamic because multiple variables both internal and external to an organization will change throughout a program's life span (Goodman et al., 1988). In a number of instances, capacity building is approached as an effort to change members of an organization or community from being passive recipients of a new program to being active participants in program implementation. Crisp and colleagues (2000) referred to this approach as a "community-organizing approach," which is "based on the notion that the most successful programs are those which are initiated and run by the members of the local community" (p. 103). However, Crisp and colleagues (2000) noted that the community-organizing approach is best suited for situations in which community members possess the motiva-

tion, leadership skills, and time to lead program implementation.

Spoth and colleagues (2004) discussed the important role of partnerships between schools, universities, and communities in increasing capacity for program delivery in public education systems. Such partnerships allow stakeholder groups to coalesce their respective resources and build upon existing infrastructures within each part of the system. The use of partnerships for capacity building requires careful attention to factors that can enable or hinder the development and continuation of the partnership. Israel and colleagues (1998) pointed out numerous facilitators and barriers to professional partnerships between researchers and community organizations. Examples of facilitators include jointly developed operating norms, goals, and objectives; democratic leadership; having a community organizer; involvement of a support staff or team; clear identification of professional roles and necessary skills; and prior history of positive working relationships between the partners. Examples of challenges include lack of trust and respect between partners, unbalanced distribution of power, conflicts, intensive time commitments, and lack of clarity on who or what represents the community.

Connecting Organizational Change and Capacity Building to CSPAP Sustainability

Taken together, these various perspectives of organizational change and capacity building underscore the importance of considering additional resources beyond the school, which can help to support changes in teachers' practices and leverage the school's capacity for implementing and sustaining a CSPAP. The partnership model by Webster, Beets, et al. (2015) highlights three partnership approaches—community-based participatory research (CBPR), communities of practice (CoPs), and service learning (SL)—that can bridge internal resources (existing within the school) and external resources (existing outside of the school) to cultivate organizational change and increase organizational capacity for CSPAPs. CBPR involves collaboration between researchers and other stakeholders (e.g., school professionals) within the community to develop contextually sensitive strategies for program implementation and sustainability (Israel et al., 1998). Ideally, this approach would support organizational change and capacity building for CSPAPs in terms of appropriate program planning, developing a state of readiness for school change, understanding key contextual factors, decreasing restraining forces in the change process, increasing program routinization, and being responsive to changes in inner (school-based) and outer (university- or community-based) contexts, including internal and external capacity, over time.

According to Webster, Beets, and colleagues (2015), CoPs and SL can build upon CBPR to further increase capacity for CSPAP implementation and sustainability. A CoP is a physical or virtual network designed to connect a group of professionals in ways that enhance their professional knowledge and skills, leading to the fulfillment of both individual and shared goals (Cambridge et al., 2005). SL is defined as "the integration of academic material, relevant community-based service activities, and critical reflection in a reciprocal partnership that engages students, faculty/staff, and community members to achieve academic, civic, and personal learning objectives as well as to achieve public purposes" (Bringle & Clayton, 2012, p. 105). Both CoPs and SL have the potential to offer continuous professional development for in-service and preservice teachers while also shifting some of the responsibility for community organizing (i.e., CSPAP implementation) from school professionals to university personnel and other stakeholders.

Initial research supports using these partnership approaches in a number of CSPAP contexts. Several studies found CBPR to be an effective strategy to increase PA promotion in after-school programs (Beets et al., 2014; Weaver et al., 2014), physical education, and general education classrooms (Weaver, Webster, Egan, Campos, Michael, & Crimarco, 2017; Weaver, Webster, Egan, Campos, Michael, & Vazou, 2017). Preservice and in-service classroom teachers indicated they had positive experiences with using virtual CoPs to learn and implement how to integrate movement into regular classroom time (Vazou et al., 2015; Webster, Zarrett, et al., 2017). SL provided numerous stakeholder groups (e.g., school-aged youth, teach-

ers, and university students) with a wide range of CSPAP-related benefits (Carson & Raguse, 2014; Michael et al., 2018; Webster, Nesbitt, et al., 2017; Webster, Weaver, et al., 2017), including increased engagement in PA (Galvan & Parker, 2011). While there is still much to be learned about how best to capitalize on internal–external partnerships to implement and sustain CSPAPs, much of the available evidence shows that building an infrastructure that expands beyond the school's immediate environment to combine resources from within and outside of the school is a sustainability approach that is well worth continued investigation.

For School Staff

While principals, assistant principals, teachers, and other professionals within the school building should work together to marshal their current resources with respect to CSPAP efforts, school professionals also must reach out to other organizations and agencies within the local community for external support of the program. A school-based CSPAP champion can serve as a liaison between the school and community partners. The CSPAP champion should be someone who is passionate about the program and wants to devote significant time and energy to its development and sustainability. This could be a physical education teacher, a classroom teacher, a school principal, a parent, or another person with a strong commitment to the success of the program.

One of the major functions of the CSPAP champion would be to construct a CSPAP committee that includes internal (school-based) and external (beyond the school) representatives from multiple stakeholder groups (e.g., school administrators, physical educators, classroom teachers, parents, teacher educators, and researchers). The committee could create a strategic plan for program implementation and sustainability, and the plan would incorporate strategies that combine internal and external resources. For example, the committee might decide to pursue a professional development school (PDS) partnership between the school and a local university that has teacher education programs. The PDS model is well established and includes a formal commitment from both the school and the university to collaborate on teacher training and research initiatives. Within such a partnership, school professionals would be responsible for hosting teacher candidates for student teaching internships and other on-site field experiences (e.g., teaching physical education, integrating movement in general education classrooms, or promoting PA during recess) as well as supporting and engaging in CSPAP research.

For Community Partners

For school–community partnerships to work, organizations and agencies surrounding the school must be receptive to partnership requests from schools. Furthermore, not all schools will take the initiative to seek external support from others in the surrounding community when attempting to implement or sustain a CSPAP. Thus, potential external partners also should offer their assistance to schools. State departments of education and local school districts can play a critical financial role in supporting CSPAPs by providing the funding needed to compensate the CSPAP champion for his or her work. Just as teachers often receive a stipend for certain extracurricular duties, such as athletic coaching, the CSPAP champion should be remunerated for leading the school in its progress toward establishing and meeting the goals of a CSPAP. Other forms of financial assistance could be hiring someone to take over part of the CSPAP champion's teaching load or assisting the CSPAP champion with administrative tasks related to the program (e.g., scheduling, record keeping, and data management).

Using the previously mentioned example of a PDS partnership, university faculty and graduate assistants would be responsible for organizing field experiences for teacher candidates and training candidates to successfully implement new PA opportunities within the school. The university should provide a liaison who works directly with the CSPAP champion to ensure a clear line of communication is maintained between the university and the school. Some of the major roles of the university liaison would be to evaluate teacher candidates during field experiences, provide CSPAP-related professional development for teachers at the school, serve on the CSPAP committee, and conduct and coordinate research initiatives at the school. Webster, Beets, and colleagues' (2015) three partnership approaches, discussed earlier (CBPR, CoP, and SL), could be integrated as part of the overarching PDS framework. The lines between research, teaching, and service would blur because the university liaison, other university faculty, graduate assistants, and teacher candidates all contribute to the way the CSPAP is designed, implemented, evaluated, enhanced, and sustained. Regardless of the resources they can provide, it is vital for community partners to remember that no program model should be viewed as a one-size-fits-all solution to increasing PA through schools. Each school environment must be understood for its unique strengths and limitations, and the implementation and sustainability of a CSPAP should be allowed to develop organically with continuous communication between all members (internal and external) of the partnership.

SUMMARY

Sustainability remains ignored in the recommendations and research related to CSPAPs. The broader literature on sustainability, capacity building, and organizational change specific to public health initiatives, particularly within schools, can serve as a guiding framework for future CSPAP research. Partnership approaches that bridge school-based resources to resources available in the surrounding community, such as university personnel within preservice professional programs, merit increased consideration and investigation in efforts to develop sustainable CSPAPs. Given the transient nature of many school communities, in which administrators, teachers, and families can frequently relocate, the life span of any CSPAP will depend on the bonds formed with external stakeholders who have deep and lasting ties to well-established institutions with vested interests in the education and health of school-aged youth.

QUESTIONS TO CONSIDER

1. What might school principals do in collaboration with external partners (e.g., community organizations, colleges and universities, or local government agencies) to increase the sustainability of CSPAPs?

2. In what ways might a CSPAP undergo change across multiple years of implementation, and what implications would these changes have for program planning and evaluation?

3. How could the lessons learned from sustainable programs, such as SPARK and CATCH, be drawn upon to increase the sustainability of CSPAPs?

4. What skills would be most important for physical education teacher candidates to learn related to sustaining CSPAPs?

5. What would a well-designed CoP look like if its primary aim were to increase CSPAP sustainability through collaboration between school professionals and community partners?

CASE EXAMPLE: STARTING AND SUSTAINING PA PROGRAMMING BEYOND SCHOOL HOURS

Kevin Brabham
Physical Education Teacher, Jesse Boyd Elementary School
Spartanburg, South Carolina

Our school is about 60 to 65 percent free and reduced lunch and mostly middle class families. We have a very diverse ethnic group. We have a decent-size gym; because it rarely gets used for something other than physical education, I don't get interrupted very often. Over the past eight years, I have been able to phase out a lot of old, broken, outdated equipment and buy new equipment, such as a 40-foot (12 m) rock climbing wall, scooters, cup stacks, balls, tennis and badminton equipment, stability balls, poly spots, cones, footballs, and numerous other stuff. My students know that being physically active is important to me, and now they think the same way. I go to some of their sporting events outside of school, offer extra physical education classes for various things during my planning periods throughout the year instead of our principal giving out popsicles or pizza, bring my two young boys to walk and bike to school days, and really encourage them to play different outside school sports or activities. One thing that I have taught our students since my first day of teaching is just because you love this game or sport doesn't mean everyone does, so that is why we do a variety of games. My students realize that they may not like the game or activity but it might be another student's favorite, so they participate fully. It took some time to teach this to our students, but they do a great job of having fun with every game we play.

Starting a PA program outside of normal school hours can seem like a daunting task. During my first year of teaching, I was lucky enough to have a coteacher who was in his 15th year of teaching and was a great mentor for me. It also was his first year at our school, and we decided to have an extra physical education class before school that we called PE Club. We already had extracurricular duties assigned to us every morning from 7:00 to 7:20. So we began by going to the cafeteria at 7:25 each day, picking up students who had already eaten breakfast and were at school early, and bringing them to the gym for a lesson or just to exercise. What started with about 20 to 25 students quickly grew to over 60 students. By the third or fourth week, we had to separate our club by grade level and reserve one day per week for each grade level to come to the club. The club went until 8:00, and we would walk the students to their homeroom classes afterward. We averaged about 30 students each day. The program has continued for the past eight years in numerous iterations, all of which have been successful. I like changing certain aspects of the program every year to keep the students (and me) excited about it. We currently call the program Fit Kids, and this year, it is a workout type of class. We use a great app called Sworkit, which gives us different workouts each day.

When my coteacher and I started on this journey, our first hurdle was getting support from our administration. When we approached our principal with the idea, his response was "Yes!" He originally thought that by allowing us to take the students out of the cafeteria, it would result in fewer students for him to watch in the mornings. But once he saw the substantial increase in students arriving early to school, he realized that PE Club actually filled a gap in our school programming; our kids needed a PA program before school. That was when our principal gave us the green light to expand PA opportunities even more. We started an after-school intramural program for our fourth- and fifth-graders. It starts right when school gets out and ends at 3:15. We have four different "seasons," which are aligned with what we are currently learning in physical education. During intramurals, we emphasize teamwork and sportsmanship. Students do have to sign up for intramurals, and I limit it to only 50 students because I am the only staff member involved with intramural days. However, I put students who are not able to participate on a waiting list for the next season.

Having successful before- and after-school PA programs requires support from administration and commitment from the physical education teacher or club sponsor. After my first year of teaching, my coteacher moved to a different school. I was nervous about whether I would be able to handle my regular duties as a physical education teacher as well as my new roles with the before-school club and the after-school intramurals, not to mention my responsibilities as a coach at the high school. I decided to have students sign up for PE Club in the mornings and limit it to 20 students per day and do it only three days a week. I limited intramural sign-ups to only 30 students. I thought to myself, "This will work out fine . . . for me." I had a lot of students and parents email and call me about why their child couldn't be in PE Club or intramurals. I quickly learned, it's not about me. I was cheating my students out of an opportunity to be active because it was easier for me. Before the winter holidays that year, I reopened PE Club to our whole school and added 20 people to the intramurals program. Once again, PE Club and intramurals began to flourish.

Sustaining these programs takes a lot of work for the physical education teacher, club sponsor, or whoever is in charge of the program. For me to be able to continue to provide opportunities for our students, I had to find funding. I would apply for grants here or there and occasionally get one. We received a BOKS [Build Our Kids' Success] grant and did BOKS as a substitute for PE Club one year. It was great. But coming up with $1,000 the next year to continue the program was hard, so we went back to PE Club. About five years ago, I decided to give a reward for the intramural champions each season. I decided I would give students shirts that said "Intramural Champions" on them. It was a great idea, but shirts cost money. I realized that for me to have successful programs, I needed to do some fund-raising. After a lot of discussion, I came up with the idea of doing a color run for our school. Within the first two weeks of registration, people from all over our community wanted to participate, so I quickly dubbed the event the Hub City Color Run and got a corporate sponsor. Over 300 people signed up. We made over $5,000 that first year, and it was incredible. I was able to buy equipment for our physical education classes, shirts for intramurals, and equipment for an active classroom. We now have done the Hub City Color Run the past five years and made enough money every year to support our programs, buy equipment for our classes, and provide funding for other school activities. I have found that external rewards are not necessary to encourage student participation, but our kids enjoy receiving T-shirts and extra physical education.

One problem I ran into was that a lot of students wanted to participate in either PE Club, now Fit Kids, or intramurals but couldn't get to school early enough or get picked up on time after intramurals were over. Last year, I had planning time scheduled for the last 30 minutes of school every Friday, so I decided I would start a club during this time. I wanted to do some type of running club and found a grant for Marathon Kids, and we received funding. I got permission from my principal, and we started Marathon Kids on Friday afternoons and had 50 students participate. It was a great time, and students earned prizes for completing each marathon. This club was so successful that my principal decided this year to make every Friday club day for the whole school, and every teacher has a club now and every student participates. This year, my club is garden club, and we are currently growing kale, lettuce, collards, and cabbage and already have had one huge harvest and are ready for our second. Our other clubs include yoga, cheer, running, knitting, cooking, and many more.

I didn't receive any formal training for CSPAPs. A lot of what I have done has been learn as you go. It would have been helpful to have had preservice and in-service preparation for the CSPAP roles I've taken on. Having a firm foundation for this kind of work would have given me a great head start. As you get further along in your career, though, you continue to learn more about what works for your own teaching style and your students. I think you have to learn what works and what doesn't work at your school. Most of the grants I have received have been pretty easy to write, but they do take time; fortunately, we have resources at our school and in our district to help. Being motivated to make a difference is key. When I was doing my student teaching internship, my cooperating teacher's passion for giving her students a chance to be active and find an activity they love to do was contagious. When I started teaching, I really wanted to incorporate fitness into every unit I taught as opposed to just teaching skill development. I wanted students to be able to take their locomotor skills and movement concepts that we review each August and see how they can be applied to sports and games. I viewed the expansion of PA opportunities beyond physical education lessons as a natural progression in my school's programming.

My principal and others in my school community bought in to ideas like PE Club, intramurals, and other new opportunities for our students because the benefits of the extra PA quickly became obvious. Over time, classroom teachers at my school have become more involved with PA promotion. We have two fourth-grade teachers who do Girls on the Run and now also do a running club. Another teacher started a walking school bus program with the help from Partners for Active Living. My district provides professional development workshops every nine weeks, and the physical education teachers across schools meet to share ideas, teach each other new games and strategies, and develop new programming. We are in the process of discussing the development of a district-wide summer physical education program. Working closely with the other physical education teachers in my district fuels my motivation to continue learning as a teacher and to provide new experiences for my students.

Beyond the support within my school and school district, our school has formed many partnerships with outside organizations to help implement and sustain our programming. Some of our partners include PAL (Partners for Active Living), Healthy Eating Decisions, and Safe Routes to School. In addition, the Mary Black Foundation has given our county funding for the SPARK and CATCH curricula. Lowes and Home Depot have donated materials to us for the Color Run as well as for class. For instance, they donated 4-foot by 8-foot (1 m by 2 m) sheets of plywood for us to make Ping Pong tables, which we have used now for four years, and they donated soil and vegetables for us to start a school garden. In sum, a motivated physical education teacher, the solidarity of the school principal and other teachers, and a supportive network of outside stakeholders have enabled our CSPAP to grow and prosper.

Social Psychological and Motivational Theoretical Frameworks for CSPAP Intervention

Megan Babkes Stellino, EdD
University of Northern Colorado

Spyridoula Vazou, PhD
Iowa State University

Lyndsie M. Koon, PhD
University of Illinois at Urbana-
Champaign

Katie Hodgin, PhD
University of Northern Colorado

Well-understood theoretical frameworks that account for social influence and motivational factors from the psychology of sport, exercise, and PA literature provide an ideal foundation for guiding CSPAP intervention research and practice. Explanations of human-motivated behavior that afford not only a basis for prediction but also understanding of CSPAP-related endeavors are essential, and thus relevant, to the focus of this text. In particular, the social and psychological factors that contribute to successful promotion of PA in schools warrant attention to sustain these efforts. In this chapter, we review the most prevalent theoretical frameworks for CSPAPs used to date and the associated findings across CSPAP components from school PA investigations guided by them; propose knowledge claims based on findings from the theoretically guided CSPAP interventions; identify knowledge gaps and propose recommendations for future research and intervention efforts framed within social psychological and motivational theoretical frameworks; suggest practical implications from the extant research for practitioners, researchers, and policy makers; and provide two case examples of successful integration of theoretically derived components into CSPAP interventions. By conducting research and practice from an evidence-based, theoretical foundation, CSPAPs will be more successful in terms of understanding how, why, and what mechanisms work for implementation and may better facilitate consistent outcomes of increased PA in the future.

Review of Theoretical Frameworks for CSPAP Research and Intervention

This section includes brief overviews of the five most prevalent theories applied to CSPAP to date: social cognitive theory (SCT), theory of planned behavior (TPB), competence motivation theory (CMT), self-determination theory (SDT), and ecological systems theory. Each theory is introduced with an emphasis on how the constructs within each theory are applicable to CSPAP and how the theoretical framework can be used to guide implementation of effective CSPAPs. While these theories are introduced separately, they do not operate exclusively from one another in use and application. Constructs from different theories can work harmoniously to form a potentially valuable combined theoretical foundation for CSPAP, which may better serve our endeavors to understand, explain, and predict intended PA promotion.

Social Cognitive Theory

Social Cognitive Theory (SCT; Bandura, 1986) suggests that individuals' thought processes, or cognitions, and behavior are reciprocally determined by their social and environmental context. Individuals are influenced by who and what are around them and vice versa. The SCT describes how individuals learn certain behaviors via important others' positive modeling of those actions. For example, as Donnelly and colleagues (2009) found, students' PA increased significantly when their teachers participated in, or modeled, more classroom PA. According to the SCT, social and environmental support is imperative for behavior change. Teachers' modeling PA is highlighted when considering PA promotion because engage-

ment in PA is frequently in social contexts and, therefore, individuals can theoretically benefit from the support of role models and access to resources in the environment (e.g., open space and PA equipment). Evidence of these theoretical contentions exist in that social support from parents (Silva et al., 2014), peers (Fitzgerald et al., 2012), and teachers (Eather et al., 2013) has been found to be a strong influence on PA participation among youth. In other words, these theoretically based research findings suggest that physical education teachers as well as all PA champions in the schools can make quite an impact through their own consistent modeling of PA and healthy living.

A central component of the SCT is self-efficacy, which involves the confidence one has in his or her ability to perform certain behaviors and achieve specific goals (Bandura, 1977). Self-efficacy has consistently been linked to youth PA (Sterdt et al., 2014) across ethnically diverse student populations (Shilts et al., 2009). The strongest source of self-efficacy is performance accomplishments, which means that by modifying the difficulty level of the tasks and making the tasks challenging (not too easy and not too hard), students are more likely to experience success, which will strengthen their self-efficacy for future participation and effort. Many school-based intervention studies focus on increasing students' self-efficacy levels to meet the PA guidelines (see table 5.1). As it relates to CSPAP, the concept of self-efficacy is also relevant to the adults (e.g., teachers, parents, and PA champions) involved in promotion, interventions, and programming of PA in schools. As research shows (see table 5.1), the more efficacious the physical education teacher is in implementing an after-school intramural program or a classroom teacher is in integrating movement breaks, the more likely students will benefit from, engage in, and experience more opportunity for school-based PA.

Theory of Planned Behavior

To better predict human behaviors, it is important to recognize what immediately precedes a behavioral decision. The theory of reasoned action (TRA; Fishbein & Ajzen, 1975) was developed based on the idea that cognitive self-regulation is an important aspect of one's behavior that occurs prior to decisions to act. The TRA postulates that one's attitudes (how one feels about a behavior) and subjective norms (how one believes important others feel about a behavior) lead into one's intentions, which then lead to behavior. According to the TRA, the greater one's intentions are to perform a PA behavior (e.g., be physically active during recess) because he or she likes PA or a teacher thinks PA is important, the more likely he or she will actually engage in that behavior (being active at recess).

The theory of planned behavior (TPB; Ajzen, 1985) builds upon the TRA by adding the element of perceived behavioral control, or the degree of one's belief that he or she has control over performing a behavior. Perceived behavioral control is similar to self-efficacy and, according to the TPB, in conjunction with attitudes and subjective norms, leads to behavioral intentions.

To apply the TPB to CSPAP implementation, positive attitudes toward and about PA at school should be strengthened (e.g., sharing knowledge about the academic and health benefits of movement for students and staff), and perceptions of behavioral control should be increased (e.g., providing PA resources). In addition, PA in school should be accepted and normalized, which could be done by showcasing teachers or other staff members who participate in PA with students and promoting PA in the school environment (e.g., hanging posters or signs with PA messages). Research findings have shown that, although not often recognized as the main motivator, adolescents' perceptions of peers' judgment and performance of PA establish positive subjective norms about PA, which in turn significantly contribute to their own increased PA behaviors (Fitzgerald et al., 2012; Priebe & Spink, 2011).

Competence Motivation Theory

Harter's (1978, 1981) competence motivation theory (CMT) is a framework that is particularly well suited to be the basis of intervention and examination of CSPAP and PA promotion. A central aspect of the CMT is the fundamental role of domain-specific self-perceptions of competence and control as they relate to motivational processes. Students who believe that they are competent at PA and have control over their PA behaviors

are theoretically predicted to be more intrinsically motivated to pursue optimal challenges (e.g., more miles during before-school mileage club or longer bouts of moderate-to-vigorous PA [MVPA] during recess). The contentions of CMT further emphasizes the profound role of significant others (e.g., teachers, parents, and peers) in the development of youth perceptions of competence, control, intrinsic motivation, and affect.

Critical aspects of the CMT that are relevant for successful CSPAP intervention follow:

- Individual perceptions of competence (e.g., beliefs about being good at physical activities) and perceived control (e.g., beliefs about how, where, when, and why to be physically active) are not only crucial outcomes of opportunities to engage in PA but also influence one's affective response to PA (e.g., liking or disliking) and subsequent choice, effort, and persistence at PA behavior (competence motivation).

- The role of important others (e.g., teachers, peers, and parents) is paramount because their approval, reinforcement, modeling, and feedback provided on challenging tasks (e.g., MVPA during recess, participation in before- or after-school PA programs) theoretically predict a positive or negative trajectory toward subsequent engagement in the task.

- Harter (1981) considered enjoyment as central to motivated behavior, such as PA.

- The CMT is a developmental perspective that accounts for changes in actual competency, accuracy of perceived competency, and sources of information used to assess competency as individuals age. Of particular relevance to CSPAP promotion are the aspects of youth competency that include both skill-based competencies (e.g., running efficiently and throwing or kicking in a mature developmental pattern) and the broader competency of being able to successfully engage in PA.

It is important to emphasize that individuals evaluate their competence (i.e., feeling that they are good at or not so good at various skills) in two ways: (1) based on how well they perform the activities compared to previous personal performance or the level of effort they exerted (task-involving orientation) and (2) based on the outcome, for

TABLE 5.1 CSPAP Interventions Grounded in Relevant Theoretical Frameworks

Author and year	Primary PA area (additional areas)	Intervention name, dose, and design	Sample	Associated theories and frameworks	
Boyle-Holmes et al. (2010)	PE	Michigan's Exemplary Physical Education Curriculum (EPEC) 2 years, 2x/week Quasi-E	n = 1,195 (600 I, 595 C) 16 schools (8 I, 8 C) Grades 4 and 5	Perceived competence and self-efficacy, attitudes, perceived support, enjoyment	
Dishman et al. (2004); Pate et al. (2005, 2007); Saunders et al. (2006)	PE (HE, staff, and community)	Lifestyle Education Activity Program (LEAP) 12 months RCT	n = 2,744 girls 24 schools (12 I, 12 C) Grade 9	SCT (self-efficacy about participating in PE), enjoyment of PE and PA, self-monitoring, support SEM	
Lonsdale et al. (2013); Rosenkranz et al. (2012)	PE	Motivating Active Learning in Physical Education (MALP) 1 PE lesson RCT	n = 288 M_{age} = 13.6 years 16 classes (4 I(a), 4 I(b), 4 I(c), 4 C)	SDT: perceived autonomy support from PE teacher	
Stock et al. (2007)	PE and HE	Healthy Buddies 21 weeks, 2-3 hours/ week Quasi-E	n = 228 I (100 K-3, 128 4-7) n = 131 C (61 K-3, 71 4-7)	SCT: peer modeling, perceived competence, perceived body image	
Jamner et al. (2004); Schneider & Cooper (2011); Schneider et al. (2007)	PE (HE)	Project Fitness and Bone (FAB) 9 months, 60 min (40 min active), 5 days/week Quasi-E	n = 122 low-active girls (63 I, 59 C) Grades 10 and 11	Affective responses to exercise, enjoyment, self-monitoring, goal setting, problem solving	
Pangrazi et al. (2003)	Classroom (school environment)	Promoting Lifestyle Activity in Youth (PLAY) 12 weeks, 15 min/day Quasi-E	n = 606 Grade 4 (35 schools) 185 PLAY + PE (10 schools) 178 PLAY (10 schools) 150 PE (9 schools) 93 C (6 schools)	Attitudes, self-monitoring, modeling, motivation (enjoyment)	
Bartholomew & Jowers (2011)	Classroom	Initiatives for Child Activity and Nutrition (Texas I-CAN!) 6 months, 1 lesson/day RCT	n = 25 I teachers (4 schools) n = 22 C teachers (4 schools) Grade 3	TPB: attitudes, perceived behavioral control/self-efficacy (teacher)	

Intervention content	Affected stakeholders	Outcomes (relevant for chapter)	Summary of primary findings
PE curriculum was developed to focus on teaching progression in FMS to improve student confidence and values of PA for health and enjoyment.	PE teachers	PA (self-report), FMS competency, and fitness	Significant improvement in FMS competency for all students as well as in PA levels and motor skill efficacy for 4th-graders in I compared to C.
Changes in PE instructional practices with focus on improved self-efficacy and enjoyment of girls by gender-separate activities, expanded choice of PA favored by female students, deemphasis on competition, absence of elimination during play, promotion of small-group interactions, emphasis on moderate-to-vigorous rather than higher-intensity activities, inclusive instruction. The LEAP HE lessons taught self-management skills for adoption of active lifestyle. School staff provided a supportive environment by role modeling and increasing communication and promotion of PA.	LEAP team (a group of school personnel), a LEAP champion (who taught the PE lessons), school staff, and family and community involvement	PA (self-report), self-efficacy, and enjoyment	Girls in high-implementing schools had greater PA levels by participating in one or more blocks of vigorous PA/day, an effect that was maintained when the girls were in the 12th grade. Changes in PA were partially mediated by self-efficacy and enjoyment.
Modified teaching strategies by (1) explaining the relevance of activities and making connections between skill development, games, and social interactions (relevance group); (2) providing opportunities for students to make choices during lesson, mainly during warm-up and organizing games near end of lesson (providing-choice group); and (3) providing extra equipment without further instruction (free-choice group).	PE teachers received 20 min training on how to modify the PE lesson	PA (accelerometer), sedentary behavior, and motivation during lesson	PA significantly increased in the free-choice group, and sedentary behavior significantly decreased in both the free-choice and providing-choice groups. Student motivation did not change, but perceived autonomy increased during both choice-based interventions.
Students in grades 4-7 were paired with students in grades K-3 by acting as role models and peer educators for healthy living (PA, nutrition, body image). Older kids delivered HE lessons and spent two 30-min, structured aerobic fitness lessons per week in the gym with their buddies.	Teachers and PE teachers	PA (self-report), BMI, fitness, perceived competence, body image, attitudes, and social acceptance	Grades 4-7 I students had a significantly smaller increase in BMI and significantly higher health behavior compared to C. I students of all grades had significantly greater increase in health knowledge and health attitudes compared to C.
Changes in PE instructional practices with focus on improved enjoyment of girls: exempted from mile-run requirement, excused from wearing uniforms during PE, offered variety of activities, allowed input into the choice of activities, offered modified activities at preferred intensities and difficulty level. One HE lesson was devoted to self-monitoring and goal setting.	PE teachers	PA (self-report) cardiovascular fitness, bone mass, and composition	Improvements in cardiovascular fitness and vigorous PA were significantly larger for I compared to C. Average daily minutes in moderate PA remained stable for I and significantly declined for C. Bone mineral content for the thoracic spine significantly increased for I. Within I, girls with low-baseline enjoyment significantly increased vigorous activity from pre- to postintervention.
Intervention focused on developing attitudes about PA and promoting self-monitoring by students to develop awareness of a variety of PAs as well as the amount of PA performed each day. Teachers were trained to model PA active behavior. Students were encouraged to select PAs they enjoyed most and to self-direct their activity to reach 30 min or more of PA independently of the teacher.	Classroom teachers	PA (pedometer) and BMI	I (PLAY only and PLAY + PE) was effective at increasing number of steps per day, especially for girls, compared to C (no treatment). No changes in BMI.
Intervention focused on increasing classroom teachers' level of confidence in their ability to incorporate PA into lesson plans through teacher training and the development of an easy-to-use curriculum.	Classroom teachers	PA (pedometer and accelerometer), teacher self-efficacy, perceived barriers, time on task, and academic performance	A significant difference between groups, with I students increasing PA by more than 300 steps and C students reducing their steps by nearly the same degree. For I, about 20% of lessons were spent at MVPA. Teacher self-efficacy was associated with percentage of lessons completed during I and perceived barriers. Time on task was significantly higher for I compared to C.

(continued)

TABLE 5.1 CSPAP Interventions Grounded in Relevant Theoretical Frameworks *(continued)*

Author and year	Primary PA area (additional areas)	Intervention name, dose, and design	Sample	Associated theories and frameworks
Donnelly & Lambourne (2011); Donnelly et al. (2009); DuBose et al. (2008); Gibson et al. (2008)	Classroom	Physical Activity Across the Curriculum (PAAC) 3 years, 90 min/week RCT	n = 4,905 (26 schools) Grades 2 and 3 followed for 3 years	Self-efficacy (teacher)
Mantis et al. (2014); Vazou & Skrade (2016)	Classroom	Move for Thought 8 weeks, 3x/week Quasi-E	n = 106 I n = 118 C Grades 4 and 5	SDT: need satisfaction (autonomy, relatedness, competence), perceived competence in math
Norris et al. (2015, 2016a, 2016b)	Classroom	Virtual Traveller 6 weeks, 3x/week RCT	n = 264 8- and 9-year-olds 10 grade-4 classes	Behavioral change wheel model: capability, opportunity, motivation (teacher)
Springer et al. (2012)	During school (PE, recess, family, and community)	Marathon Kids 6 months Quasi-E	n = 511 Grades 4 and 5 8 schools (5 I, 3 C) Low SES	Self-efficacy, social support, self-monitoring
Hyndman et al. (2014)	Lunchtime	Lunchtime Enjoyment Activity and Play (LEAP) 7 weeks and 8-month follow-up Quasi-E	n = 275 (123 I, 152 C) 5 to 12 years old	Enjoyment of PA and lunchtime activities SEM
Annesi (2004, 2006); Annesi et al. (2005, 2007)	After school	Youth Fit for Life (YMCA) 12 weeks, 3x/week, 45 min Quasi-E	n = 570 5 to 12 years old	SCT, self-efficacy theory, self-concept, social support
Wilson et al. (2005)	After school	Student-centered PA I 3x/week for 2 hours after school RCT	n = 48 (28 I, 20 C) 11 to 14 years old	SCT: self-efficacy, self-concept SDT: enjoyment, motivation for PA
Story et al. (2003)	After school (family)	Girlfriends for KEEPS (Keys to Eating, Exercising, Playing and Sharing) 12 weeks, 1 hour 2x/week Quasi-E	n = 54 8- to 10-year-olds and their caregivers or parents	Self-efficacy theory, enjoyment
Cliff et al. (2007)	After school (family)	SHARK (community-based program) 10 weeks, 2 hours/week Quasi-E	n = 13 Overweight or obese 8- to 12-year-olds	CMT

Intervention content	Affected stakeholders	Outcomes (relevant for chapter)	Summary of primary findings
Intervention focused on increasing classroom teachers' level of confidence in their ability to incorporate PA into lesson plans through teacher training sessions and goal setting.	Classroom teachers	PA (accelerometer), BMI, and academic achievement	Schools with more than 75 min exposure to I showed significantly less increase in BMI at 3 years compared to schools with less exposure to I. I had significantly higher PA levels during school day and on weekends compared to C. I had significant improvement in academic achievement over the 3 years compared to C. Students in I were significantly more active in classroom with teacher participation.
Intervention included 10-min physically active lessons integrated with math. Lessons were developed to promote satisfaction of the needs for autonomy, competence, and relatedness by emphasizing choices and active participation in learning, positive peer interactions through teamwork, and no emphasis on winning and interindividual competition.	Classroom teachers	PA (accelerometer), math perceived competence, need satisfaction, enjoyment, and math performance	Significant difference in MVPA during I days compared to C. I group had significantly higher math performance compared to C. I lessons were perceived as need satisfying. Perceived competence in math and satisfaction of need for competence from integrated lessons significantly predicted posttest math performance.
Intervention included 10-min physically active virtual lessons integrated with English and math content. Integrated lessons included Google Earth videos delivered through interactive whiteboards. Teachers received a 30-min training session.	Classroom teachers	PA (accelerometer) and on-task behavior	I students demonstrated significantly less sedentary behavior and more light-to-moderate and vigorous PA and significantly better on-task behavior during lessons (weeks 2 and 4) than C. No difference in outcomes was found at 3-month follow-up.
Program for children and their families that promoted running, walking, and healthy eating through structured school running times (e.g., recess, PE) at school, at home, and in the community. Additional elements included behavioral tracking, celebratory events in public venues (e.g., university, stadiums), and rewards.	Staff (mainly PE and classroom teachers), community members (mayors, entertainers, and athletes), and family	PA (self-report), BMI, self-efficacy, support, athletic identity, and outcome expectations	Significant improvement of PA, self-efficacy, athletic identity, and PA outcome expectations for I compared to C. For a 1-unit increase of participation, a 4%-8% increase in running, walking, and F&V intake. No differences in perceived support and BMI.
Playground was equipped with movable and recycled materials with no fixed purpose that are not typical play materials for children at schools (e.g., milk crates, swimming noodles, cardboard boxes, exercise mats, buckets). Five materials were introduced the first week and two additional each week throughout 7-week intervention. Enjoyment was targeted through novel and unpredictable new additions of playground materials that stimulate imagination throughout intervention.	School playground teacher supervision (yard duty)	PA (pedometers and direct observation), quality of life, and enjoyment of PA and lunchtime activities	I had significantly greater mean steps and distance per minute and significantly higher vigorous PA than C, both after 7-week and 8-month follow-ups. Significant differences in enjoyment of PA, enjoyment of intrapersonal play, and physical health quality of life after 7 weeks between I and C (but not after 8-month follow-up).
Included noncompetitive games and cardiovascular tasks; resistance training using resistance bands; and self-management skill sessions with goal setting, self-monitoring, self-talk, and recruiting social support.	After-school counselors	BMI, fitness, mood, self-appraisal, and self-efficacy	Significant improvement in exercise self-efficacy was found in 9- to 12-year-old girls.
Student-centered intervention emphasized intrinsic motivation and behavioral skill development for PA, including self-monitoring, goal setting, and developing strategies for engaging in PA with family and friends.	Trained graduate students	Exercise, self-efficacy, self-concept, enjoyment, and motivation for PA	Participants in I showed greater increases in motivation and self-concept toward PA relative to C.
Included nutritional education and PA engagement (dancing, double-dutch jump rope, relay races, tag, active African American games, and step aerobics). The intervention goals were to (1) increase frequency of MVPA; (2) decrease time spent in sedentary activities; and (3) experience feelings of enjoyment, physical competence, and self-confidence.	Trained African American Girls Health Enrichment Multisite Studies (GEMS) staff	PA, BMI, fitness, motivation for PA, and self-efficacy	Significant improvements in the expected direction in self-efficacy for healthy eating and positive expectancy and self-efficacy for PA.
Participants received a wide variety of PAs to develop FMS in a fun context. Group sessions were based on TARGET structure (task, authority, reward, grouping, evaluation, and timing) to develop a learning environment based on a mastery goal orientation. At-home skill challenges were encouraged.	Staff (not specified), family, and parents (at-home challenges)	PA, BMI, FMS, perceived competence, and self-perception	Posttest and follow-up test results revealed significant improvements to motor development, perceived athletic competence, and perceived global self-worth.

(continued)

TABLE 5.1 CSPAP Interventions Grounded in Relevant Theoretical Frameworks *(continued)*

Author and year	Primary PA area (additional areas)	Intervention name, dose, and design	Sample	Associated theories and frameworks	
Webber et al. (2008)	Multicomponent (PE, HE, lunchtime, before and after school, staff, community, and policy)	Trial of Activity for Adolescent Girls (TAAG) 2 years RCT	n = 1,721 (baseline) Grade 6 F n = 3,504 (post) Grade 8 F	SCT: outcome expectations, self-efficacy Operant learning theory: reinforcement with positive messages Organizational change theory: link school and community Diffusion of innovation model SEM	
Cohen et al. (2015); Lubans et al. (2012)	Multicomponent (lunchtime, recess, staff, family, and community)	Supporting Children's Outcomes Using Rewards, Exercise and Skills (SCORES) 12 months RCT	n = 460 M_{age} = 8.5 years 25 classes low-income communities (4 I, 4 C schools)	SDT: autonomy, competence, relatedness, need satisfaction CMT: perceived competence, enjoyment, self-esteem SEM	
Neumark-Sztainer et al. (2003a, 2003b, 2010)	Multicomponent (PE, staff, family, and community)	New Moves 16 weeks,[#] 4 days/week, 2 years[@] (RCT)	[a] n = 201 F M_{age} = 15.4 years 6 schools (3 I, 3 C) [b] n = 356 F 12 schools	SCT: self-efficacy, peer support, body image, enjoyment, goal setting Transtheoretical model	
van Beurden et al. (2003)	Multicomponent (PE, staff, and community)	Move It Groove It (MIGI) 18 months Quasi-E	n = 1,045 Grades 3 and 4 18 schools (9 I, 9 C)	SCT: supporting teachers and creating supportive environments	
Ahamed et al. (2007); Naylor et al. (2006, 2008)	Multicomponent (PE, classroom, school environment, family, and community)	Action Schools! BC (AS!BC) 11 months, 15 additional min of PA/day RCT	n = 515 9 to 11 years old 42 teachers 10 schools (3 I champion schools, 4 I liaison schools, 3 C schools)	SCT: support of teachers SEM	
Weaver et al. (2017)	Multicomponent (PE, classroom, and community)	Partnerships for Active Children in Elementary Schools (PACES) Quasi-E	n = 229 Grades K-5 3 PE teachers, 12 classroom teachers 4 schools (3 I, 1 C)	SCT: supporting teachers Goal-setting theory	

BMI = body mass index; C = control group; F = female ; FMS = fundamental motor skill; F&V = fruit & vegetable; HE = health education; I = intervention group; M_{age} = median age; MVPA = moderate-to-vigorous physical activity; PE = physical education; quasi-E = quasi-experimental design ; RCT= randomized controlled trial; SEM = social-ecological model; SES = socioeconomic status.

Intervention content	Affected stakeholders	Outcomes (relevant for chapter)	Summary of primary findings
Promote more opportunities for PA; improve social support and norms; and increase self-efficacy, outcome expectations, and behavioral skills. Achieved by environmental changes inside school (one of the two HE lessons was offered as PE; PE increased promotion of MVPA outside of school; lunchtime included a dance program) and outside of school (before- or after-school programs). PE teachers were trained in class management strategies, skill-building activities, and providing equipment and choices. Community partners included YMCA, local health clubs, and rec centers. Promotions included school-wide messages for PA.	PE teachers, staff trained as program champions to sustain program after intervention	PA (accelerometer) and percent body fat	Girls in I had significantly more PA (1.6 min daily MVPA) than C schools. No differences in percent body fat.
FMS through self-monitoring tasks (certificates and rewards for goals), support from significant others (e.g., parents), and feeling of a sense of control over PA experiences were expected to increase enjoyment and PA behavior. Provided student leadership to promote PA and FMS during lunchtime and recess to receive awards. SAAFE principles were implemented: supportive environment (teaching instructions), active lessons (maximum participation), autonomous (choices, reflective challenges), fair (experience success, lack of interindividual competition), and enjoyable (age-appropriate tasks, variety, no punishment). Classroom teacher training focused on instruction, time model behavior, management, and feedback.	Classroom teachers, student leaders, school staff and principals, and parents (newsletters and events). School–community links (support from local sporting organizations)	PA (accelerometer), FMS competency, and cardiovascular fitness	I maintained MVPA and improved FMS competency and cardiovascular fitness significantly more than C.
Enhanced PE curriculum focused on making girls feel good about themselves and comfortable with their body, regardless of size or level of PA. Incorporated nutrition, social support, and self-empowerment sessions; counseling sessions with motivational interviewing; lunch get-togethers; parent messages; and new fun PAs (dance, kickboxing) introduced through community.	PE teachers, parents, community, and New Moves coaches (school staff)	PA (self-report), BMI, self-efficacy, enjoyment, and self-worth	Significant decreases of sedentary behaviors, unhealthy weight control behaviors, body image, and self-worth for I compared to C. Social support, self-worth, and self-efficacy were associated with change in PA, with support being the strongest factor along with time constraints. No significant differences in BMI.
Strategies used for support were school project teams; a "buddy" program, which connected preservice teachers with practicing classroom teachers; professional development for teachers (four workshops on teaching FMS and project updates); a project website (with resources for teaching and environmental and policy changes); and funding for purchase of equipment. No changes in PE hours per week.	School principals, teachers, parents, university students (preservice teachers as "buddies"), health workers, and student leaders	PA during PE (observations), FMS, and PE lesson context (proportion of lesson spent in instruction, FMS, and fitness games)	Significant improvement in every FMS for both genders for I compared to C. Small but significant increase in vigorous PA in favor of I.
Teachers received training and resources to select plans from six action zones (PE, family, classroom, school environment, school spirit, and extracurricular). Champion schools were given training, resources, and support to champion teacher. Liaison schools received additional mentorship and support from PE specialist through weekly contacts in the classroom.	Two PE specialists as program facilitators, classroom teachers, school committee members (teachers, administrators, and parents)	PA delivered and PA levels (self-report), satisfaction and perceived support, and academic performance	Boys in liaison I group had significantly more steps/day than C. PA delivered by teachers in I groups was increased by 47 min/week. Significant change in academic performance for I but no significant difference at posttest between I and C.
Teachers were supported through an online community of practice for educators, service learning, and community-based participatory research. Teacher training included goal setting based on LET US principles (lines; elimination; team size; uninvolved children; and space, equipment, and rules) to maximize participation in PA and avoid elimination.	PE teachers, teachers, university students (preservice teachers), and community (of teachers through web)	PA (accelerometer)	The percentage of boys and girls in I achieving 30 min of MVPA/day increased from 57.5% to 70.7% and 35.4% to 56.9%, respectively, compare to C, which decreased from 61.5% to 56.4% and 52.6% to 41.9%, respectively.

example, whether they were first or last compared to others (ego-involving orientation; Ames, 1992a; Nicholls, 1984). Research results have shown that individuals who judge their competence based on personal criteria enjoy participating in PAs, have higher self-esteem, and are more persistent and more likely to adhere to PA programs. If the focus is exclusively on the outcome (e.g., outperforming others), individuals are more likely to experience feelings of anxiety, avoid participation, or drop out of PA programs (for a review, see Duda, 2001). Just as social environment is crucial in shaping motivation, so too is it important for creating perceptions of competence. The motivational climate created by significant others (e.g., teachers, peers, and parents) can be formed based on expectations, cues, and feedback and can promote a task- or ego-involving climate. To be more precise, children are more likely to perceive higher levels of competence and adhere to PA when teachers and peers behave in a manner that emphasizes individual effort and learning and exhibit support and involvement regardless of the actual skill level of each child and mistakes are accepted as part of learning (Harwood et al., 2015).

Contexts that are likely to create a task-involving versus an ego-involving motivational climate have been provided through Epstein's TARGET framework: task (providing variety and diversity are more likely to facilitate an interest in learning and task involvement), authority (students should participate actively in the learning process by choosing tasks, setting up equipment, and monitoring and evaluating their own performance), recognition (reasonable use of incentives, rewards, and feedback), grouping (the criteria used for the formation of students into groups affect their motivation), evaluation (avoid evaluation that is linked to ability assessments and is public or emphasizes social comparison), and time (the pace of instruction and the time allocated for completing tasks should reflect the needs of the students; Epstein, 1989).

Self-Determination Theory

Another valuable framework for understanding and predicting PA motivation and behavior is the self-determination theory (SDT; Deci & Ryan, 1985; Ryan & Deci, 2000a, 2002). Central to the

SDT is the contention that all motivated behavior exists on a self-determination continuum (Ryan & Deci, 2000b). The motivation continuum ranges from amotivation, which involves lack of intent and relative absence of value, competence, and contingency associated with activity or behavior (Ryan & Deci, 2000a), to intrinsic motivation, which is considered to be the most autonomous involvement in an activity or behavior for reasons entirely from within the individual and for the purpose of doing the act for its own sake. Between these ends of the continuum are four forms of extrinsic motivation, which range from non–self-determined extrinsic factors (rewards or punishment) to internalization of these more self-determined external factors (e.g., guilt) as reasons for behavior. According to the SDT, satisfaction of three basic psychological needs—autonomy, competence, and relatedness—is furthermore theoretically essential for self-determined motivated behavior, optimal functioning, and development (Deci & Ryan, 1985, 2000). The need for *autonomy* represents the innate desire to perceive one's thoughts and behaviors as freely chosen and that thoughts and behaviors originate from one's own control and as agents of one's own means (Ryan & Connell, 1989). *Competence* need satisfaction reflects the desire to view interactions with the environment and behavior as effective (Deci, 1975). The need for *relatedness* is the desire to experience a sense of belonging and perceptions of feeling connected to others (Baumeister & Leary, 1995). The degree to which these individual psychological needs are met or thwarted by contextual factors theoretically predicts individual and social psychological outcomes, such as motivation.

Furthermore, the extent to which factors in the environment are experienced as autonomy supportive, rather than as controlling, theoretically predicts levels of individual satisfaction of basic psychological needs, particularly competence and autonomy, which in turn predicts where on the self-determination continuum an individual will be in engaging with a behavior or experience (Mageau & Vallerand, 2003; Ryan & Deci, 2002a). Salient social contextual factors include general influence from teachers, parents, and coaches and the perceived interpersonal style demonstrated by these significant others (see Amorose, 2007). The presence, timing, and distribution of rewards, recognition, and feedback as well as negative consequences are also meaningful aspects of the context that create a controlling or autonomy-supportive environment.

The SDT (Deci & Ryan, 1985, 2000) has been established as a relevant framework for research in CSPAP component contexts. Standage and colleagues (2005) found that students who are more intrinsically motivated in physical education report higher need satisfaction and perceived their teachers as more autonomy supportive in their teaching style. Babkes Stellino and Sinclair (2013) found that children's intrinsic motivation to be physically active during recess was significantly predicted by their reported satisfaction of competence, autonomy, and relatedness in the recess context. Actual recess PA levels were positively and significantly predicted by competence need satisfaction for female and overweight children and autonomy need satisfaction, for males and healthy weight children. Evidence has also been established that the levels of perceived autonomy support, rather than control, for PA during recess from physical education and classroom teachers significantly relate to students' recess PA motivation (Babkes Stellino et al., 2015). While the research to date has examined only physical education and recess contexts in relation to constructs and contentions of the SDT, its premises are entirely applicable and relevant to other components of the CSPAP model.

Ecological Systems Theory

While the theories introduced thus far focus on the strong interdependence of psychosocial constructs in predicting PA, frameworks that consider the importance of multilevel influences, such as culture and policy, on human behavior, such as PA, are also relevant. A theory germane to CSPAPs that not only addresses the idea of how individual behaviors are influenced through multiple spheres of influence but has also been highlighted as a guide for the CSPAP conceptual framework for research and practice (Carson et al., 2014) is ecological systems theory (EST; Bronfenbrenner, 1977; Bronfenbrenner & Morris, 1998). Emmons (2000) specified the ecological perspective on health promotion by focusing on the social context. The resulting social-ecological

model (SEM) characterizes the influence of the levels of intrapersonal (individual), interpersonal (social), organizational and environmental (community), and policy (culture) factors on health behavior (Emmons, 2000).

As described in chapters 3 and 18 of this text, these SEM levels of influence align with the CSPAP conceptual framework. Individual *student PA* is considered the intrapersonal, or epicenter, and the *CSPAP component level* is reflected in the SEM level of interpersonal (or social influence) that comes from the context (e.g., in physical education or recess) as well as the impact of organizational and environmental *facilitators*, such as available resources and safety considerations (Carson et al., 2014). Further, the CSPAP *leaders* level of influence includes community, such as teacher leadership and supportive administration, and the outermost sphere of influence, *culture*, , reflects normative behaviors and policy-level decisions (e.g., district- or even state-level decisions about required time allotted for recess as an opportunity for PA; Carson et al., 2014). Ecological systems theory stresses the interdependent relationship between these levels, allowing for an understanding that individuals have a multitude of influences that affect their behavior, such as participation in PA (Spence & Lee, 2003). This perspective helps describe the reciprocal interactions between the individual, family, neighborhood, community, and culture that develop over time. CSPAPs, then, are likely to initially directly benefit the individual student or staff member but subsequently affect the school and community as a whole.

From a CSPAP perspective, ecological systems theory informs the separate and interactive processes that may influence the success of PA promotional efforts. Langille and Rodgers (2010) found that multilevel, school-based practitioners perceived both policy and culture as significant contributors to their school's implementation of PA initiatives. In addition, key stakeholders at the interpersonal level who were identified as playing a significant role in their school and students' PA behaviors included the principal and teachers who have knowledge and interest in health-related topics (Langille & Rodgers, 2010). Other research provides support for PA interventions based on the SEM. Simon and colleagues (2014) concluded that a PA intervention based on a social-ecological framework prevented long-term excess weight gain and predicted higher exercise intentions in adolescents. Ecological systems theory is well suited for school-based efforts to improve PA because it recognizes the importance of the relationship between an individual (e.g., student or teacher) and his or her larger context (e.g., school or community).

Description of Theoretically Guided Efforts Across CSPAP Components

Table 5.1 summarizes the several PA interventions on one or multiple CSPAP components, which employed one of the five previously reviewed theories. All constructs that comprise the theory are rarely measured or considered within an intervention. For example, the SCT has often been identified as the main theoretical framework in many studies, but often, only the construct of self-efficacy or social support has been measured or manipulated during the intervention. Use of a particular theory also has often been based on the age or developmental level of students or the target sample. For example, the CMT is considered more appropriate for understanding and applying to younger students (i.e., less than 12 years old), and the TPB is used more often with older students and adults. Regardless of the theoretical framework, the main approach for changing the PA behavior of students was through self-efficacy or perceived competence, followed by increased enjoyment for PA, social support, self-monitoring skills, and goal setting. Changes implemented at many levels (e.g., student, teacher, school, and community) were included in several studies and provided evidence of using a social-ecological framework to guide intervention. In addition, to help translate the theories into practice, the main principles utilized in the studies were the SAAFE principles (supportive environment, active lessons, autonomy, fair, enjoyment), based on the SDT and CMT (Cohen et al., 2015; Lubans et al., 2012), and the LET US Play principles (lines; elimination; team size; uninvolved children; space, equipment, and rules; Weaver et al., 2017).

Overall, 22 intervention studies with some

theoretical foundation applied to CSPAP were identified by a combination of searching electronic databases, previous reviews, and meta-analyses of the school-based PA promotion literature. The inclusion criteria were intervention studies published after 2000 that targeted a PA behavior or cardiovascular risk factors, such as obesity. Five studies were concentrated primarily on physical education; five, on classroom PA; one, on recess PA; one, on lunchtime PA; four, on after-school PA; and six, on PA employing multiple CSPAP components. The majority of the interventions (16 out of 22) focused on elementary school students. Four out of the six interventions with adolescents targeted only females through physical education modifications in order to make girls feel confident and enjoy PA participation. In addition to the promotion of PA among youth, a focus on the outcome variables of fundamental motor skill competency was identified in four interventions; fitness, in five interventions; and body composition or body mass index, in nine interventions, across all CSPAP components. The following sections focus on descriptions of how the theories previously introduced have been used to specifically examine each of the five CSPAP components.

Physical Education

While physical education was the sole component in only five of the intervention studies, it was a central element for CSPAP interventions overall because it was included in some way in half of the theoretically framed intervention studies (11 out of 22). The targeted age during physical education varied from kindergarten to 11th grade. Nine of the 11 interventions that included physical education used the SCT, one used the SDT, and one focused on modifying the affective responses to exercise in low-active adolescent girls. Four out of the five intervention studies that focused exclusively on physical education incorporated changes in the instructional practices to increase students' self-efficacy, enjoyment, and perceived support by focusing on teaching progression, deemphasis on competition and very high intensities, absence of elimination, and provision of choices as well as a variety of activities during the physical education lesson. Self-monitoring and goal-setting skills were provided in two interventions through health education, whereas one intervention included peer educators for healthy living, delivered through health education.

During School: Classroom PA Integration

PA interventions that occurred in the academic classroom were implemented with only elementary school children. Consistently emphasized in five of the seven interventions that focused solely on classroom PA were ways to increase classroom teachers' self-efficacy and perceived competence for incorporating PA into lesson plans. The most common approach was to provide training as well as easy-to-use curricula that integrated PA within academic content (e.g., counting while doing jumping jacks). One of the interventions included interactive videos (Norris et al., 2015, 2016a, 2016b), and the other provided continued support to classroom teachers through an online community of practice (Bartholomew & Jowers, 2011). Students' enjoyment, perceived competence, and need satisfaction were targeted to a smaller extent compared to other CSPAP components.

During School: Recess and Lunchtime

Few interventions targeted changes during recess or lunchtime within a clearly identified theoretical framework, and those that did were delivered through a multicomponent approach. Three out of the four interventions that were aimed to increase students' PA levels during recess or lunchtime were framed in the SCT and focused on increasing students' self-efficacy through self-monitoring tasks, rewards, and enhanced social support. Out of the four interventions, two targeted changes in enjoyment, one promoted a supportive environment and a sense of control over PA experiences (Springer et al., 2012), and one provided novel and unexpected playground material throughout the intervention (Hyndman et al., 2014).

Before and After School

Five theory-inspired after-school PA interventions, including one as part of a multicomponent intervention, were identified. No theoretically based interventions were found with a focus on before-school PA. All interventions focused on

targeting students' self-efficacy or perceived competence as well as students' enjoyment, motivation, and self-perceptions. The most common approach was through self-monitoring skills and goal setting, followed by increased knowledge on health benefits and social support.

Staff Involvement

Some interventions targeted the school staff members directly related to the specific CSPAP component area (e.g., physical education teachers for PA in physical education or classroom teachers for classroom PA). Five multicomponent interventions and one physical education–specific intervention also included a broader group of staff (e.g., principal and health educators) as a support group for policy implementation and for coaches and leaders. Promotion of staff wellness was not directly targeted in any of the identified interventions; however, training and support for teachers to appropriately instruct and promote PA inside and outside of school and to be role models through engagement in their own PA were offered in half of the interventions.

Family and Community Engagement

Social support from family and community in promoting youth PA was included in all six multicomponent interventions as well as in two after-school and two physical education interventions (total of 10 out of 21 interventions). The connection between schools and family was achieved with increased communication about the PA program and enriched information about the health benefits related to PA. Support from family and community was also targeted through a number of approaches, including sporting and celebratory events, opportunities for students to participate in fun community programs (e.g., kickboxing and dance), and counseling sessions as well as by encouraging parents to participate in walking and running events with their children. Connections with the university, researchers, and program facilitators were also noted because in two interventions, general classroom teachers were partnered with preservice teachers in order to receive support and training to successfully promote PA opportunities.

Knowledge Claims

The following knowledge claims were generated from the review of pertinent social psychological theories and the related research synthesized in the preceding sections:

- Numerous viable theories exist to frame CSPAP interventions and better understand the mechanisms (the who, what, why, and how) that predict and explain school-based PA. Examples include the extant research that has revealed substantial evidence of theoretical contentions of SCT that support better physical education practices and the SDT's emerging as a meaningful guide for predicting students' actual PA and motivation for PA during recess.

- Grounded in theoretical perspectives, youth self-perceptions, particularly beliefs about physical competence and ability, physical self-efficacy, and satisfaction of competence needs, are important factors associated with actual PA levels in the school context.

- Youth satisfaction of autonomy needs, or the opportunity to exercise choices, and perceived control is a salient theoretical construct strongly connected to increased motivation for PA and PA behavior.

- Social influences (e.g., teachers, parents, and peers and, to a lesser but relevant extent, administrators and other staff, such as paraprofessionals and recess monitors) have a very important, theoretically based, strong impact on youth behavior and, therefore, should be highly considered in promotion of youth PA within the CSPAP model.

- Environmental factors, such as how autonomy supportive or controlling the context is, are essential to promote youth PA in school-based programs. All five theories (SCT, TPB, CMT, SDT, and SEM) reviewed earlier provide a foundation for modifying the environment of all five CSPAP components to better support increased student PA.

- Use of research findings from studies of theoretically based CSPAP interventions should serve as a guide for determination of which factors (e.g., student perceived physical com-

petence and teacher efficacy for implementing PA in the classroom and parent modeling of PA behavior) are worthy of consideration in future school-based PA promotion endeavors.

Knowledge Gaps and Directions for Future Research

Many gaps in our current knowledge base exist, warranting further investigation to address the use and integration of social psychological and motivational theoretical frameworks in CSPAP implementation and research. Addressing these gaps and conducting systematic future research to answer these questions will establish an imperative foundation for CSPAP intervention and research efforts rooted in valid and relevant theoretical frameworks from the related field of social psychology. Following are some of the most relevant and current critical gaps in using social psychological theoretical frameworks to guide and implement CSPAP efforts. Limited CSPAP interventions and research are grounded in relevant theoretical frameworks. While meaningful research has been conducted, efforts have been far too limited in both grounding and evaluating CSPAPs in evidence-based social psychological and motivation theories.

- Based on extant youth PA and sport literature, achievement goal theory (Nicholls, 1984) and the related perspective on motivational climate (Ames, 1992b), as well as the transtheoretical model of health behavior change (Prochaska & Velicer, 1997), hold potential as frameworks that are applicable to theoretically guided CSPAP. Neumark-Sztainer and colleague's (2003a, 2003b, 2010) and Norris and colleague's (2015, 2016a, 2016b) examinations of classroom PA and multicomponent interventions, respectively, provide examples of the potential utility of these other theoretical frameworks (see table 5.1 for details).

- Continued CSPAP intervention and research efforts should focus specifically on the social (e.g., teachers), psychological (e.g., perceived control), and affective (e.g., enjoyment) factors identified in theoretical frameworks to explain and predict variations in PA behavior.

- No theoretically framed research or intervention efforts exist to date that are focused on before-school PA.
- Promotion and examination of staff wellness and involvement as leaders of PA in schools from a theoretically based perspective are conspicuously absent from the literature. Theories introduced in this chapter, as well as many other relevant frameworks, could be used to explore how and why school staff members engage in their own PA as well as how their own PA affects CSPAPs and students under their leadership.
- Multicomponent CSPAP efforts could be facilitated successfully using any one or more of the relevant social psychological and motivational theoretical frameworks.

Evidence-Based Recommendations and Applications

Based on the previous detailed descriptions of the relevant social psychological and motivation theories with connections to CSPAPs, we propose the following recommendations and applications categorized by two constituent groups: school staff and community partners. School staff pertains to any personnel directly involved in the delivery of CSPAPs to youth, whether or not they are employees of the school. Community partners include individuals and organizations that work with schools to deliver CSPAPs (universities, researchers, policy makers, youth organizations, parents, and families).

For School Staff

- Because theory affords explanation and prediction of outcomes, CSPAP interventions can more effectively increase student school-based PA if the development of specific programs is informed by theory.
- CSPAP stakeholders (e.g., school staff and administrators) should be sure to consider integration of factors that promote favorable

youth physical self-efficacy, perceived physical competence and ability, and satisfaction of competence needs within interventions because these psychological constructs are critical mechanisms known to predict increases in PA motivation and behavior.

- CSPAP stakeholders (e.g., school staff and administrators) should also work to facilitate satisfaction of youth autonomy needs and perceived control in school-based PA contexts because they are also important theoretically based constructs strongly connected to increased motivation for PA and PA behavior.
- Adults in the CSPAP context (e.g., teachers and parents) should be informed and educated about the powerful theoretical social influence they have on youth PA in school contexts.
- School staff (teachers, administrators, and paraprofessionals) invested in delivery of CSPAP should be aware of the impact that environmental factors, such as presentation of rewards and incentives, opportunities for individual decision making, how youth are grouped, availability of equipment and space, and quality of feedback and encouragement, have on youth PA because the context is theoretically essential to consider in promotion of youth PA in school-based programs.

For Community Partners

- Evaluation of CSPAP implementation efforts by community stakeholders should integrate relevant theoretical perspectives to better assess whether mechanisms (the who, what, why, and how) associated with PA levels are accounted for and understood. This will afford replication of effective programming.
- CSPAP stakeholders (community partners) should be sure to consider integration of factors that promote favorable youth physical self-efficacy, perceived physical competence and ability, and satisfaction of competence needs within interventions because these psychological constructs are critical mechanisms known to predict increases in PA motivation and behavior.

SUMMARY

The review of the five most prevalent theoretical frameworks (SCT, TPB, CMT, SDT, and SEM) used to date in CSPAP efforts and the associated findings across CSPAP components described in this chapter was intended to serve as a foundation for continuing to inspire social psychological and motivational theoretically guided CSPAP interventions. We further identified knowledge gaps and proposed evidence-based recommendations and applications for future research and intervention efforts framed within social psychological and motivational theoretical frameworks. The hope is that by conducting research and practice from an evidence-based theoretical foundation, CSPAPs will be more successful in terms of understanding how, why, and what mechanisms work for implementation and will better facilitate consistent outcomes of increased PA in the future.

QUESTIONS TO CONSIDER

1. What can teachers do to satisfy and avoid undermining students' needs for competence, autonomy, and relatedness as a mechanism to promote PA participation according to the SDT?

2. What types of classroom PA (e.g., movement breaks) would school leaders be most comfortable engaging in with their students to promote positive PA modeling that results in greater activity engagement by students, as suggested by the SCT?

3. What are some strategies, according to the CMT, that physical education teachers could consider when rewarding effort and individual progress, as opposed to recognizing winning and outperforming others, within the context of a physical education class?

4. How can theoretically based constructs that are important for promoting youth PA, such as the ones discussed in this chapter, be used to encourage PA among CSPAP-involved adults, such as teachers and administrators?

5. Based on the efficacy of multilevel theories of health promotion, such as the SEM, how might the school environment and policies be modified to promote positive attitudes toward PA and actual PA behavior before, during, and after school?

CASE EXAMPLES

Two real-life examples follow to illustrate how social psychological theoretical frameworks and constructs serve as an effective basis for recommendations and applications for implementation in CSPAPs. The first example describes how theoretical contentions of SDT can be evident in the curriculum and application of the before-school PA program Build Our Kids' Success (BOKS). The second example highlights how social psychological and motivational theory serves to inform the practice of fitness testing in physical education.

Linking the BOKS Program and Self-Determination Theory

Megan Babkes Stellino, EdD
University of Northern Colorado
Lyndsie M. Koon, PhD
University of Illinois at Urbana-Champaign

BOKS is a before-school PA program for elementary students. The goal of the program is to bring various social agents (e.g., parents, teachers, school staff, and local volunteers) from the immediate community together to offer before-school PA. BOKS programming includes free play and aerobic activities as well as an introduction to and practice of skilled motor movements and game-based PAs for students to boost the body and brain before the start of a long day in the classroom. The NIOST (n.d.) pursued a three-year investigation of the effect of the BOKS program and reported that significant improvements were found in the students' nutritional knowledge as a result of the BOKS Bits section of the program, participants showed a significant decrease in 400-meter mean run time, and cognitive functions (working memory and shifting) significantly improved among the students participating in BOKS compared to their non-BOKS peers.

Although the BOKS program was not developed with a theoretical framework in mind, implementation of this program serves as an opportunity to infuse aspects of the SDT (Deci & Ryan, 1985) to better predict effectiveness in promoting PA for the students involved and understand why youth accrue significant cognitive and physical benefits from participation. As previously discussed, SDT posits that to foster greater self-regulation for an activity, the environment should aim to satisfy the three basic psychological needs: autonomy, competence, and relatedness.

During the BOKS program, the need for relatedness is promoted when the students are given opportunities to engage in free play with other students prior to the start of the organized program activities and then again during the group games, in which communication, cooperation, and social engagement are required to be successful. Furthermore, relatedness needs are potentially satisfied between youth and adults because implementation of BOKS requires getting multiple individuals in the community, including but not limited to school staff, parents, and other volunteers, to come together to provide the before-school program in a safe and effective manner.

Autonomy-need satisfaction is also fostered by offering BOKS as an optional before-school PA program for students, without any negative repercussions for not attending. Youth participants also have choices about how to modify activities and games and make individual decisions about intensity, duration, and frequency of many of the physical activities incorporated in any given BOKS session.

Student needs for competence are intentionally promoted and supported with the integration of novel motor and movement skills within the BOKS curriculum. When newly learned motor skills (e.g., proper plank form), which are incorporated into the subsequent physical activities (e.g., doing push-ups), become the basis for active games, participants also experience a platform for gaining and displaying competence through skill mastery. The curriculum and instruction of motor skills and how adult leaders guide students to incorporate mastery into active games are cornerstones of the BOKS program and further evidence of SDT contentions at work.

As theoretically anticipated, it is evident that BOKS participants' reasons for participation on a daily basis are connected to the extent to which their needs for relatedness, autonomy, and competence are satisfied; those participants who experience connections with peers through activities, make individual choices, and improve physical skills are more self-determined, or intrinsically motivated, to engage in the BOKS program. Alternately, students who do not experience learning or increased competence in motor skills and connection with peers and are unable to make individual decisions within the BOKS program depend, as theoretically predicted, on rewards; incentives; and other externally regulating, non–self-determining factors to continue attendance and participation.

The BOKS program is a great example of an applicable CSPAP that fosters theoretically self-determined experiences among those involved. Although the program was not designed with the foundation of a social psychological theoretical framework, it inherently implements various techniques that satisfy the basic psychological needs of relatedness, autonomy, and competence and subsequently the nature of participants' self-determined motivation for involvement. Student participation in BOKS has great potential for resulting in positive affect and improved cognitive function; nutritional knowledge; and physical fitness levels, especially when premises of the SDT (Deci & Ryan, 1985, 2000) are acknowledged and used as a guide for effective implementation.

Theory-Based Manipulation of Fitness Practice in Physical Education

Spyridoula Vazou, PhD
Iowa State University

It is widely known that fitness practice and testing during physical education are two of the most controversial topics regarding their benefits for students' health and impact on students' motivation to be physically active. Advocates of fitness testing believe that it can educate children about health-related fitness, promote PA, and inspire lifelong participation (Welk, 2008). On the other hand, skeptics have pointed out that because of the way fitness practice and testing are implemented, students perceive a lack competence and experience negative emotions. As a result students may avoid participation in fitness lessons, which contributes to reduced motivation for regular PA (Silverman et al., 2008; Wiersma & Sherman, 2008). It is reasonable to suggest that the methods used to implement fitness practice can determine its effectiveness. Empirical research on how modifications to either the practice for fitness testing or the testing itself might improve the participants' experiences is scarce. Therefore, this example highlights an ecologically valid field experiment (Vazou et al., 2015) that shows how theory-based and empirically supported pedagogical and psychological principles can be implemented in fitness lessons during physical education. This example is further intended to describe how infusion of theoretically and empirically based principles can enhance students' experiences about fitness and potentially motivate them to adopt and maintain physically active lifestyles.

In our study, a sample of 148 students in grades four to six (52 percent females) participated in two fitness practice lessons during physical education, in a counterbalanced order. Fitness practice in both lessons included aerobic (two times five minutes) and muscular endurance (~six minutes) tasks. One lesson, called "traditional," included the PACER (aerobic exercise) and curl-up and push-up tasks and was delivered according to the standard format and instructions specified in the manual of the FitnessGram battery. The workload-matched lesson, named "novel," included the same components of physical fitness (aerobic exercise, curl-ups, and push-ups), but the structure of the tasks were modified in order to (1) replace exposure to interpersonal comparisons with positive cooperative interactions between students, (2) contain variety in practice, (3) promote autonomy and individual preferences, and (4) include upbeat and engaging music and animated videos (Vazou et al., 2015).

We made the aforementioned changes to positively affect students' pleasure and enjoyment. Specifically, we focused on positive peer interactions (element 1) because when children interact with and help and support each other, without focusing on interindividual competition and winning, their perception of competence is not threatened and they enjoy the activity (Vazou et al., 2006). We provided variety in practice (element 2) because repetition is boring, whereas the element of experimentation and variety keeps the interest high (Sylvester et al., 2014). We provided choices and autonomy (element 3) because research shows that, when people are given the option to self-regulate the intensity of exercise, they will not necessarily exercise at a lower intensity but they will enjoy it more (Stych & Parfitt, 2011). Lastly, we introduced engaging music and video (element 4) because they can work as a distraction and people can continue to feel good without focusing on the bodily stimuli from exercise (Jones et al., 2014), plus the variety of images and sounds can be enjoyable (element 2).

Following are the structural changes that we conducted in the novel lesson compared to the traditional lesson. First, in the traditional lesson, students practiced the PACER, meaning that they were asked to line up and run from one side of the gym to the other, based on the externally paced PACER cadence. This structure potentially promotes an ego-involving climate because students can compare and evaluate competence based on how fast everyone is running. In contrast, in the novel lesson, the students were running in all directions and interacted with their peers by giving high fives. Throughout the aerobic exercise, upbeat music and an animated video were playing. Second, the curl-up and push-up tasks were practiced in the traditional lesson with all students lined up but without any interactions between them. Instead, in the novel lesson the same tasks were practiced through partner games in stations (e.g., passing a beach ball during curl-ups and tapping their partner's hands from a plank position during push-ups) and with the option to practice alone.

Even though the workload of both lessons was identical, as measured with activity monitors, not surprisingly, the traditional lesson led to a significant pre-to-post decrease in positive affect, unlike the novel lesson. Further, the students enjoyed the novel lesson significantly more than the traditional lesson and perceived having higher levels of competence and more autonomy and reported a higher interest in repeating it compared to the traditional lesson (Vazou et al., 2015). Therefore, as this example shows, by relying on advances in psychological research, it is possible to have changes in fitness practices that are easy to implement and free or low cost and that positively affect students' experiences and motivation to be physically active.

PART III

Research on Program Effectiveness

CHAPTER 6

Quality Physical Education

Kim C. Graber, EdD
University of Illinois at Urbana-Champaign

Chad M. Killian, MA
University of Illinois at Urbana-Champaign

Amelia Mays Woods, PhD
University of Illinois at Urbana-Champaign

Five components of a CSPAP exist to help students achieve the recommended 60 minutes of daily PA and develop the knowledge, skills, and confidence necessary for a lifetime of healthy movement (Centers for Disease Control and Prevention [CDC], 2013). Although each component contributes uniquely to these objectives, it is quality physical education that lays the foundation for an effective CSPAP (SHAPE America, 2015a). Physical education is the primary learning environment where students develop the knowledge and skills necessary to be physically active for a lifetime. The formalized instruction embedded within physical education makes it a unique element of a CSPAP. Therefore, it is essential to the success of any CSPAP to have a quality physical education program at its core. This chapter will provide a brief review of research of CSPAPs, the characteristics of effective programs, examples of curriculum and appropriate instruction, and the role of physical education teacher education (PETE) in helping future teachers to better understand and facilitate an effective CSPAP. Finally, directions for future research and a case study are provided.

Review of Research

A primary goal of a CSPAP is to provide a variety of school-based physical activities to enable all students to participate in 60 minutes of moderate-to-vigorous PA (MVPA) every day (CDC, 2013). Physical education is an ideal environment for providing students with opportunities to be physically active in the school setting (Erwin et al., 2013), and students engage in more MVPA on days when they have physical education class than on days when they do not (Alderman et al., 2012).

The amount of MVPA students receive in physical education classes is a key indicator of the quality of the program (Sallis et al., 2012), and quality programs engage students in learning primarily through movement-based experiences. These learning experiences should be designed to increase physical literacy and optimize health-related fitness. Although students should spend *at least* 50 percent of physical education time engaged in MVPA, unfortunately, it is common for students to be physically engaged for far less time.

Promoting the development of physical literacy is another objective of a quality physical education program and the second primary goal of CSPAPs. Physical literacy is defined as the combination of knowledge, skills, and confidence necessary to enjoy PA across the life span (SHAPE America, 2013). Acquiring these competencies can be an outcome of high levels of MVPA being integrated into physical education classes (Erwin et al., 2013). Therefore, when elevated levels of MVPA are combined with appropriate instructional experiences, students' physical literacy may improve.

Characteristics of Quality Physical Education Programs

Physical education is evolving to become the foundational component of a broader school-based physical literacy development and activity promotion program. Although many schools in the United States do not have a CSPAP in place because of teacher indifference, inadequate knowledge of how to properly implement a CSPAP, or lack of a certified physical education teacher to implement the model, an increasing number are adopting the model as a mechanism for addressing the childhood obesity epidemic, enhancing cognitive performance in the classroom, improving student behavior, and providing in-school PA opportunities for students (Trudeau & Shephard, 2008). For CSPAPs to be optimally successful, the physical education program must be of high quality and support the goals of the CSPAP, which include (1) opportunity to learn, (2) meaningful content, (3) appropriate instruction, and (4) student and program assessment (SHAPE America, 2015a). The key determinants of quality physical education then become policies, curricula, instructional practices, and evaluations that support high levels of MVPA, physical literacy development, and PA promotion.

A variety of policy and environmental factors exist that can support or inhibit students' opportunity to learn in physical education. These factors have the potential to contribute to the learning environment and overall climate of a program. For example, national, state, and district policies that mandate school-based PA opportunities, such as physical education, play a fundamental role in the promotion of childhood wellness and prevention of childhood obesity (Agron et al., 2010). Policies, however, are often ineffective because of minimal compliance oversight (Graber et al., 2012) and very few schools adhere to these types of guidelines for many reasons (Lee et al., 2007). For example, state legislation related to physical education is commonly ambiguous regarding curricular and instructional mandates. Without clear guidelines, schools interpret the laws and policies in a way that is achievable for their situation (McCullick et al., 2012), which inevitably creates wide variability in schools across the nation.

Despite the challenges associated with policy development, enactment, and compliance, it is necessary for states to develop clear child wellness policies that establish and promote accountability for quality physical education and support CSPAP goals. In fact, SHAPE America (2016) recommends that states mandate daily physical education for all students in grades K-12. At the elementary level, at least 150 minutes of physical education instruction is suggested in addition to free and supervised play. At the middle and high school levels, 225 minutes of physical education per week or 450 minutes per 10-day block schedule is recommended (SHAPE America, 2015b).

Unfortunately, many states allow schools to issue physical education exemptions or waivers for students involved in sport or select extracurricular activities, such as marching band and ROTC. While a primary goal of quality physical education is to promote PA outside of the gymnasium, activities not directly taught by a certified physical education teacher often do not offer the same standards-based instructional opportunities and, therefore, should not qualify for physical education credit. For that reason, the National Association for Sport and Physical Education (NASPE, 2006) advised against granting waivers to students.

Other policy and environmental factors can support quality physical education and provide opportunities for students to learn. For example, ample equipment, adequate facilities, and appropriate technology for activity implementation are necessary for enabling students to engage in a variety of movement experiences and track their progress (SHAPE America, 2010). Class size that is modest and comparable with other content areas contributes to the safety of students and allows for appropriate instruction to occur (SHAPE America, 2009).

A key factor in determining the quality of students' physical education experiences is the instructor, and all individuals responsible for teaching physical education should be certified in the subject matter. Certified teachers have the pedagogical knowledge, content knowledge, and professional disposition that enable them to develop and implement instruction that maximizes and promotes MVPA and facilitates the development of physical literacy (Napper-Owen et al., 2008). The NASPE (2007; now SHAPE America) describes qualified physical education instructors as individuals who (1) implement instruction based on the National Standards for K-12 physical education; (2) develop an environment that encourages cognitive, psychomotor, and affective learning through appropriate practice opportunities and PA promotion; (3) use formative and summative assessments to drive instruction and curricular evaluation; (4) demonstrate professional and ethical behavior in the learning environment and act as advocates for healthy living within the school and community; and (5) engage in reflective practices to continually improve cur-

riculum, instruction, and assessment and strive to develop as a professional through the pursuit of extraprofessional learning opportunities, such as attending and presenting at professional conferences, enrolling for continuing education credits, and networking with physical education teachers employed in other schools. These characteristics enable physical education professionals to adopt and implement current best practices and establish high-quality learning experiences for their students that support the goals of quality physical education and CSPAPs.

Curriculum

Teachers employed in quality physical education programs advocate for and wisely use their instructional time. These individuals use the SHAPE America national physical education content standards as their guide to develop appropriate curriculum (SHAPE America, 2013) and achieve physical literacy. Although a variety of physical education curricular models exist that help teachers achieve the national standards and outcomes in their classes, Health Optimizing Physical Education (HOPE; Metzler et al., 2013a) is the best model for supporting the overarching CSPAP goals of promoting lifelong participation in PA through physical literacy development and high levels of MVPA. It comprises eight strands (see table 6.1), most of which are aligned closely with CSPAP guidelines (CDC, 2013) and are referred to as "teaching and learning areas" (Metzler et al., 2013a, p. 44). Some strands might occur as more traditional content units, whereas others serve as supplemental PA opportunities or HOPE promotional and training events for community members or teachers. Each strand addresses specific learning outcomes, target learners, particular learning activities, and focused assessments.

The design of the HOPE curriculum is comprehensive by providing specific guidelines for the creation of a coordinated physical education and PA program designed to help students develop lifelong PA habits. School policy and community contexts vary considerably, however, and the authors were mindful of that fact when they developed the model. All HOPE learning outcomes are broad enough to allow for context-specific content development and implementation. Metzler and

TABLE 6.1 HOPE Model Program Strands

Strand 1	Extended PA programming—before, during, and after school
Strand 2	Sport, games, dance, and other movement forms
Strand 3	Family and home education
Strand 4	Community-based PA programming
Strand 5	Health-related fitness
Strand 6	Diet and nutrition for PA
Strand 7	PA literacy—consumerism, technology, and advocacy
Strand 8	Integration of HOPE across all school subjects (including recess)

Data from Metzler, McKenzie, van der Mars, Barrett-Williams, (2013a).

colleagues (2013a) advised that student-learning experiences be chosen based on their ability to provide students with high levels of MVPA and that traditional content that involves few opportunities for MVPA (e.g., softball and bowling) should either be modified to include higher levels of MVPA or eliminated from the curriculum.

Effective Curricular Interventions

Several evidence-based physical education curricula and program interventions have been developed to achieve multiple goals (e.g.,, social, cognitive, and motor skills) while ensuring that students receive high levels of PA. For example, Sports, Play, and Active Recreation for Kids (SPARK) has been shown to significantly increase student MVPA and energy expenditures during elementary classes (Sallis et al., 1997). The intervention has also resulted in positive outcomes related to student fitness, motor skills, academic achievement, and quality of instruction (McKenzie et al., 2009). Several strands of the HOPE curriculum model include elements of SPARK instruction. The Coordinated Approach to Child Health (formerly the Child and Adolescent Trial for Cardiovascular Health; CATCH) intervention has also resulted in positive outcomes. In one study, student levels of MVPA increased 39 percent overall and above 50 percent of total physical education time during CATCH implementation (McKenzie et al., 1996).

The Middle School Physical Activity and Nutrition (M-SPAN) intervention is another program that focuses on increasing student levels of PA in physical education. Researchers advocating

for this model sought to raise teachers' awareness about the need for activity-based physical education and assisted them in developing and implementing adequate instruction to achieve higher levels of PA. This intervention resulted in students spending an additional three minutes engaged in MVPA per lesson without increasing lesson length (McKenzie et al., 2004), representing an 18 percent increase in MVPA.

Motor Skill Development

While the health benefits of PA are well documented, there has been considerable debate concerning whether physical education should emphasize increased levels of PA at the expense of skill development. Some scholars strongly believe that motor skill competence is the cornerstone of lifelong engagement in PA (Ennis, 2011), and a distinct association between motor competence (perceived and actual) and health-related fitness has been reported (Robinson et al., 2015). There are indications that the relationship between motor competence and health-related fitness increases from childhood to adolescence and is strongly linked with weight status. It seems reasonable, then, to emphasize the value of promoting motor skill development in quality physical education programs, primarily elementary physical education because it facilitates a foundation of skillfulness for lifelong PA and the development of physical literacy (Stodden et al., 2008, 2009). Effective teachers can promote motor skill development while engaging students in high levels of PA. For example, instead of asking students to stand in place while practicing ball dribbling skills, students can be encouraged to dribble while quickly moving throughout the gymnasium or playing field. This promotes PA while facilitating skill development because students must look ahead instead of at the ball to avoid contact with others.

Health-Related Fitness Knowledge

Providing adequate health-related fitness knowledge instruction is also an important aspect in the development of physical literacy. It is an aspect of quality physical education that plays a vital role in helping students achieve learning standards and adopt active lifestyles beyond the school day (e.g., Angela & Hannon, 2012; Chen et al., 2017; Dale & Corbin, 2000). Furthermore, it helps individuals become committed to achieving high levels of PA beyond high school graduation and well into their adult years (Dale & Corbin, 2000; Shephard & Trudeau, 2000). Health-related fitness knowledge may also be related to students' fitness levels (Williams et al., 2013). Therefore, it is important for physical education teachers to integrate cognitive objectives into their curricula and provide intentional learning opportunities designed to support student acquisition of health-related fitness knowledge. Of course, it is also important to provide students with other forms of knowledge during physical education. For example, to be successful when engaging in different sports, students need to acquire knowledge about game rules, tactics, and strategies.

Appropriate Instruction

A quality physical education curriculum is largely dependent on the content it emphasizes, how it is delivered, and how the teacher uses the content to instruct (McKenzie & Lounsbery, 2013). Appropriate instruction within a quality physical education program should be consistent with the goals and outcomes of a CSPAP, and instructional decisions should be based on increasing MVPA, developing physical literacy, and promoting PA to maximize student health. Further, teacher effectiveness and appropriate instruction need to be evaluated by teachers and administrators according to the extent to which they achieve positive student health outcomes, such as improved fitness levels (McKenzie & Lounsbery, 2013).

MVPA Levels

Student MVPA levels vary widely in physical education and are largely dependent on a variety of instructional and contextual factors. Activities that focus on health-related fitness, skill development, and gameplay tend to facilitate PA, whereas class management and knowledge instruction tend to hinder PA (McKenzie et al., 2000). This is illustrated by the fact that students tend to engage in more MVPA in physical education as their grade level increases (Levin et al., 2001) possibly because of less time spent on instructional and management tasks (McKenzie & Lounsbery, 2013). Developing efficient routines, planning concise task presentations, and establishing a positive learning environment can increase the amount of time students have to engage in MVPA at all grade levels. For example, instead of asking students to wait in line to retrieve a ball from an equipment basket, balls can easily be spread throughout the room so that students can immediately begin engaging in activity without having to wait in line for their turn.

Skill Development

The fundamental motor skills, such as running, skipping, hopping, and jumping, are the "ABCs in the world of physical activity" (Stodden et al., 2008, p. 291). If children cannot perform prerequisite motor skills, then they will have limited opportunities for successful engagement in PA later in life. Motor skill development is foundational to the development of physical literacy and should, therefore, be a principal objective in designing a quality physical education program. Motor skill competence plays a highly significant role in supporting PA behaviors, and teachers must invest instructional time teaching motor skills to see increased levels of PA (Stodden et al., 2008). It is also important to understand how children learn motor skills and to know the developmental stages that underpin the process (Gallahue & Ozmun, 1998).

PA Promotion

The current state of physical education within the schools makes it difficult for physical education teachers to provide the recommended 60 minutes of PA per day. Large class size, lack of equipment, inadequate facilities, and physical education teachers who lack effective teaching skills are factors that contribute to lower levels of MVPA. A report from the Institute of Medicine (2013) suggested that at least half of students' daily PA should occur in a physical education context and the remainder, through other components of a CSPAP program, such as before-, during-, or after-school PA programs. This means that PA promotion in non–physical education environments is both necessary and a fundamental responsibility of all school personnel, not just of physical educators.

Instructional Effectiveness Tools

The System for Observing Fitness Instruction Time (SOFIT) is a tool designed to assess the effectiveness of physical education instruction within a public health context (McKenzie et al., 1991). It provides data on student activity level, lesson context, and PA promotion or general teacher involvement. Decisions related to each of these SOFIT coding categories can contribute to the overall effect of physical education lessons on student health. Results from SOFIT data can help teachers identify areas of strength and improvement to ensure students maintain high levels of MVPA throughout each lesson.

The Physical Education Observation Form (PEOF) is a rating scale comprising a variety of items thought to be associated with the promotion of PA in physical education, which can be used to rate teacher behaviors, indicate the inclusion of a warm-up and cool-down, take note of PA prompts during the lesson, record positive feedback related to student participation, rate perceived student enjoyment, indicate the quality and accessibility of the equipment used during the lesson, indicate the appropriateness of group sizes for activities, and record teacher enthusiasm (McKenzie & Lounsbery, 2013).

While the SOFIT observation is a valid and reliable instructional quality and assessment tool (Rowe et al., 1997, 2004), it is important to have proper training protocols and consistent materials to maintain the reliability of the instrument (McKenzie & Lounsbery, 2013). Teachers who lack training can ask individuals such as district physical education curriculum coordinators to evaluate their teaching using this instrument.

Thus, teachers and affiliated school personnel can use the components of SOFIT and the PEOF to guide their instructional decision making and maintain a public health–focused curriculum.

Assessment

A broad range of beliefs exist about assessment in physical education, especially related to how it is conducted. Assessment can be a time-consuming process and is sometimes difficult to implement efficiently, particularly for teachers with large class sizes. Perceived time constraints and concern about management issues when conducting assessments have contributed to the lack of overall evaluation within physical education (Rink, 2014). Nevertheless, assessment provides valuable information about individual student learning and overall program effectiveness, and techniques exist for making assessment a more manageable task, such as asking classroom teachers to assist. Data collected from assessments should be used to help students and teachers understand student progress toward program outcomes and guide teachers' instruction. Thus, it is important to inform students of the assessment criteria being used and communicate the results so that students can receive individualized feedback to make targeted improvements (Kniffin & Baert, 2015).

Role of PETE

Quality physical education within a CSPAP is a relatively recent model for helping students to engage in high levels of PA throughout the school day. The implementation of quality physical education within a CSPAP requires a different and more focused knowledge base than what is required in traditional physical education (Metzler et al., 2013b). Teachers who implement the model must have knowledge about the overarching goals of both quality physical education and CSPAPs, which places greater responsibility on PETE faculty to inform future teachers about the different components of the model and provide adequate practicum opportunities in schools that have demonstrated success implementing both quality physical education and the CSPAP model. Metzler and colleagues (2013b) recommended PETE curricula be redesigned to include content and pedagogical knowledge associated with public health–related physical education and CSPAPs. The extent to which quality physical education in CSPAPs is successful is largely dependent on faculty members building their "PETE program around HOPE as a central theme and accompanying knowledge base" (p. 30).

Teacher Knowledge and Skills

Webster and colleagues (2015) recommended that PETE programs provide learning experiences during teacher education related to school, community, and family PA programming; advocacy efforts to promote PA; health behavior theory; and PA measurement and evaluation. It is also suggested that future physical education teachers acquire certification in PA promotion from organizations, such as the American College of Sports Medicine (Bulger & Housner, 2009), to enable new teachers to successfully incorporate PA throughout the school day and help them understand that physical education is only one component of a multifaceted effort to optimize students' health (Metzler et al., 2013b).

Implementing a quality physical education program as part of a CSPAP requires skills and knowledge that are not always addressed in more traditional PETE programs. Therefore, to optimize the chance that new teachers will be successful, they must acquire knowledge during teacher education about managing PA opportunities outside of physical education time, using social media and marketing to promote PA, and advocating for quality physical education within the broader school context (Metzler et al., 2013b). Advocacy efforts can include a variety of strategies, such as promoting PA throughout the school day, helping classroom teachers to integrate movement time into their classes, and teaching recess games in physical education early in the school year (Beighle et al., 2009).

Field-Based Learning

Field-based experiences are an important way to expose students to quality physical education and help them become more confident in their ability to create and support a quality physical education program as part of a coordinated school PA effort. Metzler and colleagues (2013b) outlined efforts by Arizona State University to provide field-based opportunities to undergraduate PETE students as part of their initial teacher certification program. These opportunities include assigning groups of PETE interns at the high school level to assist in implementing broad PA-focused physical education programs. The interns encourage secondary school students to engage in PA before and after school and during lunch by providing verbal prompts and experimenting with social media marketing. They are also required to design and maintain a web page promoting PA that links to the school's website. The interns attend a weekly PETE seminar focused on quality physical education skills and are evaluated on the percentage of the high school student body who attend non–physical education PA environments, percentage of students in extra–physical education PA environments who engage in MVPA, frequency of interaction with high school students, and use of a variety of marketing tactics. These criteria encourage outcomes that align directly to HOPE and help interns gauge their success.

Knowledge Claims

Based on the research reviewed in the previous section of this chapter, the following claims can be made about the available evidence for quality physical education.

- Physical education is the foundation of an effective CSPAP.
- Students should be engaged in MVPA for at least 50 percent of a physical education class.
- Physical literacy is an important goal of a CSPAP.
- Physical education should be taught by teachers certified in the subject matter.
- Class size and adequate facilities are important considerations that can influence whether a CSPAP has the most potential for being effective.
- High levels of PA and motor skills development are equally important goals of physical education.
- Data collected from assessments should be used to help students and teachers understand student progress toward program outcomes and guide teachers' instruction.

Knowledge Gaps and Directions for Future Research

Initial evidence demonstrates the potential for the CSPAP model to increase the amount of MVPA that students receive throughout the school day. Large gaps exist, however, in the knowledge base that need to be addressed. For example, relatively little is known about which elements of a CSPAP model are most effective at increasing MVPA throughout the school day and which elements have a lasting effect on retaining a commitment to engage in PA throughout the life span. Short-term and longitudinal investigations that are large scale in nature need to be conducted, both of which will likely require external funding to support studies. In addition, it would be helpful to understand how different forms of technology can facilitate the effectiveness of quality physical education and CSPAPs and whether a CSPAP is sustainable when existing teachers who were committed to the model leave the program and new faculty members are employed. Finally, investigating the effect of asynchronous instruction (where students acquire physical education content knowledge through online instruction prior to class) on MVPA is timely and may demonstrate that one of the most effective ways to increase PA levels during class is through online instruction prior to class.

Evidence-Based Recommendations and Applications

Quality physical education programs provide students with enriching movement opportunities throughout the school day and facilitate the development of knowledge, skills, and attitudes necessary for active living. Both school staff and community partners can contribute to the successful implementation of physical education, and recommendations for each group are suggested.

For School Staff

Physical education curricula should be grounded in state and national physical education standards (SHAPE America, 2013). The content should be designed sequentially to encourage developmen-tally appropriate progression through grade-level outcomes (SHAPE America, 2009). Activities should reflect the mission of quality physical education and CSPAPs by including high levels of MVPA and a focus on skills that can be applied in a variety of movement contexts. Health-related fitness knowledge and PA promotion must be embedded throughout the entire curriculum to encourage students to make healthy choices and engage in PA outside of school. Regular curriculum evaluation and revision should occur to ensure that instructional practice is evidence based.

Instructional strategies must promote a positive learning environment where students can safely engage in high levels of PA. Clear and efficient task presentations should enhance student learning and support the quality of students' physical education experiences. Teachers should intentionally plan their class routines and instruction to ensure skills are demonstrated clearly, concepts are described accurately, and activities are explained thoroughly and efficiently.

Quality physical education programs should include student-centered, developmentally appropriate assessments that motivate students to engage and understand their progress toward physical literacy. These evaluations should be based on student learning and not on attendance, participation, or class preparedness. Teachers must assess students regularly to provide appropriate learning opportunities, especially at the elementary level, where students' developmental levels vary widely. Because assessments, such as fitness and motor skills tests, take time, physical education teachers can ask classroom teachers to assist during the assessment process by keeping students who are not completing assessments actively engaged in other tasks or assisting with the collection of assessment data.

There are many components to a quality physical education program, and most of them are driven by the physical education teacher. It is important that school district administrators support physical education teachers' efforts by providing time for faculty to meet for program development and to attend state and national conferences that expose teachers to best instructional practices. Professional development opportunities for physical education teachers are critical for ensuring students receive current, evidence-based content, instruction, and assessment experiences.

For Community Partners

For students to engage in health-enhancing PA and achieve learning standards, state and national policies must be enacted to ensure students receive adequate, appropriate learning opportunities. Elementary students should be engaged in at least 150 minutes of weekly physical education, and secondary students should receive 225 minutes. Only certified physical education teachers should be allowed to teach the subject matter; they should be provided the space and equipment necessary to implement instruction effectively, and their class sizes should be comparable to classroom-based subjects. Unfortunately, some schools do not have adequate funding to meet these recommendations. Thus, it takes coordinated efforts in which parents, students, classroom teachers, and community leaders collaborate to educate school board members and legislative policy makers about the importance of the subject matter and encourage policy change.

Parents, community members, and local businesses can also contribute by providing students with adequate PA opportunities that are meaningful, developmentally appropriate, and aligned with physical education grade-level outcomes (Webster et al., 2016). Even local businesses can contribute to the effort by providing free space for children to engage in PA. For example, a YMCA or local roller rink might allow students to partake in activity without charge at certain times or on particular days of the week. Directors of park districts can contribute by facilitating shared space agreements. Community members and parents can also assist by volunteering their efforts to help the physical education teacher during instruction or when collecting assessment data.

SUMMARY

This chapter provides an overview of the components of quality physical education and the role it plays as the foundation of CSPAPs. Quality physical education should support the goals of CSPAPs by providing adequate opportunities for students to engage in MVPA and develop physical literacy. Physical education is the primary environment during the school day where students can be physically active and acquire the knowledge, skills, and dispositions necessary to participate in lifelong PA. Supportive policies and learning environments are essential to afford physical education teachers time and space to implement curricula and instructional practices that promote PA. In turn, appropriate assessment practices that evaluate student knowledge, skills, fitness, and dispositions toward PA are instrumental in determining teaching effectiveness and making improvements to curricula and instructional practices. PETE programs can support preservice teacher knowledge and skills related to implementing CSPAPs by organizing instructional and field-based experiences around the objectives of public health–oriented physical education and the CSPAP model.

QUESTIONS TO CONSIDER

1. What role should physical education teachers play in encouraging the adoption of a CSPAP model in a school where one does not currently exist?

2. What are some strategies for encouraging physical education teachers who adopt traditional teaching practices to implement instructional strategies that promote higher levels of MVPA in their classes?

3. How can physical education teachers better engage students in high levels of PA when they are employed in a school with limited equipment and large class sizes?

4. Should physical education teachers be held accountable for implementing quality physical education? If so, how should they be rewarded for implementing quality instruction or penalized when students do not achieve learning outcomes?

5. What is more important, engaging students in high levels of MVPA or teaching basic motor skills? Defend your response with at least three points.

CASE EXAMPLE: DEVELOPING A QUALITY PHYSICAL EDUCATION PROGRAM

Richard is a novice elementary school physical education teacher (K-6) in his third year of teaching at an urban school near Chicago. His first year of teaching was discouraging because his school had an outdated curriculum, limited equipment, and students who were less motivated to be active during physical education than he anticipated. Because he had acquired knowledge about quality physical education and CSPAPs as an undergraduate enrolled in the PETE program, he decided to update his curriculum during his second year as a teacher to include more developmentally appropriate activities and instruction. He began to adapt the curriculum to include units and lessons that would be enjoyable but engage students in increasingly higher levels of MVPA. He was intentional about developing units that focused on fundamental motor skills that also facilitated high levels of PA, and he was careful to include instruction that helped students develop their health-related fitness knowledge.

The curriculum he developed over the course of the school year and summer was standards based and designed to address the national grade-level outcomes for physical education, just like he was taught in his PETE program. He even decided to attend the national conference that is sponsored annually by SHAPE America to learn what other physical education faculty and researchers were doing nationally and internationally. He was intentional about connecting with motivated professionals and scholars to acquire new ways of engaging students to be active and develop physical literacy. He shared what he learned with the other physical education teachers in his district during professional development days, and he felt invigorated. Although a few colleagues were not interested in the ideas he shared, several others suggested revising the district-approved curriculum. The group began meeting weekly to plan how to improve the physical education curriculum in all elementary schools in the school district.

Richard also discovered many new evidence-based instructional strategies by reading journals that accompanied his professional memberships, and he did his best to integrate some of these strategies along with technology into his classes. He also developed new instructional routines where students could engage in PA promptly upon entering the gym, and he had his older students set basic goals at the beginning of each unit. He encouraged them to reflect as they progressed through the learning activities. He also integrated formative and summative assessments, such as FitnessGram, knowledge tests, and skills assessments, into the curriculum at appropriate grade levels to monitor students' progress and help them understand how they were improving. By using teaching reflections, suggestions he received during an evaluation from his principal, and feedback from students, he continued to make positive adjustments to the physical education curriculum and his instruction.

Richard has tried hard not to be discouraged when lessons do not always proceed as well as he anticipated because developing a quality physical education program is a process that requires adjustments. Because of the knowledge he acquired in his PETE program, he understood there are many factors that contribute to the quality of a program. He tries to be patient, and he continues to work independently and with colleagues to improve the program and overall district curriculum. He continues to adjust his instruction to include content that encourages high levels of MVPA, and he started a before-school PA program and after-school running club. Currently, he is considering using online instruction for fifth- and sixth-grade students so they can acquire lesson content prior to class and spend in-class time engaged almost exclusively in high levels of activity. He learned that with patience and the support of others in his school, community, and profession, change is possible.

CHAPTER 7

Physical Activity During School

Aaron Beighle, PhD
University of Kentucky

Heather Erwin, PhD
University of Kentucky

Collin A. Webster, PhD
University of South Carolina

Michelle A. Webster
Rosewood Elementary School

Beyond physical education, PA during school at the elementary level typically takes place during either recess or classroom PA integration. At the secondary level, PA during school may be offered via walking breaks, recess after lunch, classroom PA integration, and drop-in events. Individuals who promote PA opportunities for students, staff, and the community (e.g., PA directors, PA champions, or directors of PA) are encouraged to take advantage of every possible opportunity throughout the school day to offer PA (Erwin, Beets, et al., 2014). The evidence is clear that PA offered during the school day affects both health and cognition, including improved bone and cardiovascular and metabolic health, reduced weight gain, and reduced symptoms of anxiety (Centers for Disease Control and Prevention, 2018). In addition, it enhances attentiveness, boosts concentration (Norlander et al., 2005), and diminishes behavior problems (Mahar et al., 2006), all of which are factors known to influence learning. This chapter contains a review of research on PA during school, knowledge claims based on this research, knowledge gaps and recommendations for future research, practical recommendations and applications based on the existing research, and three case examples of PA promotion during school.

Review of Research

PA during school encompasses PA opportunities at recess and in the classroom. This section will first examine the literature related to recess PA, including studies examining current recess PA patterns and research associated with "what works" in recess interventions. A review of the research associated with classroom-based PA will then follow.

Recess

Recess has been a part of the school experience for many generations. While it was thought to be part of early schools, limited documentation of recess exists prior to the late 1800s. Until recently, recess was typically seen as a break, or "recess," from learning in the classroom and was often provided to students immediately after lunch. In 2001, Waite-Stupiansky and Findlay (2001) presented the notion that recess is fundamental to learning and should be considered the "Fourth R" in education. Research has examined the role of recess in PA promotion (Beighle et al., 2006; Erwin, Abel, et al., 2012; Ickes et al., 2013). Still, other research has examined the role of recess in social development for youth (Jarrett et al., 1998; Pellegrini & Bohn, 2005).

Recess is best defined as "scheduled outside of class time and allows students to engage in physical and social activities of their choice" (Beighle, 2012, p. 2). A key component of this definition is the element of choice. This definition is of particular importance when examining the use of recess as punishment in schools. Some schools use policies that state that recess cannot be taken away as a consequence of misbehavior during the school day or missing work. On the surface, this seems like a noble policy; however, if recess is not defined as Beighle defined it, students can be made to walk laps during recess. For instance, a teacher might require a student to walk five laps because he or she talked in the classroom. By defining recess as it is here and implementing a policy that recess cannot be taken away, schools are ensuring that children get ample time to be physically active in a way they choose.

Despite the well-known benefits of recess, including the social, cognitive, physical, and emotional aspects, the support for recess is surprisingly low (Pellegrini & Bohn, 2005; Strong et al., 2005). A survey from 2016 found that 65 percent of districts require regularly scheduled recess (SHHPS, 2016). However, recess policy is primarily left to schools, as evidenced by only 12 percent of states having requirements for daily recess. At the district level, 57 percent require and 33 percent recommend daily recess (Beighle, 2012). Even more alarming is the data examining the recess offerings for students at risk for obesity. In 2005, the Center for Education Statistics (2018) suggested that youth who attend schools in big cities, in the southeastern United States, or with a high percentage of lower-income families are the least likely to have recess. The same holds true for schools with high percentages of minorities.

While recess is typically thought of as a great place for PA, data examining student PA levels during recess is mixed. Beighle and colleagues (2006) used pedometry and found that boys were active 78 percent and girls 63 percent of recess time, with a significant gender effect but no grade effect. Ridgers and colleagues (2005), on the contrary, found that boys were active 33 percent of recess time, whereas girls were engaged in PA only 23 percent of recess time. Erwin, Abel, and colleagues (2012) \ found that a 15-minute recess contributed from 17 to 44 percent of students' school-day PA. When looking at PA over an entire day, recess contributes 8 to 9 percent of daily PA for elementary students (Brusseau et al., 2011; Tudor-Locke et al., 2006). Combined, this information suggests that approximately 20 minutes of opportunity for PA can provide valuable amounts of PA for youth.

An expanding body of research suggests that recess can provide as much as 40 percent of a child's daily PA (Erwin , Abel, et al., 2012). However, it is important to note that the PA levels during recess can range from 16 to 68 percent for boys and from 15 to 52 percent for girls (Beighle et al., 2006). These percentages indicate that some intervention is needed to maximize the effect of recess on student PA levels. Effective strategies for maximizing PA during recess have included training teachers and staff and providing equipment, painting playground markings, and creating activity zones to provide a semistructured recess environment that still allows for free choice (Erwin, Ickes, et al., 2014).

As with most experiences in schools, adults can play a key role in the recess environment. Specifically, recess supervisors, whether staff or teachers, have great potential for increasing PA in schools. All too often, recess environments are littered with benches for supervisors to sit and become disengaged with the students. At times, even at recess, students enjoy adult interaction, and sadly, they need adult assistance in finding PA opportunities. Some evidence has suggested that untrained supervisors can be counterproductive and may actually reduce student PA opportunities for students (McKenzie et al., 1997). For instance, some students may simply "hang out" with the supervisor. If the supervisor is not encouraging students to be active, recess time is not being optimized. Conversely, training staff to teach simple games during recess promotes PA and increases activity during recess. Further, when staff members are trained to interact with students, PA can be increased during recess (Huberty et al., 2011). In the Huberty study, recess supervisors were identified and trained in general activities and activities that were popular in the specific school. In addition, the physical education teacher taught recess-appropriate activities early and periodically throughout the school year. While this latter point was not researched, anecdotal comments from the supervisors suggested that exposing the students to new activities during physical education made teaching the activities during recess easier.

The sustainability of recess PA without equipment is difficult. That is, students are likely to become bored with a large grassy area for play unless equipment is provided. "Equipment" here refers to low-cost recreational equipment, such as balls, jump ropes, cones, and hoops. Large playground structures, while attractive and visually appealing, are typically cost prohibitive; thus, providing less expensive equipment may provide more variety. Verstraete and colleagues (2006) increased student PA 13 percent by providing equipment such as hoops, jump ropes, beanbags, and flying disks. Interestingly, while the authors were not clear why, student PA in the control group decreased by 11 percent during the study.

A relatively novel approach to increasing PA during recess is to paint playgrounds. The paintings in this approach can take the form of murals on walls (e.g., a forest, fort, or dinosaur) or lines for recreational games (e.g., hopscotch or wall ball). One study examined student PA before and after painting the playgrounds and found that students were engaged in PA 50 percent of the recess time after paintings (Stratton & Mullan, 2005). This was up 12 percent from before the paintings were created. Further research found that the increased PA levels persisted for six months after the paintings (Ridgers et al., 2007). This information is of particular importance given that the resources available for recess interventions are often limited. Simply painting lines and murals can have an effect that lasts almost an entire school year.

More recently, activity zones have been examined as an approach to increase PA during recess. Activity zones involve "zoning" off areas of the playground space for specific activities (Gopher Sport, 2017). Examples of zones include soccer, jump rope, dance, basketball, four square, a learning zone where a new activity is taught each week, a walking trail, and a choice zone where equipment is provided and students select the activity. Research on this approach, albeit limited, did not find significant increases in PA levels, but the researchers provided promising strategies for future implementation and research (Huberty et al., 2011).

As with most PA interventions in schools, an attractive approach is one that is cost effective and borrows from other evidence-based practices. Two studies have examined the effect of multiple low-cost interventions on recess PA. Loucaides and colleagues (2009) examined the effect of activity zones, painting, and equipment on student PA as measured by pedometry. In a 20-minute recess, students in the experimental group accumulated 300 more steps than those in the control group. Another study found that students accumulated 4.5 more minutes of PA during a 20-minute recess when the combination of staff training, equipment, and activity zones was utilized (Huberty et al., 2011).

Classroom-Based PA

Similar to recess, the integration of PA into the classroom, referred to as movement integration (MI), offers great potential for increasing daily

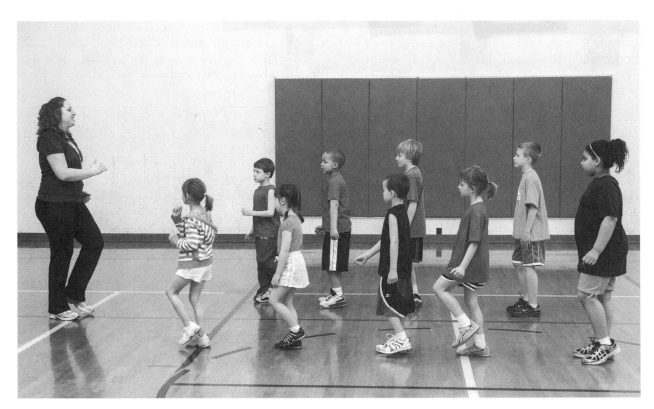

PA during regularly scheduled class time can occur in the classroom or in other school contexts when available. Here, a teacher uses the school's gym to lead her class in a movement opportunity.

PA and reducing the amount of time spent sitting during school hours (Webster, Russ, et al., 2015). Webster, Russ, and colleagues (2015) defined MI as "infusing PA, at any level of intensity, within general education classrooms during normal classroom time" (p. 304). MI can take numerous forms (Russ et al., 2017). Teacher-directed PA opportunities include leading PA breaks during academic lessons, using PA to teach academic content, or incorporating PA during transitions between lessons. Classroom-based PA opportunities can also occur as a result of the physical environment, such as when classroom seating promotes PA (e.g., pedal desks) or the placement of materials around the room requires students to move more to get what they need. Further, PA can be integrated into the classroom simply by selecting learning experiences that have students out of their seats. Teachers may also choose MI options that rely on technology. For instance, numerous websites (e.g., YouTube and GoNoodle) provide video-based activities designed to lead students in movement that either links with academic content

or simply provides a chance to get some extra PA (Russ et al., 2017).

The most recent systematic review revealed there was a 2 to 16 percent increase in classroom-based moderate-to-vigorous PA (MVPA) during classroom time and a 2 to 12 percent increase in school-day MVPA across MI interventions (Watson et al., 2017). These results suggest that MI can make a meaningful contribution to the overall goal of a CSPAP, which is to help children and adolescents achieve the nationally recommended 60 minutes of mostly MVPA each day. However, because the goal of MI encompasses increasing light PA too (Webster, Russ, et al., 2015), it is important to consider research-based strategies that have resulted in increased PA at any level of intensity.

Intervention studies have tested a wide range of curricula and prepackaged programs for MI (Webster, Russ, et al., 2015). Several curricula and programs that have an academic focus (e.g., TAKE10, Move to Improve, and Promoting Physical Activity and Health in the Classroom) or are primarily designed for movement breaks (i.e., not explicitly linked to academic content, for example, Instant Recess, Activity Bursts in the Classroom, and Promoting Physical Activity and Health in the Classroom) have increased students' classroom-based PA (Dunn et al., 2012; Erwin et al., 2011; Pangrazi, Beighle, & Pangrazi, 2009; Katz et al., 2010; Kibbe et al., 2011; Whitt-Glover et al., 2011). For instance, Erwin, Abel and colleagues (2011) provided simple activity cards for teachers to use when they sensed the students needed a break or the activity fit with the academic content being taught. Another effective strategy for increasing classroom PA is working with teachers to modify or create academic lessons with the intention of integrating PA. For instance, Donnelly and colleagues (2009) helped teachers to combine content from the TAKE10 program with existing teacher-developed lessons, whereas Erwin and colleagues (2011) collaborated with teachers to modify existing lesson plans or to create new lesson plans that infused PA with core math content (Erwin, Abel, et al., 2011). This was accomplished by meeting with the teachers to brainstorm strategies, implement those strategies, and make modifications as needed prior to making activity cards.

When it is available, using special classroom equipment is an alternative approach that can also be effective for increasing classroom PA (Webster, Russ, et al., 2015). Fedewa and colleagues (2017) found that adolescents on stationary bicycle desks spent more time in MVPA and less time being sedentary compared to a control group. At the middle school level, it was observed that when using sit-to-stand desks, students chose to stand 59 percent and sit 37 percent of the time. The remaining time (4 percent), they were considered walking, or more so, "bouncing" (Erwin et al., 2017). They were very positive about their experiences with the desks. Stability balls are another alternative to a sitting approach in the classroom. While PA levels during time on the stability balls has been shown to decrease with children when compared to those sitting in chairs (Erwin et al., 2016), the balls have demonstrated improved in-seat time and on-task behavior over the course of 15 weeks (Fedewa & Erwin, 2011). It is believed that stability balls may have this effect because they require the use of core muscles to

stay upright, which causes the users to focus on balancing themselves as opposed to using energy for other purposes, such as being off task.

School–university partnerships are another way to increase classroom-based PA. Children in elementary classrooms who received university support in the form of a virtual community of practice, community-based participatory research, and service learning demonstrated an increase in MVPA and a decrease in sedentary time (Weaver et al., 2017). The community of practice was a website designed for preservice and in-service classroom teachers where participants could interact via a discussion board as well as adopt new MI strategies and activities. Community-based participatory research involved members of the university research team meeting with the teachers to set context-specific MI goals, identify suitable strategies to meet those goals, and monitor successes and challenges in MI implementation. For the service-learning component, university students learning about MI completed assignments that involved conducting MI in the elementary classrooms participating in the study.

When aiming to increase students' PA during classroom time, it is important to consider whether changes in classroom-based PA have an overall positive or negative effect on total school-day PA. It is possible that being more active during class time could lead to a decline in students' PA during other periods of the school day because of a lack of energy. Few studies have specifically examined the effects of classroom PA on students' engagement in PA in contexts where they often can choose to be active or not (e.g., recess and after school). In the study by Weaver and colleagues (2017), children's MVPA increased not only during classroom time but also during the remaining hours of regularly scheduled school time. Based on these results, it would seem that MI does not have a negative effect on overall daily PA and that students do not compensate for increases in classroom PA by engaging in less PA at other times when they have the opportunity to be active.

The benefits of MI can extend beyond increasing students' PA to increasing students' academic performance. Numerous studies and reviews have shown positive or no effect or both of MI on academic outcomes, such as achievement, behavior, and cognition (Erwin, Fedewa, et al., 2012; Watson et al., 2017). Thus, implementing movement in the classroom does not necessarily detract from student learning and may enhance learning in certain instances. In one of the longest-term studies to date, Szabo-Reed and colleagues (2017) found that elementary children who participated in physically active academic lessons accrued more MVPA than children in a control group in each year of a three-year intervention. Children in the intervention group also spent more time on task following classroom PA, and PA was positively associated with time on task.

While numerous strategies for increasing PA during the secondary school day have been put forth, the research in this area is limited. A study surveying school administrators and students in 8th, 10th, and 12th grades showed that PA breaks offered in secondary schools differed greatly by school size, socioeconomic status, region, and student race (Hood et al., 2014). Those middle schools offering breaks demonstrated lower odds of overweight and obese students. Regarding high school facilities, schools with more indoor and outdoor facilities demonstrated a 19 to 42 percent greater odds of MVPA for their students (Hood et al., 2014). Lorenz and colleagues (2017) examined the effect of a lunchtime intervention at a junior high school and found that providing students with access to space and the opportunity to be active increased the PA levels of students. Practically, this suggests that simply opening the gym for students to be active has great potential. As suggested previously in this chapter, research on bikes in a high school classroom found that students were more active with the option of the bikes than without (Fedewa et al., 2017), and research on students in middle school who had the option of using sit-to-stand desks chose to stand over half the time when using them (Erwin et al., 2017).

Knowledge Claims

Recess offers an excellent opportunity for students to engage in meaningful, health enhancing physical activity. However, as the evidence presented in the previous section suggests, policies and other variables impacting the offering of recess can be complex. Similarly, simply offering recess may not result in students being physically active. This section provides several assertions based on the evidence presented related to recess.

- Very little is known about the activity levels of students during recess, how seasonality affects recess activity, and activity patterns students typically exhibit during recess.

- The benefits of regular recess are not limited to physical benefits. Mental, social, and cognitive benefits are also demonstrated in the literature.

- There are several evidence-based approaches to increasing PA during recess, many of which are cost effective. These approaches include activity zones, active supervision, and providing equipment.

- MI can take numerous forms; a veritable menu of options exist for classroom teachers to provide movement opportunities for their students.

- Several MI approaches can increase classroom-based PA, including a range of MI curricula and programs, teacher-designed lesson plans, special classroom equipment, and school–university partnerships.

- Although more research is needed, it appears that classroom-based PA does not lead to declines in students' PA during other periods of the school day.

- MI can have academic benefits for students and has not been shown to negatively influence academics.

- More research is needed to examine the effect of interventions to increase PA during the secondary school day.

Knowledge Gaps and Directions for Future Research

While the evidence continues to mount supporting PA during school, some key gaps in the literature need to be addressed in future research. Despite the overwhelming support for PA in schools, the uptake of administrators and teachers in using this valuable teaching tool has been slow. As discussed in chapter 9 of this book, research examining why some administrators and teachers choose to integrate PA and some do not is essential for advancing the integration of PA into schools. Additional warranted research questions specific to recess and classroom MI are abundant:

- Recess
  - How active are students at recess?
  - What is the prevalence of recess? How is recess implemented?
  - What is the optimal timing of recess? Is recess before lunch more effective?
  - Are two recesses more effective than one long recess on PA levels? Classroom behavior?
  - Are students more active in one 30-minute recess or when recess is divided into two 15-minute recesses?
  - Is goal setting an effective tool for increasing student activity levels during recess?
  - How long are interventions effective in increasing PA? That is, is there a reactive effect that wanes over time?
  - How does the effect of recess interventions vary by age? Gender? Demographics? Other student characteristics, such as obesity?
  - Can secondary schools implement novel approaches, such as drop-in activities during lunchtime or student-selected recess time, to affect student PA?
  - What is the feasibility and effect of indoor recess activities during inclement weather?
  - Can recess be established in middle and high schools? What are student, teacher, and administrator perceptions of providing recess for these students?
  - What is the feasibility and practicality of implementing walking programs at the elementary and secondary school levels?
- Movement integration
  - What are teachers' rate of MI adoption, the rate of MI diffusion across a school, or the sustainability of MI as a new part of a teacher's classroom routines?
  - What does observational research regarding MI tell us?
  - Which MI strategies are most commonly used?

- What patterns may exist in the timing and frequency of MI?
- Are there differences in MI use by teacher, school, and community characteristics?
- What are optimum MI strategies to increase secondary students' PA?
- How does classroom-based PA support PA engagements among youth and adults in other educational settings, such as preschools, universities, correctional facilities?
- How can PA be integrated into the secondary classroom? And what effect do these strategies have on student PA levels?

Evidence-Based Recommendations and Applications

Despite known gaps in the knowledge base related to PA during school, the existing research on effective strategies for promoting PA during recess and regular classroom time has implications for practice, both for school staff and community partners. Staff behaviors, equipment options, playground design, scheduling, professional trainings, and university support are some of the key factors that merit resource allocation and increased attention in efforts to translate research to best practices in promoting PA during school.

For School Staff

In most schools, educators acknowledge the utility of recess and the many benefits of recess time. However, simply offering recess is only a start; it is essential that the time spent during recess be maximized, with students engaging in as much health-enhancing PA as possible. In short, simply sending students to the playground does not ensure PA. The recess environment must be intentional to maximize student PA.

Recess supervisors are key personnel in efforts to increase recess PA. To this end, many are not familiar with the numerous strategies available to them. For instance, the simple message that active supervision, as opposed to sedentary supervision, is critical. Supervisors can be trained to set

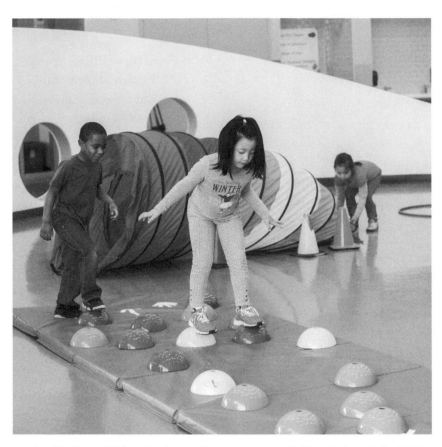

Recess environments should allow children to choose from various activities that peak their interest and keep them motivated to stay physically active. Here, children participate in different indoor recess activities.

up activity zones or provide activities that foster movement in some other manner. They can be trained to motivate students and help them find activities they enjoy. In many cases, just being a smiling, friendly face willing to play for a minute is all it takes.

Most activities that students enjoy require equipment. Thus, the provision of recreational equipment (e.g., balls, hoops, jump ropes, music, beanbags, and cones) is recommended. While there is some cost to this, the relative cost of providing this equipment is quite low and paramount to helping students engage in PA during recess. Many schools have created checkout systems for equipment to minimize equipment loss and develop student responsibility.

As discussed earlier in this chapter, several studies have examined the effect of activity zones on student PA. While structured recess in which all students engage in the same activity (e.g., kickball) is not advised because this takes the

choice and freedom away from students, setting up zones that students can freely move to is an effective strategy. Zones require some setup, but volunteers, playground staff, or even older students can set up these zones quickly. Considering the known effect, it is worth the time.

Introducing new recess activities at the beginning of the year and throughout the school year can be an effective strategy (Babkes Stellino et al., 2010). One simple strategy is to spend the early part of the physical education curriculum each year teaching students activities for recess. As the year progresses, more games can be added and taught in five minutes at the end of a physical education lesson. Some people call these new activities the Recess Activity of the Week, or RAW. An activity zone can easily be established as the RAW zone and two evidence-based strategies can be combined into one. As an example, one teacher created a short video of the RAW and played it on the wall during lunch. Students received this quick review tutorial while eating and, thus, knew how to play the activity at recess.

Intramurals are traditionally thought of as team sports that involve some level of administrative cost. Student-run intramural leagues are a great way to integrate student responsibility and show students that intramurals are not exclusively about team sports. Disc golf, roundnet, and jump rope can all be used. Students are given the responsibility to be inclusive of everyone and to create teams, set up and clean up, and track statistics. The activity changes often, and the recess supervisor provides direction on a limited basis. Again, intramural leagues combine several evidence-based approaches, are relatively cost effective, and work to maximize student PA.

Lastly, increasing the frequency of PA offerings is warranted. That is, add more recess. Beets and colleagues (2016) proposed a theory of expanded, extended, and enhanced opportunities for PA. Here, "extended" applies in that simply adding more opportunity for recess holds the potential to increase PA. That is, rather than one 30-minute recess after lunch, schedule a 20-minute morning recess and a 20-minute afternoon recess. Research is currently being conducted with schools to determine teacher and student perceptions and the effects of multiple recess periods during the day. Anecdotally, teachers and students alike are overwhelmingly in favor of the notion because of a variety of positive outcomes, including student focus on and participation in class discussions and benefits for students socially. However, it is not common practice in many schools because, often, administrators and teachers believe adding time for PA cuts into instructional time. Additionally, several school districts do not consider recess as instructional time, and some teachers believe that recess elicits fights and bullying behaviors along with safety concerns.

In many instances, classroom teachers feel that MI is valuable for their students, yet they struggle to include PA opportunities (see chapter 9 of this book). Part of the issue for some teachers may be that they believe MI has to provide MVPA for students, whereas other teachers believe they have to substantially alter their current approach to teaching. Given the range of MI options, professional development for classroom teachers should include examples of each option and make it clear that learning to integrate movement can be progressive. Teachers who are new to MI could simply try arranging their classroom furniture and materials to promote more light-intensity PA or ensuring certain management routines (e.g., transitions) include PA opportunities. These MI strategies require little effort and afford multiple classroom-based occasions for PA each day. As teachers become increasingly comfortable with students moving more within classroom space, they can try more-ambitious MI strategies, such as teaching academic lessons with embedded PA. For example, they may teach lessons integrating movement that is specifically tied to academic content, such as math: "Complete the math problem in your head, and do jumping jacks to represent the correct answer."

For Community Partners

Universities have numerous resources that can be used to support MI in many schools (Webster, Beets, et al., 2015). Teacher education programs should be viewed as a natural resource for school–university partnership building. Student teaching internships and courses that include field experiences offer prime opportunities to incorporate recess and MI-based PA promotion practice opportunities for teacher candidates. Ideally, such opportunities can be framed using principles of service learning so that schools most in need of extra support are prioritized. University programs may also offer additional support for recess and MI via research initiatives grounded in the principles of community-based participatory research (Israel et al., 2003). Research using this approach capitalizes on the active engagement of school professionals as key contributors to the research team, thus promoting research objectives, methods, and reporting that are in line with the priorities and needs of the school community. Finally, university faculty and students can develop communities of practice to provide teachers with resources and increased opportunities for collaboration. Such communities are either conducted via face-to-face meetings or online and may be organized at multiple levels, such as within a grade level at a school; across an entire school; or even between schools, school districts, states and territories, or countries. An example of a virtual community of practice for MI is Move for Thought (https://moveforthought.ning.com), which Weaver and colleagues (2017) used as part of their pilot intervention study and is free to join. At the time of this writing, the community has over 650 members from Australia, Belgium, Canada, Croatia, Cyprus, Denmark, England, Estonia, Greece, Norway, Scotland, Senegal, Spain, and the United States (23 states).

SUMMARY

PA accumulated during the school day has the potential for making meaningful contributions to the daily PA of youth. Specifically, recess and in the classroom are common locations for PA. The evidence for approaches known to maximize PA levels during these opportunities is prevalent in the literature. Using this evidence, a variety of ideas for practitioners are needed to meet their varied circumstances.

QUESTIONS TO CONSIDER

1. Discuss the current PA levels of youth during recess.
2. Provide evidence-based strategies for increasing PA during recess.
3. Explain three evidence-based strategies for increasing PA in classroom settings.
4. Present two benefits of utilizing partnerships with organizations outside of schools to promote PA during the school day.

CASE EXAMPLES

This chapter includes three case examples that highlight strategies to implement PA in schools.

Recess: Tabor Valley School

My name is Faith Jackson, and I serve as the headmaster of Tabor Valley School in England. We implement what I believe to be an effective strategy for managing equipment that not only teaches student responsibility but also decreases equipment cost. At the beginning of the year, we require students to pay a small fee to receive their equipment token for recess periods. Our parent organization and school budget supplement for students who cannot pay the fee. Money from the token fees is used to purchase playground equipment. We store the playground equipment in a small shed located on the playground. Each week, a specific class is assigned to manage the equipment shed. This means students from that class are assigned shifts to work in the shed. During recess, all equipment must be checked out of the shed using the token system. For instance, if Louis wants a jump rope, he gives his token, with his name on it, to the shed worker, who in turn gives him the jump rope. When Louis is finished, he returns the rope and gets his token back. At the end of recess, any missing equipment can be accounted for with the tokens.

Recess: Maize Field Elementary School

My name is Hope Martinez, and I serve as the physical education teacher at Maize Field Elementary School, which is located in eastern Nebraska. The school was involved in a study, after which we decided to take the recess intervention to the next level. We have added the RAW component that was discussed in this chapter. I incorporate an activity within my physical education lesson each week, and then, I am sure to include any and all equipment required with the recess equipment pack so students can engage in that activity during recess. I also more frequently add activities via short lunchtime videos so students will be reminded of the activities available to them. To enhance PA despite difficult climates, in the winter months, students voluntarily bring in shovels to clear snow from the blacktop areas during recess. We allow students to bring small sleds to slide down a hill at recess as well. If proper attire is not available for students who want to participate, our school works with local community organizations to find resources to get the appropriate clothing. We usually have no issues with finding organizations or businesses to donate.

Classroom MI

Michelle A. Webster
Rosewood Elementary School

I am in my 18th year as an elementary classroom teacher and, in 2015, was Teacher of the Year at my previous school. For most of my teaching years, I have taught second grade. This year is my first time teaching third grade. When I first started teaching, I was reluctant to have my students leave their desks because I felt I would lose control of my classroom if I allowed children to move too much. But over the years, my attitude toward classroom movement opportunities has changed. Now, I understand how critical PA is to classroom management and students' academic performance. In fact, I often assign special leadership roles that involve more movement to students who tend to stray off task the most. I have these students pass out materials to the rest of the class.

While MI helps with classroom management, classroom management also helps with MI. I establish a strong management system at the beginning of each year. My students know my expectations, which include how to behave during movement opportunities. Even though some years I have had students with physical disabilities in my classroom, I have never found it impossible to provide movement opportunities for all of my children. One year, I had a student with brittle bone disease who was in a wheelchair. He was still able to participate in PA while in my classroom because I made sure the other students understood that they needed to give him his own space and avoid touching him. My students love it when they get to be active during class, and I am able to incentivize good classroom behavior using PA as a reward.

One of my goals as a teacher is to make sure my students never sit too long; I estimate that my students spend about half of their time in my classroom out of their desks. I use a wide range of strategies to incorporate PA into my classroom routines. A lot of movement time is transition time from one lesson or activity to the next. I try to transition my students every 10 minutes or so. I'll tell them to free dance to the carpet or back to their seats, and they love coming up with their own movements. My classroom setup promotes more movement during transitions because I arrange the desks in pods (groups of four or five desks), which affords more space than putting the desks in rows. I also store materials in different places around the classroom. Students must travel around the room to get the things they need during the day.

Another way I get my students moving is by integrating PA into academic lessons. I like to use songs with accompanying movements in science and social studies. For example, we sing songs about the water cycle (condensation, precipitation, and evaporation) and move our bodies to illustrate these concepts. In English language arts, my students perform reader's theater, in which they act out a story while practicing fluency. During math class, I like using task cards with math problems (e.g., multiplication and division) to review units. I tape the cards on the walls around the room, and each student and a partner walk to the different cards to solve the problems. I place the cards at different levels on the walls so students have to bend or stretch to read the problems.

My students usually show signs of losing focus in the afternoon after lunch and recess. They either fidget or slump more and need movement to keep them going during the last two hours of the school day. So we do lots of different kinds of movement breaks. We use video-based breaks from GoNoodle, and I find lots of helpful resources on websites, such as Teachers Pay Teachers. Much of the time, however, I find that my students prefer to create their own movements as opposed to following along with someone else's. My experience has taught me that students want autonomy as learners and enjoy learning more when they can choose how to move. They also like being able to decide when to stand and work instead of sitting at their desks. Many teachers desire autonomy too. I have a better time at school when I am free to teach the way I want to. In spite of all the free resources and prepackaged ideas out there for MI, my most successful strategies to help children stay active during school have been those I came up with myself.

CHAPTER 8

Physical Activity Programs Before and After School

Brian Dauenhauer, PhD
University of Northern Colorado

Megan Babkes Stellino, EdD
University of Northern Colorado

Collin A. Webster, PhD
University of South Carolina

Chuck Steinfurth
South Carolina Alliance of
    YMCAs

Schools have been recognized as important contexts for PA promotion (Institute of Medicine, 2013), yet a pervasive emphasis on academic achievement has eroded opportunities for PA during the school day. According to the School Health Policies and Practices Study, less than 4 percent of American schools require daily physical education for the entire school year and less than half provide regular PA breaks outside of physical education (Centers for Disease Control and Prevention, 2015). In response to restrictions on PA during the school day, public health advocates have turned toward out-of-school-time opportunities, including before- and after-school programs, to help youth acquire the recommended 60 minutes of PA per day (U.S. Department of Health and Human Services, 2008).

Before- and after-school programs occur during out-of-school time and are designed for school-aged youth 5 to 18 years of age. They can occur on campus through school-sponsored programs and shared-use agreements or off campus in partnership with community recreation centers and faith-based organizations. Examples include after-school childcare and enrichment programming, PA clubs, intramural and interscholastic sports, active transportation, and before-school programming. Before- and after-school programs are well positioned to promote PA in schools because they can utilize resources, such as space, equipment, student access, and personnel, without interfering with time dedicated to academic endeavors.

The purpose of this chapter is to provide a review of research on the effectiveness of programs held either before or after school at increasing the PA of children and youth, with the goal of informing best practices for program implementation. First, the most common and viable programs that target PA promotion after or before school are introduced. The research on PA programs and interventions within these settings is then reviewed and critiqued. Overall, knowledge claims and gaps in the research are subsequently identified, followed by evidence-based recommendations for policy and practice. The chapter concludes with two case examples: one that focuses on after-school programming and another that addresses before-school programming. Both examples emphasize essential features of before- and after-school PA programs in an effort to highlight recommendations for policy makers, school professionals, and other school stakeholders.

Review of Research

While this chapter addresses both before- and after-school programs, it is important to recognize that before-school programs are often coordinated and delivered independently of after-school programs and may occur as part of separate initiatives with distinct purposes and unique resources. A great deal more research has focused on after-school programs, which will be reviewed first, followed by findings from studies of before-school programs. Out-of-school-time programs, which can occur before or after school, are not necessarily time dependent and will be reviewed last.

After-School Programs

According to the Afterschool Alliance (2014), over 10 million youth attend after-school programs in the United States. They occur in the hours immediately after school (e.g., 3:00 to 6:00 p.m.) and are frequently offered through partnerships with community organizations, such as the YMCA or the Boys & Girls Clubs of America. A traditional after-school program is held five days per week or every school day and is available to all children in a school community. Although program schedules and available opportunities vary, many include a designated homework time, enrichment activities, and time for structured or unstructured play. A subset of after-school programs, PA clubs, also occur in the hours immediately after the school day but typically meet only two or three days per week and are more targeted toward specific populations (e.g., girls) or activities (e.g., soccer).

Guidelines for PA in After-School Programs

In 2010, the National Institute on Out-of-School Time (NIOST, n.d.) published expert recommendations for PA promotion in after-school programs that consisted of both program- and staff-level recommendations (Beighle et al., 2010). At the program level, recommendations included allocating 50 percent of program time for PA, scheduling PA in 15- to 20-minute increments throughout the program, keeping student-to-staff ratios low (i.e., 15:1 or less), and providing ample space and equipment for PA. At the staff level, experts suggested the use of active supervision, effective instructional and behavioral management strategies, and the provision of both structured- and free-play opportunities in an autonomy-supportive environment (Beighle et al., 2010). One year later, the National AfterSchool Association (2011) adopted standards for healthy eating and physical activity (HEPA) in out-of-school-time programs that aligned closely with NIOST's (Beighle et al., 2010) recommendations.

According to HEPA guidelines (National After-School Association, 2011), after-school programs should devote at least 30 minutes of daily program time to PA, and 50 percent of that time should be spent in moderate-to-vigorous PA (MVPA). Researchers and other professional organizations have suggested that after-school programs should provide up to 30 minutes of MVPA during program time (Beets, 2012b; SHAPE America, 2013). Research shows that policies related to the volume and intensity of PA in after-school programs vary dramatically from state to state (Beets et al., 2010), but it appears that many experts have converged on the 30 minutes of MVPA criterion. If assessed via pedometry, this equates to 4,600 steps (Beets et al., 2012).

Several studies have evaluated the extent to which programs meet after-school PA policy guidelines. A survey of 595 after-school program site directors found that 60 percent were aware of the HEPA guidelines but only 43 percent used them for program planning, indicating a potential gap between policy and practice (Wiecha et al., 2014). Other studies have revealed that very few programs achieve the 30-minute MVPA criterion (Beets, Weaver, et al., 2016; Brazendale, Beets, et al., 2015; Trost et al., 2008). For example, a study of 25 after-school programs in South Carolina and Nebraska found that only 16.5 percent of children met the 4,600 steps per day guideline and, at that rate, children would need to spend 3.4 hours per day in after-school programs to achieve the criterion (Beets et al., 2012). It appears that programs typically provide 8 to 24 minutes of MVPA or 2,600 to 3,200 steps per day, boys tend to be more active than girls, and achievement rates of the 30-minute MVPA target range from 0.3 to 27 percent (Beets, 2012a; Beets, Shah, et al., 2015). In short, children who attend after-school programs accrue a wide range of PA minutes but often fall short of meeting guidelines (Beets, 2012b).

Research on After-School Interventions and Programs

Researchers suggest that the after-school PA environment is influenced by complex ecological systems, ranging from policies at the national, state, and local levels to the unique individual characteristics of the youth enrolled (Beets, Webster, et al., 2013; see figure 8.1). It is suggested

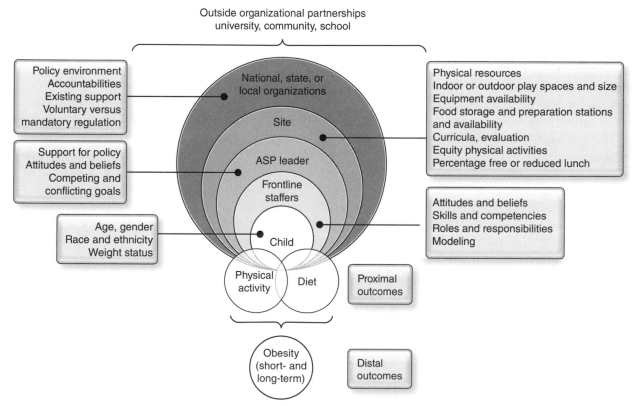

Figure 8.1 Conceptual framework to prevent childhood obesity through policy-level initiatives in after-school programs.

Reprinted by permission from M.W. Beets, C. Webster et al., "Translating Policies Into Practice: A Framework to Prevent Childhood Obesity in Afterschool Programs," *Health Promotion Practice* 14, no. 2 (2013): 228-237.

that "leverage points" (p. 229) exist within each of these levels, which can be identified to improve policies and practices related to HEPA. Experts recommend developing working partnerships with community stakeholders and considering local contextual factors to tailor interventions to community needs (Beets, Webster, et al., 2013).

After-School PA Policies and Practices

At a policy level, evidence suggests that PA implementation is stronger in sites where the director or program leader is aware of and using the HEPA guidelines (Wiecha et al., 2014), but the effects of having a written policy in place are equivocal. A study of 39 after-school programs in South Carolina and Nebraska found positive associations between the presence of a written PA policy and pedometer steps (Ajja et al., 2012). However, a subsequent study of 20 programs in South Carolina found no associations between the presence of written policy and MVPA or sedentary time measured via accelerometry (Ajja et al., 2014). Furthermore, Beets, Huberty, Beighle, Moore, and colleagues (2013) found that a written PA policy was associated with greater sedentary time and lower MVPA when PA was measured via accelerometry in 18 after-school programs. It appears that the presence of a written PA policy may be necessary, but not sufficient, for PA promotion in after-school settings.

Regarding time allotments for PA in after-school programs, evidence suggests that simply allocating more time for PA in the schedule can be an effective strategy for increasing PA accrual (Beets, 2012a; Beets, Huberty, Beighle, Moore, et al., 2013; Beets, Weaver, Turner-McGrievy, Moore, et al., 2016). The highest MVPA observed in one study was for programs that allocated 60 minutes or more for PA time, but no additional benefits were observed for programs that offered more than 75, or even 105, minutes of PA (Brazendale, Beets, et al., 2015). As a result, 60 minutes of scheduled PA time is often recommended. A study of 20 after-school programs found that an average of 66 minutes of PA was offered but the range of scheduled PA opportunities was broad (15 to 150 minutes), so many programs still need to address the time allocation issue (Weaver, Beets, Huberty, et al., 2015).

Staff behaviors have also been found to be important in encouraging PA in after-school programs. Huberty and colleagues (2013) found that, when staff engaged in PA with children and verbally promoted PA and PA was organized with equipment available, MVPA was higher. The presence of three or more of these characteristics led to a 25 to 30 percent increase in MVPA (Huberty et al., 2013). Weaver and colleagues (2014) also found that when staff played with children and provided choices of activities, PA participation was higher. Unfortunately, evidence indicates that program staff members do not consistently apply PA promotional strategies without appropriate training (Weaver, Beets, Huberty, et al., 2015).

Interventions to Improve the PA Environment in After-School Programs

Experts have adopted a collaborative, community-based environmental change approach to improving the PA climate in after-school programs, which includes policy review, professional development and training for staff, technical assistance, booster sessions, and ongoing evaluation support (Beets, Weaver, Turner-McGrievy, et al., 2014; Cradock et al., 2016; Gortmaker et al., 2012; Hughey et al., 2014; Weaver, Beets, et al., 2016). Three existing frameworks build on this approach and are available to help guide program improvement efforts. The LET US Play principles provide a guiding framework for positive staff behaviors in relation to PA promotion (Brazendale, Chandler, et al., 2015; Weaver et al., 2013; see table 8.1). They provide simple and easy-to-remember guidelines for how activities can be structured to maximize PA opportunities in after-school programs. Another approach, the 5 *M*s, describes how a clearly defined organizational *mission* around PA promotion, a *motivating* environment, properly *managed* activities, and closely *monitored* PA behaviors can *maximize* the amount of PA youth acquire in after-school programs (Weaver et al., 2012). Lastly, the STEPs framework, based on Maslow's hierarchy of needs, details a continuum of strategies that programs can use to integrate more PA opportunities for children. Early steps in the continuum focus on getting a consistent schedule in place that includes at least 60 minutes of allocated PA time. Later steps emphasize quality PA opportunities that include a variety of structured and unstructured activity options, activities that are appealing to both genders, and games that conform to the LET US Play principles (Beets, Weaver, Moore, et al., 2014).

These frameworks and principles have guided many of the interventions that have been conducted to increase PA in after-school programs. Researchers with the University of South Carolina, Arnold School of Public Health's Policy to Practice in Youth Programs initiative have conducted a number of interventions and randomized controlled trials that have investigated the effects of staff development efforts. Findings indicate that staff behaviors can be improved with intensive and sustained training (i.e., workshops, booster sessions, or ongoing technical assistance; Hughey et al., 2014; Weaver et al., 2014; Weaver, Beets, et al., 2016) and that greater staff implementation of PA promotion strategies is associated with greater PA participation among children (Beets, Huberty, & Beighle, 2013; Brazendale, Chandler, et al., 2015; Hughey et al., 2014; Weaver, Beets, Hutto, et al., 2015; Weaver, Moore, Huberty, et al., 2016; Weaver, Moore, Turner-McGrievy, et al., 2016). Results of a randomized controlled trial of 20 after-school programs (Beets, Weaver, Turner-McGrievy, et al., 2014) indicated that children enrolled in programs with staff receiving STEPs training were 2.4 times more likely to meet the 30 minutes per day MVPA guideline (Beets, Weaver, et al., 2015). The percentage of boys meeting the guideline during the first year of the study increased from 36 to 47 percent, and the percentage of girls meeting the guideline in year two went from 13 to 19 percent (Beets, Weaver, Turner-McGrievy, Huberty, et al., 2016). Other studies conducted within this initiative have reported similar findings (Beets, Weaver, Moore, et al., 2014).

Comparable efforts to improve the PA environment in after-school programs have been conducted by researchers with the Harvard School of Public Health's Out of School Nutrition and Physical Activity (OSNAP) initiative. Initial results suggested that an environmental change approach to professional development, including educational activities and parental engagement, led to more MVPA for children (Gortmaker et al., 2012). More recent findings suggested that policy changes related to PA are difficult to achieve (Kenney et al., 2014) and that collaborative workshops and ongoing technical assistance may have a limited effect on PA participation (Cradock et al., 2016).

After-School Programs and Clubs

In addition to interventions targeting the broader PA environment, a number of structured programs and clubs have also been developed to promote PA in after-school settings. For example, CATCH (Coordinated Approach to Child Health) Kids Club was developed as an after-school program for children in grades K-8 and is commonly delivered in conjunction with existing after-school programs. Early research suggested that children in CATCH Kids Club accumulated more MVPA than controls (Kelder et al., 2005), but follow-up studies revealed more mixed results (Dzewaltowski et al., 2010; Slusser et al., 2013). The most extensive evaluation of CATCH Kids Club, conducted in 330 after-school programs in Canada, indicated no PA differences between intervention and control sites at baseline or two-year follow-up, but all programs had high levels of MVPA at both time points (Sharpe et al., 2011).

The Sports, Play, and Active Recreation for Kids (SPARK) After School curriculum, also delivered through existing after-school programs, includes cooperative, fitness, sport, and skill-based activities

TABLE 8.1   LET US Play Principles

L	Shorten or eliminate *lines* so children are not waiting for their turn.
E	Eliminate *elimination* games.
T	Reduce *team* sizes and use small-sided games instead.
U	Reduce the number of *uninvolved* children and adults.
S	Modify games for maximal PA involvement by adjusting *space,* equipment, and rules.

Data from Brazendale et al. (2015); Weaver et al. (2013).

along with staff training. It is an extension of the SPARK Physical Education (PE) curriculum, and although extensive research has been conducted on SPARK PE, only two studies have examined the effects of SPARK After School. Herrick et al. (2012) compared three intervention and three control sites and found no differences in MVPA after five months of intervention. In contrast, Iversen et al. (2011) examined SPARK After School combined with a nutrition education program (Fun 5) and found improved self-reported PA and nutritional behaviors.

Similar to CATCH Kids Club and SPARK, Youth Fit for Life is an after-school PA program that is often delivered through YMCA programs and is based on social cognitive theory. It consists of sessions focused on fitness activities, nutrition education, and self-management skills and includes a staff training component. A study conducted in 14 sites with primarily African American children found improvements in body composition, muscular strength, and muscular endurance with implementation of Youth Fit for Life (Annesi et al., 2005). Follow-up studies demonstrated similar results along with increased voluntary PA participation outside of the program mediated by social cognitive theory constructs (Annesi et al., 2007, 2009, 2017).

Beyond PA programs that are integrated with existing after-school programs, there are also PA clubs that typically meet fewer than five days per week and are targeted toward specific populations, such as sedentary girls. The Bristol Girls Dance Project is an after-school PA club designed for middle school girls that includes two dance classes per week. Initial results found that girls in the dance group accumulated 5 to 12 minutes more MVPA compared to controls but showed no differences when compared to girls who attended a one-day dance workshop (Jago et al., 2012). A follow-up randomized controlled trial (Jago et al., 2013) revealed no differences in MVPA between intervention and control groups (Jago et al., 2015). It appeared that program attendance was a challenge and many girls preferred a drop-in style program instead of two day per week sessions (Edwards et al., 2016; Sebire et al., 2016).

A similar PA club, Girls on the Move, was designed for sedentary, urban, middle school girls and included PA sessions combined with motivational counseling by school nurses. Robbins et al. (2012) found no significant differences in MVPA between intervention and control groups; however, a five-year longitudinal follow-up study has commenced that also includes interactive iPad sessions with virtual female PA role models (Robbins et al., 2013). Preliminary results reveal that girls accumulated 22 minutes of MVPA during daily sessions and experienced high levels of participant satisfaction, but similar to the Bristol Girls Dance Project, attendance has been a challenge (Robbins et al., 2016).

Two other programs, GoGirlGo! (GGG) and Girls on the Run (GOTR), were also designed for sedentary girls and contain a life-skills educational component. In a study of GGG implementation in nine after-school programs, Huberty and colleagues (2014) found that girls accumulated three additional minutes of MVPA on GGG days compared to non-GGG days and experienced improvements in PA self-efficacy and enjoyment with program participation. Studies of GOTR suggested that self-reported PA increases with program participation and girls who have completed the program report greater PA participation later in life (DeBate et al., 2009; Galeotti, 2015).

Because of the wide range of after-school PA opportunities, systematic reviews and meta-analyses have been conducted to determine the broader effect of after-school programming on PA-related outcomes. For example, Beets and colleagues (2009) conducted a meta-analysis of 13 articles describing 11 after-school PA programs and found positive effect sizes for PA, fitness, and body composition with intervention. However, other systematic reviews have documented mixed findings with only half of studies reporting positive effects on PA in one review (Pate & O'Neill, 2009) and only three of nine studies reporting positive effects for PA in another review (Atkin et al., 2011). A meta-analysis conducted by Mears and Jago (2016) reported an additional 4.8 minutes of MVPA per day at follow-up and concluded that after-school interventions have varied effectiveness in terms of the extent to which MVPA increases. Likewise, a recent "review of reviews" suggested considerable differences in conclusions drawn, with overall modest effects of after-school programs on PA levels of youth (Demetriou et al., 2017). Many barriers, including transportation issues; lack of support from school administration; and students trying to balance other obligations, including academics, make participation in after-school PA programs challenging, especially in urban, high-poverty settings (Garn et al., 2014; Goudeau et al., 2014; Maljak et al., 2014). Researchers suggested that youth are more likely to participate in PA programs when activities are culturally relevant, there are desirable social opportunities embedded within the program, and the leaders are caring and enthusiastic (Garn et al., 2014; Whalen et al., 2016).

Before-School Programs

Before-school PA programs consist of opportunities for children to be active prior to the start of the school day (e.g., before 8:00 a.m.). One of the most unique and appealing features of before-school programs is that they have the potential to prepare children's brains for learning. In *SPARK: The Revolutionary New Science of Exercise and the Brain*, Ratey (2008) outlined how exercise stimulates brain cells and facilitates the development of neural connections. The author asserted that PA opportunities scheduled right before challenging academic content may contribute to improved student learning. The Zero Hour PE program in Naperville, Illinois, is highlighted as an example of how programs could be implemented, with anecdotal evidence of positive effects on academic outcomes (Ratey, 2008). Unfortunately, minimal empirical research has been conducted on the topic to date.

Research has focused primarily on two types of before-school PA opportunities: one type consisting of a formal curriculum with a structured schedule (e.g., Build Our Kids' Success [BOKS]) and one consisting of less structured opportunities for walking and running before school (e.g., mileage clubs). The current body of evidence related to the effectiveness of these programs is still in its infancy, so a variety of sources are drawn upon to gather early insights.

BOKS

BOKS is a before-school PA program designed for elementary school children that typically meets two or three days per week before the start of the school day. Structured sessions include a warm-up, an aerobic activity, a skill of the week, game time, and a cool-down with a nutrition message. Preliminary findings reveal improvements in aerobic endurance and body composition when comparing BOKS children to controls (Westcott et al., 2015). Additional evaluations conducted by the NIOST (n.d.) suggest that children in BOKS obtain approximately 1,800 steps and 17 minutes of MVPA during sessions, with promising outcomes related to working memory, executive function, attitudes, and HEPA behaviors. Conference proceedings likewise suggest that children accumulate 2,100 steps and 20 minutes of PA during BOKS sessions (Babkes Stellino & Dauenhauer, 2015), with promising effects on classroom behavior (Babkes Stellino et al., 2017). A clinical trial currently under way is examining the effects of BOKS in relation to fitness, psychosocial outcomes, and academic achievement (Pojednic et al., 2016), so stronger evidence of program effectiveness is expected to be forthcoming.

Mileage Clubs

Mileage clubs consist of walking and running programs that occur before school hours in which children walk or run laps around school campuses and log mileage using scanners or tally marks. Commercial programs, such as the 100 Mile Club, are available, but many schools develop their own programs (see before-school case example at the end of this chapter). Existing research indicates that 15- to 20-minute mileage club sessions result in 8.5 to 10 minutes of MVPA and 50 to 57 percent of time spent in MVPA, with boys accumulating more PA than girls (Stylianou, van der Mars, et al., 2016). Related studies suggest that on-task behavior is consistently higher in the first 45 minutes of the school day on days when children attend mileage club versus days when they do not (Stylianou, Kulinna, et al., 2016). One study conducted within an American Indian community found that elementary school children accumulated 0.6 to 1.0 mile per day through participation in a mileage club and teachers had positive perceptions of the program (Stylianou et al., 2014).

Out-of-School-Time Programs

A few programs exist and are delivered both before and after school that serve as opportunities to promote PA for youth. These programs include interscholastic and intramural sports as well as various forms of active transportation. Brief descriptions of these programs and interventions and relevant extant research on the effect of these programs are noted in the sections that follow.

Interscholastic and Intramural Sports

Interscholastic sports, also called varsity sports at the high school level, are competitive sport programs targeted toward skilled athletes. Because of Title IX (1972), an equitable number of interscholastic sport programs must be offered to boys and girls in public schools in the United States. Practices are typically held before or after school, and games take place after school and on weekends. Similar to interscholastic sports, intramural sports provide a competitive sport experience for youth before or after school but, in contrast, tend to remain open to all skill levels. They include a variety of sport offerings and usually consist of some form of league play followed by a culminating tournament experience.

According to the National Federation of State High School Associations (NFSHSA, 2016), over 7.8 million youth participated in interscholastic high school sports during the 2015-2016 school year. The sports with the highest participation rates for boys were football, track and field, and basketball and for girls, track and field, volleyball, and basketball (NFSHSA, 2016). At the middle school level, studies suggest that 83 percent of schools offer interscholastic sports and 69 percent offer intramural sports (Young et al., 2007). Participation rates tend to be lower for intramural sports (19 percent) than interscholastic sports (38 percent), and rates decline as children transition from middle school to high school for intramurals but not for interscholastic sports, likely caused by reduced offerings (Johnston et al., 2007).

Sport participation is associated with numerous health benefits. Pate and colleagues (2000) found that high school boys and girls participating in sport programs were more likely to eat fruits and vegetables and engage in regular vigorous PA compared to their nonsport counterparts. Participants also reported less frequent smoking behavior and reduced use of drugs, such as marijuana and cocaine (Pate et al., 2000). Perkins and colleagues (2004) found that participation in sport as a child

or adolescent significantly predicted participation in sport and fitness activities in young adulthood, with high participation rates in adolescents being associated with an eight times greater likelihood of being involved in sport as a young adult (Perkins et al., 2004). Similarly, Dohle and Wansink (2013) found that out of 18 demographic, behavior, and personality characteristics examined, participation in high school varsity sports was the strongest predictor or PA involvement after the age of 70. Studies have also documented positive effects of school sport participation on academic achievement (Trudeau & Shephard, 2008) and myriads of other psychological and social outcomes, such as self-esteem and depression (Eime et al., 2013). Regarding school offerings, a study of 154 Canadian schools found positive associations between the number of varsity sports offered in a school and self-reported PA participation among students (Nichol et al., 2009).

Notwithstanding the benefits of interscholastic sports, some experts have argued that intramural sports are an underutilized PA opportunity and may be an effective supplement to varsity sports (Bocarro et al., 2008; Edwards et al., 2014; Kanters et al., 2008). Studies comparing intramural and interscholastic sports have found that overall participation rates are higher in intramural-only schools compared to interscholastic-only schools (Edwards et al., 2011; Kanters et al., 2013). Evidence also suggests that PA accumulation is greater in intramural programs (Bocarro et al., 2012, 2014) and may lead to a more positive effect on long-term sport participation intentions (Kanters et al., 2008, 2012). Intramurals appear to play a particularly important role in promoting PA among children from lower-income families and racial minority groups (Johnston et al., 2007; Kanters et al., 2013). One simulation study suggested that adding intramural sport programs alongside interscholastic sports in North Carolina middle schools could add 43,000 sport participants per year and increase the number of disadvantaged participants by 37 percent (Edwards et al., 2014).

Active Transportation to and From School

Active transportation is defined as the use of human energy as a means of travel, such as walking or biking to or from school, in contrast to passive means, such as riding in a car or school bus. Active transportation is a key opportunity for before- and after-school PA because it requires minimal resources and can cut down on the costs of travel, reduce congestion around schools, and contribute to better air quality. However, since the 1960s, rates of active transportation in the United States have declined substantially. In 1969, 41 percent of children aged 5 to 18 relied on active transportation to get to or from school, but by 2001, that figure had dropped to just 13 percent (McDonald, 2007). Similar results from the Trial of Activity for Adolescent Girls (TAAG) indicated that only 20 percent of middle school students walked or biked to school (Young et al., 2007), and recent data from the 2014 School Health Policies and Practices Study suggests that 10 percent or less of children walk or bike to school in a majority of U.S. schools (61.5 percent; Jones & Sliwa, 2016).

Active transportation can have robust protective health effects in adults, with Hamer and Chida (2008) estimating through their meta-analysis an overall cardiovascular risk reduction of 11 percent. Systematic reviews have also revealed positive associations between active commuting and overall PA levels in children and adolescents (Davison et al., 2008; Faulkner et al., 2009; Larouche et al., 2014; Lee et al., 2008), with evidence that children can accumulate approximately 20 minutes of MVPA through active transportation each day (Bassett et al., 2013; Davison et al., 2008; Faulkner et al., 2009). Biking to school, in particular, seems to have an added cardiovascular benefit for children (Larouche et al., 2014; Lee et al., 2008).

The strongest predictor of active transportation is distance between home and school (Davison et al., 2008; Pont et al., 2009; Wong et al., 2011). One Australian study suggested that children living within half a mile of school were five times more likely to actively commute than those who lived farther away (Timperio et al., 2006). Two large systematic reviews, one including 38 studies primarily in the United States and Australia (Pont et al., 2009) and one including 65 studies in North America, Europe, and Australia (D'Haese et al., 2015) suggested additional correlates of active transportation, including walkability (e.g., the presence of walking and biking paths), residential density (e.g., land use primarily for homes), and

general traffic safety (e.g., lower speed limits). The influence of these factors appears to be mediated by parental attitudes toward active transportation (Yu & Zhu, 2016). Overall, empirical findings suggest that ethnic minorities, boys, families with lower incomes, and families with fewer vehicles are most likely to actively transport to or from school (Davison et al., 2008; Pont et al., 2009).

Two active transportation programs for youth, Safe Routes to School (SRTS) and the Walking School Bus (WSB), have been implemented and empirically evaluated. SRTS is a program that "works to make it safe, convenient, and fun for children to walk and bicycle to and from schools" (SRTS National Partnership, n.d.b). It has served more than 17,400 schools and 6.8 million students since 2005 (National Center for Safe Routes to School, 2015). The program is founded upon six principles, referred to as the Six Es, which detail how school communities can systematically design and implement effective walk and bike to school programs (SRTS National Partnership, n.d.a). Available research indicates that SRTS can improve safety when students walk or bike to school (Chaufan et al., 2012; DiMaggio & Li, 2013) and can effectively increase the number of children actively transporting to or from school (McDonald, 2015; McDonald et al., 2013, 2014; Stewart et al., 2014).

In a parallel manner, WSB is designed for a group of children to walk to or from school with one or more adults. Because safety is a major concern of parents and a predictor of active transportation behavior (D'Haese et al., 2015; Pont et al., 2009), WSB allows children to be supervised as they actively commute. WSB interventions have been shown to effectively increase the number of children actively commuting to or from school (Heelan et al., 2009; Mendoza et al., 2009, 2011), and studies have found that children participating in WSB can obtain 2 to 18 minutes more MVPA compared to controls (Heelan et al., 2009; Mendoza et al., 2011). A systematic review of 14 studies including both SRTS and WSB programs suggested that almost all interventions resulted in increased active transportation, but there was a wide range of increases (3 to 64 percent) and most studies had small effect sizes (Chillón et al., 2011).

Knowledge Claims

Based on the research synthesized in the preceding sections, the following knowledge claims have been generated:

- Before- and after-school programs have the potential to make substantial contributions to youth PA accrual because of current participation rates and existing systems and infrastructure.
- Before-school programs, after-school programs, and active transportation each can contribute 20 minutes of MVPA to a child's day.
- Youth do not consistently meet the recommended 30 minutes of MVPA during after-school programs.
- Similar to broader societal trends, boys tend to be more active than girls in before- and after-school programs and are more likely to engage in active transportation.
- After-school PA program interventions, especially those targeting girls, have only modest effects on MVPA.
- Policy changes alone are not sufficient to positively affect after-school PA.
- Allocating sufficient time for PA and training staff in effective PA promotion strategies helps increase PA accrual in after-school programs.
- Intramural sports are a promising source of PA for adolescents, especially historically underserved populations, but tend to be broadly underutilized.
- Active transportation is positively associated with higher amounts of PA in children.
- Active transportation interventions, such as SRTS and WSB, have been shown to effectively increase walk and bike to school participation rates.

Knowledge Gaps and Directions for Future Research

Gaps in our current knowledge base exist, warranting further research to address the following questions about before- and after-school PA programs:

- Why are girls less active than boys in before- and after-school settings, and how can this disparity be addressed?
- How and why do before- and after-school PA preferences change as youth transition from childhood to adolescence?
- How can schools effectively overcome common barriers to before- and after-school PA programming, particularly in urban, high-poverty communities?
- How does MVPA accumulation vary by type of interscholastic or intramural sport?
- What are the barriers (e.g., facility availability and staff supervision) to offering intramural sports in conjunction with interscholastic sports at the secondary level?
- What is the effect of before-school PA on classroom behaviors and academic performance, and how long do any potential effects last?
- What strategies can be used to encourage additional participation in active transportation to or from school?
- What are the long-term health and behavioral effects of participation in before- and after-school PA programming?

The answers to these questions will help drive improved practice and allow before- and after-school programs to meet the PA needs of youth.

Evidence-Based Recommendations and Applications

Based on the available scientific evidence, we feel confident in proposing the following recommendations for best practice in before- and after-school PA programming. The recommendations are organized into school staff and community partners. In the context of before- and after-school PA programs, school staff includes any staff members delivering programming to youth, whether they are employees of the school or not. Community partners include organizations that work with schools to deliver before- and after-school programming and the leadership of those organizations specifically.

For School Staff

Staff who are delivering before- or after-school PA programming should ensure that a variety of structured and unstructured activities are offered that appeal to both boys and girls. Often, girls are less active than boys, both within and beyond the school context, so explicit attention needs to be focused on providing attractive PA options for girls. One way to understand the interests of girls (as opposed to assuming that girls are interested only in dancing and jumping rope) is to conduct a simple survey. A survey can identify activities of interest based on the unique desires of girls in the school community and can facilitate buy-in for subsequent activities. Staff members facilitating PA programs should also consider ways in which sports and activities can be organized so that boys do not dominate the games and make girls feel unwelcome or uncomfortable. One strategy is to offer multiple fields or courts of play so that some are competitive and others are recreational. That way, all children can self-select the level of play that is appropriate for them and feel comfortable engaging in PA.

Staff members facilitating before- and after-school PA programming should be enthusiastic PA participants with youth and consistently encourage children to be active. An engaged adult can motivate children to move by increasing the fun factor of activities and serve as a role model for healthy PA. Staff members should also ensure that developmentally appropriate equipment is available and structured games and activities align with the LET US Play principles (see table 8.1). Simple modifications to the design of games can maximize child engagement and, thus, PA accrual over time.

When considering PA clubs, it is important to solicit child-level input so that offerings can be matched to PA interests and any potential barriers to participation can be identified ahead of time. Surveys allow children to share their opinions and, as mentioned previously, help secure buy-in for subsequent PA offerings. Surveys should include basic demographic characteristics, such as grade level and sex, so that a variety of PA club opportunities can be considered for different segments of the school population. Once the data has been collected and analyzed, child interests can be matched with staff leadership interests to determine which clubs to offer. Children should also be asked about any anticipated barriers to participation, such as timing, conflicts with other extracurricular activities, or transportation concerns. By soliciting child-level input in the development of PA clubs, documented challenges with implementation can be addressed in a proactive manner.

Intramural sports should be offered as a supplement to interscholastic sports at the secondary level and an option for before- or after-school PA at the elementary school level. Not all children and adolescents are interested in highly competitive athletics, but many may be open to more recreational involvement in school sports. Staff should work with other members of the school community, including coaches and administrators, to divide space and time equitably among sporting options and consider other time segments during the school day (e.g., off periods or lunch) to provide intramural sport opportunities.

Lastly, school staff should encourage and promote active transportation to or from school through educational efforts, communication with parents, and environmental modifications. Teachers can integrate walking and biking safety into classroom lessons so that children are prepared to engage in active transportation in a safe manner and they can teach children about the benefits of walking and biking to or from school. Administrators can share information with parents about safe routes to school and encourage them to participate in special events and other structured walking and biking programs. This can keep parents informed and possibly alleviate some of the concerns parents have about safety. Finally, school staff should ensure that the school environment is conducive to active transportation by installing bike racks, keeping walking and biking paths free from debris, and providing crossing guards at busy intersections. These strategies remove simple obstacles to active transportation and can also alleviate parental safety concerns.

For Community Partners

Community partners, including after-school care providers, recreational organizations, and volunteer supporters, should be aware of HEPA standards and ensure that policies and practices within their programs are aligned with national guidelines. For example, after-school programs should try to allocate at least 50 percent of program time (ideally, 60 minutes) to PA, keep staff-to-child ratios low, and ensure ample space and equipment are dedicated to PA. Organizational leaders should also be aware of contextual factors that may influence PA participation in school environments and provide staff with ongoing training in effective PA promotion strategies. An educated and informed staff is much more likely to facilitate positive and enjoyable PA for youth.

For the last recommendation, community partners should support active transportation initiatives by ensuring that neighborhoods surrounding schools are conducive to walking and biking behaviors. This could include designating safe paths in multiple directions around a school campus, posting lower speed limits for traffic in the neighborhood, and providing crossing guards at locations farther away from the school campus. Interested community partners can also coordinate and facilitate more structured walking and biking programs for youth, thus further reducing safety concerns for parents.

SUMMARY

This chapter summarizes the research that has been conducted on before- and after-school PA programs and provides key recommendations for practice. The volume of research that has been conducted on after-school programs far outweighs the research that has been conducted on before-school and other out-of-school-time programs, but results tend to support similar outcomes. Both before- and after-school PA opportunities, including intramurals, interscholastic sports, mileage clubs, and active transportation, can provide meaningful amounts of PA accumulation for children and adolescents and should be considered as integral components of CSPAPs. There are challenges associated with maximizing PA engagement among certain segments of the population, especially females and lower-income urban youth, so more research is necessary to identify barriers and overcome these challenges. In addition to examining the research, this chapter also provides practical considerations through case examples for those individuals interested in leading or supporting before- and after-school PA programs. These strategies can supplement the evidence-based recommendations and hopefully assist in the delivery of high-quality, successful before- and after-school PA programs.

QUESTIONS TO CONSIDER

1. How can before- and after-school programs be structured to maximize PA participation?
2. What specific strategies can program staff members use to encourage PA engagement?
3. How can before- and after-school PA programs be tailored to the unique needs and interests of children in the school community?
4. How do interscholastic and intramural sports differ from one another, and what are the distinct benefits of each?
5. What resources are available to encourage active transportation to or from school?

CASE EXAMPLES

Empirical research can provide valuable evidence to guide program planning efforts and professional practice, but often, published studies leave out some of the practical lessons learned regarding implementation. The following case studies, written by individuals who have substantial experience with before- and after-school programming, are provided to supplement the research summarized in this chapter with practical strategies for implementation.

After-School Program

Chuck Steinfurth, After School Experience Executive
YMCA of Florida's First Coast
Former Statewide HEPA Coordinator
South Carolina Alliance of YMCAs

I have had the opportunity to work closely with over 100 after-school programs across South Carolina that are operated by YMCAs. These programs range from serving fewer than 20 children to over 200 children. Some programs are based in schools, and others are in a YMCA facility or community building. Some of the programs have very limited indoor and outdoor space, whereas others have ample room for activities to occur. Even given all of these variables, there are some common trends I have observed at programs that excel at providing children with high levels of quality PA.

The first best practice I have seen in programs that promote PA is having a detailed weekly activity schedule. Detailed activity schedules that I have seen prove to be effective for keeping everyone on task. They include specific times, locations, and supplies needed for each activity during the day. When staff is given a clear outline of the afternoon, it leaves less open for interpretation. For example, rather than say "4:15-5:00 is games," a detailed schedule says "4:15-5:00 is tag game: Cranes and Crows (and a printed description of the activity would also accompany the schedule). When the schedule is not specific and uses just broad activity names, such as "games," staff members are not always prepared to lead a game, and it becomes less structured. From what I have observed, there is a higher chance all children will engage in PA when staff members are ready to lead games based on a schedule.

Another practice I have seen in after-school programs that do an above-average job promoting PA is understanding that PA time does not have to be only one designated time on your daily schedule. In other words, most programs have about three hours each afternoon. If you allot only one 30- or 45-minute part of your day for PA, it will be harder to reach any activity goals. Programs that exceed goals recognize the importance of utilizing the full three hours, with smaller opportunities to accumulate more PA. An after-school program at a YMCA in Columbia, South Carolina, provides children with 15 to 20 minutes each day with different game opportunities as they are arriving to the program. Before they are asked to sit for homework and snack, children are able to play structured or unstructured games. In addition, PA is also prevalent during transitions. While most programs keep children seated during homework and snack, this program gets the students up and moving for staff-led exercises, which may last only 5 or 10 minutes, but it breaks up periods of being sedentary. By the time the group is ready for an organized activity later in the afternoon, they have already received potentially up to 30 minutes of additional PA.

When it becomes time for organized, staff-led games, another common characteristic of programs that excel at PA is being intentional with leading games that encourage all children to participate. When staff members are aware of games that include a lot of standing around or games with elimination, they can make conscious choices to modify those games to ensure all children have the chance to play. Programs that tend to play traditional games, such as kickball or dodge ball, end up losing the interest of the children more quickly because they either get bored or "out." When staff members make changes to include everyone in the games, the children stay engaged and, as a result, receive higher levels of PA. I have also seen that, when staff members are willing to play games with the children, the children are more responsive and willing to play themselves. The opposite of this would be a staff member just rolling out equipment and letting the children lead their own games. When I see programs doing the latter, I often see greater levels of inactive children.

The single most important factor I have seen in programs that are successful in meeting PA goals is having a committed site leader. When the staff member who oversees the program understands the importance of getting the children moving and works with his or her staff team members to give them tools to better implement these ideas, the quality of the program improves greatly. The common characteristics I have observed in programs that promote PA all exist regardless of program size, space, or budget. When staff members are committed to making a detailed schedule each week that includes activities for all participants, the outcome will always be healthier children.

Before-School Program

Megan Babkes Stellino, EdD
University of Northern Colorado

Over the past five years, I have endeavored to integrate my work as a professor at the University of Northern Colorado with researching social psychological predictors of PA and sport, taking an interest in community- and school-based PA programming, and engaging as a mom to cultivate and maintain ample opportunities for my two elementary school–age boys and their peers to be physically active. To satisfy this venture, I took the initiative to develop and implement Tiger Miles Club, a before-school mileage club program, at Rolling Hills Elementary School in Aurora, Colorado, in the interest of providing an opportunity for elementary school students to be physically active prior to starting the school day. This program started as a grassroots effort that I organized and led with the support of other parent volunteers. Tiger Miles Club took place for 22 weeks of the school year, two days per week for 45 minutes each morning before school for the past three years. Involvement in Tiger Miles Club was available for free to all students (over 600), teachers and staff, and family members in the elementary school community. There are numerous essential components for before school–based PA programs of any kind to thrive. The following are a few of the best practices and recommendations from my experiences running Tiger Miles Club that I believe are requisite considerations for before-school programs to successfully promote PA for youth.

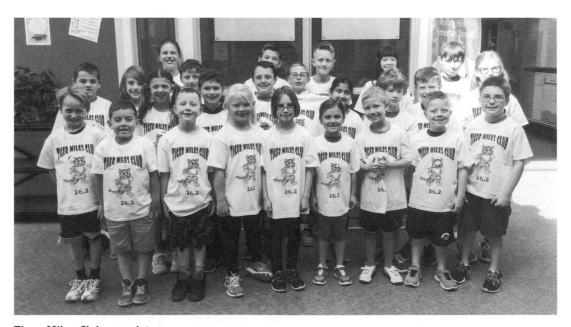

Tiger Miles Club completers.

Before-School PA Programs Should Be Approached as Works in Progress

While there are turn-key programs with evidence-based curriculums (e.g., BOKS), no one-size-fits-all program model works for all schools or communities without site-specific modifications. A program's sustainability is dependent on the extent to which it is tailored to fit the particular school, demographics of the students, and culture of the community in which it is being implemented. Use of a constantly evolving and adaptable process to implementing, evaluating, obtaining constituent feedback, reimplementing, reevaluating, and continuing to modify the way in which a program is designed and implemented is recommended to remain centered on the goal of promoting youth PA.

Quality-Invested Leadership Is Imperative as a Best Practice for Before-School PA Programming

It is not necessarily most relevant who provides the leadership; it could easily be the physical education teacher, a member of a school wellness team, or even a dedicated parent or community member. As a self-designated leader of Tiger Miles Club, my dedication was unmatched regarding ensuring that the program was offered in a manner to promote as much PA to as many children as possible in a safe, developmentally appropriate, and productive manner. My leadership in disseminating information about the importance of youth PA and the value of before-school PA in particular was highly regarded in the school community and further contributed to the reliable involvement of other parent volunteers. This best practice and recommendation is simply that persistent, dedicated leadership that can harness further school, family, and community volunteer engagement and the promotion of youth PA opportunities in the form of before-school PA programming is essential.

Fostering Both the Collective Group and Individual Participant Motives for Initial and Sustained Engagement in Before-School PA Programming

The reasons that youth participate in before-school PA programming are extremely varied. To induce actual and substantially meaningful PA among youth, a program needs to include elements that appeal to the various motives. Some youth are motivated by rewards, some by enjoyment of movement, some by social connections, and some by a combination of all these or different motives all together. My knowledge of motivational factors afforded appreciation and support for youth completing numerous laps or miles and ultimately getting a lot of PA because they love being outside and moving their bodies, because they had an opportunity to race their friends, and because of the mileage-based rewards available as well as a multitude of other reasons all simultaneously part of the same program.

Exceptional Organization Is an Essential Best Practice for Successful Before-School PA Programming

The why, when, where, what, and how of a program must be proactively created and tailored to the specific school and youth parameters of those who will be served by the program. This information must be conveyed unambiguously within the school community so that the focus can be on unimpeded promotion of youth PA. For example, with each new year of Tiger Miles Club, decisions had to be made about which specific days the program would run, whether the grass field or around the school perimeter sidewalk would be used, what the incentive program associated with mileage would be, and numerous other parameters. Consideration of school and student constraints, such as school start time and beginning mileage club with adequate opportunity for sufficient PA, accommodating students receiving breakfast at school, and meeting the needs of students with disabilities as well as facilities and space available and aspirations for number of youth intending to serve are all extremely relevant factors that must be accounted for and organized in an effective program.

These recommendations certainly do not represent an exhaustive list of best practices for effective before-school youth PA programming; however, the descriptions and examples are given to inspire and guide continued efforts to provide successful opportunities for youth school-based PA.

CHAPTER 9

Staff Involvement

Collin A. Webster, PhD
University of South Carolina

R. Glenn Weaver, PhD
University of South Carolina

Martha Carman
Ashburn Elementary School

Lee Marcheschi
Ashburn Elementary School

Athanasios (Tom) Loulousis
Edison Park School

Spyridoula Vazou, PhD
Iowa State University

Tan Leng Goh, PhD
Central Connecticut State University

Russell L. Carson, PhD
University of Northern Colorado

A CSPAP is conceptualized as a coordinated effort involving all school professionals and others who lead youth in settings where PA can be promoted. The staff involvement component of a CSPAP focuses on two variables deemed important to successful program implementation and long-term maintenance: staff wellness and staff promotion of youth PA. This chapter reviews research on these variables; highlights knowledge claims based on this research; identifies knowledge gaps and proposes recommendations for future research on staff involvement; suggests practical implications from the existing research for staff, staff supervisors, staff educators, and policy makers; and provides two case examples of successful staff involvement initiatives. Given the central emphasis of the school environment within a CSPAP, the chapter focuses on school staff but also provides some perspective related to staff in out-of-school-time contexts.

Review of Research

While the CSPAP model places staff wellness and staff PA promotion within the same component, most research has addressed these areas of focus separately. Therefore, this section of the chapter is divided into two parts: research on staff wellness and research on staff promotion of PA.

Research on Staff Wellness

A teacher's work is often stressful, and burnout is a ubiquitous problem in the teaching profession (DeFrank & Stroup, 1989). Burnout is an indicator of ill health and is defined in terms of emotional exhaustion, depersonalization, and reduced personal accomplishment (Maslach & Jackson, 1986). In teaching, higher levels of emotional exhaustion were found for women and elementary teachers compared to men and secondary teachers, and higher levels of emotional exhaustion and depersonalization were found for teachers who work in schools located in socioeconomically underprivileged neighborhoods (Vercambre et al., 2009). Moreover, high job demands, such as physical exertion (e.g., high physical effort, having to stand for long periods of time), are associated with teacher burnout (Griva & Joekes, 2003; Kittel & Leynen, 2003; Rasku & Kinnunen, 2003).

Curry and O'Brien (2012) proposed that teachers who demonstrate wellness are better able to manage job-related stress and are also more likely to promote wellness with their students. Approaches to defining wellness can be categorized generally into either a deficit-based or an asset-based perspective. A deficit-based perspective views wellness as a lack of illness, whereas an asset-based perspective views wellness as the attainment and maintenance of health (Lau et al., 2008). The difference between these perspectives is that the first emphasizes pathologies and their treatment, whereas the second emphasizes illness prevention and sustained well-being through health promotion. Contemporary definitions tend to align with the latter, the asset-based perspective. For instance, Corbin et al. (2016) defined wellness as "the positive component of optimal health" (p. 16). Furthermore, most experts agree that wellness is multidimensional and achieved via a developmental and self-determined process (Lau et al., 2008).

The National Wellness Institute emphasizes that attaining wellness requires "an active process of becoming aware of and making choices toward a more successful existence," and it identifies six dimensions of wellness: emotional, occupational, intellectual, physical, spiritual, and social (see www.nationalwellness.org for more information). The way teachers conceptualize their own wellness emphasizes its multidimensionality and highlights the importance of understanding wellness as holistic (e.g., more than just physical fitness), autonomously driven, and socially supported (Lauzon, 1992).

According to the most recent evidence, the prevalence of comprehensive school employee wellness programs in the United States is low (Eaton et al., 2007), and many school districts do not provide faculty and staff with recommended wellness program funding or services. For example, the percentage of districts that provide faculty and staff with funding or services for weight management, PA and fitness counseling, and stress management education is 34.9, 22.2, and 17.9 percent, respectively (Demissie et al., 2013). Furthermore, evaluations of interventions to improve teacher wellness are scarce (Erwin et al., 2013). Programs that have been evaluated were developed decades ago and included multiple components (e.g., individualized counseling, wellness screening, educational classes, and exercise sessions) and were reported to be effective at increasing morale (Allegrante & Michela, 1990); improving self-reported vigorous exercise, physical fitness, weight loss, blood pressure, general well-being, and stress management (Blair et al., 1984); and reducing absenteeism (Blair et al., 1986). These results echo the more extensive research on comprehensive worksite wellness programs in the private business and industry sectors, which have achieved numerous benefits for staff (e.g., Pelletier, 1996, 2011). Moreover, reviews of worksite nutrition and PA programs found positive effects on employee body weight (Anderson et al., 2009), PA, fitness, lipids, anthropometric measures, work attendance, and job stress (Conn et al., 2009). There is also some evidence that staff wellness programs can be cost effective. In the school setting, studies have reported cost savings for school districts due to reductions in hiring substitute teachers (Blair et al., 1986) and filing health insurance claims (Kaldy, 1985). However, given the limited number of high-quality studies, the overall economic effect of employee health and wellness programs is inconclusive (Lerner et al., 2013).

Based on syntheses of published research, there are several key characteristics of effective staff wellness programming. Programs should last for at least one year, to increase the chances of reducing employee health risks, and be in place for at least three years to obtain useful measures of program outcomes (Goetzel & Ozminkowski, 2008). Cognitive-behavioral strategies may be particularly effective for reducing stress management in the workplace (Richardson & Rothstein, 2008). Such strategies are "designed to educate employees about the role of their thoughts and emotions in managing stressful events and to provide them with the skills to modify their thoughts to facilitate adaptive coping" (p. 67). Health screening with feedback is another important component of wellness programming, but it is likely to be most effective if the feedback is personalized and proceeded by follow-up support (Anderson & Staufacker, 1996; Task Force on Community Preventive Services, 2009). Similarly, in the context of comprehensive programming, individualized strategies tailored to the needs of high-risk employees are recommended (Heaney & Goetzel, 1997; Pelletier, 2001). Other components of effective staff wellness programming include having

- support from organizational administrators;
- an individual who serves as a program champion and promotes the program;
- alignment between the program and other organizational goals;
- strategies to increase staff participation in the program (e.g., offering incentives, making the program accessible, or offering a menu of program engagement modalities);
- self-care and self-management support (e.g., personalized goal setting, reflective counseling, or motivational interviewing),
- social support within the organization;
- a simultaneous focus on multiple aspects of wellness;
- annual data to monitor program outcomes; and
- the ability to create a culture of wellness within the organization (Goetzel & Ozminkowski, 2008).

The use of comprehensive staff wellness programs that embody the previously mentioned characteristics may help to diminish known barriers to effective programming. Barriers exist at multiple levels within and surrounding an organization. For instance, employers may be reluctant to support staff wellness programs for a number of reasons (e.g., they are opposed to interfering with their employees' personal lives and wellness habits, they are dubious about being able to demonstrate positive program effects to senior-level administrators, or they feel their organization lacks the resources to provide the program; Goetzel & Ozminkowski, 2008). Staff members themselves may also present an obstacle to successful programming. Some employees are fearful of breaches in confidentiality and having their health risks exposed; this may, in turn, lead to low participation in the organization's wellness program (Task Force on Community Preventive Services, 2009). Even for award-winning staff wellness programs, the average reported participation rate was only 60 percent (Goetzel et al., 2001). Low participation rates have been a pervasive challenge in school wellness programs for faculty and staff (Erickson & Gillespie, 2000; Johnson et al., 2010; Resnicow et al., 1998; Woynarowska-Solden, 2016). Reasons for lack of teacher participation include family responsibilities, time constraints, and lack of support (Erickson & Gillespie, 2000). Several other factors also could influence the success of a staff wellness program. At the organizational level, school health, school climate, and overall teacher job satisfaction may moderate the effectiveness of teacher wellness programs (Cullen et al., 1999). Furthermore, Johnson and colleagues (2010) reported that bad weather, cancellations of program sessions because of instructor issues, inappropriate space provided by the school, and lack of time because of standardized testing were challenges to implementing a wellness program for teachers.

Research on Staff Promotion of Youth PA

It is clear that school professionals and staff in other community-based organizations can make a positive difference in youth PA behavior (Holt et al., 2013; Lonsdale et al., 2013; Weaver, Beets, Turner-McGrievy, et al., 2014). Staff involvement with promoting youth PA can be broadly conceptualized

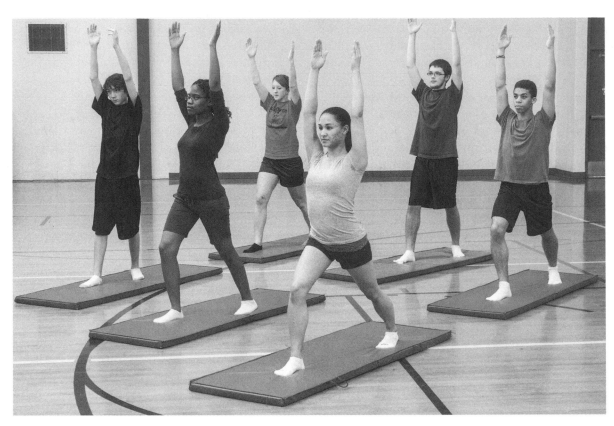

Through the involvement and support of all school staff, students can have multiple opportunities to participate in their preferred physical activities before, during and after school.

in terms of the direct and indirect actions staff members take to increase the concomitant or future amount of PA in which youth engage. Sometimes, there is a direct and immediate effect from staff members' behaviors on a child's level of PA, such as when a teacher assigns active games during a physical education class (Brazendale et al., 2015). At other times, staff members' behaviors may have an indirect and delayed effect on youth PA, such as when a teacher supports the student's PA learning needs and, in turn, the student is motivated to participate in more PA during his or her leisure time (Hagger et al., 2003). Certain staff behaviors, such as teaching children fundamental movement skills, may produce particularly durable changes in PA behavior that last into adulthood (Lai et al., 2014; Lloyd et al., 2014). All of these types of PA promotion are important to the overarching goal of a CSPAP to help youth achieve 60 minutes of PA each day.

There is a paucity of surveillance research on staff promotion of youth PA in schools and other relevant CSPAP settings. A recent study in

the United States, using nationally representative data, found that 71.7 percent of elementary schools used classroom lessons with integrated PA and 75.6 percent of schools used classroom activity breaks (Turner & Chaloupka, 2017). These rates were lower for majority-Latino and lower-socioeconomic schools, respectively. At schools where activity breaks were used, less than half of the teachers used them, and even fewer teachers used them at larger schools. Staff PA promotion in other CSPAP contexts may also be limited. For example, students often do not engage in recommended levels of PA during physical education classes (Cheval et al., 2016; Fröberg et al., 2017; Racette et al., 2015) or in after-school programs (Brazendale et al., 2015).

In contrast to the limited intervention research on school employee wellness (see previous section of this chapter), there has been a plethora of field trials involving staff promotion of youth PA. Numerous programs have been tested in a variety of CSPAP contexts, including physical education, general education classrooms, and out-of-school-time program settings. While the common feature of these programs is their focus on increasing staff PA promotion behaviors in order to increase youth PA, approaches used to increase staff promotion have varied across programs. For example, a frequently employed approach is to train staff to use a particular curriculum or prepackaged set of materials (Annesi et al., 2010; Dzewaltowski et al., 2010; Gortmaker et al., 2012; Herrick et al., 2012; Iversen et al., 2011; Kelder et al., 2005; Sharpe et al., 2011). This approach has had mixed results, with some studies showing increases and other studies showing no increases in youth PA. Possible limitations of the approach are that the curricula or materials often permit little flexibility in their use and staff are usually expected to implement them with high fidelity even though schools, community centers, and other organizations that serve youth are characteristically dynamic settings. An alternative approach is to train staff in PA promotion skills and strategies (Beets et al., 2014, 2015, 2016; Kelder et al., 2005). This approach is more ecologically valid because it allows for more flexible implementation of PA promotion behaviors and has tended to more consistently lead to increases in youth PA.

Unfortunately, in many cases, evaluations of PA promotion programs involving staff lack descriptive information about staff trainings or behaviors (Beets et al., 2009; Lander et al., 2017; Russ et al., 2015). This lack of information makes it difficult to identify strengths and limitations of the trainings and specific ways in which interventions have changed staff PA promotion. More regrettably, it is often unclear as to whether certain promotion behaviors are being adopted more than others. Little is known about which aspects of provided curricula, materials, or competencies staff use more or less, what ways staff members may adapt what they learned in trainings to satisfy the specific affordances and constraints of their given work setting, and which behaviors are to be credited for increases in youth PA.

Recent studies have validated systematic observation instruments to measure the PA promotion behaviors of physical education teachers (Weaver et al., 2016), classroom teachers (Russ et al., 2016), and after-school program staff (Weaver, Beets, Saunders, et al., 2014). These instruments categorize a range of behaviors that make it pos-

sible for an observer to systematically and reliably document the various ways staff members engage youth in PA. The development of these instruments has made it clear that staff behaviors used to promote youth PA are multifaceted and manifest in different ways depending on the context. Incorporating such observational techniques into field-based research on staff PA promotion, especially within intervention studies, will help to generate useful information that can be used to design effective programs and best practice recommendations to guide the work of interventionists, teachers, teacher educators, and out-of-school-time program leaders and their staff members. For example, the System for Observing Staff Promotion of Activity and Nutrition (SOSPAN) was used to evaluate the effectiveness of a competency-based professional development training for after-school program staff (Weaver, Beets, Saunders, et al., 2014). The training focused on PA and healthy eating promotion behaviors that SOSPAN is designed to measure. Results indicated positive changes in 17 of the 20 observed behaviors from baseline to postintervention. This study demonstrates the uptake of certain PA promotion behaviors more than others and has implications for future trainings.

While descriptive research on staff PA promotion behaviors is just emerging, a more robust research base has evolved to uncover variables that may influence the extent to which staff members promote PA. Much of this research stems from studies conducted with elementary classroom teachers. Overall, classroom teachers value PA for their students (Huberty et al., 2012; Stylianou et al., 2016) and are willing to promote PA during regular classroom time (Parks et al., 2007). However, teachers tend to perceive barriers to promoting PA. Lack of time is the most often cited barrier (Allison et al., 2016; Brown & Elliott, 2015; Cothran et al., 2010; Dinkel et al., 2016; Gately et al., 2013; Huberty et al., 2012; Langille & Rodgers, 2010; McMullen et al., 2016; Patton, 2012; Stylianou et al., 2016; Webster et al., 2017). Other important factors in classroom teachers' PA promotion can be traced to several theories of behavioral and organizational change. From a social learning perspective, self-efficacy, outcome expectancies, perceived competence, personal identity related to PA, satisfaction with one's own experiences in K-12 physical education, personal PA participation, and professional training are linked to teachers' self-reported PA promotion in the classroom (Allison et al., 2016; Cothran et al., 2010; Mâsse et al., 2012; Webster, Buchan, et al., 2015). Variables situated within the diffusion of innovations theory, specifically policy awareness, domain-specific innovativeness, and perceived attributes of PA promotion (e.g., relative advantage, compatibility, and complexity), also are relevant factors in teachers' implementation of PA promotion behaviors (Mâsse et al., 2012, 2013; Webster et al., 2013). Studies using organizational change theories and social-ecological frameworks point to the importance of the school environment, school-level support, and level of institutionalization as key factors in teachers' PA promotion (Langille & Rodgers, 2010; Mâsse et al., 2012; Webster et al., 2013).

There may also be additional factors that mediate or moderate classroom teachers' PA promotion. Using self-determination theory, Vazou and Vlachopoulos (2014) found that classroom teachers, physical education teachers, and other school personnel were autonomously motivated to implement one-minute PA breaks and participate in wellness events to promote children's PA. Furthermore, support from community partners has been shown to facilitate and increase teachers' use of classroom activity breaks (Delk et al., 2014). Staff wellness is another factor that could play a key role in classroom teachers' PA promotion behaviors. Having a faculty and staff health promotion program was a key factor that distinguished high-implementing schools from low-implementing and control schools in the Lifestyle Education for Activity Program (LEAP) study, which focused on changing instructional practices and the school environment to increase PA in high school girls (Saunders et al., 2006). This finding, coupled with studies that have linked classroom teachers' personal PA to their PA promotion with youth (Cothran et al., 2010; McKenzie et al., 1999; Webster, Buchan, et al., 2015), provides some evidence that efforts to improve school employee wellness could have a positive effect on the extent to which staff members become involved with promoting youth PA.

In the out-of-school-time setting, after-school program leaders and staff believe they can provide quality PA experiences (Hastmann et al., 2013), and staff members have demonstrated a willingness to modify games and adopt new games, as long as they have been sufficiently trained in how to do that (Sharpe et al., 2011; Weaver, Beets, Saunders, et al., 2014, 2016). Further, staff members see the benefit of providing quality PA experiences for children and believe children can develop skills, confidence, and a sense of belonging through active play with others during after-school programs (Zarrett et al., 2012). Yet as with integrating PA into general education classrooms, there are substantial barriers to increasing after-school staff members' implementation of PA opportunities. The most commonly recognized barrier in the after-school context is high rates of staff turnover (Cavanagh & Meinen, 2015; Dzewaltowski et al., 2010; Gortmaker et al., 2012; Hastmann et al., 2013; Kelder et al., 2005; Weaver et al., 2015, 2016). Typically, staff members are either high school or college students who are hired on a part-time basis and paid hourly. The position is temporary, filled by people who are in transition from one life phase to another.

Because of the short-term nature of staff positions, it is difficult to ensure that staff members acquire the necessary skills to do a good job with PA promotion. Staff members often have limited skills specific to managing physically active environments (Hastmann et al., 2013; Zarrett et al., 2012), promoting PA within those environments (Hastmann et al., 2013), and providing developmentally appropriate activities for children of different ages (Thomas et al., 2011). Moreover, because the majority of after-school program staff members are part-time employees (Thomas et al., 2011) with limited hours and little commitment to their role, attendance at staff trainings to improve these skills is often low (Hastmann et al., 2013). Another barrier to staff promotion of PA is the lack of priority placed on PA by staff, program leaders, and upper-level administrators (Hastmann et al., 2013). Often, staff members indicate that the goal of after-school programs is for children to finish their homework and have fun, not to provide children PA. This is a challenge that is particularly troublesome for incorporating PA curriculum into after-school programs because staff members often perceive that children do not like the games included in the curricula and prefer unstructured play time (Hastmann et al., 2013; Sharpe et al., 2011; Zarrett et al., 2012). Adding more scheduled time for PA may also conflict with the goal of children finishing their homework.

Surprisingly, little research has examined factors that could be associated with physical education teachers' PA promotion. While numerous recommendations call for physical education teachers to provide students with moderate-to-vigorous PA (MVPA) during physical education lessons as well as to lead, direct, or champion CSPAPs (Beighle et al., 2009; Carson, 2012; Castelli & Beighle, 2007; Heidorn & Centeio, 2012; Sallis et al., 2012), few studies have investigated possible enablers and barriers to having physical education teachers fulfill these roles. Teacher attitude was consistently the strongest predictor of physical education teachers' intentions to teach physically active lessons in a series of studies by Martin and colleagues that were framed using social cognitive theory and the theory of planned behavior (Martin & Kulinna, 2004, 2005; Martin et al., 2001). Centeio and colleagues (2014) examined the characteristics and attitudes of 10 elementary physical education teachers while the teachers worked toward becoming certified directors of PA. The teachers had positive attitudes toward being involved with the implementation of a CSPAP but had different opinions about how and to what extent physical education teachers should be involved.

In a dissertation study investigating 17 elementary and secondary physical education teachers' perspectives of the factors that influence their implementation of CSPAPs, Berei (2015) found that although the teachers had little knowledge of CSPAPs, most of them were involved with implementing all components of the model. However, there were mixed views as to whether physical education teachers should serve as leaders of CSPAPs. The teachers perceived several facilitators and barriers to CSPAP implementation. Facilitators included getting support from grants and other people in the school community, collaboration with others in the school community, advocating for and creating awareness of CSPAPs, and providing CSPAP resources and training to others. Barriers included lack of funding, additional academic requirements, inadequate facilities and equipment, and other obligations.

Knowledge Claims

Considering the research reviewed in the previous sections of this chapter, the following claims can be made about the current evidence-based knowledge related to the staff-involvement component of CSPAPs:

- High job demands, including physical exertion, are associated with teacher burnout.
- Women, elementary teachers, and teachers who work in lower-socioeconomic schools may be particularly susceptible to burnout.
- Improving employee wellness can improve work performance and lead to positive changes in health outcomes that are linked to burnout.
- Wellness is a multifaceted concept; as such, comprehensive workplace wellness programs are particularly effective at improving numerous health outcomes for employees.
- Although few wellness programs for school staff have been evaluated, such programs appear to have similar benefits as other worksite wellness programs.
- Effective worksite wellness programs are (1) based in behavioral theory, (2) include wellness screening with follow-up support, (3) target multiple components of wellness simultaneously, (4) incorporate program leadership and support, (5) offer opportunities for self-direction, (6) provide incentives to increase participation, (7) use data-based monitoring, and (8) are aligned with organizational goals.
- Barriers to implementing employee wellness programs can exist at multiple organizational levels and can include employer perceptions, staff perceptions, and overall organizational health and climate. Lack of time and space are additional barriers identified in research on teacher wellness programming.
- Teachers and other staff who work in CSPAP settings can increase youth PA.
- Surveillance research on staff promotion of youth PA is limited, but available evidence suggests interventions are needed to increase staff PA promotion in multiple CSPAP contexts.

- A multitude of programs involving staff promotion of youth PA have been tested in the field. Programs that train staff in adaptable PA promotion skills and strategies appear to be more effective at increasing youth PA than programs that train staff to use prepackaged curricula and materials with fidelity.

- Studies have provided little information about staff training and promotion behaviors. The recent development of new observation systems has the potential to improve staff training and the reporting of program implementation processes to better inform intervention design.

- Many staff members in schools and after-school programs understand the importance of promoting youth PA and are willing to play a role in such promotion.

- Physical education teachers may disagree about their specific roles within a CSPAP.

- A robust research base describes factors that could serve as facilitators and barriers to staff PA promotion. In the school setting, many studies focus on classroom teachers, but few focus on physical education teachers. Lack of time is the most common barrier for classroom teachers. Theories of behavioral and organizational change are useful in understanding teacher PA promotion behavior.

- Barriers to staff PA promotion in after-school programs include high rates of staff turnover, limited skills related to PA promotion, limited time dedicated to professional development, and competing program goals.

Knowledge Gaps and Directions for Future Research

Little is known about the effectiveness of faculty and staff wellness programs in increasing school employee wellness. Further exploratory investigation is needed to operationally define teacher wellness by drawing upon previous research that has uncovered multiple dimensions of the construct (e.g., Hattie et al., 2004; Lauzon, 1992). Correlational studies examining the association between teachers' work experiences and different dimensions of wellness also are needed to understand how job demands in teaching relate to teacher wellness. The results of correlational research can be used to design theoretically sound and comprehensive wellness programs that can be field tested in interventions using appropriate experimental designs. This will lead to a richer evidence base on faculty and staff wellness programs that are effective in reaching program goals.

Additionally, little attention has been given to the personal PA behavior of staff as a variable in staff promotion of youth PA. How physically active are teachers and after-school program staff in the absence of faculty and staff wellness programming? What factors influence staff PA behavior? What is the relationship of staff wellness to staff PA promotion behavior and youth PA? Which aspects of personal wellness are associated with staff PA promotion behavior, and what explains these associations? What kinds of PA promotion are healthier or well staff members involved in compared to less healthy or well staff members? Does a program that improves staff wellness also increase staff promotion of youth PA and, ultimately, increase youth PA?

The biggest limitation of current research on staff involvement is the lack of useful information available about staff PA promotion training and behaviors (Beets et al., 2009; Lander et al., 2017; Russ et al., 2015). In reports of intervention studies, authors often gloss over the specifics regarding how staff members were trained to promote PA and provide little to no implementation data. In instances where implementation data is reported, subjective staff reports are often used in place of objective measures. Without sufficient or accurate details about the intervention and how staff members used what they learned from training, it is impossible to know whether any changes in youth PA, or lack thereof, are attributable to the intervention and staff involvement. Program evaluations should include careful monitoring and reporting of staff training as well as systematic observation of staff promotion behaviors to provide an objective account of program delivery and implementation processes.

The research base on factors that could influence staff PA promotion provides important insights into the reasons staff, particularly elementary classroom teachers, may be either more or less involved with promoting youth PA.

However, few interventions have drawn upon this research base to design programs for implementation in elementary classrooms (Webster, Russ, et al., 2015). Trainings for classroom teachers may be more effective if they target variables found to be important to classroom PA promotion in previous research, especially research grounded in behavioral and organizational change theories. Furthermore, given that lack of time is a prominent and pervasive issue classroom teachers face when trying to promote PA, approaches that reduce time pressures related to PA promotion must be a priority in future interventions to increase classroom-based PA opportunities.

Even though physical education teachers are often viewed as central protagonists in CSPAPs, there is an unexpected dearth of research on factors that might enable or hinder physical education teachers as PA promoters. Essential questions about how realistic it is to expect physical education teachers to lead, or even support, a CSPAP must be addressed. Large-scale survey studies as well as in-depth qualitative studies are needed to build a descriptive research base that outlines key factors and useful theoretical perspectives that should be considered in efforts to involve physical education teachers in roles such as increasing MVPA during physical education lessons and collaborating with other school professionals to implement school-wide PA programming.

In after-school program settings, studies that have adopted a multicomponent, ecological approach have successfully increased staff PA promotion behaviors (Beets et al., 2014, 2015, 2016; Gortmaker et al., 2012). However, these studies have had less success in changing the structure (i.e., policy adoption and schedule adjustments) of after-school programs. Barriers to PA promotion cited by staff hint at why this may be the case, with competing priorities of finishing homework and the reluctance of staff to change programming for fear that it may encroach on children's enjoyment of the after-school program (Hastmann et al., 2013; Sharpe et al., 2011; Zarrett et al., 2012). Future research should attempt to address these barriers by creating interventions that do not encroach upon after-school program priorities and emphasizing the importance of promoting PA in the after-school program setting.

Certain types of staff members who could play key roles in CSPAPs have received little investigative attention. While before-school programs are recommended as part of the CSPAP model, virtually nothing is known about the PA promotion of staff who work in such programs. Moreover, teachers have cited organizational support as an important factor in their PA promotion (e.g., Langille & Rodgers, 2010; Mâsse et al., 2012), but few studies have examined the perceptions or behaviors of school administrators with respect to CSPAPs. In elementary schools, more PA opportunities may be tied to role modeling of PA by school principals (Barnett et al., 2009). Studies focusing on school leaders at the district and state levels are also needed because these individuals tend to make policy decisions that affect what school principals prioritize. Likewise, increased staff-involvement research on site leaders, staff supervisors, and staff educators is needed to better understand how to develop effective staff training in out-of-school-time programs. A key question for future research is whether interventions to increase staff PA promotion should be geared more toward top-down approaches (i.e., targeting higher social-ecological levels, such as policy, to influence staff behaviors) or bottom-up approaches (i.e., targeting lower social-ecological levels, such as staff beliefs and competencies, to influence staff behaviors).

There are also a number of other limitations of existing staff-involvement research. Few studies have been conducted in secondary school settings, even though adolescents are much less physically active than children (Troiano et al., 2008). Additionally, only a small number of studies have investigated programs that use specially designed classroom equipment and environmental design, which can be effective at increasing youth PA (e.g., Ayala et al., 2016; Benden et al., 2014; McCrady-Spitzer et al., 2015; Sudholz et al., 2016) and may be relatively easy for teachers to use. One issue with such equipment, however, is its cost. The cost effectiveness of PA equipment for the classroom and other CSPAP contexts and the willingness of organizational leaders to purchase this equipment are questions that must be addressed in future research. Finally, few multiyear evaluations of interventions involving staff have been conducted. The majority of PA interventions have lasted for one academic school year or less (Gortmaker et al., 2012; Kelder et al., 2005; Sharpe et al., 2011; Slusser et al., 2013). Researchers must give equal priority to questions regarding both effectiveness and sustainability for the scientific foundation of staff PA promotion trainings to make a durable effect on staff implementation and youth PA.

Evidence-Based Recommendations and Applications

School employee wellness programs have the potential to benefit the health of faculty and staff, improve work performance, and even increase faculty and staff promotion of youth PA. While such programs may have an indirect influence on PA promotion, strategies explicitly designed to nurture the PA promotion practices of faculty and staff are needed too. School professionals and community partners share the responsibilities of implementing school employee wellness programs and advancing the work of faculty and staff aimed at increasing youth PA.

For School Staff

Given the high rate of burnout among teachers and the need to maximize staff involvement with youth PA promotion, staff wellness programs merit increased attention among school administrators. Principal support must be a targeted priority in developing an implementation plan for the program because the program will fail to gain traction if it is not aligned with other organization-level goals of the school. Additionally, school professionals must be involved in helping to plan, lead, and support the program so that it is optimally responsive to the needs of faculty and staff. Program planners should incorporate multiple strategies that can be used to increase staff participation in the program. Offering a range of educational delivery platforms, such as group classes, online tutorials, and brochures; giving staff individualized feedback and counseling with tailored recommendations for maintaining or

improving wellness; supporting staff autonomy in making wellness choices; and providing activities designed to improve multiple aspects of wellness will help to increase staff buy-in to the program. When possible, schools should partner with universities or other external organizations that can help to design, implement, monitor, and evaluate the program.

To increase teachers' promotion of youth PA, principals should work with external partners (e.g., other schools and universities) to provide professional development workshops that focus on PA promotion strategies. It is important for teachers to have ongoing opportunities to explore and adopt strategies to increase youth PA before, during, and after school. Physical education teachers should plan to use active warm-ups; lead-up games; movement breaks; and transitions, especially in lessons with learning tasks that require less movement. For example, young children learning to catch a ball may need to practice catching while standing still before catching while walking or running. The teacher can start the lesson with an "instant activity" that gets children's hearts pumping, inject short MVPA breaks throughout the lesson, and modify transitions between tasks to increase PA intensity.

Physical education teachers also can follow the LET US Play principles (Brazendale et al., 2015; Weaver et al., 2013) to increase youth PA during class. LET US stands for *lines* (avoid lines); *elimination* (avoid playing elimination games); *team size* (use small-sided teams); *uninvolved teachers* (actively monitor activities and occasionally join in); and *space*, equipment, and rules (maximize use of space, equipment, and rules). These principles are just as relevant for staff PA promotion in out-of-school-time programs. Furthermore, program leaders should incorporate both structured and unstructured PA time into program schedules. Recommended skills and strategies for classroom teachers to increase youth PA include taking advantage of naturally occurring transitions, strategically placing materials on different sides of the classroom, starting the day with movement, scheduling movement breaks into daily routines, establishing classroom

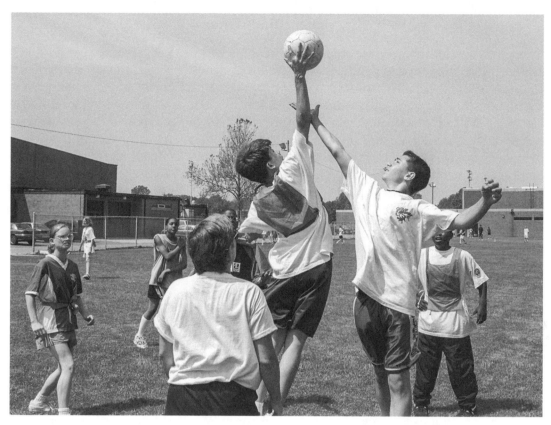

The LET US Play principles include making sure team sizes are small to allow for greater student participation, PA, and learning.

management systems that permit and encourage student movement, using PA as a reward, and planning academic lessons that integrate PA opportunities.

For Community Partners

University faculty, graduate students, teacher candidates, and undergraduate interns across the allied health fields can create and implement professional development workshops for schools. Workshops can be designed to educate principals and teachers about the known personal and professional benefits of a healthy lifestyle, provide examples of school faculty and staff wellness programs, and demonstrate strategies for promoting youth PA. University personnel also can organize opportunities for school employees to engage in wellness screening; offer activities designed to improve employee wellness; and lead movement experiences for children and adolescents before, during, and after school.

An important focus of professional development for teachers, as well as for preservice training for teacher candidates, is reducing perceived barriers to promoting PA. Workshop content should emphasize easily modifiable PA promotion skills and strategies that allow for flexible implementation and can be integrated into routine managerial and instructional practices. Teachers should be encouraged to use goal setting and self-monitoring related to their PA promotion so they stay motivated to keep students active and continue to improve in their role as PA promoters. Ongoing training is needed to ensure issues such as staff turnover do not become barriers to effective and sustainable implementation of PA opportunities, particularly in out-of-school-time programs.

SUMMARY

In conclusion, staff involvement focuses on two aims within a CSPAP: increase staff wellness and staff promotion of youth PA. Staff wellness is multifaceted, and there is a dearth of recent research on effective interventions to increase wellness outcomes for staff. In contrast, a growing body of research is available to guide intervention work related to increasing staff promotion of youth PA. Future efforts to garner the involvement of school professionals, after-school staff, and others in youth PA promotion will benefit from research that more closely investigates the connection between staff wellness and staff PA promotion; better documents implementation processes in intervention studies; and expands the focus of CSPAP research to school principals, district superintendents, and other key decision makers who influence school programming and practices.

QUESTIONS TO CONSIDER

1. Should schools be accountable for staff wellness?
2. What data might be collected to provide information to school administrators about faculty and staff well-being?
3. When developing a staff wellness program for teachers, how could the program planners ensure the program will be successful?
4. What strategies could physical education teachers use to increase the amount of PA children accumulate in general education classrooms?
5. What would a well-designed workshop on youth PA promotion for after-school staff look like?

CASE EXAMPLES

Following are two case examples of staff involvement initiatives from Chicago Public Schools (CPS). In the first example, Tom Loulousis (physical education and health teacher) describes how his school adopted a pilot PA promotion program called 30+20+10, which is run by school staff. In the second example, Martha Carman (physical education teacher) and Lee Marcheschi (classroom teacher) detail the many ways their school staff provides PA and the key factors that have facilitated PA promotion.

Implementing a Pilot Program

Athanasios (Tom) Loulousis
Ashburn Elementary School
Chicago, Illinois

In 2012, CPS formed the Office of Student Health and Wellness (OSHW), a department that assumed responsibility for overseeing everything from designing our physical education scope and sequence to securing vision and dental screenings for our entire student population district wide. Ashburn Elementary was approached by the OSHW to pilot a new program called 30+20+10. The concept of 30+20+10 is straightforward: The pilot schools were asked to provide 30 minutes of physical education, 20 minutes of recess, and 10 minutes of classroom PA every day for all of our students.

The physical education program was already in place for most of our students, but it was challenging to work out how we would implement the 30-minute requirement. Our school schedule changed numerous times during the year to try to meet the requirement without stepping on the toes of other school subjects. We eventually made it work through trial and error, which is sometimes the best way to solve a problem. The fact that our administration and teachers were willing to support this process in spite of how frustrating it was at times speaks volumes about our school's commitment to making PA a priority. When there is a group of people who are eager to come together and work toward a solution, everyone benefits.

The 20-minute recess and the 10-minute classroom PA requirements were completely different from each other when it came to implementation. Ashburn already had daily recess for our students, so it was just a matter of scheduling supervision and securing grants to purchase equipment the students could use outside. But how does one sell having to prepare a 10-minute, daily PA lesson to a room full of classroom teachers whose days are already scheduled with their own lessons, student progress monitoring, meetings about reading and math data, assessments, standardized tests, counseling students, resolving conflicts, and a dozen other responsibilities? This was not an easy task. Our solution came from the OSHW leaders, who discussed the idea of having a PA leader (PAL) at each school. This would be a classroom teacher who would be provided professional development and whose goal would be to work with the physical education teacher and administration to increase classroom teachers' participation in helping the school to meet the daily classroom PA requirement.

With that, Fitness Friday was born at Ashburn. Every Friday during our morning announcements, our PAL would send her students into all our classrooms to lead activities she had organized for the teachers the day before. The OSHW then provided our schools with a playbook of easy-to-use classroom activities, and teachers began to see the benefits of students completing a vigorous workout—so much so that they found it much easier to carve out 10 minutes during their day for classroom PA.

Our school has also done a number of other things to promote PA. We were fortunate enough to gain a partnership with the Chicago Blackhawks organization, which comes every year to do a hockey clinic. We also work with student-athletes from the University of Chicago, who speak to our students about their collegiate experiences. Moreover, we've incorporated movement breaks during our assemblies.

Advocating for our school-wide increase in PA has become very important. Generally, when hearing about more physical education and recess, parents want to know why their children are not spending more time in a classroom or computer lab instead. It was essential to promote the benefits of daily PA as well as offering engaging movement opportunities to our students. We invited parents to come out to see what was happening throughout the school day to showcase the progress we were making. Using our website to show our parent community the events at school was another valuable resource.

Since the conclusion of the 30+20+10 pilot, CPS has taken tremendous strides to reinforce physical education and ensure that all students have access to a healthy school environment throughout the district. Our OSHW leaders have spearheaded the effort to provide continuing professional development for all stakeholders regarding PA. They have been an essential resource in the scheduling process and providing technical support for staff and funding and grant opportunities for schools. Currently, all CPS schools are required to provide physical education for a minimum of 30 minutes a day, to all students.

Building Staff Support for PA Promotion

Martha Carman and Lee Marcheschi
Edison Park Elementary School
Chicago, Illinois

Edison Park Elementary School (EP) is a CPS that serves over 600 students from preschool through eighth grade and employs roughly 40 teachers and staff members. Other public schools in the vicinity were overcrowded, so EP was designed to take a small population of students from each of those schools in 2008. A bonus to opening a brand new school is that it allowed the administration to create a school culture that places value on educating the whole child, including emphasizing physical fitness and making healthy lifestyle choices.

It all began with our first principal, Pete Zimmerman, who held the belief that healthy kids learn better and that giving them PA during the school day would improve classroom performance and behavior. He held the vision that the school should serve as a community center for interscholastic sports (grades 5-8) and other fitness-related activities (grades K-8) after school hours, and he strived to provide PA opportunities for students, staff, parents, and community members during this time.

Our culture has always supported and encouraged health and wellness for our community. However, our success was not something that happened overnight. Instead, it was carefully developed by a small group of individuals who led by example and slowly persuaded the community to buy in to the idea that a school is not just a place to learn academics but also a place to educate the whole child and nurture healthy development. The following details describe how we got to where we are now.

Having Administrative Support

Administrative support is crucial to a successful CSPAP. This support can come in the form of providing time and space during the school day for PA, use of professional development days for health- and wellness-related development for staff, or allocating funding to health and wellness activities and supplies. Mr. Zimmerman allowed our school to participate in the 30+20+10 pilot program (see the first case study). He allowed the entire school's schedule to be changed to accommodate daily physical education in our primary grades. He allowed the physical education teachers to present PA break ideas and strategies to classroom teachers during professional development days along with providing research that proved that the brain was more active after PA.

Our principal not only supported health and wellness during the school day but also supported programs that took place after the last bell. He allowed the building to stay open late for Fit Friday Fitness Club for kids; a boot camp for parents; a Family Fit Night, which provided fitness activities for families; open gym for Dads Club basketball games; Itty Bitty Dance Classes; and intramural and interscholastic sports, and he even opened the building on the weekends for a Saturday basketball camp and a community 5K (which he would also run).

Providing Teachers With Options

One of the most fundamental things that can be done to implement PA in the classroom is to provide teachers with options for what they can do with their students. The key to success is that these activities should not create additional work for teachers. We made sure teachers had access to necessary equipment, such as projectors, speakers, and laptops. One activity that was particularly successful at EP was FitDeck Exercise Playing Cards. Ten sets were purchased (using grant money) for classroom teachers' use. The cards focused on three areas: yoga, resistance tube, and fitness junior. A teacher would shuffle the cards, choose one, and instruct the students to complete the activity specified on the card. Some cards could be as simple as jumping in place or as advanced as a side plank. Another way teachers would use the cards was by distributing the cards, having students perform different activities for a short amount of time, and then switching cards.

Our school was able to develop a relationship with a local yoga studio (a parent on the Wellness Committee taught at this studio). Through this partnership, we were able to get a donation of a set of yoga mats. Teachers were able to use these mats in their classrooms to go along with activities from children's yoga videos on YouTube, Yoga Kids instructional cards, or Calm Classroom yoga series to instruct the students in basic yoga poses. Teachers also learned how to use yoga to get desired results from their students—energize, destress, or increase focus and concentration.

Through another grant, we were able to purchase stability ball chairs for our primary classrooms. Stability balls work great for students to sit on in place of chairs, and they double as a piece of equipment to use during PA breaks. The balls help students with high amounts of energy focus while their bodies are unknowingly moving the ball, which transfers otherwise disruptive behaviors away from the learning environment.

Our school has a flat-screen television on a rolling cart with an Xbox. Teachers are allowed to use the Xbox as a reward for the students. Programs such as Dance Dance Revolution are great to get students active while they are also having fun. Some teachers create a classroom rotation and use the Xbox as a center since a limited number of students can use it at one time. Some teachers have also been known to dance along with their students!

Last year, we were a part of a GoNoodle campaign in Illinois. GoNoodle is a website that contains hundreds of videos that encourage PA in the classroom and at home. Teachers were given a GoNoodle account and encouraged to use the program in their classrooms. Videos could be as short as 90 seconds or as long as 15 minutes. Many of the videos contain an academic component as well, such as multiplication facts and spelling activities.

Obtaining Teacher Buy-In

To have a successful PA program during school hours, teachers need to buy in to the program. They must believe that taking the time for activity breaks and participating in fitness in the classroom will help make them more effective educators and will benefit their students. When we showed teachers the research that PA helps promote an active brain, we provided a side-by-side picture of brain scans. Gasps were heard when the staff members saw the pictures. It was clear that the visual helped persuade them that PA could improve student learning.

Teachers also need to feel confident that they are implementing PA properly. The last thing a teacher wants is an injury. At our school, we led teachers in 20-second "instant activities" during a professional development presentation. This was helpful in modeling the activities so teachers saw how they worked and were ready to use them. Another thing that can boost teacher confidence is showing teachers how to properly manage movement in the classroom. Showing teachers how to use music to guide movement and establish start and stop signals, as well as giving teachers ideas on how to best manage movement in their space, can make them more comfortable leading activities. We also made suggestions such as taking the long way from the cafeteria to the classroom or taking a bathroom break in another area of the school as simple ways to increase movement during the school day.

Having a Health-Promoting School Culture

The school's culture needs to promote a healthy lifestyle for everyone and support staff wellness. We have a very active wellness team, which is able to keep wellness as a priority during all school activities. Our Wellness Committee is made up of parents and teachers who keep our school focused on making health and wellness a priority. We created opportunities for teachers to come together and engage in movement. One day a week during the teachers' lunch period, teachers would meet in the gym for a midday workout. They would complete boot camp workout videos, circuit training, weight lifting, or yoga. Students would love peeking in the gym windows to see their teachers getting some exercise. The teachers were setting the example for our students by being active role models for participating in PA. Additionally, every January, we hold the Wellness Challenge, which begins with the start of a new year and New Year's resolutions. Staff could earn points for eating healthy, drinking water, and logging PA time. The staff member with the most points earned at the end of eight weeks was the winner. It was great to motivate each other in this challenge.

Our school created policies that discourage unhealthy celebration and encourage healthy ways to celebrate and provide PA as a reward. We wanted our students to lose the idea that sugary foods are a reward and PA is a punishment. To change this mindset, we started by asking parents not to supply items such as cupcakes for student birthdays. We provided alternative ideas, such as donating a book to their student's classroom library or passing out pencils or stickers. We also provided teachers with the idea of giving their classes an extra recess for great behavior. Students no longer associate a peer's birthday with a dessert and, instead, ask for extra recess.

We created connections with the community to bring activities to our school that the district did not fund, such as yoga, a running club, taekwondo, and bowling. When our district cut all after-school sport programs, we held fund-raisers to get the money needed for coaches and referees so we could play against other schools in the area. We also provide a host of other PA opportunities. We have an annual walk-a-thon, held traditionally on Halloween, to provide extra PA to counterbalance the candy students will later collect while trick-or-treating. Students love challenging themselves to walk more laps and enjoy walking with their teachers at the event. We have a Family Fit Night, which gives families a chance to see physical activities in the area, such as local gyms and fitness, yoga, and dance studios. Each winter during physical education, students participate in a Jump Rope for Heart event. They learn about their hearts and the importance of staying active while raising money for the American Heart Association. In the spring, our school hosts Pound the Pavement, a 5K that takes runners and walkers through the neighborhood, starting and ending on the school's campus. It's amazing how many students, parents, and teachers complete the race! In June, we hold our annual Field Day, where students participate in activities such as tug-of-war, sack races, relay races, kickball games, and obstacle courses. These activities that happen during the year help to keep students and staff excited about PA.

CHAPTER 10

Family and Community Engagement

Gregory J. Welk, PhD
Iowa State University

Joey A. Lee
University of Colorado at
Colorado Springs

Schools provide an ideal setting for coordinated youth PA programming, but comprehensive approaches are clearly needed to optimize effectiveness and sustainability over time. Social-ecological models of health promotion have long emphasized the need to target multiple settings and the importance of the environment (both physical and social) on health behaviors. These principles are clearly consistent with the specific recommendations for family and community engagement in CSPAPs. School-based programming can influence youth during the school hours, but for optimal effectiveness, programming must build connections and support networks to facilitate PA behaviors at home and in the community.

The standard PA recommendations for youth also directly reinforce the importance of shared responsibility for youth activity promotion. The stated goal is that half of children's weekly PA (150 minutes) should occur at school with the other half occurring at home or in the community. Schools may decide to focus their efforts on only the school contribution, but engaging parents and community partners can establish a shared vision for promoting and supporting children's PA. Messages and programming directed at families can help communicate and establish this shared vision while also building advocates and support for school-based programming.

Parents (and families) serve as gatekeepers who influence youth behaviors at home as well as the effect of school-based programming on children's attitudes and behaviors. For example, parents can either reinforce or negate messages or attitudes shaped by teachers and programming at the school. The availability of community support and resources can also influence the likelihood that youth will achieve (or have the opportunity to achieve) the goal of accumulating 60 minutes of PA a day. To increase the likelihood of achieving the 60-minute goal, it is essential to incorporate intentional and targeted efforts to promote PA at home and in community settings. As shown in figure 10.1, family and community engagement (FCE) can synergistically amplify CSPAP applications while also promoting sustainability.

The focus of this chapter is on reviewing research and best practices related to effective FCE in CSPAP applications. The first two sections review past research and describe the basis for inclusion of FCE in CSPAP applications. The next two sections introduce gaps and priorities in research and provide strategies for improving FCE in future CSPAP applications. The final section describes methods and approaches used in an ongoing CSPAP-based project called SWITCH (School Wellness Integration Targeting Child Health). Emphasis in this final section is placed on the system-based approaches currently being used to promote school and family engagement in the programming.

Review of Research

FCE is central to CSPAP, but separate realms of research have examined the nature of parenting

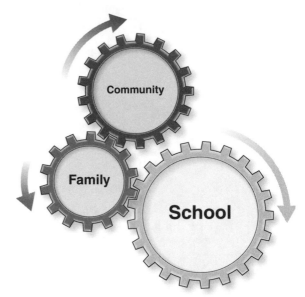

Figure 10.1 Conceptualized benefits of FCE in a CSPAP.

on youth behaviors as well the effect of community environments. This section will provide an overview of the foundation for including FCE in a CSPAP followed by a summary of studies that have specifically targeted these components within CSPAP frameworks.

Foundations of FCE in CSPAPs

Foundational principles for FCE have been proposed in school programming well before the formal launch of the CSPAP (Sanders, 2001). Epstein (1987), for example, proposed a useful theory to explain how schools, families, and communities collectively interact to socialize and educate children. The central principle in this model is that positive outcomes are best achieved through cooperative action and support. Epstein and Sanders (2006) later defined school–community partnerships as the "connections between schools and community individuals, organizations and businesses that are forged to promote students' social emotional, physical and intellectual development" (p. 20). The paper included a comprehensive evaluation conducted through a network of more than 400 schools to elucidate the different types and features of school–community partnerships. While this work was aimed at broad educational reform, there are many insights that are directly relevant to current challenges in promoting a CSPAP and whole-school programming. In fact, the inclusion of FCE in CSPAP applications may have been justified in part on the documented importance of FCE in these broader education goals.

Parenting practices and family influence are also known to have a strong influence on youth PA behaviors (Garriguet et al., 2017; Langer et al., 2014; Rebholz et al., 2014). Families largely influence the PA and healthy eating environments and opportunities that students are exposed to on a daily basis. Although evaluations of the influence of family involvement in school wellness programming have been somewhat equivocal, there is evidence that PA behaviors of children and parents are highly intertwined (Lee et al., 2010). Review studies have also clearly documented that targeting family and youth in combination leads to better outcomes than targeting youth independently (Van Sluijs et al., 2007).

Parent engagement has been operationalized within CSPAPs as a mechanism to support students' PA behaviors at home and to provide a path for involving parents in school health programming (Centers for Disease Control and Prevention [CDC], 2013). Parent engagement in CSPAP applications is envisioned to help schools support wellness programming through volunteer efforts and integrating parent expertise in school wellness initiatives (e.g., nutrition education, leading before- and after-school programming, and grant writing). Community engagement, in turn, is viewed as a strategy to capitalize on local resources and establish partnerships with local organizations (e.g., shared-use agreements, professional development for staff, and student wellness programming). The definitions and descriptions in this seminal document lay out a clear vision for FCE, but challenges lie in operationalizing these ideas. Promoting FCE in a CSPAP is especially challenging because it necessitates efforts and actions outside of the school building. It also requires a significant investment of time in pursuing, establishing, and maintaining relationships as well as the requisite communication and interpersonal skills needed to do this. In this powerful quote, Epstein (1995) directly linked family engagement with the school's overall philosophy about education:

The "WAY" schools care about children is reflected in the way schools care about the children's families. If educators view children simply as students, they are likely to see the family as separate from the school. That is, the family is expected to do its job and leave the education of children to the schools. If educators view students as children, they are likely to see both the family and the community as partners with the school in children's education and development. Partners recognize their shared interests in and responsibilities for children, and they work together to create better programs and opportunities for students. (p. 701)

A separate document released by the CDC provides specific guidelines to help schools implement strategies for promoting parent engagement (CDC, 2012). The guide provides a compelling rationale for schools on the importance of parent engagement and specifically references an important study on parental influence (Epstein, 2010) that emphasized the value of parents and school staff working together to support and improve the learning, development, and health of children and adolescents. However, the CDC (2012) guidebook extends this notion in ways that speak more directly to the relevance of FCE in CSPAP applications:

Parent engagement in schools is defined as parents and school staff working together to support and improve the learning, development, and health of children and adolescents. Parent engagement is a shared responsibility in which schools and other community agencies and organizations are committed to reaching out to engage parents in meaningful ways, and parents are committed to actively supporting their children's and adolescents' learning and development. This relationship between schools and parents cuts across and reinforces children's health and learning in multiple settings—at home, in school, in out-of-school programs, and in the community. (p. 6)

The CDC's (2011) *School Health Guidelines to Promote Healthy Eating and Physical Activity* provides schools with strategies to consider for developing and implementing FCE initiatives. Recommended strategies include (1) establishing multiple methods for communicating health messages to parents, (2) involving parents on the school health council, (3) developing and implementing strategies to motivate families to participate in school-based health programs, (4) providing access to community wellness resources, and (5) demonstrating cultural awareness toward healthy eating and PA initiatives.

A separate report by the CDC (2012), titled *Parent Engagement: Strategies for Involving Parents in School Health*, provides a more comprehensive document with specific action items and steps that schools can consider utilizing to optimize FCE. The document promotes a three-step process (connect, engage, sustain) for engaging parents (and community members and organizations) in school wellness. The document also provides a detailed process of how schools can connect and communicate with parents and provide them with support, foster learning at home, and encourage and invite parents to be a part of the decision-making process at school. In addition, strategies for collaborating with the community are also provided. This resource can serve as a foundational document for schools that are looking to enhance FCE and for researchers who are looking to develop a protocol for evaluating the influence of FCE on PA in CSPAP interventions. However, putting these guidelines into practice remains challenging. The next section will describe key knowledge gaps that need to be addressed to advance research on FCE integration in a CSPAP.

Effectiveness of FCE in CSPAPs

A number of studies have sought to integrate school and community programming, but there are few examples of programming strategies that can be readily used for CSPAP applications. A systematic review of controlled studies emphasized the importance of multicomponent interventions that targeted both school involvement and FCE, although evidence was supportive only for studies with adolescents (Van Sluijs et al., 2007). Separate Cochrane Reviews have also been done on community involvement and school-based interventions,

so brief summaries are provided here for context.

Baker and colleagues (2015) Cochrane Review provided an update of findings from a 2011 review that yielded largely equivocated findings. The updated review included four new studies that were rated as being of high quality, but none were shown to promote gains in population levels of PA. Environmental changes were found to promote gains in segments of the population (e.g., gains in more people walking), but the gains were thought to be too small to create a measurable population effect. The review concluded that broad community trials may not effectively reach a sufficient segment of the population and that combinations of more integrated strategies may be needed. This is clearly the concept behind CSPAP applications. While community interventions may not be effective on their own, it is possible that school-based programs with clear community connections (i.e., whole-community approaches) may be more effective, at least for youth.

The specific Cochrane Review of school trials (Dobbins et al., 2013) concluded that school-based PA interventions are effective in increasing duration of PA and reducing time spent watching television. In fact, the authors reported that children exposed to school-based PA interventions are three times more likely to engage in moderate-to-vigorous PA during the school day than those not exposed. However, it is hard to distill the features in the specific studies that contributed to the effects. As described in the implementation science literature (Brownson et al., 2012; Leeman et al., 2015; Remington & Brownson, 2011), another limitation of highly controlled school-based studies is that they can rarely be disseminated into real-world settings.

An advantage (and challenge) of CSPAP applications is that the studies are typically designed to be conducted under more real-world conditions. This improves the external validity of the findings, but the downside is that it is often more difficult to control and assess the fidelity of implementation. In a comprehensive review of CSPAP applications (Russ et al., 2015), 14 studies that included at least two CSPAP components were reviewed. The authors concluded that there is currently a lack of evidence supporting multicomponent CSPAP interventions. Interestingly, all 14 studies in this review were categorized as having an

FCE component. While this shows that parent and community components are commonly included in CSPAP applications, it also indicates that the FCE methods currently being used in CSPAPs are not having the intended effect. The nature of the parent engagement strategies in these studies varied widely, with strategies ranging from education events and health fairs to simple communication strategies and newsletters. The diversity of approaches and designs makes it difficult to draw conclusions, but it is clear that the parent components in current CSPAP applications have not been designed or delivered in effective ways. Cipriani et al. (2012) recently highlighted the need for more attention on FCE in CSPAP applications. The tagline to their paper bears repeating as a guide for the present chapter: "The least implemented component of a Comprehensive School Physical Activity Program—engaging families and communities—may be the most important" (p. 20).

Interestingly, the statement is somewhat in contrast to the Russ et al. (2015) review, which reported that FCE was the most commonly implemented component in CSPAP applications. However, this may speak more directly to the degree of significance and comprehensiveness of the approaches used to successfully engage parents and community members. For instance, one study prompted parent engagement by sending notecards to participants' homes every two to three weeks (Neumark-Sztainer et al., 2010), but it is hard to determine the intensity or effect of this modest communication strategy. Thus, studies included in the review could have implemented low-dose FCE components or may not have included sufficiently robust process or outcome evaluations to fully understand the effect of FCE.

The limited evidence base has led to a more concerted effort to improve the structure, rigor, and approaches for CSPAP applications. Recent CSPAP papers have provided conceptual frameworks for designing and implementing studies (Carson, Castelli, Beighle, et al., 2014; Webster et al., 2015); summaries of theory-based best practices (Carson, Castelli, Pulling Kuhn, et al., 2014; Hills et al., 2015; Webster et al., 2015); descriptions of potential barriers and facilitators (based on interventions that mimic elements of a CSPAP; Hills et al., 2015); and reflections on other mul-

ticomponent, school-based PA interventions that could be viewed as CSPAP applications (Russ et al., 2015). However, there is limited evidence about the specific mechanisms that may underlie the role of families in school-based PA interventions (e.g., CSPAP applications). A recent meta-analysis (Brown et al., 2016) emphasized the importance of goal setting and reinforcement as well as the inherent value of families spending time being physically active together. Building these concepts into theory-based, CSPAP applications with robust evaluation plans will help to advance work in this area.

Qualitative analyses may be particularly important for understanding FCE integration because parents and community partners are external to the school system. School leaders may not know how to effectively engage families and community partners. Families may also not understand the significance of their role in protecting the health of students or how they can be involved in doing so through school systems. One study (Patino-Fernandez et al., 2013) clearly captured the disconnect between parents' and teachers' expectations about each other's role in youth's nutrition education and PA offering. Utilizing focus groups, the study reported themes related to parents' and school staff members' perspectives on the division of the roles of providing nutrition education and PA opportunities. Although there was a high level of concern from both parents and school staff for supporting healthy behaviors in school, each group implicated the other as the one holding the primary responsibility for addressing the issue with students. Despite contrasting views, parents and school staff agreed there was a need to implement comprehensive school-based efforts to support student health.

Another study by Deslatte and Carson (2014) utilized qualitative approaches to document how engaging parents in school PA programming enhanced support for CSPAPs. The study demonstrated the value of parent engagement through the eyes of physical educators in schools attempting to implement full-scale CSPAPs. The following quote from the study provides a particularly insightful look into the importance of FCE components for building interest and support for CSPAP applications from a physical educator's perspective:

Excitement for the PE program also spreads to the parents through students' stories of PE class or parent-teacher orientation meetings, where parents are able to realize the programs in place are not like what they had "when they were in school." Parents demand the activity and are more willing to support programs, such as before and after-school activity programs, once they see the excitement of the students. (p. 15)

Despite the intuitive logic, few school-based studies have specifically sought to influence parenting practices in efforts to promote positive youth outcomes. One exception is a recent study (Straker et al., 2012) that used motivational interview techniques to guide parents and youth to set short- and long-term behavior-change goals each week (child for himself or herself; parents for supporting child health). The use of goal setting and reflecting on goals was thought to help with forming habits and providing reinforcement of positive behaviors for both parents and children. This application provides a good example of how parent involvement can be enhanced; however, a limitation is that this one-to-one approach is intensive and time consuming.

This brief review demonstrates both the importance and challenge of engaging families in CSPAP applications. School leaders may assume that parents know what goes on in school or that simple communications are sufficient; however, the reality is that direct, coordinated, and intentional communication strategies are needed to promote effective FCE.

Knowledge Claims

The following list summarizes interpretations and conclusions based on the available literature in this area. Because of the limited work done in this area, the conclusions are informed by evidence but are not necessarily evidence based.

- Family involvement is associated with positive youth development, adoption of healthy lifestyles, improved academic performance, and lower odds of students engaging in risky behaviors.

- Family engagement in school programming is strongly recommended and valued, but existing strategies are difficult to implement.
- Curricular demands leave little time for schools to focus on engaging parents.
- School leaders are not trained on how to engage parents and community members in CSPAP initiatives.
- Providing staff with professional development targeting how to engage families and community members may be effective.
- Approaches to engaging parents in CSPAPs vary widely across studies (both in strategy and dose), and this has made it hard to evaluate the overall effect of FCE.
- Both teachers and parents report a lack of time as a significant barrier to engaging parents or engaging in CSPAP initiatives, respectively.
- Establishing a welcoming and inviting school environment for parents and community members can make it more comfortable for them to participate in CSPAPs.
- To accommodate parents, schools should provide clear instructions for how parents can engage in CSPAP efforts.
- Providing a variety of opportunities for parents to engage in CSPAPs is important for accommodating a variety of times and skills to ensure all parents have an avenue for engagement.
- Communication should be delivered to parents using multiple platforms (e.g., email, school website, social media, and phone calls).
- Parents and community members should be included on the school wellness team to ensure these groups have a voice in developing the school's wellness vision.
- Future research on FCE in CSPAPs necessitates more attention on process and outcome evaluation assessments.

Knowledge Gaps and Directions for Future Research

Important gaps remain to be filled in this line of research. Although a large number of studies have incorporated FCE components in CSPAP applications, few have effectively evaluated the effect that these factors have had on youth's behavior change or precursors to change. There is also a need for more creative ways to engage parents in school activity programming. School leaders often report that it is difficult to engage parents in school programming because pf lack of time (crowded curriculum), resources, and training. Parents indicate that engaging in school programming is difficult because of a lack of time (competing priorities) or understanding what kind of role they could play and how they would get started (Patino-Fernandez et al., 2013). Finding effective ways to engage and invite parents to participate in school PA initiatives is integral to successfully implementing FCE in CSPAPs.

Informational and educational packets and newsletters are the most commonly utilized component to engage families in CSPAP programming. However, there is little objective data on whether parents read newsletters or newsletters influence aspects of CSPAPs (e.g., child participation in CSPAPs, child and family health knowledge, motivation, and child and family behavior changes). Another prevalent strategy of engaging families in CSPAP programming is family and child "homework" assignments. Similar to newsletters, there is no objective data available to inform whether family homework assignments are effective at modifying health-related attributes at either level (child or family). Although studies have integrated this approach (Luepker et al., 1996; Williamson et al., 2007; Young et al., 2006), no study has demonstrated how these tasks specifically influence students' PA.

School seminars, family fitness nights, and health fairs are other frequently used strategies, but attendance is typically low and effects are unclear and difficult to document. The common approach to understanding the "effect" of these events has been to take attendance for students and parents, but it is unclear if attendance alone is effective at facilitating behavior change and how significant or long-lasting any effect might be. One study reporting on family participation and perceptions of family engagement events (Caballero et al., 2003) reported that parents indicated enjoying learning about healthy behaviors at family fun nights and reported that 58

percent of families participated in the events, on average, over a three-year period. This information provides evidence that fun and educational events focused on engaging families in healthy activities may be a useful and effective element of FCE in CSPAPs, but further evaluation and understanding are needed. While in-person events may provide more opportunities for discussion and establishing relationships, online seminars might provide more flexibility to accommodate schedules and reach those parents who may not be likely to attend in-person events.

Research comparing the relative advantage of different strategies to engage parents is particularly important in advancing FCE integration in CSPAPs. In a formative evaluation (Welk et al., 2015), the relative advantages of print versus online communications to promote parent engagement in a school activity promotion project were systematically evaluated. Youth were tasked with completing weekly self-monitoring worksheets of their lifestyle behaviors, but the method of delivery to the home varied. The advantage of the print-based materials (sent directly home) is that parents had them directly available. The advantage of the electronic delivery (through newsletters) is that it was possible to provide reminders and keep parents informed. Results demonstrated higher "tracker" return rates from the print-based schools but no significant differences in parent and child interactions or reported behavior change. This study revealed the challenges of promoting parent involvement and provided an example of a structured comparison that helps to advance understanding of parent engagement methods.

While there is value in additional work with these traditional methods, it would seem timely to prioritize exploration of more contemporary communication channels for engaging parents (e.g., email, social media, and text messaging). Fundamental research is also needed to understand how to build capacity of school leaders to promote parent and community engagement. Research conducted by Epstein and Sanders (2006) pointed out that school leaders are not well trained in how to promote parent engagement. A comprehensive example of how school leaders may be better prepared to interact and engage parents in school programming is provided by Epstein and

Sanders (2006). There are needs for both preservice instruction for new teachers and in-service instruction for existing teachers to promote skills in parent engagement.

The lack of evidence to support the current emphasis of FCE components demonstrates that there is a need for more effective evaluation and implementation methods. The gap could be because of incomplete theories as well as inadequate application of theories to practice. The next section summarizes strategies for applying theory to practice in promoting FCE.

Evidence-Based Recommendations and Applications

Schools want (and need) evidence-based programming to help operationalize and enhance school wellness programming. However, traditional school- and family-based intervention studies rarely get adopted and used in real-world settings. Focused efforts on training schools to implement CSPAP applications have also not proven to be highly effective (Russ et al., 2015). This section provides guidelines and suggestions for more effectively promoting FCE in CSPAP applications. We will first introduce principles of social-ecological models because these models underlie the rationale for targeting multiple levels of influence to have a larger effect. We will then introduce principles of systems theory because they provide a useful way to conceptualize how to promote change in complex sociological systems. Specific suggestions are provided for school staff and community partners because their perspectives, influence, and roles are different.

Social-Ecological Foundations of CSPAP Applications

The use of social-ecological models is widely endorsed in community and public health applications, and it is also the foundation of effective CSPAP applications. Ecological models of health behavior posit that behaviors are influenced by intrapersonal, social and cultural, and physical environmental variables and that targeting multiple levels provides advantages for changing health

behaviors (Sallis & Owen, 2015). The principles of targeting multiple settings and a focus on changing social and physical environments are clearly foundational elements of CSPAP applications; however, it is challenging to operationalize social-ecological models in school-based studies (Elder et al., 2007). Interestingly, the five CSPAP components are typically depicted as five separate entities rather than as an integrated system (CDC, 2013).

The Youth Physical Activity Promotion (YPAP) model provides a useful framework for conceptualizing how school, family, and community influences can harmonize to directly affect youth behaviors (Welk, 1999). The model was based on social-ecological principles and employs constructs from the PRECEDE-PROCEED planning model to enable constructs to be operationalized in flexible ways depending on the setting or application. The predisposing factors are viewed as the primary individual drivers of behavior and include two related constructs from social cognitive theory, which are operationalized as "Is it worth it?" and "Am I able?" Individuals who have positive perceptions related to these constructs would be expected to be predisposed to PA; however, the model also includes direct and indirect pathways from reinforcing and enabling factors (see figure 10.2). Reinforcement can come from a variety of sources, including parents, peers, teachers, and coaches, so the model captures multiple sources of influence on youth behaviors. The enabling factors capture access to resources and environments that are conducive to PA, so the model can capture the independent contributions from school, home, and community environments.

Previous studies have supported the hypothesized links in the YPAP model (Rowe et al., 2007) as well as the overall utility for understanding youth PA behavior (Schaben et al., 2006). Emphasis has been placed on operationalizing and evaluating the predisposing factors, but studies have also directly supported the direct and indirect influences from parental reinforcement on youth activity behavior (Silva et al., 2014; Welk et al., 2003). While not developed with CSPAP applications in mind, the YPAP model provides a useful framework for planning behavior-change programming because it enables factors to be linked in a logic model format. Examples of how the model has been applied in practice are provided in the final section of this chapter.

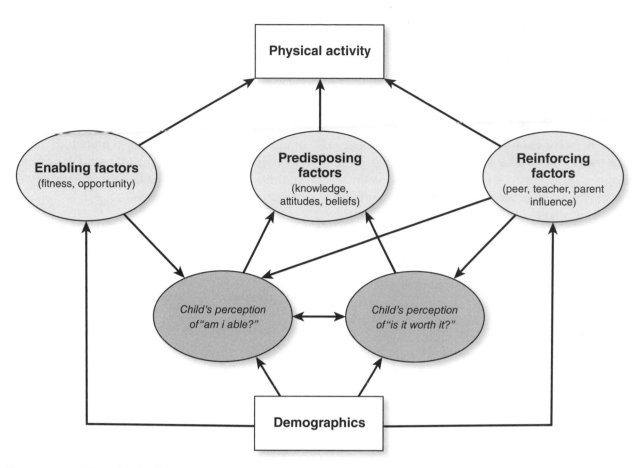

Figure 10.2   Hypothesized interactions between predisposing, enabling, and reinforcing factors in the Youth Physical Activity Promotion model.

Adapted from G.J. Welk, "The Youth Physical Activity Promotion Model: A Conceptual Bridge Between Theory and Practice," *QUEST* 51, no. 1 (1999): 5. Reprinted by permission of the publisher (Taylor & Francis Ltd, http://www.tandfonline.com).

An important caveat about the YPAP model is that, like other models, it only provides a road map to guide the programming. Specific applications of theory are still needed to build the causal paths that lead to behavior change. Specific theory-based strategies that may help to activate the FCE components of CSPAP applications are the focus of the next section.

Application of Systems Theory for Understanding and Enhancing CSPAP Applications

Many applications of social-ecological theory have simply sought to include programming at multiple levels, but the real goal of CSPAP is to promote integration across levels. Thus, rather than independent strategies at multiple levels, it may be more effective to develop effective implementation strategies that can affect multiple levels. This type of approach has been referred to as an "ecological systems perspective" because it captures the dynamic factors that influence complex systems, such as families, schools, and communities, as a whole. Rather than targeting isolated changes, the focus is on linkages, relationships, feedback loops, and interactions among the system's parts (Hawe et al., 2009).

Understanding the context and relationships within a system is the first step to changing it. For example, a system application at the family level (i.e., family systems theory) provides a useful framework to explain how a family system can influence health behaviors (Kitzman-Ulrich et al., 2010). This adaptation suggests that modeling, support, and reinforcement interact within the family system to influence behaviors. However, the nature and strength of relationships are thought to mediate or moderate the influence of support and encouragement of behaviors within the family. As described by Kitzman-Ulrich et al. (2010), behaviors of any one family member may influence the behaviors of any other family member (e.g., a child can influence adult behavior or an adult can influence another adult). Few studies have directly examined family systems theory, but research conducted by Gunawardena and colleagues (2016) provided evidence of the potential for children to act as change agents within families. The results indicated that youth within the study were influential in decreasing weight and increasing PA of their mothers. This application provides a foundational justification for efforts to encourage and empower children to act as change agents in family lifestyles.

While the family systems theory specifically emphasizes interactions within a family, the principles of systems theory can be readily extrapolated and applied to more complex systems, such as schools. In essence, the same elements proposed within the family systems theory can be applied at the school level (e.g., modeling, support, and reinforcement). In families, parent–child and child–sibling relationships are likely stronger (because of genetic factors, culture, and family bonds); however, similar relationships and influences clearly operate within schools. For example, peer influence is important between students in a class as well as between teachers in a school. As adult leaders, teachers also reinforce, enable, and support youth behavior in ways similar to parents'. Thus, to extrapolate the family systems theory to a more general "systems theory" approach, additional tiers simply need to be conceptualized. The "school-level" tier would emphasize the effect of teacher and staff modeling, support, and reinforcement of students' PA behaviors at school (similar to the parallel constructs of family systems theory). Similarly, a "student-level" tier incorporates the effect of students as role models (at school and at home) as well as peer support and reinforcement.

An advantage of systems theory is that it helps explain how small, isolated efforts can contribute to broader change in the system over time. These concepts can be leveraged to drive parallel changes in home and community settings. Social and cultural shifts through these efforts may be hard to detect, but they can have profound effects if they take root. By promoting FCE, schools implementing CSPAPs can capitalize on the added support from families and community partners while also fostering healthy behaviors in home and community settings. The use of systems theory provides a viable approach to developing programming that reaches and influences multiple levels emphasized in social-ecological models. Separate sections follow that explain how schools and community partners can each use this information to enhance CSPAP applications.

Applications for School Staff

Schools clearly value and appreciate involvement from families and community partners but, as described earlier, may not know how to effectively engage or reach them. Families may also not understand the significance of their role in protecting the health of students or how they can be involved in doing so through school systems. By adopting a systems approach, schools can take active steps to create a positive school climate with strong parent and community involvement. Formalized efforts to improve communication with parents is one simple way to promote family engagement, but this can be amplified through intentional efforts to enhance the school and home environment. Schools can train staff to model, support, and encourage healthy PA habits at school and create avenues for incentivizing engagement for students and staff. Schools can also implement programming to train students to model healthy behaviors (to peers and younger students) to encourage others to be active and reinforce positive PA behaviors. Logical extensions would also aim to target community involvement. By incorporating an integrated approach that works through multiple (critically important) ecological levels, interactions can potentially synergize to produce a larger overall effect.

Applications for Community Partners

Research groups and community partners often seek ways to facilitate and support school wellness programming. However, too often the strategies provided are top down and provide little autonomy for schools to coordinate programming in ways that work best in their environment. Adopting a systems perspective can establish a more participatory approach for working with and through schools. Sixteen school-based interventions were reviewed and scored on the degree of capacity building and partner involvement as part of the evaluation (Krishnaswami et al., 2012). Interventions that built local capacity and created equitable partnerships were found to have better outcomes than those that did not embrace those principles. According to Hawe et al. (2009), an intervention "is an event in a system that either leaves a lasting footprint or washes out depending on how well the dynamic properties of the system are harnessed" (p. 270). The point is that traditional top-down interventions have no chance of succeeding unless they are built from the bottom up and in ways that complement and enhance the existing system. The focus of this chapter is on family and community impact and broad systems-based approaches that can help understand the forces that shape and influence connections with both families and community partners. From an evaluation perspective, the model can also aid in understanding the influence that specific intervention elements may have on students' PA behaviors. Applications of FCE and school-system change are described in the following case study on the SWITCH initiative.

SUMMARY

This chapter covered the importance of promoting FCE for CSPAP applications. It also presented systems-based strategies that may prove helpful in both understanding and promoting engagement.

QUESTIONS TO CONSIDER

1. What synergies and motivations may drive parents to want to make a difference in their child's schools?
2. How can students be prompted and empowered to be change agents in their families and communities?
3. What role can parent–teacher organizations play as facilitators or drivers of CSPAP applications?
4. What motivations drive teachers and school leaders to take the extra step to more fully engage parents in the education process and in school activities?
5. What type of community partners and what degree of engagement can best complement school wellness programming?

CASE EXAMPLE: THE SWITCH PROJECT

The previous section summarized the relevance of social-ecological models for CSPAPs and the value of adopting a systems-based approach to creating and supporting change in schools. In this section, examples and insights are given of how systems-based approaches are used to facilitate the adoption, implementation, and maintenance of an evidence-based program called SWITCH. Specific emphasis will be placed on how SWITCH promotes family and community involvement.

Background and History of SWITCH

SWITCH is a multicomponent youth obesity prevention program based on social-ecological principles (Gentile et al., 2009). While not originally developed as a CSPAP application, it clearly incorporates principles consistent with CSPAPs (CDC, 2013) and broader whole-school programming models (Institute of Medicine, 2013). The programming is coordinated through schools, but specific emphasis is placed on affecting both the home and community environments (Eisenmann et al., 2008). Through SWITCH, schools help children to "switch what they do, view and chew." Thus, the programming targets three behaviors: increasing PA, decreasing screen time, and increasing daily consumption of fruits and vegetables.

The original controlled efficacy study demonstrated potential of the SWITCH program for childhood obesity prevention (Gentile et al., 2009). Compared with children in control schools, children in treatment schools had significantly larger reductions in screen time and greater increases in fruit and vegetable consumption at the postmeasurement and six-month follow-up (compared to children in control schools). However, the high cost of the program modules ($60 per child) imposed limitations on any dissemination efforts. Formalized partnerships with regional YMCA hubs were explored as a potential strategy to facilitate implementation in schools, but a limitation of this approach was that schools (and teachers) tended to rely on the YMCAs to run the program and never really bought into the programming. Not surprisingly, results from a formative evaluation demonstrated that more engaged schools had stronger outcomes (Welk et al., 2015). To promote broader dissemination, it became apparent that new approaches were needed. Through a US Department of Agriculture–funded study, the focus shifted to an emphasis on building and supporting school engagement so that schools can manage SWITCH programming on their own. Schools are still provided with resources to run SWITCH, but their priority with this rebranded version is to build capacity for system change.

The logic model used to guide the dissemination of SWITCH is shown in figure 10.3. Consistent with the YPAP model described earlier, youth behaviors are targeted for change through specific predisposing, enabling, and reinforcing factors. The FCE components of this CSPAP application are primarily from the reinforcing factors (parent and teacher encouragement) and enabling factors (healthy home and school environments). The desired synergy between the school and home environments is depicted with the dark, double-headed arrow. The arrow is intentionally double headed (i.e., reciprocal) because the home and school components should reinforce each other to create stronger overall effects. As previously described, few multicomponent CSPAP applications have been shown to produce additive benefits, but this may be because of a lack of integration in these components. In the present iteration of SWITCH, school engagement is expected to drive parent engagement, and both will synergize to promote student interest and engagement in the programming.

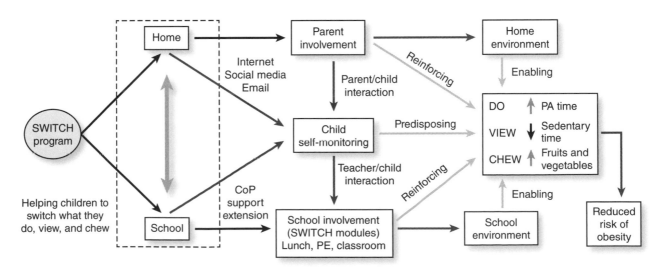

Figure 10.3 Logic model for SWITCH depicting synergistic and additive benefits of integrated school and family programming.

Application of Systems Theory to Promote School and Family Engagement

The SWITCH implementation framework is based on an established school training developed through the Healthy Youth Places (HYP) project (Dzewaltowski et al., 2009) and further refined in the HOP'N after-school project (Dzewaltowski et al., 2010). These projects predated the conception of CSPAP applications, but they used innovative methods to promote PA and healthy eating in schools. In this case, emphasis was placed on directly building the capacity of existing school leaders to create healthy environments. The SWITCH adaptation of this model involves local coordination by a team of three school wellness leaders who work within their school system to implement programming. Schools receive preliminary training on the basics of the SWITCH philosophy, but consistent with the HYP model, the focus is on building school capacity for school change.

A novel aspect of the adapted SWITCH training method is that it uses principles of motivational interviewing (MI) to promote autonomy and ownership of school-system change. MI is an established strategy widely used for individual behavior-change applications, such as health coaching. However, in SWITCH it has had similar utility for promoting school change. Through monthly checkpoint sessions, schools are encouraged to plan programming that works best within their own school system. The sessions encourage a "continuous quality improvement" approach so that schools learn from past efforts and build capacity over time. The emphasis is placed on promoting competence, autonomy, and relatedness because these constructs are fundamental predictors of intrinsic motivation. Thus, the inherent goal of SWITCH training is to promote independence and motivation to facilitate school-system change that targets improved school wellness.

Consistent with the systems theory methods described earlier, school SWITCH leaders are encouraged to work within their own school network to promote broader interest and involvement across the school. The internal promotion and organic networking within the school help to bring interest and involvement for SWITCH programming in physical education, classroom, and lunchroom settings. For example, classroom teachers are more likely to adopt and use a CSPAP aimed at classroom activity breaks when the ideas percolate up and are supported through the school rather than externally from a research team. SWITCH leaders are also encouraged to establish a youth leadership team to get students engaged and involved in the planning and promotional efforts. These youth advocacy hubs are strengthened through a formal partnership with the state 4H program, which has extensive experience in promoting positive youth development. While not a required element, the advantage of the 4H integration is that it also helps schools to tap into local county extension leaders for additional support. This helps to bring other community-based resources and energy to the programming.

The SWITCH program is still evolving, but the use of sound theories and models has been important for effectively engaging families and community partners. The emphasis on professional development and capacity building in the schools is also consistent with recommendations for promote broader community and school coordination of CSPAP applications (Webster et al., 2015). Iterative evaluation cycles will allow training methods, web tools, and implementation strategies to be refined over time. However, our experience is that efforts to promote FCE in CSPAP applications can have synergistic benefits (as depicted in figure 10.1). Consistent with CSPAP visions, the SWITCH program is managed by the school but is powered by (and dependent on) strong FCE.

CHAPTER 11

Multicomponent Optimization Strategy and CSPAP Implementation

Ashley Phelps, MPE
The University of Texas at Austin

Yeonhak Jung, MS
The University of Texas at Austin

Darla M. Castelli, PhD
The University of Texas at Austin

In 2013, education and health experts united to develop the Whole School, Whole Community, Whole Child (WSCC) conceptual model (see figure 11.1) as a collaborative approach that acknowledges learning and health (Lewallen et al., 2015). Within the WSCC model, schools develop policy and provide opportunities for students to engage in health-enhancing learning experiences, such as participation in PA that is offered through a variety of forums. Implementing a CSPAP is one approach that is supported by the infrastructure of the WSCC model because it recommends school-wide measures to increase PA opportunities for students, staff, and community members in and around the school setting (Beets et al., 2009).

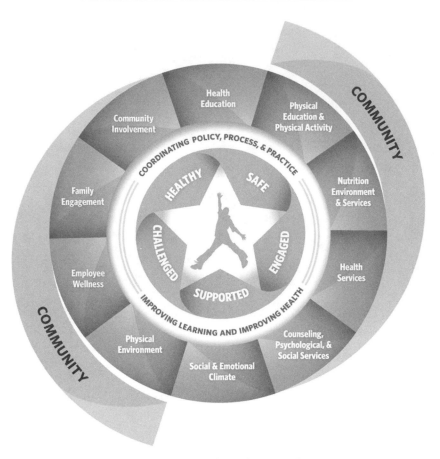

Figure 11.1 Whole School, Whole Community, Whole Child framework.

Reprinted from ASCD, 2014, *Whole School, Whole Community, Whole Child: A Collaborative Approach to Learning and Health.* Available: http://www.ascd.org/permissions.aspx.

A CSPAP is both the process of coordinated thinking and the implementation of a multicomponent approach that can be used to promote a variety of PA throughout and beyond the school day and a feasible means of increasing PA in both youth and adults. A CSPAP is intended to maximize physical education learning outcomes and provide opportunities for application. Although a CSPAP is a practical model that helps students accumulate 60 minutes or more of PA throughout the day, the status of research related to the simultaneous implementation of all five CSPAP components (physical education, PA during school, PA before and after school, staff involvement, family and community engagement) is scarce. There are, however, a multitude of studies that discuss the

implications and experiences of physical educators and classroom teachers applying one or two of the CSPAP components within their prospective schools (Chen et al., 2014; McMullen et al., 2014). Given the lack of consensus as to how to best advance implementation, teacher leaders need help in simultaneously fulfilling each of the five CSPAP components. Inevitably, barriers will be encountered and will need to be overcome.

In this chapter, we review the research, propose knowledge claims based on this research, and identify knowledge gaps. Specifically, we make recommendations for future research on the Multiphase Optimization Strategy (MOST) framework and how it can be used to help school staff and community members carry out a more efficient and sustainable CSPAP. Moreover, we make recommendations from the existing research for coordinated school health initiatives, CSPAP implementation, and barriers to overcome regarding a CSPAP by using a public health framework (MOST) that supports a CSPAP. We also provide two case examples of successful school staff and community member–led CSPAP implementation utilizing the MOST framework. Furthermore, we elaborate on MOST's application to public health behavioral change. Behavioral interventions, such as MOST, can help to address the subtleties within each of the CSPAP components by evaluating them through a variety of dynamic systems that support the delivery of the program elements. One benefit of this comprehensive framework is that it considers the ideal criterion and limitations of each CSPAP component as well as the contextual differences between schools. Before exploring this implementation model, let's review some of the evidence that supports the WSCC and CSPAP models.

Review of Research

Coordinated school health initiatives have been around since the early 20th century (Institute of Medicine, 2005, 2013). It was not until recently that the CSPAP application emerged to develop a school climate that was favorable for the promotion of PA throughout the life span by incorporating its five, essential components (Centers for Disease Control and Prevention [CDC], 2013; National Association for Sport and Physical Education [NASPE], 2008). Since the introduction of this coordinated approach, there has been an emergence of studies done on its behalf. Interestingly, CSPAP research has mainly been conducted by component; that is, to the best of our knowledge, there has yet to be an experimental study of multiple schools in which there was confirmed implementation of all five components. In the prior chapters, you have read about each of the five CSPAP components: (1) quality physical education (chapter 6), (2) PA during school (chapter 7), (3) PA before and after school (chapter 8), (4) staff involvement (chapter 9), and (5) family and community engagement (chapter 10). In this section, we will discuss the WSCC and each CSPAP component and its place

in the literature and how it has been prioritized during implementation.

WSCC Framework

The WSCC conceptual model places the child at the center of ecological change while involving families and communities to improve and maintain the psychological and physical environments that are necessary to bring about health-enhancing behavioral change. With an emphasis on coordination of policy, process, and practice, the WSCC is an advancement from previous approaches because it considers the daily routines of teachers and students in schools. The WSCC organizational structure allows for the enhanced alignment, integration, and collaboration between education and health sectors. Overall, the WSCC emphasizes a community approach to health, with schools functioning as a critical member of that society.

In a study that looked at the implementation of health initiatives through multicomponent comprehensive and coordinated school approaches, self-reported data was collected from 1,031 school administrators in a nationally representative sample. Findings indicated that only 7 percent of middle school and 1 percent of high school students attended schools offering CSPAPs (Colabianchi et al., 2015). Students who were enrolled in schools with multicomponent programs, like CSPAPs, were significantly more physically active than those students in schools that implemented only a single component. Although the prevalence of multicomponent programs is low, there is definite evidence to support the implementation of such programs. By offering at least three components, such as daily physical education, PA during school (e.g., recess, PA in the classroom), and before- and after-school programming, schools are more likely to have students who participate in the recommended 60 minutes of moderate-to-vigorous PA (MVPA; Bassett et al., 2013).

Briefly, when schools implement a multicomponent program, like a CSPAP, it provides additional benefits beyond those gained by students in schools that offer only physical education or physical education and one other component. As such, schools can elect to implement a CSPAP sequentially by adding opportunities through each component (e.g., bringing back recess and adding PA breaks during the school day) or by holistically considering the CSPAP as a process that requires a cultural shift within the school. A review of this multicomponent approach will be discussed in the following section.

Multicomponent interventions have been deemed more effective when compared to single component interventions (CDC, 2013). Moreover, although studies on multicomponent approaches utilizing a CSPAP framework are still in their infancy, there are a handful of studies that have examined the effects of a CSPAP and the implementation of all five of its components. While multicomponent approaches are ideal, they are often hard to achieve because of a multitude of factors (e.g., environmental, cultural, and structural). A review of MOST will also be discussed to help school staff and community members carry out and maintain an efficient CSPAP.

Research on Multicomponent CSPAP Interventions

In a 36-week multicomponent study, cardio-metabolic measures (e.g., triglycerides and high-density lipoproten [HDL] and low-density lipoproten [LDL] cholesterol) were taken from 217 school-aged children at pre– and post–CSPAP intervention (Burns, Brusseau, & Hannon, 2017). This study took place at five low-income elementary schools. As part of the staff, each school had a PA leader (PAL) who worked with teachers and students on how to increase PA throughout and beyond the school day. A PAL is someone who has received training in CSPAPs and is well versed on how to put PA into educational practice. Often, the PAL is the physical education teacher; however, for this particular study, the PAL was an hourly paraprofessional. Some of the PAL's responsibilities included instructing quality physical education, educating classroom teachers on the importance of PA in the classroom, and opening up the gym and facilities before and after school for students to drop in and be active. The PAL offered professional development opportunities for both classroom teachers and physical educators to ensure that the implementation of PA at school was developmentally appropriate. At the end of the intervention, HDL cholesterol

and triglycerides had statistically improved over matched control participants. Changes in health markers were attributed to the enhancement of PA throughout the school day (Burns, Brusseau, & Hannon, 2017).

Similarly, in another study, goal setting and cardiorespiratory endurance were measured in multicomponent CSPAP schools (Burns, Brusseau, & Fu, 2017). A total of 1,618 school-aged children were recruited from five urban schools. Each of the schools had adequate facilities (e.g., large grassy areas, gym space, playgrounds, and blacktop areas) for the CSPAP. A PAL was employed at each school to operationalize the CSPAP organizational structure. The PAL worked closely with the school leaders in setting district-wide goals for faculty and staff to increase PA across the day in hopes of strengthening student engagement and decreasing off-task behavior. Classroom teachers were encouraged to incorporate three 10-minute PA sessions throughout the school day. Recess included semistructured activities, like the ones taught in physical education, so students could apply the skills they learned during their quality physical education lessons. Anytime students had the opportunity to sit, they were encouraged to stand.

Goal-setting strategies included setting daily step counts while at school, standing or moving rather than sitting, and setting individual fitness goals. Step counts were measured using pedometers, and cardiorespiratory endurance was measured using the Progressive Aerobic Cardiovascular Endurance Run (PACER) test. After randomizing children into goal-setting and non–goal-setting groups, there was a significant increase in PA and cardiorespiratory endurance in children who were part of the goal-setting group compared to children in the non–goal-setting group. In conclusion, at the end of a 36-week period, the goals set forth by the PAL maximized the PA efforts of the children in the goal-setting group. More specifically, on average, sixth-graders increased their PACER results by 15.3 laps. Goal setting by a PAL within a CSPAP context leads to greater increases in school-day PA and cardiorespiratory endurance (Burns, Brusseau, & Fu, 2017).

The effects of a multicomponent CSPAP intervention on PA and health-related fitness were examined in 1,390 children utilizing a pre- and posttest design (Brusseau et al., 2016). PA measures were taken at baseline (1 week before CSPAP enactment) and 6 and 12 weeks after implementation. Each of the three schools within this study had a PAL. As soon as children got to school, they would put on a pedometer and wear it until the end of the school day (Monday through Friday). Health-related fitness measurements included body mass index (BMI) measures, PACER test, and FitnessGram push-up and curl-up tests. Before the CSPAP intervention, there were no structured activities during recess, physical education was taught within a traditional context (e.g., teacher centered and increased wait time), and there were no activity breaks or before-school PA programs. Measures at the end of the CSPAP intervention included significant increases in step counts (603.1 steps) and MVPA (4.9 minutes) when compared to baseline measures. There were also statistically significant increases in PACER laps (6.5 laps), push-ups (1.2 repetitions), and curl-ups (3.4 repetitions). Briefly, PA and health-related fitness standards significantly increased when compared to baseline.

Centeio, McCaughtry, and colleagues (2014) conducted a study that looked at overall changes in students', teachers' and administrators', and parents' PA levels at the end of an eight-month CSPAP program. Four of the five CSPAP components were delivered simultaneously across six urban elementary schools. Each school had a CSPAP coordinator, who educated school staff on the importance of PA and supported schools in their CSPAP endeavors. Physical education teachers were trained to offer quality physical education lessons across the content of the curriculum. Classroom teachers were provided with ideas about PA in the classroom and how to incorporate them into lesson content. Teachers kept a daily log of the integrated activities. Active recess was also encouraged by offering a variety of equipment for students to be active, game cards (e.g., cards that summarized what was taught in physical education), and active supervision. Each of the six schools offered an after-school program that included a healthy snack, walking segments, and fun games. A total of 344 fourth-grade students, 260 parents, 22 fourth-grade teachers, and 12 administrators participated in this study. Student

PA measures were collected using accelerometers, and adult PA measures were self-reported by completing the International Physical Activity Questionnaire (IPAQ). Comparison of before and after data resulted in a significant increase in child MVPA (by 58 percent) as well as a significant increase in daily metabolic equivalent (MET) for teachers (17 percent) and parents (57 percent), thus evidencing improvement in both child and parent behaviors.

The multicomponent studies reviewed thus far have taken place during the school year. One study examined the effects of summer break on PA in children from CSPAP schools (Fu et al., 2017). Measures of school-day PA, BMI, and PACER were analyzed. It was anticipated that summer break might affect PA behaviors in children because of hot temperatures and the lack of direct support for PA opportunities, thus hindering or regressing the health benefits acquired from those who attended CSPAP schools. Participants included 1,232 school-aged children from a total of three schools. Measures were collected at the end of the first CSPAP year and the beginning of the second CSPAP year. Daily, pedometer step counts decreased over the summer by 484 steps, and PACER laps decreased by 5.4 laps. Overall, the benefits gained from a multicomponent CSPAP intervention may be lost during the summer months when children are out of school. Before data collection, this CSPAP intervention increased PA by four minutes per day, steps by 600 per day, and PACER laps by 6.5 laps. Results from this study indicated that long-term adherence to a CSPAP and its health benefits might be at risk during summer breaks (Fu et al., 2017). Collectively, these studies suggest that CSPAP implementation is influenced by the context as well as the ability to deliver direct support for PA opportunities; as such, the public health intervention approach of MOST is worthy of consideration.

Using MOST to Overcome Barriers to CSPAP Implementation

At the beginning of this chapter, we briefly introduced a public health framework that systematically optimizes multicomponent interventions. Specifically, adherence to a framework determines what should be revised, replaced, and discarded.

The MOST can help both school staff and community members identify barriers related to various CSPAP components and attempt to include or modify them by looking at the need for and the success of the component. Moreover, the MOST is a framework for developing, evaluating, and optimizing field-based behavioral interventions (Collins et al., 2005, 2011, 2014). The origin of this underlying principle came from engineering science. To produce prototypes, engineers typically first conduct experiments to investigate how to solve a problem (e.g., reduced air quality might require better ventilation). Ultimately, the investigation is intended to build prototypes (e.g., create a low-cost self-test kit for air quality) and increase the efficiency of the response (e.g., what are the options now that we know there is poor air quality). With continued trials, the best and most promising approaches emerge. Application of the MOST approach might help school staff to facilitate a cultural shift to one that is more health-oriented by hosting a series of events or trying new events to see how well they fit in the context (e.g., lunch before recess; a walking school bus; or a Zumba, bike, and broccoli wellness day) before fully committing the resources required to embed an idea as part of the school curriculum.

Analogous to the CSPAP implementation, the development of smaller prototypes might mean that teachers try to integrate one or two smaller ideas at the beginning of the school year, as opposed to attempting to address all five components of the CSPAP at once. For example, students get to bring bags of equipment out to recess and play student-led games that they have already learned during PE. If a barrier is encountered, then a school staff or community member could help to overcome the barrier (e.g., equipment was used once and lost or broken and parent–teacher organization [PTO] purchases equipment for each classroom). At the end of the year, the teachers or parents decide if the activity, representing the CSPAP component of during-school recess, was worth the investment. This example is one possible starting point regarding how to apply the MOST framework. Since the MOST process has been utilized for years in areas of engineering, manufacturing, and public health (Baker et al., 2016; Collins et al., 2007, 2011; Pellegrini et al., 2014; Strecher et al., 2008), we believe the MOST

can be applied to CSPAP components to establish which activities or components in the entire comprehensive PA plan are most practical and optimal in a given school or context.

MOST interventions are meant to be both broad and convenient because what constitutes a CSPAP can vary by school. The strategy is a sequence of steps to help teachers, administrators, and community members make decisions about resources and needs with the ultimate goal of discovering the most appropriate program within a given context. The MOST approach is intended to affect efficacy, effectiveness, and cost effectiveness. The latest version of this comprehensive framework has three phases of implementation: preparation, optimization, and evaluation (Collins et al., 2014; figure 11.2).

Preparation Phase

The objective of the preparation phase is to lay the groundwork for multicomponent implementation and optimization of a PA intervention. Conducting a literature review, identifying related health theories, and examining existing data (e.g., FitnessGram data from students) should be undertaken in this phase. If the teachers are not used to completing these tasks, then a school–university partnership could be formed, whereby the university faculty carries out the initial steps in this phase. Teachers can visit another CSPAP, contact teachers who are already implementing a CSPAP, and participate in online forums. As a professional development activity, the teachers could use the *Let's Move!* Active Schools Assessment Guide (Active Schools, 2014) to evaluate the current degree to which the CSPAP is being implemented.

The preparation phase determines which components of the CSPAP, beyond quality physical education, will be implemented. During preparation, teachers should conduct a self-assessment to identify the following information: What are school staff already doing that fits into the CSPAP structure? What school traditions should be kept? Who should be involved in the school–university partnership? What PA program do the students like the most? After the "keepers" are identified, a critical analysis must be conducted to pinpoint what needs to be changed or added to the CSPAP. Teachers can do this by asking the following questions: Which program components are coun-

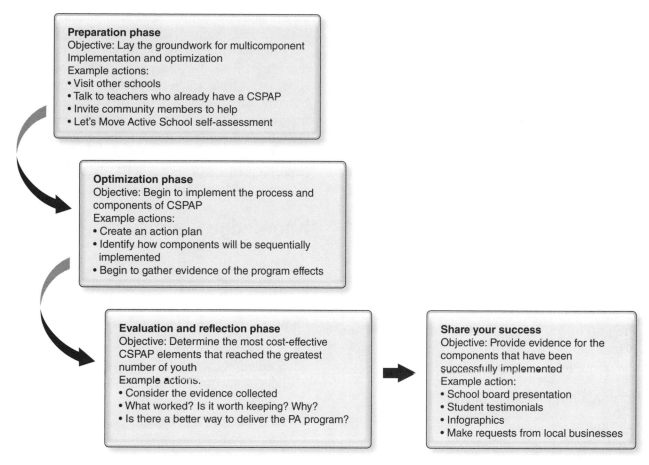

Preparation phase
Objective: Lay the groundwork for multicomponent
Implementation and optimization
Example actions:
• Visit other schools
• Talk to teachers who already have a CSPAP
• Invite community members to help
• Let's Move Active School self-assessment

Optimization phase
Objective: Begin to implement the process and
components of CSPAP
Example actions:
• Create an action plan
• Identify how components will be sequentially
  implemented
• Begin to gather evidence of the program effects

Evaluation and reflection phase
Objective: Determine the most cost-effective
CSPAP elements that reached the greatest
number of youth
Example actions.
• Consider the evidence collected
• What worked? Is it worth keeping? Why?
• Is there a better way to deliver the PA program?

Share your success
Objective: Provide evidence for the
components that have been
successfully implemented
Example action:
• School board presentation
• Student testimonials
• Infographics
• Make requests from local businesses

Figure 11.2 Phases of the MOST.

Modified from Collins et al. (2007); Collins et al. (2014).

terproductive and should be discarded? Which programs are underenrolled or too costly? What concerns did the classroom teachers have about PA in the classroom? The implementation team needs to identify the main reasons that children in this context do and do not participate in PA.

Although there are grand tendencies to reconstruct educational systems, the application of the MOST for implementing a CSPAP is intended to be practical, not burdensome. The first phase of MOST can be enacted by an individual within school, by a group of physical education teachers in a school district, by a school wellness team, or through a newly formed school–university partnership. The makeup of the group does not matter as much as the considerations and determinations that need to be decided before a CSPAP can be implemented. Often, teachers see something new and want to implement the activity in the next lesson. Applying a CSPAP is a process, not

a single event. As expressed previously in the existing research, early adopters of the CSPAP identified planning, supportive administration, and sustained passion as keys to successful implementation of a CSPAP.

Optimization Phase

The optimization phase involves finalizing the selection of PA opportunities within a given component and developing an action plan for subsequent implementation. This is a time to gather evidence of the effectiveness and quality of CSPAP components that are already in place. The physical education teacher and critical community partners need to create an action plan and timeline for implementing the PA events by component. Once this is complete, the teacher, with help from others, needs to gather evidence of the program's effectiveness (e.g., How many students participated in the program? How did the classroom teachers respond to the PA break request? What barriers did the teachers and students face?).

When a teacher wanted to begin a bike and walk to school program, she first contacted the director of the Safe Routes to School program in her city. Together, they began an active transportation program that included a walking school bus, an annual bike and helmet safe day, a bike rodeo, parent crossing guards, and a microchip check-in program. The governmental agency had the data and some resources to share, and the teacher could gain access to parent volunteers. Together, the partnership resulted in neighborhood children participating in PA before and after school. The teacher recorded the average number of bikes in the bike racks, informally interviewed students at the bike rodeo, and presented the results of the program at the end of the year to the school board. In return, the PTO gave the teacher more resources for the program's continuation.

Evaluation and Reflection Phase

The question is, did the program accomplish what it set out to accomplish? The objective of the evaluation and reflection phase is to identify what the most cost-effective, meaningful tenets of the CSPAP are. Simply put, which activities have the most reach and work the best? Reflective thinking is a critical element of our professional practice because this deliberation brings about new learnings (Danielson, 2009). In accordance with Danielson's recommendations, there are four modes of thinking, which range from lower- to higher-level thinking: (1) technological thinking (e.g., Did the PA program adhere to school district policies?), (2) situational thinking (e.g., Was PA provided at the right time? Did the theme of the field day align with the students' interests?), (3) dialectical thinking (e.g., In the moment, was it the right thing for the teacher to permit PA participation without notifying the parents?), and (4) refining the skill of reflection (e.g., What else do we need?). The final mode of reflection is meant to develop mindful decision-making habits.

Pellegrini and colleagues (2014) conducted one research example of a program evaluation in which they investigated the effectiveness of a weight loss intervention over a six-month period.

This prospective study intended to examine which of the five intervention components or component levels was the most meaningful and cost effective regarding the desired outcome of weight loss. This study was significant because it was the first field-based obesity program to use this approach. Like the practice of teaching, one needs to reflect on the effectiveness of a CSPAP. If the program is not cost effective and does not attract many students to participate in safe, positive PA, then an alternative activity should be considered.

Knowledge Claims

The research reviewed in the previous section of this chapter provides the basis for several knowledge claims about implementing multicomponent PA programs through schools.

- A multicomponent approach to children's PA promotion can lead to statistically significant improvements in health markers.
- Goal setting by a PAL resulted in significant increases in PA and cardiorespiratory endurance among children in the goal-setting group compared to those in the non–goal-setting group.
- Goal setting can maximize PA participation throughout the school day.
- When compared to baseline measures, there were significant increases in step counts and MVPA upon implementation of a multicomponent CSPAP.
- HRF measurements increased significantly when compared to measures taken before the implementation of a multicomponent CSPAP.
- Significant increases in PACER laps, push-ups, and curl-ups were observed.
- In schools that incorporated four of the five components, student MVPA increased with a CSPAP intervention.
- Teachers and parents also significantly increased their overall MET per minute, which resulted in a bidirectional effect with students.
- Time out of school during the summer may hinder the long-term benefits of a CSPAP intervention.

- Time out of school during the summer was attributed to a decrease in steps and PACER laps.
- The MOST approach can be analyzed to develop, evaluate, and optimize a multicomponent CSPAP.
- The MOST can be applied to each of the CSPAP components for optimal PA behaviors because it can identify critical points in which PA can be increased and promoted within a CSPAP framework.
- The MOST approach consists of three implementation phases: preparation, optimization, and evaluation and reflection.

Knowledge Gaps and Directions for Future Research

Regarding the application of a CSPAP, there are still gaps in our knowledge that need to be addressed. Specifically, we need to secure empirical evidence about (1) how best to prepare future physical education teachers and teacher educators to embrace their evolving roles; (2) the format and delivery of professional development for physical education and generalist teachers; and (3) how to inform administrators about the importance and process of WSCC models, such as a CSPAP (Goc Karp et al., 2014). Although seminal (Castelli & Beighle, 2007; Beighle et al., 2009) and targeted articles (Goc Karp et al., 2014) have been organized in several special features by the *Journal of Physical Education, Recreation & Dance* and have appeared in journals, empirical evidence of multicomponent and process implementation of CSPAPs is scarce. Even less is known about how the application of the MOST may further advance the reach and depth of comprehensive programming in schools.

Evidenced-Based Recommendations and Applications

Because the implementation of a CSPAP is complex, multicomponent approaches must be a shared responsibility of all school staff and community members (Centeio, Erwin, et al., 2014; Doolittle & Rukavina, 2014). Our recommendations surrounding the application of the evidence will focus specifically on how staff and community members can help to facilitate implementation of CSPAPs, using the MOST approach.

For School Staff

It is critical for school administrators, physical educators, and generalist teachers to promote health throughout a multicomponent CSPAP; however, school staff members may not have the time or the skills to enact the preparation and optimization phases of the MOST. A school–university partnership could facilitate implementation of a multicomponent CSPAP by providing access to evidence-based strategies through professional development (Castelli et al., 2013). One health theory that has been suggested to explain and carry out the multiple stages involved in the process of implementation is the diffusion of innovations theory (Glowacki et al., 2016). Focused on communication across all involved parties, the theory suggests that a CSPAP is perceived as a novel innovation, and then it evolves through contextually based development, adoption, and implementation, whereby sustainability can ultimately be achieved. A study of 256 health and physical education teachers suggested that the degree of CSPAP implementation was significantly predicted by a teacher's ability to promote PA to the students, other teachers, and school administrators, thus confirming the importance of the role of the physical education teacher. However, an overreliance on physical education teachers' implementing all the components by themselves is an unreasonable expectation for many teachers, particularly novices. A school–university partnership could assist physical education teachers as well as provide meaningful and relevant professional development opportunities for school staff.

Professional development comes in many forms. School–university partnerships are one way in which learning can occur among the preservice teachers (undergraduate students who are preparing to become teachers), cooperating teachers, and university faculty, alike (Castelli et al., 2012). Schools with an exemplary CSPAP could serve as a professional development venue, where educators and university faculty can visit and learn how successful implementation was achieved. Further, the notion of self-assessment of readiness and adapting the CSPAP to the contextual and cultural needs of the school community is paramount. Using the MOST may help to formalize the implementation process and lead to increased effectiveness with the application of multicomponent CSPAPs and school–university partnerships.

Shared leadership approaches also have the potential to influence feasibility, fidelity, and sustainability of a CSPAP. In a school–university partnership, preservice teachers could visit a public school to help conduct fitness assessments at the end of the school year. This data could be stored and interpreted to determine the needs of the students by grade, track student progress toward their goals, and plan future lessons. By having the preservice teachers work with the K-6 students, the objective of conducting a fitness assessment on and setting goals for all children in grades 3-6 suddenly became feasible. Because the preservice teachers were trained on how to use the FitnessGram, the assessments were valid. Figure 11.3 displays some data collected during an ongoing school–university partnership established over four years. The data was used to help the students set PA goals, which was initially part of the preparation phase but over the years has transitioned to be part of the optimization and reflection phases of the MOST approach. Practicing teachers used the data to reflect on their instructional practice about the health-related fitness of children.

Briefly, professional development and shared leadership can be fostered through school–university partnerships. Given the faculty expertise and resources available at a university, this partnership is well positioned to assist with using the MOST approach, specifically by helping with the preparation and optimization phases.

For Community Partners

Although the evidence is not quite as well established in the literature as that for school–university partnerships, the inclusion of community partners also has merit, especially when attempting to address multiple components. Like the school–university partnerships, community partners can help with implementing distinct elements of the CSPAP. Local businesses can provide equipment, resources, training, and outlets beyond the school day for individuals to participate in PA.

As previously stated, the implementation of a multicomponent CSPAP can result in significantly higher step counts and total PA among students compared to students who attend a school with one or two components or no CSPAP. Despite these gains during the school year, we know that such increases can be lost when students are out of school and in the summer, when the weather is warmer and there are fewer direct supports for children to be physically active. Youth organizations offer programs that can help to fill this void when school is not in session. By offering PA programming and safe places to be active during warm weather, organizations, such as DrumFIT, YMCA, and Boys & Girls Clubs, can also have a role in MOST approaches (see chapter 8 regarding after-school PA programs). In summary, both formal (i.e., school–university) and informal (i.e., organization) partnerships can play a vital role in providing opportunities for children to participate in daily PA.

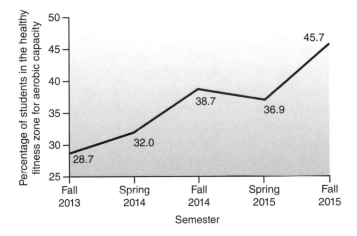

Figure 11.3   **Student data collected as part of a school–university partnership (these data are based on the 7th grade average).**

SUMMARY

As an example of WSCC, comprehensive programs, such as CSPAPs, help to coordinate thinking and increase fidelity of program implementation. Using the MOST, which outlines phases focused on preparation, optimization, and evaluation and reflection of the implementation of a new program or initiative, is intended to increase efficacy, effectiveness, and cost effectiveness. Specifically, comprehensive efforts should target the coordination between policy, practice, and student learning experiences, such as community-based opportunities to participate in PA. Sharing the responsibility of enactment across multiple stakeholders, who include pre- and in-service teachers, administrators, and community members, is a contemporary approach to offering effective physical education programming in today's educational climate.

QUESTIONS TO CONSIDER

1. Think of a school that you attended as a student. Using the MOST, consider how involving the school staff could be the first step toward implementation of a CSPAP.

2. WSCC focuses on the coordination of policy, process, and practice. How can we consider the daily routines of teachers and students in schools to best prepare them to recruit other staff and community members to get involved in the implementation of a CSPAP?

3. Because comprehensive, multicomponent approaches result in high student PA, what ideas do you have about how community members can contribute to a CSPAP at a school near you?

4. How might the MOST framework be utilized across different school contexts within a single school district? How might implementation across such schools focus on unique points of emphasis from the perspective of a community member?

5. What steps can be taken by school staff to enact a cultural shift within the school that identifies the CSPAP as a WSCC process or a health-first way of thinking?

CASE EXAMPLES

This chapter includes two case examples.

School–University Zumba, Bike, and Broccoli Wellness Day

This case represents an authentic application of the MOST approach to planning and carrying out a wellness day using a school–university partnership. Valleyview School District has 86,000 students enrolled in 146 schools, across grades K-12. During a one-day professional development workshop, the district physical education teachers decided to have a wellness day focused on PA and healthy eating. Mohamed Kou, a physical education teacher in his 10th year at Valleyview Middle School (2,500 students in grades 6-8), was identified as the host of the first event. After a model was established, it would then be rolled out in other middle schools during the same academic school year. Knowing that planning and carrying out a wellness day would require a lot of help, Mr. Kou contacted the local university, where he had attended a professional development workshop and previously hosted a student teacher. Having an established relationship with the university people who place preservice teachers for field experiences made the request easy to fill.

Valleyview Middle School is a Title I school in which 63 percent of the student body successfully passed the state standardized achievement tests last year. Only 41 percent of the students passed the language arts achievement tests because the student body had a high proportion of English language learners. Valleyview was known for having a quality physical education program, bike and walk to school programs, and strong athletic teams.

During the preparation phase, the Valleyview teachers and university faculty and students met and collectively recruited local businesses and government agencies to contribute to the wellness day (e.g., United States Dairy Association (USDA) had an office in the major metropolitan area). The preservice teachers sent an email to the USDA to invite an educational outreach representative to the wellness event. Furthermore, the local hospital was currently launching a campaign focused on healthy relationships, more specifically, how family support could enhance academic success and reduce health risks. The Valleyview and preservice teachers planned the entire event as a service learning project through a course assignment administered by the university. The single-evening event consisted of Zumba, offered by a community member; a bike rodeo; healthy eating sampler; and an exhibits area where parents could secure resources.

The optimization phase was primarily focused on the event itself. All participants were asked to check in and provide email addresses and a brief rationale on why they attended the event. Preservice teachers facilitated the event while Valleyview teachers involved their students and parents in each of the activities that were provided. In the bike rodeo, local public works and Safe Routes to School repaired bikes; taught safety lessons; conducted a bike giveaway to 10 students; and had the students participate in challenges on their bikes, scooters, and skateboards. At the end of the event, businesses and government agencies were asked if they would attend the event again and whether they had achieved their outreach goals. Gathering evidence from the perspective of all stakeholders and soliciting their recommendations for future iterations of the event are essential parts of the optimization phase.

Reflection and evaluation, as part of the final phase of the MOST, were conducted on behalf of a subcommittee of preservice teachers from the university, hospital personnel, community stakeholders, and parents, hosted by the city's Parks and Recreation Department. This phase was the most beneficial because people reflected on the quality and effectiveness of the event (e.g., it inspired people to make healthy choices, it was fun being around our neighbors, or the children enjoyed seeing their friends outside of school). While business representatives had a chance to advertise the healthy items that they had on their menus, they also had the chance to discuss new classes that they were offering (e.g., karate, judo, gymnastics, and learn-to-swim classes). This shared space and the mutually beneficial event were initiated by preservice teachers who are preparing to become the physical educators of the 21st century.

Community Members Driving Policy Supporting the Implementation of CSPAPs

In Texas, every school district is mandated to have a School Health Advisory Council (SHAC), whose members oversee the implementation of coordinated school health initiatives as outlined in the district wellness policy. The Texas legislation preceded the development of the WSCC framework and CSPAP model, but it is intended to achieve similar goals by providing opportunities for children to participate in PA. This example takes place in an urban area in Central Texas at an elementary school of 1,000 students in grades pre–K-5 and outlines by phase a factual undertaking using the MOST approach.

Ms. Tina Alverz, mother of three children who attend Peyton Place Elementary School, while volunteering at the school witnessed her son, Javier, being withheld from recess.

Javier was asked to sit on the sidewalk edge and watch his classmates playing instead of being active at recess. When Ms. Alverz inquired as to why Javier was asked to sit out, his teacher replied because he could not sit still in the classroom when he was supposed to be completing his math worksheet. Ms. Alverz and Javier accepted the consequence, without objection.

As a member of the school district SHAC, Ms. Alverz asked other parents if their children had been withheld from recess. When discovering that nearly all of the parents had had at least one child withheld during his or her elementary school experience, the SHAC reviewed data on the facilities, resources, and policies on each elementary school campus as they related to recess. As part of the preparation phase of the MOST, the review revealed that the school campuses were differential in that some campuses had playground equipment and others did not. Further, individual principals reported varying accounts of practice-related supervision, policies for withholding recess from students, the length and timing of recess, and whether recess was offered before or after lunch. Once the disparities were identified, the SHAC was charged with creating a recess policy whereby all children could be offered equitable opportunities for both structured and unstructured PA during the school day. Over the next academic school year, monthly meetings with parents, teachers, and principals resulted in the development of a district recess policy that would ensure best practice and equity across all 32 of the district elementary school campuses. After school board approval of the policy 12 months later, the SHAC began to consider each CSPAP component and how there could be policy, process, and implementation at every campus in the district.

During the preparation phase, each school formed a PA committee (PAC), which included the physical education teacher and community members. At their first meeting, they used the *Let's Move!* Active Schools Assessment Guide to identify what was already happening on each campus and what facilities already supported PA during the school day. Each PAC used this information to set goals for the annual school improvement plan, which was contextually unique for each campus. Further, some schools exhibited a greater readiness than others, so schools were encouraged to start by implementing quality physical education and then move toward quality physical education plus one CSPAP component. Of the 32 schools, 10 schools submitted a multicomponent plan. New teachers or those who were just getting started with the CSPAP visited schools that were attempting to implement multiple components.

As part of the optimization phase, teachers and school principals were asked to collect data on the existing PA programs. Like the recess data that prompted this initiative, information on enrollment, policies, and cost was gathered. In some schools, campus PACs were formed with the help of the PTO. Once in place, the PAC began initiating some of the prioritized steps. If one school wanted to paint its playground, the SHAC–PAC–PTO collaboration provided a forum for soliciting materials and workforce to get the task done. Once completed by one school, they could in turn challenge or help another school to do the same.

The final phase of the MOST, reflection and evaluation, was conducted at the school level and reported back to the district as lessons learned from the CSPAP implementation. It is important to note that the school district administration was supportive of trying new things and did not enact consequences if the implementation did not work as intended. Administrative support was an essential safeguard for teachers who may have been providing PA programs for the first time. At this phase, data related to academic achievement, PA opportunities, and physical fitness was also recorded and interpreted.

PART IV

Contextual Considerations

CHAPTER 12

CSPAPs in Urban Contexts

Sarah Doolittle, EdD
Adelphi University

Paul Rukavina, PhD
Adelphi University

Kevin Mercier, EdD
Adelphi University

For children, youth, and families living in school districts identified as "large urban" districts (Centers for Disease Control and Prevention [CDC], 2014), sufficient opportunities for quality physical education, health-related PA, sport for all students, and opportunities for family PA are among the disparities that affect public health (Yancey et al., 2007). Recent evidence on the positive impact of PA for children, youth, and families has influenced scholars and decision makers to reexamine school policies and practices for promoting and providing opportunities for PA, especially in urban schools serving low-income and minority communities. CSPAPs in these and other urban schools could offer multiple benefits for the health and well-being of children, families, and communities (U.S. Department of Health and Human Services, 2013). The purpose of this chapter is to review existing literature and evolving practices for CSPAPs in urban school environments, paying attention to limitations and potential assets that are specific to public schools in urban community contexts.

Review of Research

Studies of health disparities reveal that children and youth who live in large urban school districts, are ethnic minorities, or are from low-income homes tend to participate in PA less often than their Caucasian age mates in suburban and middle- and upper-income communities (Basch, 2011; CDC, 2014; DeBate et al., 2011; Gordon-Larsen et al., 2006; Yancey et al., 2007). Furthermore, variations in youth PA and prevalence of obesity correlate with "geography and areas of poverty, income, and violent crime. Thus, a presumed reason for racial and ethnic differences is the overrepresentation of minorities living in environments where access to safe places to engage in PA is more limited" (DeBate et al., 2011). Although personal choices do matter for PA participation, environmental influences on those choices may be more important for scholars and practitioners seeking to increase PA for children, youth, and families in urban settings.

For example, research shows that large urban schools serving minority and low-income students offer fewer PA facilities (Fernandez & Sturm, 2010) and opportunities for sport and physical education participation than schools in suburban or rural communities (CDC, 2014; Johnston et al., 2007). Barriers include limited resources (e.g., facilities, class size, teacher quality, funding for equipment, and extracurricular staffing); formal compliance issues with school district and union rules; priorities for academic testing and test prep; limited teacher and administrative support; and school, student, and family cultures that affect PA program quality (Cothran & Ennis, 2010; McCaughtry et al., 2006; Moore et al., 2010; Ward & O'Sullivan, 2006).

Conversely, studies of PA interventions for urban, minority, and low-income populations indicate that increasing access to opportunities for enjoyable PA in and through schools can positively affect obesity and associated health outcomes (CDC, 2013; Centeio et al., 2014; Dauenhauer & Keating, 2011; Garn et al., 2017; Institute of Medicine, 2013; Staurowsky et al., 2015). Many studies find that students in this demographic who participate in school-based PA and sport also gain positive psychosocial goals in areas such as self-esteem and self-efficacy as well as reductions in depression, anxiety, and high-risk behaviors, such as smoking, drug use, and violence. Positive effects in terms of school attendance, academic achievement, and improved graduation rates are also associated with regular participation in school-based PA and sport programs (Castelli et al., 2015; Centeio et al., 2018; Donnelly, et al, 2016). Thus, strong and consistent evidence supports policies to provide more PA, especially in school districts identified as "large urban." Increasing PA among children in this sector is among the most important national public health priorities, potentially yielding billions of dollars of savings in medical costs (Lee et al., 2017).

Despite these findings, developing, implementing, and sustaining programs that support health-related physical education, sport, and PA in urban schools has been a slow process. The lack of progress indicates that making changes in schools sufficient to affect public health goals is a complex undertaking. Identifying variables that influence children and youth to participate in PA and focusing on "modifiable correlates" (Moore et al., 2010) among barriers and facilitators increase the potential that changes in schooling or interventions provided at school can yield important progress toward public health goals. To this end, determinants and correlates of participation in PA and sport are presented in figure 12.1, a social-ecological framework derived from multiple reviews of research (Bauman et al., 2012; Sagas & Cunningham, 2014; Sallis et al., 2008). Figure 12.1 illustrates the interconnected intrapersonal, interpersonal, organizational, community, and policy factors that influence PA opportunities for urban children and youth. These factors are described in the next section and suggest a number of modifiable correlates that may enhance efforts to design and deliver CSPAPs in urban settings.

Intrapersonal Factors

These influences include biological and demographic variables, such as age, gender, ethnicity, socioeconomic level, and status as able bodied, all of which consistently correlate with higher or lower levels of regular PA. Psychological factors, including knowledge, beliefs, motivation, and self-efficacy, are also included at this level of the framework.

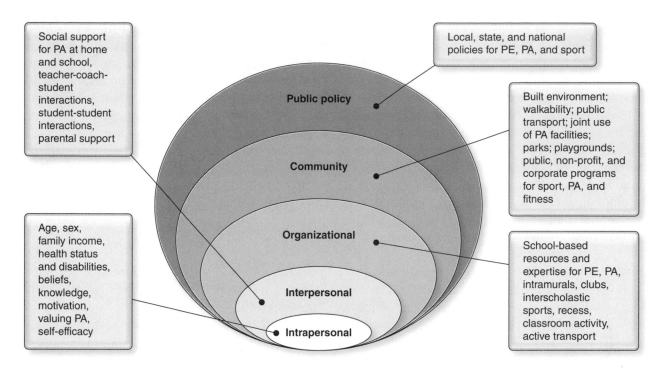

Figure 12.1 Social-ecological influences on participation in urban physical education, sport, and PA.

Adapted from Bauman et al. (2012); Sallis et al. (2008).

Demographic research related to the obesity crisis consistently presents a grim picture for children and adolescents who live in cities. Low-income and minority children, especially girls, rank highest for overweight and lowest for regular health-enhancing PA (Basch, 2011; CDC, 2014; Phillips & Young, 2009). Socioeconomic status, whether urban or rural, appears to be the more important factor over the urban environment per se in terms of influencing PA participation (Joens-Matre et al., 2008; Sterdt et al., 2014; Yancey & Kumanyika, 2007). Child and adolescent psychological factors, such as perceived competence, self-efficacy motivation, and attitudes, are positively correlated with increased PA. Behavioral and sociocultural attributes, such as participation in sport, access to facilities and programs, time outdoors, and support from parents and significant others, also consistently correlate with PA for children and adolescents (Sterdt et al., 2014). As important as these intrapersonal factors are, there is little in this level of research to modify when planning interventions. Factors in the following levels suggest more guidance for building CSPAPs.

Interpersonal Factors

Interpersonal factors, such as the influence of social support from families and friends at home and school together with cultural values for sport and PA, especially the influence of school instruction and extracurricular experiences, do affect PA participation and may be more modifiable than identifying demographic or psychological categories. Designing and delivering physical education as a valuable subject matter for students in urban schools has been a topic for researchers for many years and includes modifications at the interpersonal and organizational levels. Consistent recommendations over the past several decades include making a shift in emphasis away from individual psychological variables and toward environmental changes that could influence student perceptions and choices. Recommended changes for urban physical education programs have traditionally focused on curricular relevance, relationships, and ensuring student success (Ennis, 1999). More recently, scholars have called for culturally responsive instructional practices that shift from a perspective of student deficits toward building on strengths of students, values in their community culture, and assets available in the environments surrounding schools (Cothran et al., 1999; Culp, 2017; Garn, McCarthy, et al., 2014).

These recommendations do not mitigate the impact of limited resources, however. Decades of studies on urban physical education teachers and programs show a constant struggle for equipment and instructional resources, professional development, curricular time, and administrative support, all of which undermine efforts to deliver sound, relevant, and effective instruction (Flory & McCaughtry, 2011; Maljak et al., 2014; McCaughtry et al., 2006). Students, parents, teachers, and administrators too often fail to see the relevance and value of physical education and thus support a minimum expectation of attendance and compliance to meet state or district requirements for physical education. The lack of support for learning or achievement leads to physical education programs and policies that allow inadequate teaching expertise as well as tolerance for minimal physical education class time and large class sizes, inadequate facilities, and limited or poor-quality equipment necessary to teach. Additionally, urban schools have a long history of conflicting goals for physical education and related sport programs, with little expectation or administrative accountability for student learning (Cothran & Ennis, 2010; Ennis, 1999; Kulinna et al., 2006; McCaughtry et al., 2006; Sallis & McKenzie, 1991) and, often, an overemphasis on elite varsity sports (Lawson, 2005).

Organizational Factors

Organizational influences also help to explain the persistent limited access to PA programming in urban schools. Researchers have detailed the structural constraints limiting opportunities for school-based sport and PA (Fernandez & Sturm, 2010; Garn et al., 2017; Turner et al., 2017). They report that urban schools have less recess time and more cases of no recess time compared to suburban and rural schools because of higher enrollments, less available activity space, and more scheduled time devoted to instruction in tested subjects, such as English language arts and math. Urban, high-minority, and high-poverty schools have significantly fewer gymnasiums provided to students, and the capacity of the facilities in relation to class sizes is worse. Urban, low-income, and minority students also have inadequate playgrounds at school and less access to neighborhood recreational facilities. Thus, about 30 percent of 6- to 12-year-old students who are from homes with the lowest income (below $20,000) engage in no sporting activity, compared to 11.5 percent of those from homes with the highest income. Half as many low-income students, 34.6 percent compared to 68.4 percent of high-income students, played a team sport (Aspen Institute, 2017).

In response to decades of underperforming programs in many underresourced and urban schools, research on alternative physical education curricula, such as Sports for Peace, fitness education, and sport education, shows that quality urban physical education programs are possible (Cothran & Ennis, 2010). When teachers and administrators address the students' interests, ensure experiences with success, and attend to interpersonal relationships between teachers and students and among students, school-based physical education and PA programs can be a positive experience (Ennis, 1999; Garn et al., 2014; Griffin, 1985). Studies also show that new funding for facilities, equipment, and supervisors or coaches for physical education and PA also makes a difference (Bai et al., 2017). Large grants that provide budgets for new equipment and professional development can improve physical education and PA programs in underresourced urban schools, at least for a time (Centeio et al., 2018). Case studies of outstanding teachers and groups of teachers who have successfully found ways to deliver quality physical education and PA experiences also show ways in which physical education can be improved. The use of public facilities outside of school is beginning to attract physical education teachers, who may be able to use these resources in their instructional or extracurricular programs through joint-use agreements (CDC, 2014; Institute of Medicine, 2013; Jones & Wendel, 2015; Turner et al., 2015). For secondary level physical education teachers especially, preparing high school students for lifelong PA once they leave school requires introducing students to community programs, clubs, and other PA opportunities.

Community Factors

Community influences identified as contributing to PA participation include the built environment and programs and services offered outside of schools. Proximity and perceived access to safe and inviting parks and recreational facilities, especially those in the natural environment, and available public transport and "walkable" neighborhoods are increasingly seen as powerful correlates of PA participation for older children, adolescents, and adults (Gordon-Larsen et al., 2006; Kimbro et al., 2011). Supporting public funding for infrastructure for walkable neighborhoods and parks and recreational facilities in or near all neighborhoods and providing low-cost programs in public school gymnasiums and playgrounds, public parks, and recreation departments have a positive impact on PA for children, adolescents, and adults.

To supplement public funding in low-income communities, corporate and nonprofit agencies are increasingly providing financial support, media attention, and personnel to increase PA (Aspen Institute, 2017). ESPN, NBA, NFL, Nike, and other agencies advocate for and support the development of urban facilities, shared-use agreements, active transportation to school, and bike lanes and walking trails as well as staff support. With the research and guidance provided by nonprofit agencies, such as the Aspen Institute and Laureus Sport for Good Foundation, corporations are increasingly supporting research-informed, developmentally appropriate, and inclusive sport programs; sport-based youth development; and coach training. Ironically, at the same time, sport industry investments are pouring into video game development and competitions, "betting this is what kids want" (Aspen Institute, 2017, p. 8).

Research into the influence of the built environment to encourage PA from adults and children is gaining ground with urban planners. New development includes creating and improving public parks; bicycle paths; more-inviting walkways; and fitness, sport, or parkour resources as well as playgrounds, pools, and skate parks (Carlson et al., 2016; Davison & Lawson, 2006). Perceptions of easy access to recreational venues and safety are essential elements. Assessment and redevelopment plans for low-income urban neighborhoods

that invite and include the views of community members in planning stages provide a strong foundation for program and facility development that residents will use (DeBate et al., 2011).

In terms of implementing CSPAPs, the PA leader charged with introducing or running a CSPAP most often is assumed to be a professional from inside the school. This makes sense. As a member of the school community, this leader has existing knowledge of the characteristics and interests of the students and organizational constraints of the school as well as the capacity to gain knowledge of available programs and build relationships with the community. Internal leaders understand the intrapersonal factors that influence PA participation for their students; they use interpersonal, organizational, community, and policy influences and a level of authority to expand physical education into CSPAPs. This internal leader is frequently a school official, such as a physical education teacher or physical education administrator. Unfortunately, in large urban districts, as in other school districts, too often there is no school leader or teacher able or willing to start a CSPAP.

An alternative to an internal CSPAP leader is for schools to establish relationships with local colleges or universities to take advantage of available student interns and faculty expertise (Coppola et al., 2018; McMullen et al., 2014; Webster, Beets, et al., 2015). While these partnerships may be beneficial to both parties, it is unrealistic for all schools to have a university partner to assist in CSPAP implementation because the number of public schools in cities far exceeds the number of universities willing or able to partner with local schools. Unless a special relationship is sustained, school–university partnerships often end when grant funding runs out.

A third option for CSPAPs, unique to urban settings, is partnering schools with external community partners: corporate and nonprofit agencies that specialize in sport and PA promotion and may offer programs for child and youth development as part of their overall mission. The sheer number of corporations and nonprofit agencies located in urban environments together with their institutional commitments for community service often results in new resources, both human and financial, to support PA and sport programs for low-income schools. Thus, city schools may have access to funding and support for sport and PA that is not present in less densely populated areas. For schools without a willing school leader or a university collaboration, partnering with non-profit- or corporate-sponsored programs from outside the school may provide the best opportunity for implementing a CSPAP.

An added benefit of school–community partnerships is that organizations educate students about the opportunities and locations for PA within the local community. Health clubs, dance studios, bowling alleys, archery and golf clubs, recreation centers, and swimming pools often welcome school physical education and PA programs because after graduation, community programs will be a primary source of PA. Students and their families can learn about these organizations through school-based partnerships (Allar et al., 2017). In many of the English-speaking countries, national support is provided to community sport organizations to partner with schools to provide coaching expertise in schools, recruit students to local clubs, and encourage students and graduates to transition to local sport organizations for sport experiences schools cannot provide (Eime & Payne, 2009; Hogan & Stylianou, 2018; Wilkinson & Penney, 2016).

If physical education teachers or other school staff members are not able to lead quality PA programs and university partnerships are not available, schools may benefit from PA youth development professionals from the community. Community partner agencies may be able to push in leadership, coaching, expertise, energy, and equipment from outside the school to provide quality sport and PA programs to students in urban schools. In New York City, for example, several external nonprofit agencies have partnered with public schools to provide CSPAP-related services that schools are unable to provide for themselves. In this section, we present an overview of some of the organizations working in New York City as well as a case study showing how such organizations might be a powerful force in initiating CSPAPs when developing CSPAPs from within schools seems impossible.

In addition to well-known organizations, such as the Boys & Girls Clubs of America and the YMCA, which provide a variety of after-school enrichment programs in their own facilities as well as in schools, several national organizations have emerged that specialize in school-based sport and PA promotion. Up2Us Sports is one nonprofit leader within the United States, which is based in New York City. The organization primarily trains sport coaches to reduce youth violence, promote health, and inspire academic success. A list of their membership shows 142 New York–based organizations, the majority of which operate in the five boroughs of New York City. Many of these organizations work directly with schools to provide sport programs, PA, and other opportunities both within and beyond the school day. Additional organizations include Playworks, a national organization that has been placing coaches in 16 New York City schools during recess, as of 2016, reaching 10,800 New York City students as part of programming in over 1,200 schools and 700,000 students across the United States. Kids in the Game partners with schools to provide services such as early drop-off and after-school PA sessions, organizing and leading field day events, recess programming, evaluation and curriculum development, and family fitness events. Play Rugby USA teaches positive life skills through rugby and partners with schools to provide after-school programming. PowerPlayNYC aims to empower girls through after-school PA offerings throughout all five boroughs. I Challenge Myself offers alternative secondary physical education courses, including a cycling course in which senior high school students have an opportunity to go on a seven-day college bike tour. Harlem Lacrosse and Leadership operates in four large urban U.S. cities, including New York, and teaches lacrosse to students at risk for failing in school while providing academic support throughout the school day. As part of its programming, Asphalt Green conducts Recess Enhancement Programs (REPs) in New York with 60 schools, affecting over 28,000 students to date.

Simply providing PA or sport practice does not guarantee that PA goals for participants are being met (Bleeker et al., 2015). Kahan and McKenzie's (2018) study of a well-designed running club describes the challenges of delivering minutes of moderate-to-vigorous PA (MVPA) even when that is the clear priority of such a club. With the addition of new PA opportunities provided by external agents, research could demonstrate that they provide the intended outcomes and identify practices for staff training, but few research studies have been published that show whether community providers achieve their intended impact. One study of Reeboks' Build Our Kids Success (BOKS) program determined that children in a before-school program three days per week over 12 weeks improved body mass index (BMI) and student engagement scores. Two days per week and less did not show significant change in those two outcomes but did show some improvements compared to a control group (Whooten et al., 2018). Several studies of recess programs have shown modest improvements in PA and social outcomes (Chin & Ludwig, 2013; Massey et al., 2018). However, there are too few published studies that detail best practices and impact for PA programs conducted by community partners. While this is also true of traditional physical education and sport practices, decision makers who have evidence of impact will be able to weigh the contributions of each kind of program and choose accordingly.

Another concern regarding community providers for CSPAP programming is the organization's ability to serve all students with not only one after-school sport or PA for a single team or group but establishing school-wide services—before and during as well as after school. A second problem is the uncertain background of coaches—whether they have sufficient pedagogical training to work effectively with schoolchildren. Each of the aforementioned organizations working in the city has spent considerable time working with school administrators to establish a relationship and develop trust before gaining access to work with children in the schools. The New York City Department of Education (NYC DOE) must also approve of these organizations working within a district school or in an extended school-day setting. The challenge often facing these groups when seeking approval to work in connection with schools is convincing the schools that they have the knowledge and expertise not only of their content but also of working with children to safely deliver beneficial programming.

As in most schools, the local administrator, often the building principal, is the gatekeeper responsible for allowing organizations to provide their services at school. Gaining the principal's support is a key factor for an external agency to initiate programming within a school setting. While these community groups have had success with specific schools in offering components of a CSPAP, most commonly in the form of increased after-school PA opportunities, one New York City–based nonprofit agency, Wellness in the Schools, has developed a more comprehensive program and relationship with several schools to implement a more comprehensive version of CSPAP. This group is described in the second case example later in the chapter.

Public Policy Factors

Influences at the local, state, and national levels influence PA participation, especially in terms of funding. New policies requiring certified physical education teachers, district-supported professional learning communities, ongoing professional development, assessment of students, data reports, and school report cards are making a difference, albeit slowly, in terms of influencing quality PE and increasing PA opportunities for urban children and youth. Among the multiple pressures urban public schools face, physical education and student participation in sport and PA remain low priorities (Turner et al., 2017), but this long-standing tradition may be changing with increased public recognition of the value of PA opportunities in school.

For example, a persistent parent in California challenged his city's school district in court to meet state-mandated minutes of physical education long overlooked in his state's urban school districts. To date, more than 35 districts, including San Francisco and Los Angeles, have been forced to change (Adams, 2015). New York City and other large urban school districts have responded more proactively since this lawsuit and are now providing new funding for meeting state requirements for physical education and professional development and increased funding for after-school programs ("Evaluation of Mayor De Blasio's," 2016; "Mayor De Blasio," 2017; Office of the New York City Comptroller, 2014). With overwhelming scientific evidence supporting the benefits of PA, urban schools may have found the political support they need to strengthen physical education as well as CSPAPs. Likewise, new state and local funding for PA has encouraged policy changes, and some urban district and school administrators are making organizational changes to reinvigorate physical education, require daily recess, encourage active transport, and take advantage of available extracurricular sport and PA organizations offering cost-effective PA programs that are attractive and inclusive for all students.

At the national level, policies included in the 2015 Every Student Succeeds Act (ESSA) for the first time explicitly support physical education and school-based PA as part of a sound basic education and an important aspect of a safe and healthy school environment (U.S. Department of Education, 2017). The Whole School, Whole Child, Whole Community philosophy underpins the language and policies of ESSA. Federal funding will be distributed by states, but the language of the act allows health, physical education, and PA at school a seat at the table and a sound basis on which to be included in grants to schools. With Title I funding explicitly dedicated to underserved schools, urban school districts will be able to access new funds directly associated with CSPAP.

Knowledge Claims

Research demonstrates that among the social disparities affecting children youth and families in large urban contexts is a lack of opportunities for enjoyable PA, sport, and quality PE. CSPAPs may be one way to provide more opportunities, and a way to take better advantage of time, facilities, and human resources available in schools. But implementing the CSPAP model is not simple and will challenge existing values and priorities in schools and communities, and long-held commitments among PA professionals. The review of research presented thus far has been framed on a socioecological framework to identify constraints and assets of urban settings that might be modified if stakeholders can be persuaded to make changes. Professionals and policy makers may need to keep in mind the following research findings.

- Understanding the policy, community, organizational, interpersonal, and intrapersonal factors affecting access to PA opportunities helps explain at least some of the social disparities

of regular PA participation in urban contexts. Furthermore, a social-ecological frame of reference points to new interventions beyond the physical education curriculum and teachers' and coaches' interactions that could change the school environment so that urban children and youth could increase participation in PA. Interventions that both draw from and affect more than one level of the social-ecological framework, termed "reciprocal determinism," (Gutuskey et al., 2014) and are sustained over sufficient time (chapter 4) are more likely to be successful.

- The residential density of urban settings provides a built environment that supports PA: sidewalks; public transportation; and a wide variety of recreational and sport venues, playgrounds, parks, and exercise facilities. CSPAP leaders can take advantage of available public transportation and public recreational facilities to expand opportunities for students, especially secondary students, and encourage family participation.

- Access to medical, educational, and sport expertise through city-based hospitals, universities, and community agencies can contribute to helping urban schools develop CSPAPs. The rich mix of intellectual, social, and professional perspectives available in urban environments provides opportunities for inter-professional collaboration to deliver engaging programs and for CSPAP research and development.

- Urban political and tax structures are beginning to prioritize public health and well-being in schools, and physical education teachers who think about extending physical education and PA beyond traditional structures toward initiatives for child and adolescent health and well-being may find grant programs and other forms of public financial support.

- Mixed populations from a range of socioeconomic and educational levels—parents and community members, well-funded corporations, and local businesses—can and do collaborate to fund extracurricular PA and sport programs for children and youth.

- Barriers to increased PA for urban children and youth still remain:

- School policies and deep organizational structures, budgets, and contracts limit the potential for extensive in-house supervision of PA opportunities by school personnel.

- School PA facilities often are limited and overpopulated. Funding additional personnel and facilities must compete with many other priorities.

- Urban parents may resist unfamiliar opportunities for participation because of perceived dangers in neighborhoods, playgrounds, programs, and personnel.

- Reliance on grants and corporate donations is inconsistent and makes long-term planning uncertain. Perceptions of corporate messaging that is inconsistent with school and traditional community values discourage some professionals from taking advantage of these collaborations.

- Part-time coaches and PA supervisors who are not teachers may be poorly prepared to include all students safely and effectively in sport and PA programs. Volunteers, external coaches, and part-time workers must be vetted and supervised by school personnel familiar with CSPAP goals.

Knowledge Gaps and Directions for Future Research

CSPAP outcomes must be assessed to establish credibility. Initial studies have focused on ways to expand active transport and classroom PA because they are consistently found to increase measurable PA (Macdonald et al., 2018). Measuring the impact of recess and before- and after-school PA programs is more complex because these experiences are freighted with multiple goals other than minutes of MVPA and changes in fitness or BMI results. Reporting the effect of CSPAPs in terms of changes in school attendance, social-emotional development, positive behavior, school connectedness, and academic achievement may also support the development and expansion of CSPAPs because these are goals most school professionals embrace.

A variety of techniques have been used to identify programs and practices that meet physical, social-emotional, and academic goals. Developing effective practices has begun for in-class PA, but more work is needed to match high-impact practices for before- and after-school programs and summer programs. These evidence-based practices should be included in coach training and professional preparation.

Descriptions of PA programs and strategies that engage adolescents, girls, and marginalized students are needed. Initial studies indicate that teachers' and coaches' interactions and careful selection of program activities can engage disengaged students. Recruiting teachers, coaches, and CSPAP leaders who are willing to cast off deeply held values for elite, competitive athletes and sport programs may be necessary (Lawson, 2005).

The suggestion that CSPAPs may have a positive effect on communities points the way toward questioning how CSPAPs can contribute to urban community schools, which serve not only students but also the neighborhoods, where adults and families also need PA resources and other services related to health and well-being (e.g., Diamond & Freudenberg, 2016; Lawson, 2005). Jones and Wendel (2015) described schools as untapped resources for the community. It would be worth exploring how PA opportunities provide benefits to community members other than youth and children attending schools. The research on urban CSPAPs is in its infancy, but continued work in this area offers a more hopeful perspective for urban students and a more important role for PA professionals working in cities.

Additional studies of CSPAP leadership are needed regarding whether providers are internal school personnel or external community partners who build PA into schools. Interactive and collaborative skills are important, especially to confront and inspire changes to the deep culture of physical education and sport in many urban and other underresourced schools. Identifying strategies to take advantage of facilitators and address barriers will be necessary. Newer studies on CSPAPs are exploring ways to persuade principals and classroom teachers to buy into and implement whole-school approaches, such as the CSPAP model, and often citing limitations of time and effort by physical education teachers. It may be essential to tap into resources external to traditional school personnel if all children are to have opportunities for enjoyable extracurricular PA. Learning to manage such assets is an unfamiliar role for physical education and physical education teacher education. Studies that illustrate successful management, high-impact practices, and collaborative negotiation skills may be useful in redesigning professional preparation for teachers and community partners.

Evidence-Based Recommendations and Applications

Recent studies of urban CSPAPs are beginning to describe how schools are successfully implementing recommended physical education and PA programs despite school resource constraints and the deep cultural resistance that too often characterizes urban schools (Garn et al., 2017; Turner et al., 2015). These studies explore both barriers and facilitators to illustrate ways urban school professionals can take advantage of social and environmental assets to provide new opportunities for quality physical education and PA programming. Studies often include specific recommendations for practical action, focusing on school staff and increasingly on community partners as well.

For School Staff

Initiating a CSPAP requires leadership. Internal leaders seem best positioned to "pull in" and negotiate multiple social-ecological influences of the urban setting that affect quality programs. When internal leaders are not available, external agents from community organizations may be able to bring programs and staff to initiate some aspects of CSPAPs. Collaboration and negotiation between insiders and outsiders is essential.

CSPAPs require program management. Good program managers know the students and the community. They understand how to arrange organizational and community assets from their local environment, how to keep in mind aspects that will make it easy for students to choose to participate, and what factors concern parents so that they can support participation.

CSPAP leaders must also understand and model interpersonal relationships within programs. PA providers must be perceived as caring—concerned with positive student–student, student–teacher, and student–coach relationships. Setting goals to reach all students and inspiring staff and parents may be essential. Traditional sport coaches who focus on finding and developing elite players only may not be good CSPAP leaders.

CSPAPs take years to build. Developing successful programs is a process of beginning with one component and adding others. Multidimensional and long-term strategies must exist to incorporate changing student interests and evolving leadership and adult involvement.

For Community Partners

Every organization needs to have specific goals. Goals must be matched with data-based evidence to show how well the organization achieves its stated goals.

Look for assistance with program evaluation from local experts and organizations that provide technical assistance to nonprofit agencies. Passion for one's sport or activity is not enough. Universities with strong education, physical education, and sport programs may be able to assist with evaluation, staff training, and other areas of expertise you need. Recruit for staff positions from university undergraduate and graduate programs.

While there may be overlap in the desire to help promote development of children and youth through sport and PA, community providers seldom work together to achieve common goals. Collaborate with the existing physical education and school sport programs. Collaborate with other community partners who share your facilities and also work with your students. Keep in mind shared CSPAP goals, and work together for the benefit of your schools, students, and community.

Community agencies are often underfunded and understaffed. The selection and training of direct service providers is essential. Some coaches come to community agencies with experience as athletes and, sometimes, boundless enthusiasm for their sport. Training is often limited to child safety and basic management and organizational skills, whereas goals of programs include personal and social development that far exceeds the personal enthusiasm of a potential coach. Develop sound professional development for staff, and hold coaches accountable for meeting interpersonal and organizational expectations.

Community partners can find opportunities to engage with school through school district departments of education and health as well as through state and federal grant programs. CSPAPs depend on funding and policies that encourage school personnel and others to provide services. Community partners may be powerful advocates for public policy and funding that could expand opportunities for many schools.

SUMMARY

This chapter reviewed the literature on CSPAPs and influences on physical activity for children and adolescents in urban settings. While much of the CSPAP literature to date appears to be context free, the social-ecological environment plays an essential part in the success or failure of CSPAP implementation. Most of the successful CSPAPs described fall into two groups: those that are self-sustaining, relying on internal staff and school assets, and those dependent on university partnerships. Schools in urban contexts confront many challenges but also assets and resources beyond those provided internally or through nearby universities. Some of these resources may be unavailable in smaller, more affluent school districts. Understanding one's context from a social-ecological frame of reference may assist scholars, decision makers, and physical education and PA professionals to understand and address barriers to implementing functional CSPAPs in their schools—wherever they are located. It is especially important for schools in large urban districts to consider how external organizational, community, and policy influences interact to create both positive and negative environments for physical activity when developing opportunities for all students in school. Internal school resources alone will never be sufficient to establish and maintain functional urban school CSPAPs.

As the CSPAP concept catches on in urban schools, internal and external approaches will likely become more sophisticated. In New York City and other urban areas, public policy has engendered the development of a rich assortment of new agencies and young sport and PA professionals who can contribute to changing schools so that CSPAPs are more feasible. Cities are moving away from a long-standing, tightly held culture of providing elite or varsity sports for a few at the high school level and toward redistributing resources toward many students at secondary and elementary schools to help reduce the public health disparities that affect student success. Insiders and outsiders will need to work collaboratively to pool funds, facilities, personnel, enthusiasm, and expertise. With CSPAPs as a new way of thinking about physical education, fitness, and sport, the possibilities seem as vast as cities themselves.

QUESTIONS TO CONSIDER

1. If traditional physical education and school interscholastic programs fail to provide needed PA for all students, how should these two institutions be redesigned so that resources can support programs that deliver health and well-being to all school students?

2. How might urban school district administrators be persuaded to create a paid CSPAP leader position for every school?

3. How can measurement of outcomes help physical education distinguish itself from PA so that the instructional nature of physical education is not overtaken by PA programs?

4. How can corporate and nonprofit PA providers be regulated to ensure they deliver appropriate high-quality programs to public school children?

5. Should public schools assume responsibility for reducing public health disparities?

CASE EXAMPLES

The following section presents two cases illustrating different approaches for taking advantage of the urban social-ecological context to improve PA opportunities in urban schools. The first case is one that was initiated by physical educators who led from inside the school to implement CSPAP components. The second case was initiated by a community provider for PA from outside of schools, pushing in programs that move schools toward CSPAPs. Both cases show how school and community leaders draw upon urban resources to create more PA opportunities for students.

CSPAP Implementation From Within a School

In this case, two New York City physical education teachers recognized the need for expanded sport and PA opportunities and drew upon community resources to develop their vision of a CSPAP in a low-income, minority K-8 urban public school (Doolittle & Rukavina, 2014). This case is a clear example of an urban CSPAP developed by teachers within the school with judicious use of available community resources but firm oversight by teachers and administrators.

Outcomes

At the time of the study, this CSPAP was in its 13th year. Within this program, scheduled physical education exceeded city and state requirements, and before-, during-, and after-school voluntary physical activities were offered for all children from fourththrough eighth grade. The school administration, teachers, staff members, and parents supported daily, active 20-minute recess for K-8 students, and 26 different no-cut sports and activities for upper elementary and middle school students. The extracurricular program offered all interested students opportunities for learning, practicing, and competing in traditional steam sports, but also a wide variety of nontraditional sport and physical activities, including cross country running, surfing, skateboarding, wrestling, cheerleading, ice-skating, dance, bicycling, table tennis, Ultimate, lacrosse, bowling, badminton and the use of individual fitness machines. Because extracurricular activities were scheduled one to three days per week, many students participated in multiple sports and activities in each of the three scheduled seasons. Special events and family initiatives involve students, staff, and parents up to five times per year, and substantial grant writing, community donations, and fund-raising were organized school-wide to support programs. Coaches were classroom teachers and school staff members and were paid through the school's discretionary budget, grants, and funds raised through parents and the community.

Analysis of participation data for 2012-2013 indicated that 82 percent of the sixth-, seventh-, and eighth-grade students participated in at least one extracurricular sport and half of those students participated in two or more activities per year. Some students participated in up to 10 activities per year. Physical education teachers collaborated with an external recess and elementary after-school program and selected sport organizations to find facilities and resources necessary for multiple high-quality and active opportunities. This school's program met at least minimum levels for all components except classroom activity in the CSPAP policy continuum (CDC, 2012). The following analysis describes aspects of program implementation in relation to the social-ecological model previously described.

Intrapersonal Influences

In this low-income, multiethnic school, which was planning and delivering physical education, sport, and PA programs, teachers prioritized social-emotional outcomes, such as student attention, impulse control, problem solving, social relationships, cooperation, empathy, self-confidence, self-worth, and school success. The foundation for achieving these goals through PA is the goal of inclusion for all in each opportunity and offering activities based on student interest. All students are part of all events and can engage in multiple activities in the same season. If a group of 20 students petition to add new sports, the physical education teachers commit themselves to finding a way to staff, equip, and schedule that sport. The program emphasized transferring to high school and life beyond what is learned through quality, inclusive sport and PA participation. Teachers were conscious of differences in background and family income levels and assured that no students paid to participate.

Interpersonal Influences

Many special events celebrating sport and activities occur throughout the school year in which the philosophy of the program and the program goals are reinforced. For example, at the awards night, which occurs after each of the three seasons, parents, siblings, and some alumni attend and bring dishes to a family-style potluck dinner. The physical education teachers celebrate all students' involvement through pictures and stories of what happened over the season.

Benefits cited by the CSPAP leaders and teacher coaches included the personal and professional satisfaction of seeing students succeed in self-selected sports and physical activities, thrive as students, and make friends with a wide variety of peers despite disadvantages of poverty and difficult family circumstances. The teachers also described the satisfaction of creating and leading a positive school culture that was highly valued by the entire school community and recognized throughout the city as an exemplary school.

Organizational Influences

Working together over years, the physical education teachers redesigned physical education to get the children excited about sport and PA. Beginning in the upper elementary levels, instructional activity units in physical education operate as an introduction to sport and PA opportunities offered before and after school. The physical education teachers coached several sport teams themselves and recruited classroom teachers, administrators, and parents to coach and assist with clubs and teams. Sustained program messaging and practical coordination by the physical education teachers assured that all sports and activities were conducted within established program goals and norms of behavior were consistent.

The transformation to a CSPAP school was built one sport or activity at a time, taking more than a decade, and fraught with traditional obstacles, such as no budget, not enough gym space, and resistant administrators. Furthermore, maintaining a large and diverse program that was staffed almost exclusively by classroom teachers from their school required much time and energy beyond normal contract obligations. The physical education teachers work with administrators for budget, scheduling, and other permissions. They present a plan and budget for each season, making administrative support easy for principals.

Community Influences

A major challenge to these teachers is accessing sport and PA facilities and sufficient equipment for multiple sports. They have joint-use agreements and permits with the city for playing fields and use of a recreation center. The school partners with many sport organizations and grant-funding groups to provide equipment and coach training in wrestling, dance, swimming, bicycling, lacrosse, table tennis, running, ice-skating, bowling, and field trips to outdoor camps. They use public transportation for access to a city beach for surfing and beach volleyball as well as for interscholastic competition.

A recent initiative of the physical education teachers is to connect like-minded middle schools by creating sport leagues. When they initially started the program, middle schools in New York City did not have an extensive interscholastic sport league beyond basketball. The teachers recruited other schools and coordinated a middle school league. The league has grown to a large number of schools and is now administered through a partnership with Manhattan Youth, a New York City community organization.

In densely populated cities, there are many enthusiastic individuals, some of whom can afford or find ways to collect funds to donate equipment to schools in need. When the school budget is not available for the PA program, the physical education teachers depend on fundraising, which often includes bake sales, silent auctions, family fun carnivals, and potluck dinners. They also write grants and network for funds, equipment, facilities, and expertise.

Public Policy Influences

Taking advantage of available funding streams from the school district and other city agencies, the physical education teachers make the system work for their students. The teachers ensure that they meet all physical education requirements for the district and diligently report required fitness test results. The program is nearly self-supporting within the terms and conditions of the union and district contracts, including extracurricular pay for teachers who coach. They have convinced four successive principals and a number of district administrators to support the programs by providing evidence of benefits to the school through attendance data, applications for admission, academic success for students, and parental and community attendance at school events. Meeting policy obligations and presenting data to decision makers and funding agencies have helped sustain support. This case illustrates what consummate internal leaders can accomplish in urban settings when providing quality physical education, sport, and PA for their students is important enough.

The downside of this teacher-led program from the physical education teachers' point of view (J. DeMatteo, personal communication, December 20, 2017) is the personal cost for the physical education teachers in terms of time and energy. After 15 years of building this program, teachers are now seeking to shift more of the program management to external community partners so that one teacher can spend more time with his new family and the other teacher can take time out for health issues. Working closely with the community partners allows the teachers to unload some of the day-to-day management of the middle school sport league. In addition, partner sport organizations are now beginning to provide part-time coaches in certain of the school's sports. While still closely overseeing the program, both physical education teachers reported a need to relinquish responsibility for some parts of the program or risk burning out.

CSPAP Implementation From Outside a School

In this example, a community partner, Wellness in the Schools (WITS), initiated CSPAPs in high-need urban elementary schools. WITS is a nonprofit organization based in New York City that aims to inspire healthy eating and physical fitness as a way of life for students in public schools. Its Coach for Kids program placed a coach in each of its public schools, primarily during recess time, every day of the school year. Its parallel program, Cooks for Kids, placed a chef in schools several times a week.

Outcomes

Though the levels of success and implementation vary, WITS programs were able to address the four non–physical education areas of a CSPAP (staff involvement, PA during school, PA before and after school, and family and community engagement). WITS cooks taught the lunch staff how to prepare healthier menu options, worked to implement salad bars, developed an approved alternative menu that the school district would support, offered family cooking classes, and worked to bring local providers of fresh fruits and vegetables into the school. WITS coaches ran recess programs daily, aimed at increasing MVPA for all and decreasing inappropriate and unsafe behaviors. They led classroom fitness breaks and helped teachers learn to lead fitness breaks on their own. They organized family fitness nights and partnered with local organizations and professional teams for special school events.

WITS self-reports that its Cooks for Kids program is currently in 87 schools in New York City, working with 43,500 students, and the WITS Coach for Kids program is in 31 schools, serving 15,500 students. Since WITS started working with New York City schools, it have served 11 million meals and led 54,000 hours of PA (W. Siskin, personal communication, June 16, 2017). An evaluation of the WITS program is ongoing, with year one data showing an increase in vigorous activity during recess compared to control schools (Tisch Center for Food, Education, & Policy, 2018). Assessments for its PA program are based on SOPLAY (McKenzie et al., 2000) and an assessment of prosocial behavior, and WITS reported a decrease in incidents of unsafe or inappropriate recess behavior.

Another outcome is the positive media attention that its partnership can garner. The WITS and NYC DOE partnership has now been featured on several local and national television shows, including the *Today Show* and *Good Morning America*, highlighting the benefits for New York City children that quality WITS programming makes possible.

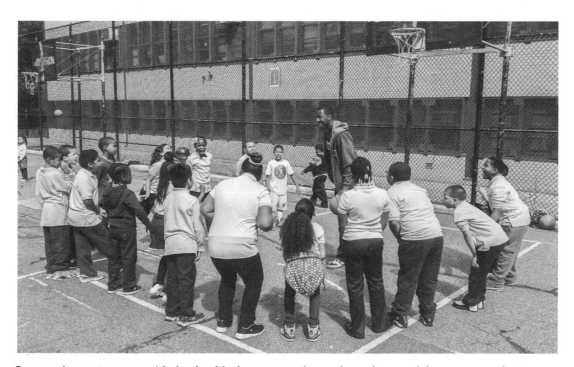

Community partners provide leadership for more active, safe, and prosocial recess experiences.

Photo courtesy of Wendy Siskin, Wellness in the Schools.

Intrapersonal and Interpersonal Influences

The WITS program targets the highest-need schools, many of which have very poor or overcrowded PA facilities and often little instructional physical education. In some cases, physical education classes are led by teachers who are not certified physical education teachers, and many students have only one physical education class per week. This pattern of poor physical education and limited PA often has a long and deep history in some schools. Bringing in a young, energetic PA coach, even if he or she works only at recess, is a welcome addition to many schools. Coaches are expected to work with physical education and other teachers, when possible, and other adults to ensure that students get their active recess period. The WITS coaches are held accountable for completing program elements. They meet together periodically for training, group-support, and problem-solving sessions. They are expected to build collaborations with other adults at school and to work at changing the culture of the school in the direction of more and better opportunities for PA for all students at recess.

Organizational Influences

Because external agencies start from outside the school system, their challenges often begin at the organizational level as they look to initiate CSPAP activities within a school environment. WITS directors negotiate with school leadership to meet program expectations and then commit to a three-year phase-out program. For the PA program, coaches section their playgrounds for different activity choices appropriate for various grade levels and number of students, sometimes up to 80 students at a time. They also teach and supervise optional playground games. They are equipped with one bag of various equipment, such as jump ropes, balls, and cones, and expected to help students learn to self-manage games and encourage all students to engage in highly active and safe recess experiences.

To convince schools of the qualifications of its staff and the quality of its program, WITS has developed a relationship with NYC DOE's Office of School Wellness Programs and with individual school-level administrators, most often the school principal. WITS shared with all parties the nature of the training the cooks and coaches received, the specific responsibilities of their employees, and the benefits of improving the nutrition habits and PA levels of their students through its programming.

Though WITS has conducted an external evaluation, to date, results have not been published in a refereed journal. Initial results, collected through appropriate and rigorous instrumentation, appear promising and provide a strong model for other community partners to emulate. Many urban community partners providing CSPAP services track PA opportunities and number of students reached. While this data may help with fund-raising, it is limited in objectively determining the quality of data, fidelity of programming, or the degree to which PA behaviors are changing.

Community Influences

Three primary community barriers for WITS in beginning its work in schools were (1) acquiring the funding to deliver its programs; (2) convincing individual schools as well as the NYC DOE of the abilities of the coaches and cooks who would be working directly with the students, staff members, and families of New York City; and (3) attracting qualified cooks and coaches. Funding was and continues to be achieved through gala benefit dinner auctions, tennis outings, celebrity chef events, grant funds, and direct donations. The amount of money raised continues to be a limitation in the number of schools that WITS can reach. Discussions among staff members and within the WITS Board of Directors are ongoing on the best ways to scale up and improve the quality of programming.

Having overcome the barriers for entrance to the schools, WITS continues to look for ways to expand to new schools and to develop the quality and effectiveness of its programming. In addition to gaining support with NYC DOE, the positive media attention has helped with interest and funding. Schools within New York City now apply to WITS for its services, and WITS has an extended wait list for schools it cannot service.

WITS has a challenge in recruiting qualified chefs and coaches for its programming. The pay for these positions is not high, especially with the cost of living in New York City. It has been able to address this situation in two distinct ways. For the Cooks for Kids program, it was able to identify restaurant owners and chefs to donate their time and help recruit other early career chefs to work in the Cooks for Kids program. To help with recruiting qualified coaches for the Coach for Kids program, WITS set up a unique fellowship program with a local university for a master's degree program with a concentration in sport-based youth development. This fellowship program helped address concerns about the educational background of coaches and to provide an incentive beyond the low salary.

Public Policy Influences

Because the NYC DOE provides funding to support community providers to work in schools, WITS and other community providers can supplement traditional physical education and sport programs in schools where there were no resources dedicated to PA. Now that community providers are vetted by the NYC DOE, schools can be more confident in allowing organizations into their schools and take advantage of new low-cost opportunities to improve recess and extracurricular PA programs for all of their students.

Community partners are currently conducting PA programs in urban schools and have been doing so for some time. Originally, their mission was to provide much-needed, low-cost after-school care. Now, they are contributing to the goals of increasing PA and leading more after-school sport programs since funding for such programs has become available. In terms of supporting CSPAPs, community providers may be essential partners for urban and other underresourced schools but should not be seen as a simple solution. Credible evidence of positive impact is rare and modest. Published reports in the literature regarding the impact of individual organizations are rare. BOKS, Playworks, and Asphalt Green have published evaluation results through refereed publications and can document positive impact and strategies for others to follow. Playworks recess programming led to an increase in the vigorous activity levels of girls compared to girls in control schools (Bleeker et al., 2015; James-Burdumy et al., 2016) and to higher rates of activity among minority students. Students from schools that took part in Asphalt Green's recess program demonstrated higher rates of vigorous PA (Chin & Ludwig, 2013). The BOKS program reports similar modest gains (Whooten et al., 2018).

It is apparent that with a growing number of community partners working on promoting PA and implementing components of CSPAPs, these partnerships should be encouraged, expanded, and further developed. Some of these organizations are actively working to collaborate with physical education teachers, who are better positioned to provide the synergy between CSPAP components and offer the best route toward continuing the programs when organizations move on. A greater level of impact could be achieved by collectively promoting the accomplishments of all nonprofits working within a sector to increase the PA levels and health of an entire community.

CHAPTER 13

CSPAPs in Rural Settings

In this chapter, the implementation of CSPAPs in rural school settings is discussed. Potential benefits to students, staff, family members, and communities are the same in rural settings as in other contexts regarding increasing exposure to physically active and healthy living messages and programming. However, as discussed in this chapter, there are many aspects of rural communities that pose additional challenges to both the health of individuals and the implementation of programs such as CSPAPs. Thus, when designing programs for rural schools, it is important to anticipate such conditions that may be different from urban and suburban settings.

Pamela Hodges Kulinna, PhD
Arizona State University

Michalis Stylianou, PhD
The University of Queensland

Kent A. Lorenz, PhD
San Francisco State University

Shannon C. Mulhearn, MS
Arizona State University

Tom Taylor, BS
HealthWorks Foundation of Arizona

Shawn Orme, MA, MS
HealthWorks Foundation of Arizona

Alan Everett, MBA
HealthWorks Foundation of Arizona

Although this chapter will canvass the topic of PA, it is key to note that, academically, rural school districts also face challenges related to improving student achievement. These challenges may include teachers' teaching a variety of subjects or multiple grade levels and high teacher turnover as well as limited school choices and tutoring options. Although rural academic disparity continues its historical trend, there is promising evidence of academic improvements, which suggests that most students (90 percent) in grade 10 from both rural and nonrural environments expected that they would attend college (Molefe et al., 2017). While this data is specific to the midwestern United States, data from the National Educational Longitudinal Study (Byun et al., 2012) indicates that, although youth from rural settings still appear to be disadvantaged (primarily because of family socioeconomic status and parental expectations), there is also a significant advantage that their rural setting provides increased access to family and social resources. These increased resources may help offset rural-setting disadvantages related to enrollment and graduation in postsecondary education.

The chapter begins with a brief overview of research related to CSPAPs in rural settings. This chapter also provides some suggestions for the future direction of research studies in this area. Finally, a real-life example is presented using a case study of a CSPAP implementation in a rural school district.

Review of Research

In this section, the intent is to provide a few examples of the types of outcomes researchers have investigated within rural settings. Readers are invited to consider what insights the research community has exposed in this area as well as what additional knowledge yet to be studied would benefit the field.

Meeting PA Requirements

School-aged children acquire the majority of their PA outside of the school day (Cox et al., 2006). This activity occurs in parks, playgrounds, community centers, and sport programming outside of school. However, according to a large study focusing on rural youth across the United States, high percentages of youth (25.9-54.5 percent, depending on the state) in rural areas do not participate in any after-school sport teams or lessons (Liu et al., 2007). Another source of accumulating PA is active transportation to and from schools, such as walking or riding bikes, which relies on safe spaces for children to travel and the necessary infrastructure (e.g., sidewalks or bike lanes). Available evidence suggests that rural children and adolescents are less likely to actively commute to and from school compared to their urban peers (Babey et al., 2009). Because many of these outside-of-school opportunities are lacking for students in rural settings (Liu et al., 2007), schools become increasingly important in their role to provide access to PA opportunities for this population. For this reason, while there is often an effort to maintain some balance between an academic focus and PA goals and opportunities in schools, this struggle seems more prominent in rural school environments.

Disease Risk

Physical inactivity and poor nutrition are associated with chronic diseases linked to most premature deaths (e.g., stroke, cancer, and heart disease). Health risks alone, however, do not appear to be adequate motivation for change, and it can be difficult to modify these unhealthy behaviors (i.e., physical inactivity and poor nutrition) for both children and adults. A study comparing the health of youth in urban versus rural contexts in Canada (Ismailov & Leatherdale, 2010) found significantly more overweight and obese youth in rural than in urban and suburban environments. Similarly, in Spain (Moreno et al., 2001), youth were significantly more overweight in rural than in urban environments. Further, in the United States, rural youth have been found to be more overweight and obese (Liu et al., 2008) than urban youth. Rural youth in the United States have 26 percent greater odds of being obese compared to urban children (Johnson & Johnson, 2015). Studies comparing the health of youth in urban versus rural contexts in Canada, Spain, and the United States (Ismailov & Leatherdale, 2010; Liu et al., 2008; Moreno et al., 2001) have found significantly more overweight and obese youth in rural than in urban and suburban environments.

It could be the difficulty in changing physical inactivity and poor nutrition behaviors in rural environments that leads to these communities being less likely to meet national recommendations (Fan et al., 2014). Rural students often fail to meet the PA and nutrition recommendations because of factors across numerous ecological levels (e.g., policy, environmental, and individual levels). For example, changing policies in rural environments poses unique challenges because of lower population rates and correspondingly fewer available resources than in suburban and urban communities (Barnidge et al., 2015). At the individual level, there also has been less access to health-care messages and health programming in rural contexts (Murimi & Harpel, 2010). Creating health-promoting environmental change can also be more challenging in rural contexts that have limited opportunities for healthy eating and PA. Limitations may include inadequate places to walk or hike and limited parks, sport facilities, and places to purchase healthy foods (Johnson & Johnson, 2015; Moore et al., 2010; Murimi & Harpel, 2010).

CSPAP Research in Rural Settings

Initial studies of CSPAPs in rural settings are available, although limited, with the majority of them having addressed only one or two of the CSPAP components. In one example investigating all five components, Jones and colleagues (2014) conducted a feasibility study of CSPAPs at 11 school sites in rural Appalachian communities, and their results supported the viability of developing CSPAPs in rural communities. Issues identified as affecting sustainability were policy and environmental changes, partnership opportunities, and existing infrastructures for programming. Both "leadership and capacity building" and increased access to PA were noted as prime facilitators of sustainability. This was evidenced by several teachers and community members being able to gain access to school facilities for new or additional programming (e.g., basketball courts), which resulted in more PA opportunities. Additionally, school personnel were successful in creating both group-level (e.g., wellness committees) and school-level leaders (e.g., PA directors). Another identified strength was the

ability of school personnel to increase access to PA and integrate it into the school climate (e.g., after-school programming with new transportation schedules or 15 more minutes of PA added in classrooms). Obstacles identified included a lack of professional development and gender differences in PA opportunities (specifically a need to provide more activities that attract girls).

Whereas Jones and colleagues (2014) studied the feasibility of all components of CSPAPs in rural Appalachian communities, Bershwinger and Brusseau (2013) focused on the during-school PA component of CSPAPs. They addressed classroom PA breaks during the school day and relationships with overall school-day PA with a group of rural children in western New York. Findings suggested significantly more physically active school days for students during weeks with PA breaks along with an extra five minutes of moderate-to-vigorous PA.

Revisiting the ecological factors mentioned earlier, one rural CSPAP, the Healthier Missouri Communities (e.g., Baker et al., 2017; Barnidge et al., 2015), targeted both PA and nutrition through environmental and policy initiatives. This project, administered by the Prevention Research Center in St. Louis, is community based and includes 12 counties in rural Missouri. In the first study (Barnidge et al., 2015), partner groups participated in an action planning process to adopt evidence-based programs. Interview data led to themes related to both benefits and challenges associated with regional partnerships and resources sharing. Dominant themes also addressed enablers and barriers to long-term partnerships and program adoption. Stakeholders indicated that benefits overshadowed challenges. Two key lessons were forwarded for future regional partnerships in rural communities. First, there is a need to have the funders involved in the partnerships developing programming at the regional levels. Second, time must be spent on relationship building. The literature on social capital suggests the important relationship building that supports any health initiative (Jordan et al., 2016).

In a second study involving the Healthier Missouri Communities, four schools in rural Southeast Missouri were represented, and stakeholder interviews along with SOPLAY observations were used to determine if PA participation related to the dissemination of the environmental and policy changes (Baker et al., 2017). Ecological factors at the individual level (i.e., interest, self-efficacy, knowledge, and skills), organizational level (e.g., support from peers and school leadership), contextual level (e.g., changes in the culture of the school to healthy and active and infrastructure for PA participation), and intervention level (e.g., project must be viewed as necessary and flexible) made a difference in schools' adopting the policy and environmental changes. Specific outcomes included less sedentary and more vigorous PA behavior during recess at rural schools. Teachers also reported improved student focus and fewer misbehaviors as a result of using brain breaks. Further, two of the schools increased walking. Involving administrators and teachers in planning and implementation was identified as promising for rural interventions and policy changes.

Another long-term project that has attempted to implement a CSPAP in a rural community is the Kearney Nebraska project (Heelan et al., 2015). This six-year study in a rural midwestern environment aimed to address childhood overweight and obesity by promoting healthy eating and extending PA participation with 2,400 elementary students from nine schools. A secondary programmatic goal was to use population dose strategies to retrospectively determine the impact dose of individual strategies used. The program extended beyond a CSPAP with body mass index (BMI) screenings, wellness groups, and food services changes. Related to the CSPAP, the intervention addressed PA professional development, improved physical education programs, and increased school-level PA programming (e.g., before- and after-school programs, classroom PA breaks, and structured recess programming). Findings showed the absolute reduction in obesity as 2.5 percent and the relative change in overweight as 7.6 percent. The highest dose scores determined were for CSPAPs (5.6-9.7 percent) because of the high reach and strength of the CSPAP model. The lowest dose score was for the BMI screening and obesity treatment program (0.6-1.6 percent). This treatment program was effective for participants; however, it involved a smaller group of students.

Knowledge Claims

The following section summarizes the knowledge claims from the literature related to healthy behaviors exhibited in rural settings.

- Children and adolescents in rural settings have fewer opportunities than their peers in other settings to engage in PA, particularly outside of school (i.e., PA, sport programming, and active commuting to or from school). Therefore, the role of the school is critical in helping rural students engage in PA.

- The role of schools in supporting PA is particularly critical when considering the significantly higher levels of overweight and obese children and youth in rural contexts in the United States as well as in other countries.

- Challenges to promoting CSPAPs in rural communities may include insufficient resources, professional development for teachers, and infrastructure for activities and sport.

- Factors at multiple levels can facilitate the success and sustainability of CSPAPs in rural settings. These considerations may include providing more access to health-care messaging and PA and sport programming at the individual level. At the policy level, developing or changing policies can lead to more available resources for rural communities. Environmental changes can also be supported in rural settings, such as providing before-school walking programs.

- CSPAPs can lead to better lines of communication, more PA, better student focus with fewer misbehaviors, and increased adoption of healthy behaviors by children and youth in rural communities.

- Programming in rural communities should consider students' preferences for CSPAPs, physical education, and sport, particularly girls' and secondary students' preferences because these groups typically have lower levels of PA participation.

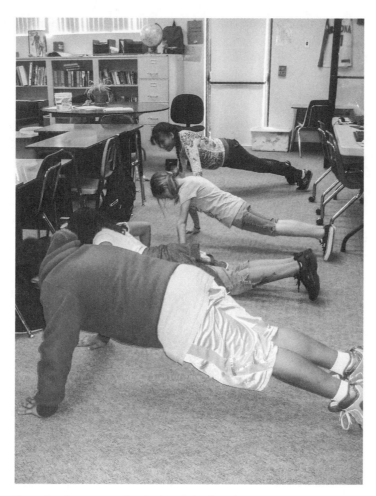

Sample classroom physical activity break.

© Pamela Kulinna

Knowledge Gaps and Directions for Future Research

Although there have been a few studies in this area, very little is known about the barriers to implementing CSPAPs in rural settings and how to overcome them. Comprehensive studies are needed (including up to all five components of the CSPAP model) on the PA outcomes of CSPAPs across stakeholder groups (e.g., school personnel, students, families, and community members) in rural settings. What structural or programming changes could be made in rural settings to make CSPAPs more widely available for students, teachers, and school personnel as well as for families and communities?

Evidence-Based Recommendations and Applications

The Centers for Disease Control and Prevention (2013) and SHAPE America (National Association for Sport and Physical Education, 2008) recommend CSPAPs for all environments, including rural communities. Documents, such as checklists to ascertain a school's readiness for the program and a template for budgeting, are available, free of cost, to help schools in implementing a CSPAP (visit the SHAPE America website at www.shapeamerica.org). While rural settings have common characteristics, the unique setting of each school and district is what should drive any CSPAP-related change. Keeping the school's individual characteristics in mind, the following suggestions can be tailored to meet the integration needs of each setting.

For School Staff

Organize professional development that includes a focus on integrating themes regarding health, such as PA and healthy eating, into content areas. Ongoing training and support are critical to building new skills and receiving quality feedback needed to explore additional modes of seamless integration (Guskey, 2002). Further, poll teachers to identify the types of professional development they are most interested in related to CSPAP implementation.

Begin staff meetings with demonstrations from teachers on campus, allowing them to model successful practices from their own classroom. Physical education teachers may act as a resource to collaborate with classroom teachers to create new content presentation involving PA and healthy behaviors (Stylianou et al., 2015).

Consider inviting staff to participate in before- or after-school walking or activity programs, or design a separate program just for staff. Potential benefits to teachers and staff include feeling more energetic, having an outlet for stress, and improved mood (Langley & Kulinna, 2018). Langley and Kulinna suggested that this type of involvement may naturally create healthy role models for students within the school.

Discuss the benefits of physical activity with your principals. Administrative support is essential to implementing new practices. A lack of administrative support or the perception of this support being absent is often noted as a barrier to integrating new, healthy behavior content or methods into classrooms (e.g., Centeio et al., 2014).

Plan fitness or sport nights that combine physical activity with other content areas. For instance, coordinate with science, technology, and math to offer a STEM fitness event.

For Community Partners

In cooperation and conjunction with school-based events, community partners and parents and guardians can get involved and support a CSPAP in the following ways.

Participate in wellness fairs or fitness nights. Participating in such events supports the school and allows parents and other community members to learn about you and your place of business.

Provide funding for physical activity equipment. As demonstrated in the case study at the end of this chapter, funding from community sources can equip schools with much-needed materials to promote movement integration within all aspects of the school day. This funding could also come in the form of gift cards or products to be used as incentives for participation in programs for students, staff, or parents.

Volunteer for physical activity events at the school, such as field days, turkey trots, or jump rope competitions. Volunteering benefits the school by providing additional adult supervision for events as well as giving you the opportunity to interact with members of the community in informal settings. Share your experts and expertise. Engage as a guest speaker for grade-level assemblies to present on being healthy in your community.

SUMMARY

In this chapter, we looked at the implementation of CSPAPs within rural school settings. Beginning with an overview of research focusing on these schools, we provided evidence supporting the need for CSPAPs and enhanced focus on PA during school, including increased risk for chronic diseases, geographic barriers to active transportation to and from school, and limited access to PA programs outside of the school day. Prior relevant research is promising by demonstrating benefits to students, staff, and community through the integration of various aspects of a CSPAP. From the Appalachians to western New York, Missouri, and Nebraska, research partnerships have demonstrated positive outcomes while also identifying important barriers to success in their programs. These results contributed to the development of the evidence-based and tailored stakeholder recommendations presented within the chapter to facilitate successful implementation of future programs within rural communities.

QUESTIONS TO CONSIDER

1. How can you engage school personnel and other stakeholders (e.g., students and community members) in the development of a CSPAP?
2. What unique challenges exist for a specific school or district, and what implications do these challenges have for a CSPAP?
3. Where and how can you enhance family and community involvement?
4. What teacher support can you provide? For how long? How will this support change over time (e.g., from group workshops to individual classroom visits)?
5. What are some policy changes that may need to be implemented? Will any policy changes need revisiting as the program develops?

CASE EXAMPLE: SOUTHWESTERN U.S. RURAL COMMUNITIES

In this case example, we present findings from the first year of a CSPAP spanning five years in a state in the southwestern United States.

The case study was initiated when a philanthropic group (HealthWorks Foundation of Arizona) of local professionals with a shared goal of improving the health of their rural community approached faculty at a large university to partner in efforts to improve children's health. These efforts centered around schools.

In an attempt to address the health-related challenges (e.g., low PA levels and increased overweight and obesity levels) youth in this rural area were facing, a CSPAP was used, which included a healthy behavior knowledge component. In this process, the case study project team members partnered with school personnel within the district and designed a unique model for the school district based on the context and stakeholders' perceptions of needs. The project design and outcomes are described in this case example.

Table 13.1 displays a brief overview of the individual components of the multifaceted intervention. The table is a quick reference for what was implemented at the school-district level. The column titled "Select outcomes" provides a snapshot of results, and the column titled "Take-home lessons" gives a summary of the lessons learned from each component. This information is described in more detail in the next section.

TABLE 13.1 METHODS OVERVIEW

	School changes	Select outcomes	Take-home lessons
Design	Expanded CSPAP, including school-wide PA integration		Customize your program to meet the needs of the individual school and community.
Curricular model	Grade-specific *Fitness for Life* elementary textbook with targeted classroom instructions		Provide support for using the resources! Just handing teachers a book does not help them make changes.
Students	173 (boys = 94, girls = 79) Grades 3-8		
Healthy behavior knowledge assessment	37-item test given at the beginning and end of the year to fourth- to eighth-grade students	On average, students improved healthy behavior knowledge 19% to 29% during the year. Significant improvements in average number of correctly answered items at time 2.	Despite improvements, we still need to focus on misunderstandings and incomplete knowledge evident through the tests at both times 1 and 2.
Interviews	Semistructured interviews with teachers, school personnel, and students	Themes: (1) change takes time; (2) need for consistency in policies and practices within the school leadership; (3) noted positive student outcomes by teachers and students themselves; and (4) stakeholders' views about the need for school, family, and community partnerships.	Feedback from all stakeholders was positive about the CSPAP. However, challenges were identified and need to be addressed.
Physical activity breaks	Integrated into all classrooms based on textbook and additional resources provided		
Pedometers—step counts at school	Compared steps during the school day for a "normal" week and a "wellness" week	Average daily steps during school for normal week was 5,366 steps versus wellness week, 6,433 steps.	A school-wide program, such as a CSPAP, can improve average daily school-day steps, in particular, during focused wellness weeks.
Pedometers during physical education	Collected data at two points in the year (before and after CSPAP implementation)	Boys' average steps increased by 486 per class; girls' steps increased by 429.	A focus on quality physical education can increase students' steps during the physical education class time.
Professional development	Four workshops focusing on classroom teachers' integration of PA in the classroom and parallel workshops for the physical education teacher. Support equipment was provided, and mentor teacher provided individualized follow-up communications.		Support the teachers. Provide many examples, and give many opportunities for them to ask questions. Provide support, demonstrating practical applications of the techniques and equipment you are giving them. Use the teachers as models; let them show what is working in their classes.
Wellness weeks	Four throughout the year	Activities included PA breaks with and without use-and-play videos, school-wide nutrition events, physical education lesson plans and activities, school signs promoting wellness, school-wide PA events, and newsletters to get families involved.	Having scheduled weeks for the whole school to focus on health and activity creates excitement for your program. It also brings the school together with a common topic and provides fun ways to cross curricular boundaries. Students and staff enjoy these.

Setting

One rural school district in the southwestern United States partnered with a local university on this CSPAP project, with 18 teachers and school personnel and the students. The school district, the Diamondbacks (pseudonym), is a K-8 district with 90 percent of its students eligible for free or reduced lunch. This small community has a population of less than 4,000 people. There is little infrastructure for PA or sport in the community (e.g., lack of sidewalks, community centers, and sport fields outside of the school district). It is situated in a mountainous region about 100 miles from the closest urban community.

CSPAP Approach Used in the Diamondbacks School District

The Diamondbacks School District adopted a CSPAP model plus a nutritional component. The case study project included the following components:

- Increased physical education class time
- A conceptual physical education curriculum (active part in gym and interactive part in the classroom) through the *Fitness for Life* curricular model
- Structured recess activities
- Classroom PA breaks
- Four wellness weeks throughout the academic year (i.e., school- and class-based special activities and guest speakers invited to the school, including Eat Well Wednesday and Get Fit Friday events)
- Professional development for classroom teachers to train them in how to integrate PA and other knowledge about healthy behaviors in their classrooms
- Food service policy and nutrition practice

What We Did in the Case Study

A mentor teacher with more than 20 years of experience was recruited to collaborate and deliver professional development for this project. Having an expert teacher on hand to help teachers was invaluable. With her help, four workshops were conducted for all participating personnel at the Diamondbacks School District across the school year. At these workshops, classroom teachers discussed and practiced ideas for providing PA breaks and integrating PA and healthy behavior knowledge into many content areas across the curriculum. The process of cross-curricular integration was considered in an effort to anticipate problems and to work together as a school team to conceptualize solutions. For example, simple suggestions for integrating health knowledge while grouping students for any content activity was to give students cards with pictures of foods and then ask them to put themselves into five groups using knowledge learned earlier about the food plate (rather than just getting into groups). A targeted workshop focusing on modifications for students with disabilities was provided to teachers working in the resource classrooms as well as to the physical education teachers.

To further support teachers as they applied their new skills, the team members set up a website with resources and had our mentor teacher communicate with (email and phone) and visit the teachers. Examples of how the mentor teacher assisted the project teachers included modeling teaching lessons; coteaching lessons; providing feedback on specific lessons; and discussing curricular, teaching, and school issues. The mentor teacher along with other research team members also worked with teachers and school personnel to develop materials (e.g., lessons and activity breaks) specific to the school's and teachers' environment. There was also a school-level leader (physical education) involved in the project to coordinate efforts at the school.

Curriculum and Resources

As part of the project, classroom teachers received relevant curricular materials from the *Fitness for Life* elementary textbook series. The textbook series targets classroom instruction. Each teacher was provided the textbook specific to the grade level taught (e.g., *Fitness for Life Elementary School Classroom Guide—Kindergarten*). In addition, the physical education teacher received a classroom set of the *Fitness for Life* physical education textbook materials appropriate to the grades taught (Corbin et al., 2007, 2010).

The physical education teacher received physical education equipment for his or her program, which was determined by a school team of administrators, teachers, and students. All teachers also received a classroom set of pedometers to use with their students on a regular basis.

Gathering Evidence About the Effectiveness of the Case Study

To collect both quantitative and qualitative data, a variety of measures were employed throughout the study. Pedometers (Yamax Digi-Walker SW-200) were used to measure steps (e.g., Brusseau et al., 2011). A knowledge test was used to gauge what students learned about healthy behavior knowledge (Teatro et al., 2013). Teachers reported their participation levels (e.g., number of PA breaks and wellness week activities implemented). Wellness week activities included PA breaks with use-and-play videos (included in the *Fitness for Life* textbooks), PA breaks without the use of videos, classroom lessons and worksheets teaching about healthy behaviors, school-wide nutrition events, physical education lesson plans and activities, school signs promoting wellness, school-wide physical activities, and newsletters to promote family involvement in school-wide events. Stakeholders (i.e., teachers, school personnel, and a number of students) shared their thoughts during and near the end of the school year through interviews with the research team (along with reflections and field notes).

Project Outcomes

- PA: PA increased in the project across the year, except for daily steps (over 24 hours). Students became more active during school, wellness weeks, and physical education classes. Secondary students in grades 6-8 were less active than elementary school students.

- Knowledge: Students overall improved their healthy behavior knowledge during the year. However, students in this case study and all known studies in the United States (e.g., Kulinna, 2004) show that K-12 students know too little about being healthy. Girls and boys had no differences in healthy behavior knowledge.

- Wellness week activities: The average number of wellness week activities that the teachers implemented across the four wellness weeks are presented in table 13.2. As the table shows, on average, teachers implemented between two and six promotional activities (e.g., sending newsletters home or using signage in hallways) and between four and eight physical activities (e.g., brain breaks, physical movement breaks, or campus walks) across the four wellness weeks.

- Themes: Four major themes emerged for the year from interviews and focus groups with the teachers, school personnel, and students. The first theme was that change takes time. For example, teachers and school personnel were much more receptive to new ideas and more resourceful at the end of the year. One second-grade teacher shared, "Initially, I had a mixed reaction, the one part of teaching, feeling kinda overwhelmed with the things that are going on, 'oh one more thing to fit in.'. . . A little hesitant in the beginning but once we got into it, I could really see the benefits of the program." The workshops and continuous support from the administration and the wellness coordinator and the student buy-in helped in getting more teachers to buy in to the project over time.

At the same time, there were constant challenges, such as time constraints, in the school district as well as some opposing effects. Policies and practices with opposing effects constitute the second theme. For example, while one administrator added a checklist item for PA breaks on the classroom observation, she also prohibited walks around the school, something that students enjoyed, because of misbehavior issues. Also, the food services director went above and beyond to prepare healthy meals, but the birthday and healthy snack policy (not allowing sugary snacks from home) was not enforced.

The third theme was positive student outcomes. Students were more active and ate better at school by the end of the year. Teachers and students also expressed their positive perceptions of the program. For example, one kindergarten teacher shared, "The kids really love it, so even after wellness week, they ask about it: 'Are we going to do it again?'" Students did, however, have incomplete knowledge about PA and nutrition despite improvements.

The final theme was the widespread perception of the need for school–family partnerships discussed by all stakeholders. This was reported as one of the biggest challenges because of difficulties in communication and low parent attendance rates at school district events and conferences in this rural community. Again, this points to some of the unique challenges faced in rural environments and the need to develop innovative, context-driven plans to include families in such environments.

TABLE 13.2   Wellness Week Accomplishments

Event/week number	Mean promotion activities* per teacher	Mean PAs** per class
1	6.03	7.55
2	2.22	3.47
3	4.62	6.42
4	5.45	5.34

*Examples of promotion activities: newsletters home and signage in hallway.
**Examples of PAs: brain breaks, physical movement breaks, and campus walks.

Lessons Learned and Recommendations for Practice

Despite the health benefits of PA, many children and adolescents do not meet the recommended guidelines (U.S. Department of Health and Human Services, 2008). Using the results from the 2016 PA report card, the overall indicator for PA levels in the United States was given a grade of D because of the low prevalence of meeting PA guidelines (Tremblay et al., 2016). Similar to findings in other communities, our project found that most of the students did not meet these recommendations and that boys accumulated more steps per day than girls.

Our data supports that the implementation of a CSPAP can positively affect students' steps while at school. Students had more school-day PA (steps) than has been previously reported for elementary students in the southwestern United States (Brusseau et al., 2011). This is a revealing finding as to the impact of a comprehensive model that targets during-school PA. Remaining aware of students' PA challenges in this rural setting outside of school, school-day steps are key to getting them close to the recommended daily average rather than counting on out-of-school hours to accomplish this.

Although this project showed a significant increase in students' healthy behavior knowledge, their knowledge levels in this area were still low. Stakeholders (teachers, school personnel, and students) expressed positive perceptions of the program; however, these school personnel discussed challenges with this project as well as in general because of their rural context (e.g., limited teacher support, fewer resources, and geographic barriers between the school and families).

Based on previous literature and this case study, recommendations for practice are subsequently addressed. First, it was constructive to include stakeholders in the design of the programs for the school district. Including stakeholders along with being flexible regarding the implementation of program details in order to align with each school's unique culture helped develop a sense of ownership over the program, gain administrative support, and enhance buy-in from school staff. Second, gaining administrative support was a key factor in teacher buy-in for the program. If teachers are to feel comfortable trying new things, which may or may not be successful in their first attempts, it is the administrators who allow flexibility to do this. It is important to remember that any change requires time for teachers to experience the new thing (e.g., curriculum, innovation, and technique). Once they are exposed and begin to see positive changes, the system reinforces itself with school personnel continuing healthy behavior activities at school. Finally, change takes time and effort, and teachers need support and follow-up to change the way they teach (e.g., Guskey, 2002), particularly related to healthy behaviors because most classroom teachers were not taught to create healthy schools (although this is changing). For this reason, it is important that administrators understand why the teachers need additional support, be willing to walk by a classroom and see students out of their seats during academic instruction, and stand behind their teachers as they work to implement new strategies.

In our project, it was important for the research team members to be patient and to focus on small but critical improvements (e.g., healthy behavior knowledge increases). Team members started by supporting (e.g., offering help) early adopters who showed initiative and were motivated to participate. In response to their success, other teachers followed suit, became more engaged, and later benefited from the project team members' customized support.

The third recommendation is to have strong program leaders (e.g., PA leaders) at the school district who will advocate for changes and provide support to teachers and staff. At this school district, the leaders included an administrator, the physical education teacher, and the nutrition director. These individuals were invaluable to changing the culture of the schools and the adoption of healthy behaviors and improved knowledge outcomes.

The final recommendation is to keep in mind that rural environments will need more support to implement models promoting PA and health. This rural school district was at a disadvantage in terms of creating healthy and active schools. Some of the factors contributing to this disadvantage included (1) fewer teachers (e.g., some teachers in multiple roles); (2) limited resources (e.g., little fitness equipment); (3) bus schedules (e.g., because the majority of students took the bus to school, before- and after-school programming was limited); and (4) food service challenges included limited availability of local fresh fruits and vegetables and a lack of food policies regarding celebrations. These challenges are important to consider in decisions about what CSPAP components can be targeted and how. For instance, before-school programming can positively contribute to students' PA and readiness to learn (e.g., Stylianou, Kulinna, et al., 2016; Stylianou, van der Mars, et al., 2016); however, this component may be less feasible to implement because of bus schedules and availability of staff who can facilitate and supervise PA opportunities before school.

CHAPTER 14

International Perspectives and Initiatives

Jaimie M. McMullen, PhD
University of Northern
Colorado

Déirdre Ní Chróinín, PhD
Mary Immaculate College

Michalis Stylianou, PhD
The University of Queensland

Tuija Tammelin, PhD
LIKES Research Centre
for Physical Activity and
Health, Finland

School-based PA initiatives are commonplace internationally, with countries around the world recognizing the position of the school as a practical venue to address public health goals associated with decreasing sedentary behaviors in young people. Consistent with recommendations made by U.S. organizations, such as the Centers for Disease Control and Prevention (CDC, 2013) and the Institute of Medicine (2013), internationally, many local authorities and organizations (e.g., Department of Education and Skills [Ireland], Sportscotland [Scotland], and Department of Education and Training [Queensland, Australia]) have encouraged schools to implement a multicomponent, whole-of-school approach to PA promotion. Although the context within which programs are operating differ from country to country and, often, even from region to region within countries, many school-based PA initiatives share common strengths and challenges.

In this chapter, we will provide an overview of research originating outside of the United States that focuses on school-based PA initiatives. We will provide an overview of international policy associated with school-based PA promotion and then discuss relevant research that provides context for specific knowledge claims. Additionally, the reader will be introduced to a variety of international school-based PA initiatives and some associated case studies. The authors would like to acknowledge the complexity and enormity of the task of outlining all international school-based PA initiatives; therefore, this chapter should not be viewed as an exhaustive review. Rather, we will provide readers with some insight into established practices being used outside of the United States. When considering terminology, it is important to highlight that the CSPAP model that is promoted within the United States (CDC, 2013) does not represent all the initiatives being implemented internationally. Therefore, this chapter will adopt a more representative term of "whole-of-school" when referring to initiatives that include goals of promoting PA beyond the curricular approaches associated with physical education.

Review of Research

The following subsections will consider literature originating outside of the United States with respect to school-based PA promotion. First, we will consider the policy landscape that influences how and why PA is promoted in schools and then provide an overview of the evidence associated with whole-of-school PA promotion.

Policy Landscape

When considering the implementation of school-based PA initiatives, it is important to consider the policy landscapes that exist at local, regional, and national levels. The *EU Action Plan on Childhood Obesity 2014-2020* (European Commission, 2014), for example, mentions the school several times with respect to the successful implementation of the plan, with one of its areas for action specifically calling for the promotion of healthier environments in schools. Another area for action—encourage physical activity—asks that focus be directed to provide families with optimal opportunities to be physically active throughout the day and suggests that the school be a venue to accomplish this. Naming the school as a venue for PA participation for the whole family is in line with a CSPAP that includes parents in its framework (CDC, 2013). At a more local level, many countries, in response to public health concerns, have developed their own national PA plans, which also highlight the importance of the school. The World Health Organization (WHO, 2015) recently produced factsheets from the various EU member states that report information such as whether there are national documents and action plans, recommendations, and goals and surveillance of PA; who takes leadership for PA promotion; and the nature of any intersectoral networks that exist. These factsheets provide an interesting snapshot of PA policy and practice from a variety of countries. Many of the country-specific factsheets represented in the sample highlight school-based PA promotion efforts. For example, in Denmark, Put the School in Motion trains teachers to infuse movement into their academic curriculum, and in Spain, the Give Me 10! initiative encourages 5- to 10-minute PA breaks and additional active teaching units throughout the curriculum (WHO, 2015).

Globally, several countries regularly participate in an evaluation process that provides report card–style grades for a variety of PA measures (Tremblay et al., 2014). The most recent global exercise included 38 countries from six continents. The countries were evaluated in the following categories: overall PA, organized sport participation, active play, active transportation, sedentary behaviors, family and peers, school, community and built environment, and government strategies and investments (Active Healthy Kids Global Alliance, 2016). When considering the school, the following indicators are assessed:

- Percentage of schools with active school policies (e.g., daily PA, recess, "everyone plays" approach, bike racks at school, traffic calming on school property, and outdoor time)

- Percentage of schools where the majority (80 percent) of students are taught by a physical education specialist

- Percentage of schools where the majority (80 percent) of students are offered at least 150 minutes of physical education per week

- Percentage of schools that offer PA opportunities (excluding physical education) to the majority (80 percent) of their students
- Percentage of parents with children and youth who have access to PA opportunities at school in addition to physical education
- Percentage of schools with students who have regular access to facilities and equipment that support PA (e.g., gymnasium, outdoor playgrounds, sporting fields, and equipment in good condition)

When considering the trends in the results, only 59 percent of the participating countries received a C grade or better. This means that 41 percent of the countries are succeeding with less than half of children and youth when it comes to promoting PA at school.

Whole-of-School PA Promotion

In line with a CSPAP, whole-of-school, comprehensive approaches to PA promotion are being implemented worldwide with a variety of national, regional, and local initiatives in place to increase the likelihood that young people will achieve internationally accepted PA recommendations. This approach to PA promotion has been commonplace internationally for some time, but there continues to be a lack of a significant body of research focused on experiences of whole-of-school PA program development and implementation in countries around the world.

In Europe, the major push toward promoting PA (and other health behaviors) in schools came in 1992 when the European Network of Health Promoting Schools was launched. The basis of the network was to encourage schools to promote health through the curriculum, environment, and wider community (Nutbeam, 1992). Published research originating outside of the United States in this area dates back to the mid- to late 1990s, for example, the work of Pühse (1995) on the Bewegte Schule, or Moving School, initiative in Germany and McBride and Midford's (1999) work on the Western Australian School Health Project. One of the challenges with learning about international whole-of-school PA initiatives is that the majority of the work is published in the native language of the country of origin, which is the case with

Pühse's work. However, more literature, published in English, that discusses implementation strategies and reports results of whole-of-school PA promotion and intervention efforts has started to emerge internationally.

In Ireland, the school's role in promoting PA was explored, and it was revealed that primary schools that implement the Active School Flag (ASF) in Ireland improved the structure and inclusivity of PA opportunities for children (Ní Chróinín et al., 2012). Further, it was determined that employing a self-evaluation and self-improvement process, which is encouraged through the ASF initiative, could lead to positive changes in school-based PA promotion. More recently, Bowles and colleagues (2017) provided insight on how engagement in the ASF processes positively affect children's engagement in PA by encouraging innovation and fostering collaborations that were empowering and inclusive.

Implementation of the first year of a two-year whole-of-school PA intervention, Physical Activity 4 Everyone (PA4E1), has reduced the decline of PA participation among young people in Australia (Sutherland et al., 2015). Implemented in disadvantaged schools, the intervention included seven school-based PA promotion strategies, which were introduced in a staged fashion. The two-year outcomes of the program revealed positive results associated with increased minutes of moderate-to-vigorous PA in adolescents (Sutherland et al., 2016). These results support the recommendations made through policy and research for multicomponent approaches to PA promotion and are promising because the participants are secondary school students. However, given that the intervention has a planned two-year implementation period, its trial may have limited ability to suggest sustainability practices.

In New Zealand, Project Energize, identified as a "through-school" program that incorporates PA and nutrition in an attempt to control obesity, has seen encouraging results related to PA, body mass index and fitness outcomes (Rush et al., 2011; Rush, McLennan, et al., 2014). Recently, Project Energize was assessed to consider the cost effectiveness of the initiative. It was determined that the project was cost effective and could help improve long-term quality of life (Rush, Obolonkin, et al., 2014). Most importantly, and something that could serve as a guide for other programs, in 2015 Project Energize celebrated its 10-year anniversary (Rush et al., 2016). This program has been sustained by funding from the local health department and has reached over 53,000 elementary school students. The positive results rendered from this initiative have not only fueled its sustainability but have also inspired the development of a sister initiative in Ireland called Project Spraoi (Coppinger et al., 2016).

Research on Finland's Finnish Schools on the Move initiative has shown positive changes in schools. For example, initial research into the program has demonstrated increased PA during recess and throughout the school day, more recess time spent outdoors, more active commuting to school during winter, and greater student involvement in the planning of school PA opportunities (Haapala et al., 2014, 2016; Tammelin et al., 2012). A survey completed by school staff saw most respondents agreeing that PA during the school day increases student satisfaction with school and contributes to a more pleasant and peaceful learning environment during academic lessons (Kämppi et al., 2013).

The international initiative with the largest published evidence base originates from the Canadian province of British Columbia. There have been a number of research publications that illustrate the benefits of the Action Schools! BC initiative. The initiative has not only been successful in increasing PA participation (Naylor & McKay, 2009; Naylor, Macdonald, Zebedee, et al., 2006; Naylor et al., 2008); it has also effectively promoted healthy eating (Day et al., 2008). Children who participated in Action Schools! BC made gains in bone mass and strength as well as improvements in cardiovascular fitness and blood pressure (Naylor, Macdonald, Reed, et al., 2006; Reed et al., 2008). Children who participated also maintained levels of academic performance similar to their peers'. Academic performance was increased for children who were performing below their grade level (Ahamed et al., 2007). The Action Schools! BC model has also been shown to be effective in promoting PA and healthy eating in First Nations and rural aboriginal populations in British Columbia (Naylor et al., 2010; Tomlin et al., 2012).

Knowledge Claims

The review of research in the previous section of this chapter gives rise to several assertions that can be made about the available evidence on CSPAPs in international contexts.

- Internationally, schools are being asked to promote PA beyond physical education by including the whole school as well as the surrounding community.
- Multicomponent initiatives can have positive impacts on PA levels, body mass index, blood pressure, and fitness outcomes.
- Although initiatives differ widely, there are consistent features of many whole-of-school programs, including PA throughout the school day and quality physical education.
- There are many short-term evaluations of whole-of-school programs that demonstrate positive results.
- Few long-term evaluations of outcomes or impact have been conducted.

Knowledge Gaps and Directions for Future Research

Given that the preceding review of school-based PA literature is not exhaustive, the reader is encouraged to consult one of several publications that originate from outside the United States and that discuss a variety of school-based PA interventions (e.g., Cale & Harris, 2006; Dobbins et al., 2013). However, based on what we do know, there seems to be several gaps that warrant consideration for future research.

The gaps in the international research relating to whole-of-school approaches for PA promotion mirror those encountered in the United States. For example, little is known about the sustainability of effective programs and whether programs are actually reaching the inactive population for which they are intended (Reid, 2009). A recent Cochrane Review of school-based PA promotion initiatives determined that there is more research to do if we are to understand the long-term impact of whole-of-school and other school-based PA interventions (Dobbins et al., 2013). There also seems to be a need to understand more fully the perceptions and experiences of stakeholders as the recipients of these school-based programs (Dyson, 2006). There does not appear to be consistent evaluation procedures within and across programs, and there is an absence of process evaluations that could provide valuable insight into the sustainability and feasibility of programs.

The reviewed research appears to support the trends in the United States, with the prevalence of whole-of-school PA programs being implemented in the elementary school setting. Given what we know about the decrease of PA as children transition to adolescents, researchers worldwide should make an effort to expand their work to include the secondary school level. When considering the role of physical educators as champions of PA promotion within the school, little is known about their perceptions of this role or preparedness to fulfill the responsibilities. Cale (2000a) confirmed that physical education teachers in central England lacked a significant amount of knowledge associated with PA promotion in schools. Although this data is more than a decade old, there is a lack of recent work describing otherwise. Funding and support are also common challenges among international programs, and although some governments are dedicating additional funding to support these efforts (e.g., Finland, subsequently discussed), others have stopped operating at the institutional level based on lack of funding (e.g., Poland's PE with Class [English translation]).

Although it is difficult to comment extensively on the effectiveness of whole-of-school approaches internationally because of limited published work, the responsibility being placed on schools worldwide means that this subject must remain a research priority. A challenge associated with identifying specific best practices associated with whole-of-school PA promotion is that it is important to consider the sociocultural, organizational, and environmental influences that exist within schools (Cale, 2000b). Schools located only a couple of miles away from each other can significantly differ contextually, so considering the differing contexts that are possible within an international landscape is daunting. However, it is important that we continue to engage in relevant research to determine the extent to which school-based PA interventions and initiatives are effectively meeting public health recommendations and find ways to share results and best practices across our international networks.

Evidence-Based Recommendations and Applications

The following section will highlight initiatives from Australia, Canada, Finland, and Ireland with the intent of providing the reader with some practical examples of whole-of-school PA promotion strategies being used outside of the United States. Given the partnership approach, which includes stakeholders across various groups, this information provided about the initiatives is relevant for school staff and community partners alike; however, some specific recommendations for school professionals and community partners is provided. Additional information on some of these initiatives, including best practices, relevant research, and areas for development, can be found in a recent issue of *Quest* (McMullen et al., 2015).

Australia: CQ Sporty Schools

According to the 2016 national report card on PA, more than half of Australian children and young people are not meeting the daily PA recommendations (Schranz et al., 2016). In this same report card, the indicator "school—infrastructure, policies, and programming" was assigned a grade of B minus. However, although schools have some PA policies and programs in place, available data suggests that recommendations from the federal government as well as from state and territory governments and other associations regarding the time allocation for PA and physical education are often not met in Australian schools (e.g., Audit Office of New South Wales, 2012).

The Physical Activity Innovation in Schools (PAIS) project was an Australian initiative created to develop, test, and share new and innovative localized and tailored approaches that make it easier for schools and teachers to regularly provide PA to students during the school day (M. McNamara, CQ Sporty Schools project coordinator, personal communication, September 11,

2015; Queensland School Sport, 2015). PAIS was developed based on the evaluation findings of the Queensland Department of Education and Training's Smart Moves Policy, which called for less prescriptive approaches to increasing PA in schools (Department of Education and Training, 2012; M. McNamara, personal communication, September 11, 2015). Further, the project was designed to capitalize on the inherent expertise within schools (e.g., classroom teachers and physical education specialists) in pursuing the preceding goal (M. McNamara, personal communication, September 11, 2015).

The project targeted primary schools in two of the seven education regions in the state of Queensland and was funded by the Queensland Government under the Queensland Healthy Children initiative, which is part of the National Partnership Agreement on Preventive Health. Hence, the project had a preventive character, which was designed to contribute to efforts to reduce the rates of chronic disease in the community. PAIS was also aligned with the Queensland Department of Education and Training's policy for Supporting Student Health and Wellbeing, which highlights the critical role of schools in providing opportunities for students to participate in both structured and unstructured PA during school time.

In Central Queensland, the PAIS project was named CQ Sporty Schools, and it focused on reinvigorating school sport (Queensland School Sport, 2015). Specifically, CQ Sporty Schools aimed to increase PA programming in Central Queensland state schools through (1) providing training to classroom teachers to enhance their competence and confidence to deliver sport and PA during school time and (2) developing partnerships with local, regional, state, and national sporting programs and organizations that share an interest in raising the levels of PA in children. These two aspects were considered critical in maximizing the value, quality, and sustainability of the project. Further, CQ Sporty Schools adopted a strengths-based approach, which acknowledges the strengths (i.e., personnel, structures, and resources) of the various school communities and attempts to use them in the best possible way to increase school sport and PA participation (Queensland School Sport, 2015).

For the purposes of the CQ Sporty Schools program, primarily physical education specialists or similarly skilled teachers were recruited to act as project coordinators for their schools. Physical education in Queensland primary schools is primarily taught by specialists; however, generalist classroom teachers typically teach physical education in primary schools across the rest of Australia (Queensland School Sport, 2015). Project coordinators, in collaboration with school administrators, worked to train their school's classroom teachers in terms of delivering PA and also worked to form partnerships with various sporting organizations and individuals, particularly from their local communities. More than 30 schools from the Central Queensland region were recruited to participate in the CQ Sporty Schools program trial with their year 3 and 4 teachers and students. Participating schools were supported by grants for purchasing equipment and securing teacher release time for professional development.

Canada (British Columbia): Action Schools! BC

Action Schools! BC is a comprehensive school health–based model that aims to integrate both healthy eating and PA into school life. Action Schools! BC supports public, independent, First Nations, and Francophone elementary and middle schools in British Columbia to make healthy choices easy for children, teachers, administrators, and the wider school community. The vision for Action Schools! BC model draws on social-ecological theory to integrate healthy living into school life by leveraging opportunities the school setting provides to contribute to students' health (MacKay et al., 2015). Engagement and empowerment of stakeholders, including educators, students, administrators, caregivers, and members of the school community, is at the core of the model. A partnership approach to social change through knowledge translation and exchange is proposed. Action Schools! BC is a whole-of-school model that promotes best practice in six action zones:

- School environment: Promoting a safe and inclusive school environment that supports healthy choices

- Physical education: Supports the delivery of physical education through professional development for teachers, leadership programs for children, and resource and planning guidance
- Classroom action: Promotes classroom-based PA and healthy eating activities
- Family and community: Promotes PA and health events and activities that connect local community members and families
- Extracurricular: Promotes opportunities for PA before, during, and after school
- School spirit: Encourages whole-of-school promotion of healthy eating and PA

Action Schools! BC provides training to teachers and students to promote inclusive and diverse PA and healthy eating opportunities across these six action zones. Professional development for teachers includes workshops focused on PA and health policy, implementation practice, and in-school mentoring support. Resources are provided to schools to support them to create a customized action plan to promote healthy living and increase PA opportunities for children in the schools. These resources include planning guides, resource lists, and practical activity ideas for implementation, and they are freely available on the Action Schools! BC website. The content of training and resources is informed by best practices and interventions through both national and international partnerships.

Action Schools! BC was developed in 2002 and initially targeted at grades 4-6 in elementary schools. The pilot included 275 elementary schools and 25,740 children in British Columbia. Pilot activities included professional development for teachers and provision of curriculum-linked resources to schools, including teaching resources and support materials. An evaluation of the pilot took place over 18 months in 2003-2004. The evaluation involved over 500 children from 10 elementary schools in Vancouver and Richmond (seven intervention and three nonintervention) in a randomized controlled trial (Naylor, Macdonald, Zebedee, et al., 2006). Findings indicated that participation in Action Schools! BC resulted in a significant, positive influence on minutes of PA. These encouraging findings from the pilot evaluation resulted in a scaling up of the initiative

supported by funding from the British Columbia Ministry of Health, and it was rolled out across the whole province. The initiative was also helped by a mandate from the provincial government of British Columbia that required all elementary schools to deliver 30 minutes of daily PA. In the ensuing years, a new middle school level was developed, and a healthy eating component was added in 2007. In 2006, a student leadership component was added, which involved provision of training and resources to older children to help them lead younger children in indoor and outdoor physical activities and healthy eating activities. By June 2012, Action Schools! BC had significant uptake across British Columbia: 1,455 (92 percent) schools were registered. Over 81,000 teachers had participated in workshops, and over 550,000 children have been involved in the program since 2004.

Demonstration of effectiveness in different settings has been recognized as a particular strength of the model (Kriemler et al., 2011). Action Schools! BC demonstrates the value of partnership with key stakeholders to enhance children's PA and healthy eating practices. The influence of support from the provincial government and significant funding provided momentum to implementation. Training and resourcing of teachers aligned with supportive school policies equipped the local school community to positively influence school-based PA and health choices.

Finland: Finnish Schools on the Move

The Finnish Schools on the Move initiative is a national action program that aims to establish a more physically active operating culture in schools. Schools and municipalities participating in the program implement their own plans to enhance PA during the school day, mostly during recess and academic lessons. However, the number of mandatory physical education lessons have not been increased on a large scale. The program supports the dissemination of the ideas and practices developed by schools through organizing professional development seminars and producing and distributing educational materials. Finnish Schools on the Move operates in close interaction with the central government and has been implemented from the bottom up and top down simultaneously. While the program has been initiated by the government (top down), each school is given autonomy to plan the activities that it believes would most benefit the development of a physically active culture (bottom up).

The Finnish Schools on the Move program began in 2010 with a two-year pilot phase involving 45 schools in basic education (grades 1-9) throughout Finland (Tammelin et al., 2012). In the second phase (2012-2015), the program expanded significantly, and since 2015, it has also been implemented in upper secondary school and higher education settings. During the third phase (2015-2018), the program became a governmental priority and is one of the key projects for developing learning environments in basic education. As stated in May 2015, "The *Schools on the Move* project will be expanded across the country to ensure school children one hour of PA each day" (Prime Minister's Office, Finland, 2015). Finish Schools on the Move is currently funded by the Ministry of Education and Culture and organized by the National Board of Education, regional state administrative agencies, and various other organizations. To support the recent actions related to the government program, 21 million euros ($25 million) have been allocated by the Ministry of Education and Culture for the program to operate in municipalities for 2016-2018. In January 2017, 77 percent (1,878 of 2,449) of all schools in basic education had registered with the program.

Municipalities and schools participating in the program implement their own individual plans to promote PA during the school day. This bottom-up approach, including implementation of these customized plans, has appeared to enhance principals', teachers', and students' feelings of ownership over the process. Specific actions have not been required from schools, but many of them have chosen to increase and promote PA during recesses and lessons and before and after school. Actions to increase PA during recess have especially been a key element. In many schools, students have been educated to act as "recess activators" for organizing PA among their peers during recess time. In schools, concrete actions have also included the investments in equipment and facilities to motivate recess activity and students in the planning of playgrounds. Additionally,

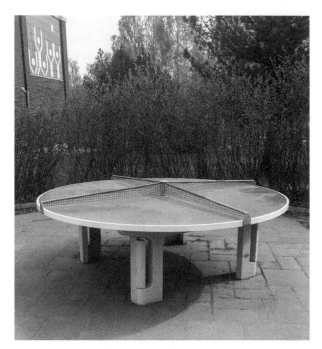

A four-person Ping-Pong table located on a playground at a lower secondary school in Finland that was designed in consultation with students.

© Jaimie McMullen

the school-day structure has changed to allow for prolonged recess periods to organize activities as well as implementing active breaks and physically active teaching methods during academic lessons.

The program disseminates schools' ideas and best practices regarding how to make the school day more active, and schools can exchange ideas by participating in local and national professional development seminars. Finnish Schools on the Move also provides materials and information about the latest research results and proven practices on the website. Schools have been offered the opportunity to get help from a local mentor. To help schools implement their plans, a guide for how to become a "School on the Move" has been published as well as a self-evaluation tool for PA promotion in schools. After completing the online self-evaluation survey, consisting of nine development areas, schools get a visual summary of their answers, making them aware of their own status of action and school culture concerning PA promotion.

Ireland: ASF

In Ireland an active school is a school that strives to achieve a physically educated and active school community. Active schools are recognized through an ASF (Active School Flag) award. The ASF is a national-level, whole-of-school PA initiative in Ireland that was developed in 2009 by the Department of Education and Skills, which continues to fund and oversee the initiative through a National Steering Committee. Primary and postprimary schools, special schools (special educational needs), and Youthreach centers (early school leavers) can all engage in the ASF process. According to the ASF website, as of January 2017, there were 655 schools with a current flag status. The voluntary nature of the ASF award means that, in many schools, an individual who acts as the ASF coordinator champions the process. To be awarded an ASF, a school must follow these steps:

- Raise whole-of-school and community awareness: All members of your school community should be informed about the ASF process and invited to contribute.
- Register and form an ASF committee: An ASF coordinator should be appointed and a committee formed, including representatives from all areas, such as pupils, teachers, parents, and the wider community.
- Complete a self-evaluation of current provision across the following four areas:
  - Physical education planning, resources, and professional development
  - PA promotion, including active travel, extracurricular activities, and PA promotion during the school day
  - Partnerships with pupils, parents, the local community, and national agencies
  - Active School Week participation as an integral part of the ASF process

Schools are then required to plan and implement improvements across the preceding four areas and demonstrate the impact of these changes on their school community. It is recommended that schools implement improvements at their own pace and monitor them for tangible impacts on the school community. The ASF is noncompetitive, with emphasis on self-improvement by considering levels of provision at the outset of the process and local factors, such as access to facilities and resources. Exemplars from other schools, support resources, and examples of activities are provided on the program's website. The ASF does not provide any direct training or resources to schools but, rather, encourages schools to access support and resources in their local communities and through national sport organizations.

Accreditation involves submission of the required ASF documentation through an online form. Submissions are compared to defined success criteria using evidence such as film clips, photographs, testimonials from children and members of the school community, and the school website. An accreditation visit is completed in the school to confirm achievement of all success criteria. Awarding of the ASF includes receipt of an ASF certificate for display in the school, an actual flag that can be flown outside the school to demonstrate recognition as an Active School, and a letter of congratulations. Usually, a flag-raising ceremony is held to celebrate the awarding of the ASF. The ASF award is for a three-year period, at which time, schools can reapply for the flag based on a similar self-evaluation process.

The levels of participation from schools, particularly at the primary level, in this voluntary initiative and the extensive positive testimonials from participating schools are indicators of success of the ASF initiative. There is, however, limited research on the impact of the initiative on PA levels and children's experiences of PA participation in schools that have adopted the physically active culture advocated by the initiative. However, as mentioned in the introduction to this chapter, Ní Chróinín and colleagues (2012) have found that engagement in the ASF processes prompted schools to prioritize and promote PA provision in ways that resulted in children's experiencing a wider range of more inclusive physical activities.

For School Staff

Based on the examples from Australia, Canada, Finland, and Ireland, school professionals should consider the following recommendations:

- Seek support from the school administrator when implementing a whole-of-school PA program.

- Complete a self-evaluation that will provide you with information about current available PA opportunities in your school.

- Learn about the resources available to you (e.g., funding, ideas, and social support).

- Develop a team or committee that includes a variety of stakeholders (e.g., students, teachers, school staff, parents, and community members).

- Consider a bottom-up approach when designing your whole-of-school PA program that considers the needs of your school community.

For Community Partners

Based on the examples from Australia, Canada, Finland, and Ireland, community partners should consider the following recommendations:

- Approach schools or accept invitations from schools to be involved in whole-of-school PA promotion efforts, particularly on committees that are dedicated to whole-of-school PA programming.

- Consider resources that you might be able to provide to schools that could support the implementation and sustainability of whole-of-school PA programs (e.g., facilities, equipment, volunteers, and advertising).

- Consider ways that you can specifically support secondary schools that are trying to develop a more physically active school culture.

SUMMARY

This chapter provides context from an international perspective for school-based PA promotion. Several successful PA initiatives are being implemented in schools worldwide, and lessons can be learned and applied from these efforts. While context differs from country to country (and even from city to city), schools, as an institution, have similar features. Therefore, we encourage readers to seek out ideas for successful school-based PA promotion not only from their local regions but also from distant places because schools are more similar than they are different.

QUESTIONS TO CONSIDER

1. How does high-level policy affect school-based PA promotion efforts within schools?

2. Why is there is so little evidence of PA initiatives within secondary schools as compared to elementary schools internationally?

3. Choose one of the PA initiatives outlined in this chapter, and provide two strengths of the initiative and two areas of development that could strengthen the program.

4. When considering the various PA initiatives outlined here, list and discuss at least three characteristics that are observed across several initiatives (e.g., partnership approach).

5. What can be learned from considering initiatives from many places? How do culture and context affect the delivery of school-based PA initiatives?

CASE EXAMPLES

The following case examples are compiled from the stories of various schools that exhibit an active school culture and are representative of scenarios that are within schools from each of the countries discussed.

Australia—Collaboration

Alpha State School is a primary school in a rural town in Central Queensland. The school serves about 700 students in years prep to 6 and has over 40 full-time equivalent teaching staff, including two part-time specialized health and physical education (HPE) teachers. Students in Alpha State School are provided with one weekly 30-minute HPE lesson as well as two daily breaks (a 40-minute lunch break and a 20-minute afternoon break), during which they can eat and be physically active. Students at this school in year 5 and higher have opportunities to participate in interschool sports.

As soon as the CQ Sporty Schools program was announced, the two HPE teachers at Alpha State School, Alison and Jon, approached the administration team and obtained approval to enroll the school in the program. Upon approval from the administration, Alison and Jon arranged a meeting with all eight year 3 and 4 teachers (female = 7; male = 1; average teaching experience = 3.9 years), who willingly decided to participate in the program with their classes (n = 210 students). Subsequently, Alison and Jon secured funding through the program and assumed the role of program coordinators at their school.

Alison and Jon were passionate about the program and sought to find ways to facilitate its success and sustainability. Upon approval from the administration, they scheduled a weekly 30-minute program session (in addition to the weekly HPE lesson) for all year 3 and 4 classes and, hence, made it part of the school schedule. Additionally, on program days, Jon and Alison set up all necessary equipment so that the classroom teachers would not need to worry about appropriate equipment or setup time. Further, Alison and Jon used program funding to secure release time for the classroom teachers, during which they engaged with various sports from both a participant and a teacher perspective under the guidance of expert community coaches. For example, they received volleyball training during two half days and also received continuous support from the volleyball coach during the period they taught the sport. Support for these teachers also included the provision of manuals with activities and games.

Because of the training they received, classroom teachers reported feeling more competent and confident in delivering sport lessons to their students and enjoying going out for the weekly sport session. Classroom teachers also took ownership of the program and, without any support from Jon and Alison, organized an all-day volleyball carnival in collaboration with the external volleyball coach. Both classroom and HPE teachers noted improved student skill levels in the sports taught through the program and enhanced cooperation and conflict management skills during sport and in the classroom. Additionally, many students joined before- and after-school clubs as a result of their participation in the program.

Ireland—Leadership and Student Voice

The following case study is compiled from the stories of various schools that have achieved the ASF award in Ireland. For real-life examples, video testimonials, and photo stories, visit the ASF website.

Abbeyview Primary School is a four-teacher primary school in a small rural village in southeast Ireland. It is the only primary school in the village. Boys and girls aged 4-12 attend the school. The school has a long association with the Gaelic Athletic Association (GAA) in the traditional Irish team invasion games, hurling, and Gaelic football. The boys in senior classes represent the school in interscholastic GAA tournaments. There is no team for the girls. Tom is involved in the GAA locally and trains the boys' school team. He is dedicated to the team and gives his time voluntarily. Tom is conscious, however, that not all children are part of this team and that there are no other opportunities for being active after school. Tom is eager to provide PA opportunities for all the children in the school. He particularly wants to find options to cater to less skilled children, who shy away from team sports. Tom suggests to the staff members that they apply for the ASF.

Tom volunteers to act as coordinator. He organizes class elections to vote children onto the ASF committee. In organizing the class nominations, he emphasizes to the children the importance of having both children involved in sport in the school already and children who are not active at school included on the committee. The committee also includes some parents and the school principal. With Tom's help, the children on the ASF committee lead a consultation process with other children in the school, which involved a survey and interviews. They asked the children what they liked about current provision and asked them to identify new activities that they would like to implement at the school.

Led by the children's ideas, Tom sourced and organized a number of new PA options based on the principles of variety and choice of activity. For example, Marie, one of the other teachers, volunteered to lead a yoga class every morning before school. All classes engaged in cycling activities as part of an active travel initiative. Rounders (similar to baseball) games were played at lunchtime in preference to the more physical game of soccer. Tom sourced new ideas around cooperative and noncompetitive activities for all the teachers to use in physical education classes. The children love the new approach to PA in their school. The yoga class has full attendance from all senior pupils every morning. The children can identify classmates who are now physically active at lunchtime when, before, they would stand around talking. The no-contact nature of rounders allows the boys and girls to play together. The "sporty" children enjoy the variety of activity and new challenges. All the children enjoy the new physical education when they get to try out new games and activities. Abbeyview Primary School was awarded the ASF in May 2014. The children nominated Tom to raise the flag at the award ceremony because of all the work he had done to help them receive the ASF. One year on the ASF children's committee is still operational, and their voices continue to shape provision of PA in the school.

Finland—The Culture of Active Transport

Central Secondary School (CSS) is a lower secondary school located in Finland that serves 580 students aged 13-16 years. Consistent with the cultural norm in Finland, the majority of students commute to and from school using active transport (i.e., bicycles). The school day starts at 8:00 a.m. and includes regular breaks throughout the school day so that students are not sitting in the same class for longer than 45 minutes at a time. The school schedule was designed purposefully to include breaks long enough to provide students with the opportunity to engage in PA. As a result, there is a break every 45 minutes during the school day, which results in five breaks throughout the school day (in addition to an extended lunch break) with break times ranging from 5-28 minutes.

This school participates in the Finnish Schools on the Move program and puts an emphasis on developing an active school culture to make the day more pleasant for students and teachers. One initiative that the school does not need to "push" is active transport. The majority of students at this school cycle (or walk) to school each day, even in the winter when there is a significant amount of snow on the ground. There is a large bike shelter at

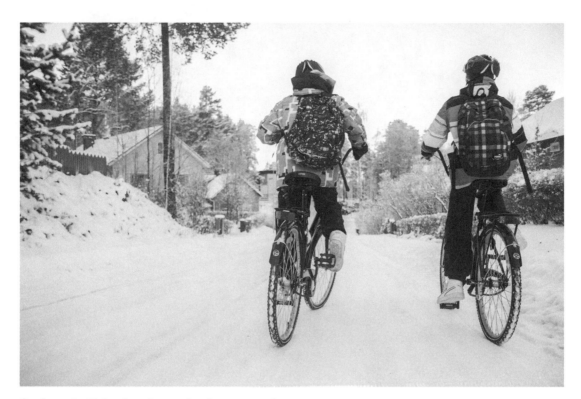

Students in Finland cycle to school year-round.

Courtesy of Finnish Schools on the Move, Jouni Kallio

the front of the school for visitors to campus. This shelter is regularly filled with hundreds of bicycles, which are left unlocked and lined up side by side. Additionally, there are several other informal bike racks across campus—grass or concrete areas where young people just leave their bikes in groups to collect at the end of the day. Students at CSS claim that it is easier to cycle to school than driving a car from their homes because the multiple bike paths leading to their school are more convenient and take less time in commuting.

Infrastructure and high-level policy in Finland facilitate active commuting as an accepted and convenient mode of transportation. Therefore, schools that participate in the Finnish Schools on the Move program are able to focus on other school-based PA promotion efforts as they work to build their active school culture.

CHAPTER 15

Implementation of CSPAPs in Nontraditional Settings

Timothy A. Brusseau, PhD
University of Utah

James C. Hannon, PhD
Kent State University

This chapter is designed to provide important contextual information about nontraditional education settings as well as strategies and suggestions for implementation of a CSPAP. Nontraditional settings include preschools, universities, special schools, alternative schools, homeschools, and youth in custody facilities. To date, there is very limited research related to CSPAPs in these alternative contexts, which opens many future research opportunities. In this chapter, we review the research on these variables; propose knowledge claims based on this research; identify knowledge gaps and propose recommendations for future research on staff involvement; suggest practical implications from the existing research for staff, staff supervisors, staff educators, and policy makers; and provide case examples of successful CSPAP initiatives.

Review of Research

This section highlights either the research that has been conducted or lack of research pertaining to preschools, universities, special schools, alternative schools, homeschools, and youth in custody.

Preschools

In the United States, 61 percent of preschool-aged children attend some type of childcare center (Chuang et al., 2017). The Institute of Medicine (2011) has recommended that preschoolers participate in 15 minutes or more of PA per hour, which equates to three hours per day. Unfortunately, data indicates that preschool-aged children are not meeting this recommendation (Bornstein et al., 2011; Reilly, 2010). A lack of adequate PA participation could be a factor associated with 22.8 percent of children aged 2-5 years being classified as overweight or obese (Ogden et al., 2014).

Given the number of children attending childcare centers, these venues offer an ideal location to affect daily PA levels. In fact, Pate and O'Neil (2012) have highlighted the recommendation that children receive 120 minutes of moderate-to-vigorous PA (MVPA) per eight hours spent in a childcare setting. However, even though most preschools are regulated by states, with the exception of Head Start programs, very few states actually have requirements for daily PA (Van Stan et al., 2013).

A limited amount of research has been conducted in preschool settings assessing the impact of PA interventions. Those studies that have been conducted indicate that the most effective programs include multicomponent interventions that have structured, teacher-led PA; involve parents; and provide ample outdoor space and portable equipment (Ling et al., 2015; Pate et al., 2013). Given the factors that have been shown to be effective in increasing PA, it would seem that a CSPAP would be ideal to implement and evaluate within childcare settings.

Colleges and Universities

Each year, 21 million young people attend college (U.S. Department of Education, 2016). Traditionally, many universities required some PA-related courses to be completed as part of the general education requirements for graduation. Over the past 20 years, many of these requirements have subsided, thus limiting the PA opportunities for many students.

CSPAPs have not been formally implemented and evaluated at the college and university level. However, we do know that the college years are a critical time of transition from adolescence to adulthood when lifestyle habits, such as PA, can be greatly influenced (Dinger et al. 2014; Gordon-Larsen et al. 2004). Data from the National College Health Assessment II suggests that meeting MVPA recommendations is associated with several positive health factors, including fruit and vegetable consumption, adequate sleep, and a healthy body mass index (Dinger et al., 2017). Many colleges and universities have a variety of support structures in place to encourage PA among students, faculty, and staff, including campus recreation facilities, outdoor recreation opportunities, club sports, intramurals, residential life, sport and PA classes, and employee wellness programs.

Evidence points to the effectiveness of many of these existing support structures. For example, participation in sport and PA classes has a positive effect on students meeting MVPA recommendations, PA enjoyment, and making students more aware of PA opportunities on their campus and in the community (Brock et al., 2016; Curry et al., 2015; Melton et al., 2015). Additionally, outdoor and campus recreation programs have been proven to have positive impacts on areas such as academic success, retention, improved mental and physical health, and development of social skills (Andre et al., 2017). University wellness programs have been shown to have a positive impact on both PA and cardiovascular risk factors (Butler et al., 2015; Haines et al., 2007).

Nontraditional School Settings

A growing number of youth attend school in alternative contexts, including special schools, alternative schools, and juvenile justice facilities. These alternative contexts generally refer to educational settings outside of conventional elementary and secondary schools. A vast majority of youth in these nontraditional schools are dealing with poverty, poor educational experiences, lack of adult supervision, and learning disabilities. They typically have poor attendance and disciplinary issues and are underperforming academically. Other schools or facilities are designed specifically for youth with a cognitive or physical disability, girls who are pregnant or parenting, or youth in custody. Juvenile justice facilities, alternative schools, and special schools are three common alternative education contexts, and each of them has unique complexities that need to be considered when planning.

Special Schools

Special schools most often include youth with a disability. Special schools may be designed specifically for youth with autism, deafness, blindness, or other disabilities. Children with disabilities are more susceptible for being physically inactive and are, therefore, often exposed to the hypokinetic diseases associated with low levels of PA (Sherrill, 1997). Rimmer and Marques (2012) found that children with disabilities are falling well short of meeting PA recommendations. More specifically, children with disabilities spend more time sedentary and are six times more likely to be obese when compared to typically developing peers (Neter et al., 2011). Certain disabilities also may be related to less PA, making it essential to understand student disabilities (Sit et al., 2007). Rimmer (2006) has also suggested that many disabilities limit youth ability to participate in normal daily activities. It is common for children with disabilities to spend limited time in organized or structured activity opportunities (Law et al., 2006). Furthermore, it is important to be aware of the location of the activity, the environment, and what social support is available because these factors will directly affect activity participation (Sit et al., 2007). PA has been shown to improve behavior in children with disabilities (Miramontez & Schwartz, 2016). Unfortunately, little is known about PA of children in special schools. Sit and colleagues (2007) found that children with disabilities accumulate little PA at school. They specifically recommended increased frequency of physical education, more PA opportunities throughout the school day, and home and community involvement. A follow-up study (Sit et al., 2008) found that both policy and the environment affected PA accumulation in physical education class and recess. More recently, Sit and colleagues (2017) found that children with disabilities spend 70 percent of their school day sedentary and children with intellectual disabilities have even lower PA. This study again highlights the need for cost-effective PA programs.

Alternative Schools

Alternative schools often serve students who are at high risk for failing or dropping out of regular school or have been expelled because of behavioral issues (Sirard et al., 2008). Alternative schools may also cater to youth who are working, pregnant, or parenting. These youth often have issues with attendance or abridged schedules, which make regular PA difficult. Kubik and colleagues (2004) found that very few opportunities and little physical space were available for PA programming in alternative schools and that teachers and administrators were very supportive of PA intervention opportunities. Sirard and colleagues (2008) explored the PA patterns of alternative high school students and suggested that PA was relatively low in this population. They continued by suggesting the importance of programming or interventions in this setting. Grunbaum and colleagues (2001) found that many alternative school students are at risk for acute and chronic health problems and that the school setting should be used to help alleviate these health concerns. Reimer and Cash (2003) identified strategies and best practices for ensuring success of alternative school students. They suggest low student-to-teacher ratios (less than 10:1), small student enrollment (less than 250), clear mission and discipline code, caring faculty with continued professional development, high expectations, program specific to students' expectations and learning styles, flexible school schedule and community involvement, and total commitment to every student's succeeding. Previous research (e.g., Raywid, 1994) has suggested that experiential learning, flexibility, and parental involvement may also be important. Lubans and colleagues (2012), in their systematic review, highlighted that PA has been shown to have a positive effect on the social and emotional well-being of at-risk youth. Martinek and Hellison (2016) have shown the benefits of PA and sport among at-risk populations by assisting in teaching responsibility. With the understanding that PA has many psychosocial and emotional benefits and alternative school youth are falling short of recommended PA, considering CSPAPs would appear to be relevant. Alternative school research has already indicated the importance of staff, community, and parent involvement in these programs, each of which is a hallmark of a CSPAP. An expansion of PA as part of student educational experiences in physical education, in the classroom, and before and after school should be targeted.

Juvenile Justice

Juvenile justice facilities house students with criminal or rehabilitation needs for between two weeks and four years. These facilities differ greatly and include school teachers, counselors, and security staff. Many times, programming in these facilities does not include regular physical education or alternative PA opportunities. To date, only a single study has explored the PA patterns of youth in custody (Brusseau et al., 2018). Findings suggested that youth in custody are falling short of PA recommendations both across their entire day and during school hours. They further found that only one in three youth was in the healthy fitness zone for aerobic fitness (Welk & Meredith, 2010). Brusseau and colleagues (in review) examined the impact of a PA program on youth PA and found some initial increases before averages reverted back to baseline data. The complexity of organizing teachers, security staff, and other personnel made it difficult to maintain the improvements.

Homeschooling

Increasingly, children are participating in homeschooling (Redford et al., 2016); specifically, more than 1.5 million children are schooled at home, where PA opportunities are often an afterthought. Wachob and Alman (2014) suggested that the health status of parent teachers was a strong determinate for children's aerobic fitness and body composition. Welk and colleagues (2004) found that homeschooled children are slightly (not significantly) less active than their public school peers. Many homeschooling situations do not include formal physical education. An examination of a community-based homeschool physical education program (Swenson & Pope, 2016) found that children spent 70 percent of their time sedentary.

Knowledge Claims

Based on the review of research in the previous section of this chapter, the following evidence-based assertions can be made.

- Sixty-one percent of children attend preschool or childcare centers. Preschoolers should participate in 15 minutes of PA each hour.
- Twenty-one million young people attend college. PA participation in college is related to academic success.
- Children with disabilities are more susceptible to inactivity. Social support is key in special schools.
- Little PA opportunity is available in alternative schools. Experiential learning is important for student success in alternative schools.
- Youth in custody are falling short of PA recommendations.
- More than 1.5 million youth are homeschooled. Children in community physical education programs are mostly sedentary.

Knowledge Gaps and Directions for Future Research

Limited research exists on CSPAPs in nontraditional school settings. The research clearly highlights the importance of PA for youth in all of these settings. Efforts in this chapter have identified ways that each component of a CSPAP can be implemented in each setting to promote PA. The lack of research and CSPAP efforts in these settings offers an exciting opportunity for practitioners and researchers who wish to promote PA in these important settings.

Evidence-Based Recommendations and Applications

This section highlights CSPAP recommendations that should be considered for preschools, colleges and universities, special schools, alternative schools, juvenile justice facilities, and home-schools (see table 15.1).

For Preschool Staff

Although CSPAPs have not been formally implemented in childcare centers, there are many similarities in K-12 settings that would allow for

a coordinated approach to implementation and evaluation of programs. To effectively coordinate a CSPAP at a childcare setting, an important first step would be to establish a PA director. Depending on the structure and resources at the childcare center, this person could be the facility director, a movement specialist, or a dedicated teacher. This person would need to form a CSPAP committee

TABLE 15.1 Recommendations and Applications for Nontraditional CSPAP Contexts

Context	Physical education	PA before and after school	PA during school	Family and community involvement	Staff involvement
Preschool	Physical education delivered by a trained specialist Physical education delivered by preschool teachers who have been trained	Drop-in morning play sessions Community and business partnerships	Classroom brain breaks (limited research) Indoor and outdoor play	Invite a parent to school day Family fun days	Active involvement of teachers during play Training teachers to engage in play behaviors
College and university	Sport and lifetime activity courses offered through kinesiology departments Mandatory fitness class for incoming freshmen (online, PA tracking, campus and community resource mapping)	Intramural and club sport programs Campus recreation Residential hall drop-in morning and afternoon exercise opportunities	Classroom brain breaks (limited research) Campus recreation center	Campus running and walking events offered to community Community use of recreation fields and gym space for PA events Family and kids activity days hosted by university	Faculty and staff wellness programs Faculty involvement in residential life and live-learning communities
Special school	Certified adapted physical education specialist Developmentally and disability-appropriate activities Modifications to equipment, time, facilities, and rules	Intramural sports and physical activities that are disability specific Morning drop-in programs to prepare students for learning	Classroom activity breaks Structured recess activities	Community programs (e.g., Special Olympics) Regular family PA	Faculty and staff wellness programs
Alternative school	Choice of activities Fitness or health club model Individualizing instruction where possible	Drop-in programming Mother and child activities	Active academics and hands-on experiences	Family and community support and encouragement of students' PA	Faculty and staff wellness programs
Juvenile justice	Choice of activities Fitness or health club model Sport education Individualizing instruction where possible	Drop-in programming Intramurals Interfacility competition	Active academics and hands-on experiences	Community support and programming from nonprofits, religious groups, and universities	Staff leadership and support Staff wellness program
Homeschool	Individualized for the student or small group Recreational or university programs	Parent teacher–led games and play Recreational programs	Active academics Activity breaks Recess opportunities	Community and neighborhood PA experiences	Parent wellness efforts

to evaluate and make recommendations based on the resources, location, and space available at the center. Potential individuals to make up a childcare center CSPAP committee include teachers, parents, community recreation professionals, and college or university early childhood movement education specialists.

Quality physical education is recognized as the cornerstone of an effective CSPAP. This would ideally be designed and delivered by a certified physical education teacher who specializes in early childhood movement. However, with few regulations requiring PA in preschool settings, it is unlikely that many childcare centers would make this level of investment in a full- or part-time position. An alternative and more cost-effective option for childcare centers is to train classroom teachers to deliver structured physical education to their students. While there is some limited evidence to support the use of prepackaged PA programs in preschools (Chuang et al., 2017; Sharma et al., 2011), more research is needed in this area before conclusive recommendations can be made. An alternative approach, while not possible in all settings, may be to partner with local colleges and universities to offer in-service training and support in early childhood physical education. In addition, there may be opportunities for preservice physical education teachers to gain experience delivering physical education within the childcare centers or for the centers to transport children to campus for physical education programming in early childhood movement laboratory settings. The ultimate decision on how best to effectively deliver physical education will need to be made by the CSPAP committee based on the unique circumstances of the childcare facility.

PA before and after school is another component of a CSPAP. Although research is lacking in this area in these settings, there are a number of potential options to consider as part of a comprehensive CSPAP in childcare settings. One option is to have early drop-off play sessions. Many fee-based preschools provide an early drop-off service. However, it comes with an additional cost, which may fall beyond the financial means of many U.S. families. Providing this option at no cost as part of a CSPAP would allow all children to benefit, not just the financially privileged. After-school PA opportunities could be provided through partnerships with local recreation programs and businesses. For example, community recreation programs could offer sessions on sport skills development, such as T-ball or soccer, at no cost and then offer families the opportunity to sign up their children for organized leagues. The same partnership could be arranged with businesses, such as martial arts studios, to provide several introductory sessions on-site for free and then provide parents with information to continue with fee-based sessions.

PA during the school day is something that is generally integrated into most childcare settings through indoor and outdoor free play as well as active learning in the classroom. However, the most effective approach is something that has been and is still being investigated by many scholars. A review of PA interventions in preschool settings suggests that the most effective programs to increase MVPA were teacher led, involved outdoor activity, and included unstructured activity (Gordon et al., 2013). Other studies evaluating the impact of teacher-led curriculum (Chuang et al., 2017; Trost et al., 2008) and design of the outdoor play space (Hannon & Brown, 2008; Nicaise et al., 2012) have found positive effects on PA levels. In addition, adequate PA participation in preschool-aged children has been shown to improve early literacy (Kirk & Kirk, 2016) and enhance cognitive functioning (Palmer et al., 2013). Given the many positive effects of PA and the recommended guidelines for daily PA among preschoolers, a preschool CSPAP should be committed to various planned in-school physical activities, such as recess and play, active academics, and PA breaks.

Staff involvement is a key component of an effective preschool CSPAP. The teachers have the most contact with the children throughout the school day and can influence PA through curricular approaches as well as during play. However, childcare center workers are often reluctant to engage in play with preschoolers (Gagne & Harnois, 2014). For teachers to feel comfortable directly engaging in PA, they must feel support from preschool facility directors, parents, and other teachers and have the space and resources available to be motivated (Gagne & Harnois, 2014). Adult encouragement is linked to increases in PA highlighting the role of teachers in promoting PA (Biddle & Goudas, 1996).

For Preschool Community Partners

Family and community involvement in a preschool CSPAP could take several forms. As noted earlier, there are various community partners, such as community recreation and private businesses, that can help create PA opportunities in childcare centers. It is also well established that parents play a pivotal role in influencing PA behavior in children (Pugliese & Tinsley, 2007). Thus, it is important to engage parents early in an effective CSPAP. Some ways that childcare facilities might consider engaging parents is to invite them in to be active with their children during scheduled outdoor play or to stay with their children during a morning play session. Childcare centers could consider organizing family fun days and set up stations with various physical activities and challenges that parents and their children can engage in together. If the center is lacking the available space, it may be able to partner with a local park or college or university to host the event.

Overall, early childcare settings are similar to elementary school settings where CSPAPs have been successfully implemented. Thus, it appears that there is potential to implement a structured CSPAP. It just takes central coordination, a strong and dedicated leadership team, and attempts to foster community and university partnerships to make a strong preschool CSPAP a reality.

For College and University Staff

Although CSPAPs have not been formally implemented at colleges and universities, the structures are in place for a coordinated approach to implementation and evaluation of programs. To effectively coordinate a CSPAP at the college or university level, an important first step would be to establish a PA director. This person (could be someone from student affairs) would be vital in bringing representatives together from across campus to coordinate activities and reduce duplication and overlap. Important members of a CSPAP committee on a college campus could include the chair of a kinesiology department, director of campus recreation, director of intramural and club sports, director of campus wellness services, or director of residential life as well as a campus vice president or dean of student success or academic affairs. These individuals would be well positioned to inventory existing programs and resources, identify resource gaps and needs, leverage university–community partnership opportunities, and develop a coordinated approach to a campus CSPAP.

At most college campuses, kinesiology departments offer a variety of team and individual sports and fitness classes, thus making them well positioned to be leaders in this area. An example of a program serving a large number of students (over 2,000 annually) is Active Auburn, offered through the School of Kinesiology at Auburn University. Auburn utilizes online learning in its PA program through which students track their PA with activity monitors; learn basic concepts of PA and wellness; and become connected to campus resources for activity, such as the campus recreation center (Brock et al., 2016). Although physical education is required at less than 40 percent of U.S. colleges and universities (Cardinal et al., 2012), given the emphasis on student retention, time to completion, and data available regarding the positive impact of PA on a variety of cognitive outcomes, there is no better time than the present to press for physical education as a requirement at all college and university campuses as part of a CSPAP.

There are many components of a CSPAP already occurring on most college campuses. Intramural and club sport programs are good examples of before- and after-school PA opportunities. The positive effects of such programming have been studied for several years and include important outcomes, such as student retention (McElveen & Rossow, 2014) and positive affect (Webb & Forrester, 2015). Residence halls are another venue with promise for before- and after-school PA. Fitness rooms can be designed and group exercise sessions can be organized so that students who do not have time to go to the campus recreation center before class can still get in a quick morning workout. However, this takes coordination and cooperation among the many constituents of a CSPAP.

PA during the school day is supported through use of campus recreation centers. In fact, the purpose of campus recreation programs is to serve all students, faculty, and staff in the college campus community. A strong recreation program is essential for a successful college or university CSPAP.

Another way to increase PA throughout the school day is with classroom brain breaks. Although most of the work in this area has been in K-12 school settings, recommendations are being made for similar applications in college campus classrooms (Ferrer & Laughlin, 2017). Brain breaks in college courses may be as simple as having an opportunity to get up and move around during lengthy lecture classes.

Staff involvement is an important component of an effective CSPAP. As mentioned earlier, campus recreation is designed to serve not only students on campus but also faculty and staff. Many colleges and universities offer wellness programs with incentives, such as reduced health-care premiums or rebates (Baicker et al., 2010). These programs often integrate various units across campus, such as health services for biometric screenings, kinesiology departments to offer faculty and staff activity classes, and campus recreation to offer similar classes or personal fitness consultations. An opportunity that may be missed is getting faculty and staff directly involved in PA with students. Residential halls and, specifically, live-learning communities offer a tremendous opportunity to connect college personnel and students in PA-related events. For a simple example, a group of students in a live-learning community are taking a physics class as a cohort. They could invite a physics professor to engage in PA with them and discuss topics such as the force velocity relationship. Similarly, students are taking a sport psychology class together. A professor could come to an event where students are competing in teams. The teams could use different precompetition visualization or relaxation techniques and then have a discussion about them after the event.

For College and University Community Partners

College campuses are also well positioned to support family and community involvement in CSPAPs. Campus organizations, such as fraternities and sororities, campus student health services, and many others, often host running and walking events on campuses to support various organizations and charities. In addition, campus recreation facilities can be rented out for community-based PA events, such as family fun days,

youth sport events, and health fairs. There are also many natural opportunities to get students' families involved in organized PA around holiday and semester break times. These are just a few of many potential ideas to support community and family involvement in a campus CSPAP.

Overall, the structures are already in place on most college and university campuses to implement a structured CSPAP. It just takes central coordination, a strong and dedicated leadership team, and a spirit of cooperation across the campus to make it a reality.

For Special Schools Staff

When designing CSPAPs in this context, it is essential to implement activities that are appropriate for the individual students and can be safely implemented by school personnel. Often, all components of a CSPAP can be implemented, assuming proper training, equipment, and space are accessible. Collier (2011) has identified strategies for adapted PA opportunities. It is important to clearly understand the etiology and characteristics of the disabilities present. Teachers must then focus on a child's learning style, strengths, and limitations. When implementing PA opportunities, it will be important to ensure the correct modifications are made, which may include equipment, rules, environment, and instruction (Lieberman & Houston-Wilson, 2009). Some examples might include simplifying the rules for children with an intellectual disability or modifying equipment for a student with a visual impairment. Class format and teaching style should also be considered to meet the needs of the students. This information suggests that it is essential to have a director of PA in special schools who is well aware of the students' disabilities and any modifications that may need to be made to meet the needs of these students.

Quality physical education is of upmost importance in this population to ensure that foundational PA skills can be developed and appropriate activities can be learned. Ideally, classes should be taught by a certified adapted physical education specialist who has experience working with children with the identified disabilities. Modifications and adaptations to equipment, facilities, rules, and time need to be made to ensure a safe and enjoyable learning experience. The use of peer tutors has been shown to help with improved PA experiences in physical education classes (Lieberman et al., 2000). The peer tutor can provide the support and interaction needed to help students with a disability successfully participate in PA.

Similar to traditional school settings, before- and after-school PA opportunities are a terrific way for youth in special schools to be physically active. Intramural programs targeting PA and sport that meet the needs of children with disabilities is essential. For example, a sport such as goal ball or beep baseball might be a program used with children who are blind. Other activities could be implemented based on the resources available and the disability of the students.

PA during school, including recess and classroom PA, is an important opportunity to be active. It can help students with disabilities with behavior and academic achievement. Developmentally appropriate classroom activity breaks as well as structured recess activities may be best to ensure that activities are safe and enjoyable.

Students with disabilities, depending on severity, may be dependent on the support and leadership from school teachers and staff to be physically active. It is important for all teachers and staff to be aware of student needs and the necessary adaptations. School wellness programs can also promote PA with school personnel. Whether it be in the classroom or lunch room or at recess, making sure that adaptations are made to include all children is essential to maximize PA opportunities and set up children for a lifetime of activity.

For Special Schools Community Partners

Family and community involvement are essential for all youth but especially children with disabilities, who often need the additional support to safely engage in PA. Programs such as the Special Olympics or other community-based disability programs are extremely important because they provide a fun and developmentally appropriate activity experience. It is important for local recreation and community centers to consider children with disabilities when offering youth sport programs. Family PA is also important to supplement the lack of activity opportunities available for youth with disabilities. This might include family walks after dinner or planned adapted sport activities.

For Alternative School Staff

Alternative school teachers and administrators have identified PA as an important part of the school day. A point person to be the director of PA should be aware of the challenges of working with this population and what types of experiences are best suited to meet the needs of these youth. Ideally, the physical education specialist will work with other teachers and staff to develop the best plan for the various groups of students enrolled in their alternative school. Providing flexibility and choice will be essential for these students.

Quality physical education centered on choice will be important. The fitness club model (Houston & Kulinna, 2014) may be best suited because students can work individually and have a choice of where and how they want to be physically active. Other approaches, such as Teaching Personal and Social Responsibility (Hellison, 2011), may be appropriate to teach respect and responsibility through PA. Providing these youth with ownership of their PA directions may have the best long-term impact. Using teaching styles centered on individual instruction and pace of learning may also be helpful. An example might be the personalized system of instruction that allows students to move through modules when they are ready (Prewitt et al., 2015).

Before- and after-school programming in the traditional sense would be challenging because of the complex schedules and interests of many students in alternative schools. The best approach may be regular drop-in activity opportunities where students have the flexibility and choice to be active when they have time. Childcare may be important at schools with young mothers to ensure that they take advantage of activity opportunities or even mother and child programming. Any intramural or group programming needs to be culturally relevant for the youth in these schools to ensure interest.

PA during school might include efforts to infuse active academics. Alternative schools have identified hands-on learning and experiences as most important for student success. Furthermore, the use of PA to engage youth in learning could be beneficial because it includes experiential opportunities. Faculty and staff wellness programs should be available to promote PA across all school personnel.

For Alternative School Community Partners

Similarly, working with community partners, school staff, and family members to promote learning is also considered important in alternative schools. Engaging these folks in the learning and PA of youth in alternative schools could provide additional support that may lead to increased PA in these schools.

For Juvenile Justice School Staff

To implement CSPAPs in these facilities, both the school staff and facility personnel must work together and understand safety issues before implementing activities. When planned for, these 24-hour facilities provide a great setting for before-school group exercise, classroom activity breaks, quality physical education, and after-school and weekend intramural activities. Adding PA promotion to the job description for security staff and ongoing training and professional development is a key to future success. Often, youth are organized into groups for such things as housing and meals. The director of PA could be the staff member who oversees these smaller communities of youth as he or she interacts with them throughout the day and the be point person for promoting PA.

Quality physical education should be included in school experiences of youth in custody. Similar to students in alternative schools, the health club model or a focus on personal and social responsibility may be an ideal curricular model in these settings. The sport education model (Siedentop et al., 2011) may also be an option because the setting allows for long seasons and often has limited available equipment. This model will allow the rotation of responsibilities and thus ensure that students of all interests and abilities may find an aspect of sport that they enjoy. It also promotes appropriate sporting behavior and rewards teams across various psychosocial, cognitive, and affective outcomes.

Before- and after-school programming (including on the weekends) is essential for youth in custody. This programming requires a commitment from facility staff to organize and supervise intramurals and drop-in activities. Support and security staff do not always have expertise in PA, so they would benefit from ongoing professional development and training. Each facility is affiliated with a school district, which may allow for the training to be done as part of regular professional development for physical education teachers. Giving youth choice and the opportunity to decide what activities they want to participate in would be best to maximize involvement and enjoyment. Student schedules are tightly regimented but could allow for early morning, after-school, and evening programming. Interfacility competition is another option to promote PA and reward students with an opportunity to interact with youth in a sport setting outside of their typical facility experience.

PA during the school day may be best suited to include active academic opportunities. Similar to youth in alternative schools, youth in custody may benefit from experiential learning opportunities. Providing the training and resources for school teachers to incorporate activity into classroom learning may have a dual benefit of promoting academic learning while also increasing youth PA.

For Juvenile School Community Partners

PA of youth in custody is dependent on the involvement of both staff members who work closely with these youth all day, every day, and community partners who volunteer their time. Resources to provide opportunities for youth to be exposed to various projects and new opportunities are also needed. Often, nonprofit, religious, and university programs are interested in serving these students. PA and health can be regular targets of these groups.

For Homeschooling Community Partners

CSPAP training and resources need to be available through homeschooling websites and easily accessible for parents, who will be the PA directors in this setting.

Quality physical education at home would have to include individual or small-group activities because most opportunities would be with the parent teacher alone or with siblings. Ensuring activities are appropriate developmentally and can be experiences with the parent or siblings of various ages is required. Recreation centers and universities often have homeschool PA programs available, which provide social interaction of homeschool students while promoting PA and health in this population. These programs often have a small fee attached that covers instructor and equipment costs.

Similarly, before- and after-school programming as well as PA at school is dependent on the parent teacher either leading such programming or ensuring the student is able to enroll in local recreational pursuits. Regular learning breaks (recess or activity breaks) as well as active academic opportunities should be considered by the parent teacher. Parent teachers need to be engaged in PA with the students and ensure community and family PA opportunities are promoted. Parent teachers are also role models for healthy behavior, and efforts should be made to engage in PA.

SUMMARY

This chapter provided important contextual information about nontraditional education settings as well as strategies and suggestions for implementation of CSPAPs. To date, there is very limited research related to CSPAPs in these alternative contexts, which opens many future research opportunities.

QUESTIONS TO CONSIDER

1. How can preschools and childcare centers infuse quality physical activity experiences into their programs?
2. What student-specific considerations need to be made when implementing a CSPAP in alternative schools or in the juvenile justice system?
3. How might we ensure positive experiences for students participating in a CSPAP in special schools?
4. How can existing college and university programming or resources be utilized to implement a CSPAP?
5. What community programs or resources are available to help with a homeschooling CSPAP?

CASE EXAMPLE

Happy State University is a midsized institution in the northeastern United States. Happy State University is a well-respected institution, known for being highly ranked as a great place to work and for having exceptional employee benefits and a content student body.

Problem

Although Happy State has been doing well, recent analysis demonstrates a major projection of an increase in health-care costs, which will be passed on to employees in the form of greater employee contributions. In addition, a recent climate survey revealed that employees are spending a great deal of time sitting in their offices and desire more campus resources and incentives to engage in PA. At the same time, the student population has been accessing student health facilities at record rates, and the university has been experiencing drops in freshman to sophomore retention as well as four- and six-year graduation rates.

Solution

Happy State administrators decided to make a commitment to be a healthy campus through developing a comprehensive university PA program. They hired a director to coordinate the program. The coordinator began by engaging key stakeholders around the campus, including the Kinesiology Department, campus recreation, food services, residential living, and human resources benefits, to form a stakeholder committee. The committee members created and distributed a survey to faculty, staff, and students to determine program interests and desires. They also planned several open-campus forums to hear directly from the campus community and engage in open dialogue. After gathering information, the committee members decided to take a two-step approach by first working to implement a faculty and staff wellness program and then implementing a student-centered program based on the lessons learned from the faculty and staff implementation. Happy State administrators created a menu of health and wellness options and provided a monetary incentive for all employees meeting a certain number of options per period. In addition, Happy State began offering fitness classes to employees in the morning, at midday, and after work to accommodate schedules. The university also worked to create a more walkable campus environment and implemented a bike share program on campus to encourage riding bikes to meetings.

For students, Happy State began requiring an online health and wellness class as part of the freshman experience. Through this class, students could learn key concepts of health and fitness, monitor and track their own PA levels, and become connected to campus and community resources for PA. Additionally, Happy State began offering outdoor adventure activities to students at a reduced rate, offset by central university resource allocations. The university also expanded its intramural sport programs and found space in all residence halls for mini-fitness rooms with 24-hour access.

Evaluation

Happy State University is conducting follow-up surveys with faculty, staff, and students to evaluate the desirability of the initiatives launched and to receive feedback on what could be improved. Committee members are tracking student visits to the health-care facility and first-year retention and graduation rates. They are also tracking employee health-care access and hope to reduce health-care costs through a healthier campus workforce.

PART V

Developing, Measuring, and Promoting CSPAPs

CHAPTER 16

Conducting a Systematic Needs Assessment for CSPAP Success

Eloise Elliott, PhD
West Virginia University

Sean Bulger, EdD
West Virginia University

Emily Jones, PhD
Illinois State University

Alfgeir Kristjansson, PhD
West Virginia University

Needs assessment is a systematic process used to identify and analyze needs and assets of communities, organizations, businesses, and schools (Kaufman & English, 1979; Witkin & Altschuld, 1995). The process typically involves the collection of multiple data sources to inform and fully contextualize the situation in advance of program planning, implementation, and evaluation. Needs assessments are regularly used and documented in health care, public health, education, instructional technology, and sociology. As outlined in the Centers for Disease Control and Prevention's (2013) *Comprehensive School Physical Activity Programs: A Guide for Schools*, a seven-step strategic process for developing a CSPAP, an early and necessary step is conducting an assessment of existing opportunities and resources. Despite the importance of needs assessments, there is limited empirical evidence to support that schools are conducting them before implementing multicomponent PA programs (Jones et al., 2014). This chapter will (1) review the literature on conducting needs assessments, both generally and specifically in schools; (2) propose knowledge claims based on the available research; (3) identify gaps presently in the literature related to conducting needs assessments in CSPAPs; (4) outline practical applications for both researchers and practitioners from the research; and (5) provide an example of an effective needs assessment in a school district.

Review of Research

Human service programs are usually created to serve a group of people or a community to facilitate improvement in health and behavior. In the development of such programs, a formal needs assessment commonly paves the way to initiate the decision-making phase in understanding whether there are needs and, if there are, how to best plan a program or intervention to meet those needs. A needs assessment will also help to demonstrate the necessity and relevance of a proposed intervention and to garner support. Funders, elected officials, policy makers, educators, program planners, and other stakeholders will require knowledge and understanding of the need for any given program and intervention proposal to support it moving forward.

The planning of a needs assessment usually begins with questions such as these: What is the problem, and what is the need for change? What approaches can best be utilized to tackle the problem? What resources, both existing and new, will be required to facilitate a positive outcome? Answering these questions requires the collection of data and analyzing and disseminating it in an understandable manner. Hence, on the front end, identifying the best available data sources to answer these questions will be a priority. These sources include existing data from official sources, such as archives, as well as the generation of new information, such as surveying school personnel, parents, students, or community members or conducting interviews with key informants. The results of a well-crafted needs assessment can improve program quality, ongoing development efforts, and evaluation (Allegrante et al., in press).

Needs assessment is applied in most areas of behavioral sciences and education. It serves as a snapshot of the current situation and seeks to address a given problem by gathering relevant information on the environmental context, target audience, supporting stakeholders, programs, resources and services, and opportunities that are already in place and those needed to improve behavior, the environment, and programming. Needs assessment ranges from determining the physical component of a given environment, such as accessibility to buildings and walking paths, to the individual behaviors of citizens. To provide a few examples, in recent years, needs assessment has been employed to evaluate the demand for PA programs in urban (Misra et al., 2016) and rural environments (Gates et al., 2016) and to improve PA opportunities for children in rural areas (Kristjansson et al., 2015). Other needs assessments conducted in schools have focused on assessing student needs and success (Page et al., 2013), teacher needs (Hursen & Birinci, 2013; Pavri, 2004), and school improvement strategies (Moore et al., 2016). This list is not exhaustive; it merely serves to demonstrate the wide breadth of circumstances where needs assessment is often used.

Theories

A common starting point in the development of a needs assessment is a theory. Theories formulate the organizing process of how and where to acquire information for a given problem, map existing resources and possible additional resource needs, and clarify the relationship between concepts and constructs. Several systematic techniques and planning models have emerged to guide needs assessment and the formative stages of intervention planning. While there are numerous techniques and models available, this chapter briefly introduces two assessment and planning models that have gained popularity: The PRECEDE-PROCEED model and the theory of community organizing (Glanz et al., 2015).

PRECEDE-PROCEED Model

Initiated in the late 1970s, the PRECEDE-PROCEED model is a theoretical road map to a specified destination (Green & Kreuter, 2005). In the context of needs assessment, the model provides a structure for the application of concepts and can be viewed as a logic model linking causal assessment and intervention planning into a framework. Its name is descriptive of the model's eight phases and their role in intervention planning, with the first four phases devoted to assessment and planning before program application and the latter four phases dedicated to implementation and evaluation. Because our discussion pertains to assessment and planning, we will limit our coverage to the PRECEDE part of the model, which stands for predisposing, reinforcing, and enabling constructs in educational diagnosis and evaluation. This part of the model concerns the educational diagnosis that precedes an intervention plan: phase 1 is social assessment; phase 2 is epidemiological, behavioral, and environmental assessment; phase 3 is educational and ecological assessment; and phase 4 is administrative and policy assessment and intervention alignment. In these phases, information and data are collected through asset mapping, literature reviews, data registries, archival records, and documents as well as prospectively at town hall meetings and with interviews, focus groups, participant observations, and surveys. Once these four phases are completed, program planners can select an intervention that aligns to the identified resource needs, organizational barriers and facilitators, and policies pertaining to program implementation. Phase 5 relates to program implementation, and phases 6 to 8 are devoted to process, impact, and outcome evaluation (Bartholomew et al., 2015). For a complete description of the model, see Green and Kreuter (2005).

Community Organizing

The theory of community organizing is another theory frequently used as a basis for needs assessment. This theory rests on the notion that individuals in communities are best positioned to bring about sustainable change in their lives and environments rather than relying on outside forces, although periodical use of external experts can often be helpful or even necessary, especially during the initial phase of change. As a result, the theory of community organizing largely concerns the empowerment of community members to engage and take control of the issues they have prioritized. Community organizing is rooted in local development and facilitates community ownership of the process and change with the goal of improving perceived control, coping capacity, and the health and behaviors of community members. In this instance, a "community" can be defined by geographic boundaries (e.g., ethnicity, religion, occupation, or sexual orientation), similar demographic profiles (e.g., gender, age, or occupational status), or units of patterned social interaction (e.g., sports, churches, or Internet-based profiles; Wallerstein et al., 2015).

The theory of community organizing includes five main concepts: participation and relevance, empowerment, critical consciousness, community competence, and issue selection. Participation and relevance concern the engagement of community members as equals. Community members create their agenda based on perceived needs, shared power and governance, and awareness of resources. Empowerment is a social process for people to gain mastery over their lives and communities to create desired changes. Group collaboration is key in this endeavor. Critical consciousness is based on mutual reflection and action in making change where community members participate in dialogue that links causes to community actions. Community competence is the ability of the community to engage in effective problem solving where community members identify issues, create consensus, and agree on strategies for change to reach selected goals. Finally, issue selection concerns the identification of winnable and specific targets of change that unify and build community strength where community members identify issues through shared participation and decide on targets as part of the overall strategy. The key attributes of a well-selected issue are that it is winnable, simple, important to many people, and part of an overarching plan (Wallerstein et al., 2015).

Common Data Collection Methods

When conducting needs assessment, many types of information and data are collected. The most common approaches include document and archival records analysis and quantitative and qualitative methods (figure 16.1).

Document and Archival Records Analysis

Most agencies and organizations maintain records in some form, and many, such as federal, state, and local governmental agencies, also collect routine data for this purpose. Such information can provide critical evidence concerning the demographic profile of the school or community, the frequency of the issue under scrutiny, how widespread a problem is, and where resources may be found to mitigate the problem. During needs assessment, archival records and governmental databases often form the initial information pool for the assessment team.

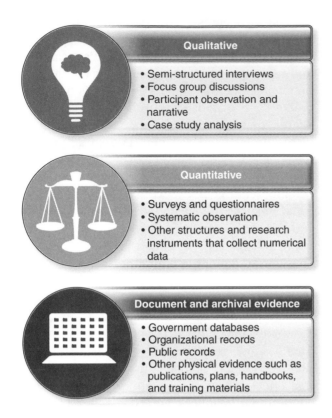

Figure 16.1 Multiple methods for data collection.

Quantitative Methods

Social surveys are often applied in needs assessment research and provide an opportunity to map phenomena of high relevance to a large group of participants. They are therefore appropriate for garnering information that is generalizable to a given population, particularly as related to basic observations, such as assessing the frequency of a problem or people's attitudes toward solutions. Surveys are usually conducted with a questionnaire that is developed and administered to a sample of people who are representative of the community. This data collection can take place, for example, at worksites, in schools, during town hall meetings, or in the general community. Common methods of collecting survey data are by phone, in person, or self-administered using paper and pencil or online. For those interested in further readings, many excellent textbooks are available on how to plan, design, and conduct surveys (see, for example, Dillman et al., 2008; Fowler, 2014).

Qualitative Methods

In contrast to the quantitative nature of surveys, qualitative approaches that operate with a small number of participants are also frequently employed in needs assessments. They offer an opportunity to gain a detailed insight into the issue because they are both flexible and focused in nature so that the problem can be studied at a deeper level than possible with social surveys (Kristjansson et al., 2015). Qualitative methods include semistructured interviews with key informants, such as managers, patients, or students; focus groups, which are conducted with a small group of individuals, usually 5 to 10 people who operate with group dynamics to engage members in a focused discussion around an issue; and participant observations where the researchers collect live data during the operation of study (Livingood et al., 2011).

Systems Thinking

As previously described, needs assessment remains an important preliminary step in understanding the context of any human services program targeting behavioral, environmental, program, and policy modification. The application of needs assessment methodology and its underlying theory represents a critical early factor in the development of a CSPAP due to the inherent difficulties in planning, implementing, and evaluating a multicomponent intervention. Schools are complex systems characterized by interdependent relationships across multiple levels of influence and inputs (Institute of Medicine [IOM], 2013; Jones et al., 2014). A system can be thought of as a structured entity made up of components that interact uniquely (Anderson et al., 1999; Hays, 2006; Laszlo & Krippner, 1998; Shaked & Schechter, 2013). For example, schools have varied goals, priorities, expectations, and accountability mechanisms that are influenced by local, state, and federal policies. The components, or subsystems, are both independent and interdependent, thus allowing the system to function in its entirety (Shaked & Schechter, 2013). When viewed as a system, schools include a range of subsystems, such as subject or content areas, developmental levels, institutional roles, and teaching units that engage administrators, parents, teachers, students, and community partners (Hanson, 1996). Systems thinking allows researchers and practitioners to examine the independent and interdependent relationship of subsystems as they work collectively toward a common goal, to facilitate the acceptance and adoption of tailored, context-specific CSPAP programs.

Transformational and Transactional Factors

Given this measure of complexity, the IOM (2013) recommended the application of systems-based approaches if school PA interventions are to move beyond behavioral science approaches to produce scalable and sustainable change. Accordingly, it is critical that organizers invest sufficient time and effort to understand the targeted system and subsystems as well as the relationships among components at an early point in the CSPAP development process (IOM, 2013; Jones et al., 2014; Shaked & Schechter, 2013). The Burke–Litwin model of organizational performance and change provides a framework for understanding the environmental factors that act upon a system to influence individual and organizational performance (Burke, 2002). Within this model, transformational and transactional factors interact to facilitate or impede change. Transformational factors include leadership, mission and strategy, culture, and external environment. Transactional factors include individual needs and values, task requirements and individual abilities, motivational levels, management practices, work climate, and organizational structure. If the intention is to facilitate systemic change, school leaders are advised to prioritize transformational factors because the modification of transactional factors in isolation often produces limited progress (Burke, 2002). Considering the significance of transformational factors, it is essential that needs assessments incorporate relationship-building approaches that engage school leaders and stakeholders, who are positioned to facilitate meaningful change regarding these bigger-picture issues (Brusseau et al., 2015). Needs assessment organizers must focus on involving key constituent groups in shared decision making by providing ongoing opportunities for input and collaboration (Blank et al., 2003). School and community partners can help to provide a deeper and better integrated

understating of local history, culture, and context needed to fully inform later decisions regarding organizational policy, programming, and practice (Warren & Map, 2011). Organized listening campaigns that engage policy decision makers, community and business leaders, district- and school-level administrators, local wellness policy committees, teachers and staff members, parent groups, and community members at large represent an important actionable step in CSPAP needs assessment (Brusseau et al., 2015). During these interactions, CSPAP developers can

- disseminate information on national and state recommendations for school PA;

- share evidence on programmatic strengths and weaknesses while collecting additional supporting evidence;

- brainstorm recommendations for school improvement to guide further decision making;

- explore other, unconsidered opportunities and possible barriers to sustainable change; and

- initiate relationships with individuals and partners who are well-positioned to contribute to CSPAP. It is also vital that these early relationship-building efforts extend beyond mere tokenism and the evidence gathered is distilled and used to inform program design transparently.

This degree of stakeholder input remains of continued importance beyond the point of needs assessment as well.

Transactional factors represent an additional area of concern during needs assessment given their potential influence as barriers and facilitators to CSPAP adoption and maintenance. Researchers have recommended the application of a social-ecological perspective to better organize the interactive levels of influence (components, facilitators, leaders, and culture) and the associated contextual factors (Carson et al., 2014). More recently, Hunt and Metzler (2017) identified the contextual factors that influence CSPAP development in a review of the related literature. The significance of these potential barriers and facilitators is likely to vary among school settings, further highlighting the importance of needs assessment during CSPAP development (Jones et al., 2014).

The determinants identified by Hunt and Metzler (2017) are reflective of multiple social-ecological influences, and CSPAP developers are advised to pay careful attention to the related interactions between and within levels:

- *Intrapersonal.* Time constraints, motivation, energy, knowledge, and confidence
- *Interpersonal.* Social barriers, teacher and staff time, and lack of leadership
- *Organizational.* School policies, schedules, facilities and equipment, competing priorities, administrative support, limited resources, staff and faculty training, and supervision
- *Community.* Logistical constraints, such as transportation, security, maintenance, and liability
- *Public policy.* State and district policies and laws and enforcement or lack thereof

Key facilitators have been found to include continuing professional development for CSPAP leaders (Beighle et al., 2009); use of conceptual models to support implementation and sustainability (Webster et al., 2015); creation of professional learning communities and school, community, and university partnerships (Brusseau et al., 2015; Bulger & Housner, 2009; Castelli et al., 2013); and overall school environment, infrastructure, and policy (Lohrmann, 2010). Despite our emerging understanding of the relative importance of these contextual issues, "future empirical research is needed to answer some of these remaining implementation and feasibility questions, many of which can be best addressed by those standing on the front lines of CSPAP implementation: the PE [physical education] teachers" (Hunt & Metzler, 2017, p. 334).

It is worth noting that while approaches to needs assessment that focus on deficiencies can produce information relevant to planning, critics argue that they also present the risk of providing a somewhat incomplete characterization given the emphasis on existent problems (Beaulieu, 2002; Sharpe et al., 2000).

Strengths-Based Approaches

Strengths-based approaches, such as appreciative inquiry and asset mapping, can also be incorporated during CSPAP development and implementation. Coghlan and Brannick (2014) posited that *appreciative inquiry* has emerged as a form of action research that is established on the basic premise that "if people focus on what is valuable in what they do and try to work on how this may be built on, then it leverages the generative capacity of metaphors and conversation to facilitate transformational action (Ludema and Fry, 2006; Bushe, 2012, p. 57)." Given the number of CSPAP components that many schools already have in place, a systematic approach that builds on strengths offers advantages, such as leveraging limited resources, facilitating buy-in and support, increasing awareness of existing programs, and focusing on program improvement.

Researchers have also proposed *asset mapping* as an effective alternative or follow-up to traditional needs assessment during CSPAP development (Allar et al., 2017; see figure 16.2). Asset mapping employs an inherently participatory and flexible framework for identifying, supporting, and using community resources with the goal of moving toward a shared vision for change (Sharpe et al., 2000). Kretzmann and colleagues (2005) indicated that program organizers can employ asset mapping to identify and mobilize five categories of community resources: (1) residents with specialized skills and interests; (2) voluntary networks, associations, and clubs; (3) public and private institutions with complementary missions; (4) physical assets, such as parks and recreation facilities; and (5) economic resources, such as business partners. During asset mapping, organizers employ a range of information collection techniques, including windshield and walking tours, key stakeholder interviews, focus groups, community resource inventories (Baker et al., 2007; Dorfman, 1998; Goldman & Schmalz, 2005), and vision casting (Sharpe et al., 2000). When applied to CSPAP development, asset mapping affords school personnel a platform for communicating and establishing connections among schools, families, and community members (Allar et al., 2017). While asset mapping does not build capacity directly, it offers an economical approach for determining hidden resources that increase organizational capability (Robinson, 2003).

Knowledge Claims

As demonstrated in the review of literature, the following knowledge claims related to needs assessments can be derived:

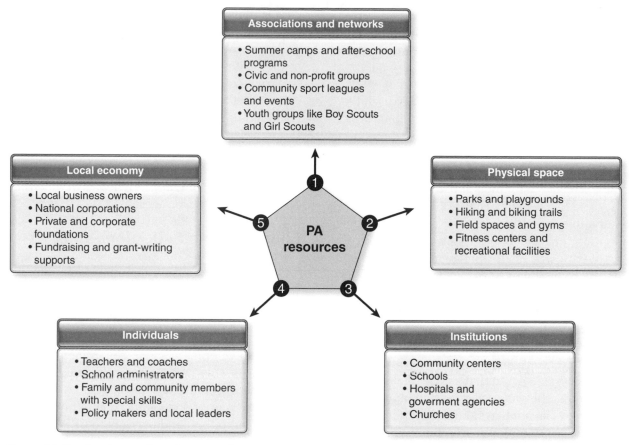

Figure 16.2   Asset mapping of community resources.

- Needs assessment is used in behavioral sciences to gather background information prior to program planning and implementation across a range of settings.

- Researchers often employ theories and models to inform the needs assessment process and guide decision making.

- Depending on the specific information needed to inform program design decisions, quantitative and qualitative methods are applicable.

- At an early point of program planning, organizers can use needs assessment to better understand the targeted system and subsystems at work in the school environment.

- Relationship-building approaches that engage school leaders and community stakeholders are critical to facilitating meaningful organizational change.

- Asset mapping and appreciative inquiry provide strengths-based alternatives to traditional needs assessment during program development.

Knowledge Gaps and Directions for Future Research

The implementation of an effective and sustainable CSPAP is dependent on the planners' understanding of the needs and strengths of the school context and surrounding community and the facilitators and barriers unique to that context. Needs assessment data can provide information to help determine priorities and identify changes that will have the greatest impact. If both researchers and practitioners have the knowledge and tools to successfully conduct a needs assessment, their efforts will be more focused on what strategies will achieve the best result.

Limited Practice-Based Evidence

Although common to public health and social science researchers, practitioners typically receive limited formal training in the area of program planning and evaluation. This lack of formal training contributes to the considerable gaps in the literature related to needs assessment during CSPAP intervention processes. A potential explanation for the lack of needs assessment data published within applied research is a discipline-wide reliance on randomized, individual, behavioral data in the development of population-based health interventions. These research-to-practice approaches involve the application of highly generalized research findings and intervention design features into settings that are not contextually compatible, resulting in often poor acceptance, adoption, and behavior change rates. Given the complexities of health behavior change, public health professionals have become critical of one-size-fits-all approaches in population-based physical inactivity initiatives (Livingood et al., 2011). Considering that research-to-practice approaches have become commonplace within applied social science interventions, Livingood and colleagues (2011) have suggested that a false dichotomy has been created between intervention planning and design and the contextual characteristics of the intervention setting, thus overemphasizing highly controlled, randomized research practices and underemphasizing the value of contextually based applied research.

As an alternative to research-to-practice approaches, Livingood and colleagues (2011) have advocated that approaches that are practice-based research or evidence be applied in the planning and evaluation of health behavior change initiatives. Practice-based evidence approaches complement systems theory and thinking because they focus on understanding contextual variables and their application to inform intervention design (Green, 2006; Livingood et al., 2011). Although not yet widely used or reported in formal empirical research findings, practice-based approaches align with and substantiate the use of needs assessment processes and protocols in the planning and development of CSPAPs. Toward the important end of lessening the existing knowledge gap of practice-based research approaches, researchers and practitioners are urged to systematically collect, report, interpret, and disseminate how needs assessment data contributes to the relevance and impact of planned and implemented school- and community-based PA interventions.

It is also recommended that future research on CSPAPs involve the use of existing tools and resources to evaluate needs, values, and assets to connect with local entities and drive practice-based research. As more researchers begin to systematically collect and use needs assessment data in the planning and development of CSPAPs, it is expected that we will see a rise in contextually based, tailored programs and initiatives that address the needs and complement the assets of the unique and wonderfully complex schools and individuals in which and for whom CSPAPs were designed.

Choosing Data Collection Protocols

Needs- and asset-based assessment protocols vary widely. There is a need for evidence-informed protocols to be established in the future so that researchers and local decision makers can use them to inform their decision making during CSPAP development. It is recommended that these protocols incorporate multiple sources from existing and new data to facilitate a deeper understanding of school and community needs, assets, facilitators, and barriers to CSPAP.

Examples of Possible Data Collection Focus Areas

- *Demographics.* Enrollment, attendance, ethnicity, gender, free and reduced-cost meals, cultural and linguistic diversity, at-risk populations, and family structure
- *School climate.* Classroom management; PA opportunities that exist before, during, and after school; administrative support for PA; equipment and resources; and facilities and play space audits
- *Student achievement data.* Formative and summative data related to student achievement each year
- *Student health data.* BMI, fitness testing, and objective PA measurements
- *School staff support and perceptions.* Professional development; staff involved in providing more PA opportunities before, during, and after school; and staff perceptions of the value of PA
- *Community involvement.* Community resources and services that strengthen school

programs and family engagement, actual PA opportunities that are provided through school and community collaboration, and existing and potential community partnerships

- *Student engagement.* Students' interests and priorities and current participation in school-related PA
- *Family engagement.* Volunteer opportunities that exist for parents, PA with the family through school-sponsored programs, and actual involvement of families in school decisions
- *Communication.* Students' and parents' use of technology and school-to-parent communication

CSPAP Data Collection Methods

- *Document and archival records analysis.* Census data, school demographic data, and strategic planning documents (e.g., school wellness and school improvement plans)
- *Qualitative methods.* Stakeholder interviews, focus groups, visits and participant observation, town hall meetings and recommendations, and community asset mapping
- *Quantitative methods.* Surveys of students, families, teachers, and community stakeholders and facilities and equipment inventory

There is a wide selection of existing evidence-informed, open-access instruments, inventories,

and databases available to measure and monitor a number of CSPAP-related variables (see table 16.1). After determining the variables of interest, careful consideration and selection of needs assessment tools and data collection strategies can be decided on collaboratively with all team members. Additional factors that teams are advised to consider while developing a needs assessment protocol include availability of needed resources; project benchmarks and estimated time to completion; steps to and politics of gaining access to key informants; and the expertise and capacity of the team to collect, analyze, and interpret needs assessment data. Teams that invest in understanding and addressing these factors can enhance their capacity to plan and execute needs assessment protocols that result in meaningful and actionable deliverables.

Regardless of the selected tool, a key component of an effective needs assessment is the capacity of the team to carry out CSPAP development and implementation. The World Health Organization's (2009) report titled *Systems Thinking for Health Systems Strengthening* outlined 10 steps to guide a systems-thinking approach to intervention planning and evaluation; the first two steps are convening stakeholders and collective brainstorming. Therefore, when possible, developers should seek to involve school staff and community leaders in CSPAP planning and development. Involving them can influence buy-in and acceptance and provide meaningful insight into the school cul-

TABLE 16.1 Examples of CSPAP Needs Assessment Inventories and Databases

Agency or organization	Resource title
SHAPE America	CSPAP Policy Continuum Inventory
	Indoor Physical Activity Space Inventory
Healthy Eating Active Living (HEAL)	Physical Activity Asset Inventory Questions Youth in the Community
Centers for Disease Control and Prevention	Behavior Risk Factor Surveillance System
	Youth Risk Behavior Surveillance System
Active Living Research	Physical Activity School Score (PASS)
	School Physical Activity Policy Assessment (S-PAPA)
National Cancer Institute	Database of Standardized Questionnaires About Walking & Bicycling
National Physical Activity Plan Alliance	U.S. Report Card on Physical Activity for Children and Youth
Centers for Disease Control and Prevention	Physical Activity Data and Statistics
	Physical Activity Surveillance Systems

ture, context, and social norms. These types of participatory efforts require a significant investment of time and a commitment to building and maintaining trust; however, systematic involvement of stakeholders can "incorporate community participation and decision making, local theories of etiology and change, and community practices into the research effort" (Wallerstein & Duran, 2006, p. 313).

Allocating sufficient time and resources (financial and human capital) to conduct a thorough needs assessment requires careful consideration, and the inherent difficulty should not be underestimated. The completion of certain needs assessment protocols can take as little as a few months, whereas others can extend across a year or more. Depending on available resources, it may be appropriate to offer incentives (financial or other) to the individuals and stakeholders who contribute information to the needs assessment (e.g., participating in interviews and completing inventories). While incentives are certainly not a required component of a needs assessment protocol, in some instances, they may prove helpful in gaining access, establishing trust, and facilitating a win-win outlook for those involved. Whether or not incentives are an option, it is advisable for CSPAP needs assessment teams to remain mindful of the amount of information that is being sought from individual sources and work to minimize burden and interruption of normal schedules and educational practices while collecting data. By minimizing the burden and interruptions, you may begin to build positive relationships among local decision makers and key players.

Critical Role of Team Interaction

Positive and ongoing interactions among researchers and practitioners is equally important to fill the knowledge gaps. Social interaction (i.e., face-to-face interactions and conversations) among the CSPAP community (teachers, administrators, students, parents, and community partners) during the needs assessment process can facilitate sharing of current knowledge and the creation of new knowledge across organizational boundaries. Without a collective desire to determine needs and share knowledge, perspectives, and expertise to implement CSPAP strategies,

initiatives are often stifled, and isolated efforts fail to be adopted or widely accepted within the community. Using community-based participatory research approaches allows CSPAP stakeholders to work alongside one another beginning with the needs assessment and continuing into implementation of the intervention. These approaches help develop trust and participation and ensure that the research efforts are truly relevant to the school and community. If researchers and practitioners have the knowledge and tools to successfully conduct a needs assessment, their efforts will be more focused on the strategies that will achieve the best result. Developing a strong CSPAP community around the context of the school can result in robust needs assessment data through the exchange of knowledge and will continue to enhance the CSPAP in the school through a higher level of trust, shared norms, and mutual exchange.

Evidence-Based Recommendations and Applications

Lessons learned from the research and implementation of the comprehensive needs assessment conducted in the case example, subsequently described, provide helpful evidence-informed recommendations. These recommendations are intended to guide school staff and community partners who wish to conduct a systematic needs assessment to make informed decisions in planning an effective CSPAP. Additional brief recommendations are mentioned for working with researchers, policy leaders, and funding agencies.

For School Staff

County and school administrators and teachers know more about their particular context than anyone else. Their knowledge and expertise are valuable to the needs assessment team, so it is essential that they be involved or take the lead. Taking the lead includes selecting and facilitating needs assessment data collection strategies, such as interviews, focus groups, student data, facilities audits, and demographic information. Other recommendations for school staff follow.

Consider Your Systems

Schools are inherently host to a wide range of subsystems, such as subject or content areas, developmental levels, and individuals with different roles and responsibilities. All those who reside within the system interact and influence one another on a daily basis. An initial step in needs assessment is to carefully examine the social structure and subsystems within your school, paying specific attention to how the context influences (positively or negatively) PA behaviors.

Organize What You Know

Carefully consider information that is already available through existing school- or district-level reporting mechanisms before gathering new data. Accessing existing databases and gathering information about your school and those who work and learn there can save you much time and effort in the information-gathering process of a needs assessment. Once you have organized what you already know about your school, identify what gaps exist, and develop a realistic and feasible plan for collecting new data.

Work Toward Your Strengths

The intentional identification of your schools' strengths can better position you to revitalize; reengage; or retool people, places, and programs to design strengths-based CSPAP programs that embrace and address the uniqueness and diversity of your school. Conduct an asset-mapping exercise to identify resources already in place that can positively contribute to your intended outcomes, such as community partners and school staff who have specialized skills and interests; clubs or organizations that currently advocate for PA; facilities and equipment that are physical assets; and economic resources, such as grant programs, that can help.

Collaborate for Sustainability

Assemble a CSPAP leadership team of individuals with unique perspectives and skills who have a shared vision regarding PA. Hold regular meetings that result in actionable tasks associated with the CSPAP and can stimulate progress, generate awareness, and contribute to the sustainability

of a CSPAP across multiple levels of influence within a school.

For Community Partners

A needs assessment that involves community members and leaders will not only strengthen the proposed actions within the schools but also help to bridge the gap between schools and communities and give community partners a voice. These stakeholders can also use the needs assessment to demonstrate opportunities for their company, agency, or organization to provide services, expertise, funding, or other contributions to their local school's CSPAP plan. Recommendations for community partners follow.

Consider Your Systems

Consider the influence of systems within your organization and community, especially how you could use the social-ecological model as a way of exploring the influence that certain organizations have on schools and vice versa. Consider how the community and school in partnership can support one another to create a win-win program that is part of a sustainable CSPAP and also meets the desires of your system in making meaningful contributions to the community. It is also important for you to recognize the unique advantages and constraints of working with teachers and administrators in the school setting and realistically set goals that meet the needs of the school's contextual environment.

Organize What You Know

Determine what information is already collected via required reporting mechanisms in your organization that may be helpful in assessing the needs of the community and, therefore, the school's overall CSPAP. Be a part of determining what data methods should be utilized for the needs assessment to inform the CSPAP, and volunteer to contribute to the data collection.

Identify Your Assets

Identify the people, places, and programs in your organization and community that can promote and support PA. Make contacts to communicate the CSPAP vision and to solicit interest and potential contributions from others in your organization and the community.

Collaborate for Sustainability

Identify individuals within your organization who will be champions for working with the school. Regular participation in CSPAP team meetings and completion of identified tasks are important to CSPAP development, implementation, and sustainability. New or existing resources are critical to sustainability, so your assistance in sharing or leveraging resources will be most helpful to a CSPAP.

Working With Others

School staff and community partners should consider the importance of including university researchers on the CSPAP team and how the needs assessment results can help to influence buy-in and support from policy leaders and funding agencies.

Researchers

University researchers can be instrumental in developing a plan for a needs assessment as well as contributing to the team in CSPAP development, implementation, and evaluation. A well-done needs assessment provides concrete evidence of strengths and weaknesses and informs decisions about interventions, programs, and policies from data collected from a variety of sources. Researchers are well suited to provide a theoretical framework and evidence-informed strategies to help justify the needs assessment as well as CSPAP development, implementation, and evaluation overall. However, researchers should never assume they know what a school system needs or wants without first listening to the people most involved at the school level. Through collaboration between the school, CSPAP partners, and researchers beginning with the needs assessment and moving forward, this multidisciplinary team provides expertise in all areas of developing a successful plan.

Policy Leaders

When local or state policy changes are considered, documented evidence related to need is critical. Needs assessment data that demonstrates the gaps between current and desired conditions helps to make the case for needed policy action. Engage a policy leader on the CSPAP team, and share the results of your needs assessment with local and state policy leaders to support change.

Funding Agencies

Many funding sources require needs assessment results to demonstrate that the proposed programs or services are in fact what are most needed. When applying for funding, the CSPAP team should be sure to include an initial needs assessment and document how the data generated will inform the proposed initiative.

An overview of the process to effectively conduct a needs assessment is highlighted in nine steps in the sidebar titled "Lessons Learned: Steps in Conducting a Successful CSPAP Needs Assessment." These steps are based on the related literature and our evidence-informed practice, and the overview includes a few questions that CSPAP developers should ask themselves when carrying out these steps.

For an intervention, program, or initiative to be perceived as valuable by those involved in the development and implementation processes, it must address a particular need that has been identified and help to provide a solution for it (Soriano, 2012). A systematic needs assessment will demonstrate a clear awareness of what schools require to develop, implement, and sustain an effective CSPAP. Additionally, the assessment will help to garner teacher buy-in and support and can best identify the needs of underserved populations and help inform decisions related to specific CSPAP components when a limited amount of resources are available. Assessing the school and community needs can provide a framework from which to plan the CSPAP and provide a baseline for program evaluation.

Lessons Learned: Steps in Conducting a Successful CSPAP Needs Assessment

- *Determine objectives.* What do you want to learn?
- *Choose collaborative partners.* Whom do you need to buy in to the CSPAP for its success? Practitioners, researchers, school administrators, students, parents, community stakeholders?
- *Choose the target audience.* Who will be determining needs and identifying strengths? Whom will you choose to be a representative sample of the target audience?
- *Determine data collection techniques that include a variety of sources.* Will you collect direct or indirect data or both? What instruments and techniques will you use?
- *Develop a management plan.* When should all the data be collected and analyzed? Who is responsible for its collection and analysis?
- *Develop partner buy-in.* Have you considered external stakeholders who represent a range of knowledge, skills, and expertise?
- *Conduct the needs assessment.* Who, what, when, and where?
- *Analyze the data.* What is required, and who will provide the analyses?
- *Data interpretation and dissemination.* How will this data inform program design and improvement? What about intervention or content selection? Who should see the results of the assessment and in what format?

SUMMARY

This chapter highlights the role of needs assessment as a preliminary step in CSPAP planning, delivery, and evaluation. The underlying goal of needs assessment remains the acquisition of new knowledge related to the internal and external factors in an organization that influence program development. The related literature, while limited, supports the potential significance of needs assessment in helping CSPAP developers fully understand the various contextual factors that will influence the effectiveness and sustainability of the CSPAP. While a range of theoretical frameworks, research perspectives, data collection methods, and recommendations for best practice were shared in this chapter, it is important to reinforce that the needs assessment process is inherently flexible and customizable to your specific school and community setting. Regardless of the particular methodology selected, though, it is critical for you to engage key school and community stakeholders, look across and within levels of influence to identify assets and constraints, and organize the findings in a way that can be easily shared for use in planning.

QUESTIONS TO CONSIDER

1. The chapter described the PRECEDE-PROCEED model and the theory of community organizing, both of which are commonly used during needs assessment. Select one of them, provide a brief summary of its defining features, and discuss how it could be used to inform the needs assessment process.

2. Organizational changes in school environments are contingent upon transformational and transactional factors. Reflect on an attempted change that you have observed in a school setting. Was it successful? What transformational and transactional factors served as facilitators of barriers to the targeted change?

3. Strengths-based approaches, such as appreciative inquiry and asset mapping, are often used to complement more traditional approaches to needs assessment. What are the primary advantages of using these types of strengths-based approaches during CSPAP planning?

4. A range of well-designed data collection instruments are accessible online. Select one of the instruments from table 16.1, and use it to collect data on your school environment. Based on the results, summarize the current strengths, weaknesses, and opportunities related to CSPAP development.

5. The McDowell CHOICES case study included resultant recommendations for school staff and community partners. Based on your experiences working with those groups, what recommendations would you add to those lists?

CASE EXAMPLE: THE MCDOWELL CHOICES (COORDINATED HEALTH OPPORTUNITIES INVOLVING COMMUNITIES, ENVIRONMENTS, AND SCHOOLS) PROJECT

The authors of this chapter developed a district-wide school-based intervention called the McDowell CHOICES Project. To begin the project, a systematic needs assessment was conducted. This case example will describe the needs assessment strategies used in the McDowell CHOICES Project.

Our team was approached by a funding agency interested in providing support for the development of a successful health intervention to schools in southern West Virginia. The identified county was designated as having extreme health disparities and lack of opportunities for improving the health of its citizens. After meeting with county school and community stakeholders to gauge their support and interest, the funders, our team, and the local stakeholders made a collective decision to pursue a needs assessment to further identify needs, interest, facilitators, gaps, and barriers. The assessment results were then used to determine the intervention strategies that would be most successful and those that would most likely not affect the environment, systems, and policy in that school district.

The comprehensive needs assessment laid the foundation for the McDowell CHOICES project, a district-wide initiative aimed to increase CSPAP opportunities for students to reach the recommended 60 minutes of PA each day. Before intervention strategies were finalized, we collected multiple sources of data to gain insights from all influenced sectors (school faculty and administrators, community members, parents, students, and county leaders). This strategic process provided the context of the 11 schools in the district and their surrounding communities and identified gaps between current practices, policies, and procedures that restricted opportunities for PA participation before, during, and after the school day. We considered the following elements most important in assessing needs associated with the CSPAP components of the schools and in determining the next steps in the CSPAP implementation process: school personnel perceptions of strengths and weaknesses, requests from family and community members, student opinions, principals' and school wellness committees' recommendations, and the current status of school environments (i.e., policies, practices, resources, and facilities; Jones et al., 2014; Kristjansson et al., 2015).

As part of the needs assessment, site visits were made by at least two researchers on our team to all schools. During the site visits, we collected data using the following approaches:

- Semistructured interviews with the principal and physical education teacher
- School facilities and equipment audits

- Physical education curriculum and equipment inventory form (sent before site visit)
- Professional development needs worksheet (sent before site visit)

A feasibility study of this data revealed important elements in adopting a successful CSPAP plan (Jones et al., 2014).

- *School leadership.* Principals and teachers who are champions for increasing physical education and PA and take the initiative to invest their own personal time to provide new opportunities, resources, and promotional activities will increase the likelihood of a successful CSPAP.

- *Access and opportunities.* For new and continued before-, during-, and after-school PA programs to exist, supporting resources must be available. These resources include qualified individuals to deliver programs outside of the regular school day, funding to pay these PA leaders, and continued professional development for physical education and classroom teachers. Additionally, transportation availability for students will oftentimes make or break a successful after-school program.

- *Equipment and resources.* Teachers must have adequate equipment to effectively offer new programs, enhance the existing physical education curriculum, and provide PA opportunities in the classroom and recess settings. After-school programming often requires new equipment to provide new and exciting opportunities for children that will motivate them to stay after school and participate.

- *Safe and usable outdoor play spaces.* Well-maintained outdoor play spaces that include a variety of activity spaces (e.g., climbing structures, running area, hard surface, and courts) are important to a successful CSPAP to allow students more opportunities for structured and unstructured play throughout the school day. These spaces can also enhance family PA after school. Schools that do not have adequate outdoor play spaces can sometimes utilize nearby community playgrounds or green spaces to help provide more opportunities for outdoor play.

- *Community collaboration.* Establishing joint-use agreements with community groups to share facilities helps to extend the PA opportunities available to both students and their families into the community and allows community members to become more involved in their local schools. Barriers that must be resolved include concerns related to liability and supervision, PA leader credentials and pay, and maintenance of the facility.

- *Asset mapping.* Using asset mapping to identify physical assets, such as community playgrounds, parks, and recreational facilities, is helpful in the needs assessment process. Data provided by the mapping allows program developers to make informed decisions about what PA opportunities are possible within a community and can be a catalyst for identifying new community and school partnerships and resources (Allar et al., 2017).

In addition to these needs assessment measures, we also conducted an online student interest survey of almost 500 students (grades 6-12) to help identify students' PA interests and motivation to participate, which could be incorporated into the school setting. We also held two town hall meetings with 80 community and family members who gave us insights into the community members' perceptions about PA, opportunities to be physically active, and facilitators and barriers to participation. Furthermore, we conducted both school personnel and community stakeholder focus groups to gain additional insights into their perceptions related to PA using a semistructured SWOT (strengths, weaknesses, opportunities, and threats) analysis framework. Lastly, we collected baseline body mass index measures on second-, fifth-, and eighth-graders and a student PA behavior survey with all fifth and eighth grades (Kristjansson et al., 2015).

The needs assessment data enabled us to better understand the context of the county, school, and surrounding communities. This information allowed for the development of a more customized approach to CSPAP implementation. The multisector collaboration through sharing of ideas, expertise, and opinions served to assist in the development of components of the project that targeted the needs and desires of specific contextual environments within the district.

Assessing School Physical Education and Physical Activity Programs: Selected Tools

Thomas L. McKenzie, PhD
Professor Emeritus, San Diego State University

Evidence matters! Assessment substantiates program value, and CSPAP professionals increasingly need to be able to justify their programs as well as their proposals for modifying them (e.g., need, space, and budget allocations for personnel, facilities, and equipment). Generating data on CSPAP program factors is important for assessing baseline levels of PA and program use, evaluating the effects of program changes and interventions, and advocating for successful program components. Thus, there is increased need for both practitioners and researchers to be skilled in using validated tools to collect, analyze, summarize, and share data.

Given the limited time and resources available to many CSPAP professionals, it is of utmost importance they have access to tools that generate data that is both usable (e.g., understood by professionals and laypersons) and generalizable (e.g., has widespread use, such as permitting comparisons beyond the local site). Toward that end, this chapter provides an overview of eight selected tools that have been previously used to assess school physical education and PA policies and practices. Their protocols are either summarized here or available publicly free of cost. The selected tools range from sophisticated direct observation strategies used by trained observers to self-reports by various practitioners. Instruments used to assess PA using mechanical and electronic means (e.g., pedometers and accelerometers) are described in chapter 21.

Each tool has its own purpose, protocol, and training needs. Some tools assess only opportunities for PA (e.g., physical education, recess, and sport practice schedules) or environmental contextual factors (e.g., reported facility types) within a school setting, whereas others use validated observation techniques to directly assess PA as it concurrently occurs. Overall, the tools can be used to assess both macrolevel (e.g., policies using questionnaires) and microlevel data (e.g., on-site assessments of PA occurring during ongoing programs). Some tools are designed specifically to generate information primarily useful for making on-site decisions; other tools, when accompanied by suitable training and study designs, are valid for research purposes.

The chapter is organized in five sections. The first section summarizes three direct observation instruments that have been used by trained, certified observers to make moment-to-moment decisions about student PA and associated concomitant physical and social factors (e.g., lesson context, instructor behavior, and child social interactions). The second section summarizes three instruments that rely on the impressions and reports of key informants (e.g., classroom teachers, physical education specialists, and school administrators), which aid in the understanding of more global school variables related to on-site PA. The next section describes the Physical Activity Program Opportunity Index (PAPOI), a tool that can be used with the previously described instruments to assess opportunities for PA (e.g., minutes per student per week) provided by a school within its various CSPAP programs. This section concludes with a description of the Physical Activity School Score (PASS), a web-based tool designed to increase awareness of evidence-based PA practices. PASS permits users to assess opportunities for children to be physically active at their local school and to make comparisons to other locations. The fourth section provides evidence-based recommendations and applications for practice. The last section concludes the chapter with two case examples of how the System for Observing Fitness Instruction Time (SOFIT) and System for Observing Play and Leisure in Youth (SOPLAY) tools were used to successfully assess physical education and leisure-time interventions in schools. Table 17.1 provides a brief overview of the tools.

Systematic Observation Tools

Systematic observation has many advantages over other methods of assessing PA (e.g., self-reports, accelerometers, pedometers, and heart-rate monitoring). These advantages include being a direct method ("what you see is what you get") that supports the simultaneous generation of information on concurrent physical and social factors in the setting where the activity occurs (McKenzie, 2016; McKenzie & van der Mars, 2015). As a direct method, it has strong internal (or face) validity and the advantages of flexibility and low participant burden (e.g., school practitioners are not asked to recall past details, wear a monitoring device, or provide a fluid sample). As well, observations can be done in locations where other assessment tactics do not function well (e.g., aquatic and wrestling environments). Nonetheless, there are disadvantages to using direct observation, including the time and costs for observing and travel, need for observer training and recalibration, and potential participant reactivity.

The use of direct observation as a reliable and valid means for assessing PA, and the contexts in which it occurs has increased recently, mirroring the rapid technological advances that support observer training and data entry, storage, and export. The availability of instructional videos for

TABLE 17.1 Summary of Instruments Reviewed in This Chapter

Name	Main users	Data source	Main focus
OBSERVATION TOOLS			
SOFIT	Researchers	Interval recording	PA in physical education, lesson context, teacher behavior
SOCARP	Researchers	Interval recording	Playground social interactions
SOPLAY	Researchers	Time sampling	Number and PA levels of area users, area contexts
SELF-REPORT TOOLS			
S-PAPA	Practitioners and researchers	Administrators and activity leaders	Characteristics of physical education, recess, other PA programs
PARC	Practitioners and researchers	Homeroom teacher	Class minutes for physical education, recess, and activity breaks
SPAS	Practitioners and researchers	Activity leaders	Characteristics of intramural, interscholastic, and club PA programs
PAOI	Practitioners	Activity leaders	School PA summary score
PASS	Practitioners	Parents and laypersons	Evidence-based PA school characteristics

instruments on the web also makes observer training both more consistent and readily accessible. As well, the design of apps for small electronic recording devices now facilitates data entry and makes file sharing easier for both practitioners and researchers.

Research considerations in selecting observation techniques and instruments and in training observers how to used them reliably in both structured (e.g., physical education and sport practices) and unstructured (e.g., recess and free play during leisure time) settings in schools have been recently described in two papers: "Top 10 Research Questions Related to Assessing Physical Activity and Its Contexts Using Systematic Observation" (McKenzie & van der Mars, 2015) and "Context Matters: Systematic Observation of Place-Based Physical Activity" (McKenzie, 2016). The latter paper emphasizes the use of observational strategies to assess group-level PA, an important consideration in open environments, where people come and go in a seemingly indiscriminate fashion (e.g., during recess and leisure time before and after school). Because PA is contextual, being able to assess the number of students (and others if assessing shared use of facilities) and their characteristics (e.g., gender and activity levels) in specific school locations is important for both public health research and helping practitioners in the design and assessment of their activity spaces and programs.

Numerous and diverse observation tools are available for assessing PA at schools. This chapter focuses on three related instruments. They were created for substantially different purposes and procedures but have commonalities, including being published and widely used, using similar PA codes that have been validated (e.g., via accelerometry, heart-rate monitoring, and pedometry) with different school populations (e.g., age groupings and special needs children), having cost-free written protocols and video training materials readily available to facilitate instrument utility and observer reliability, and being well supported by both behavior analytic principles and social-ecological theory.

Advances in portable electronic technologies have created opportunities to move from conventional paper and pencil and mechanical data collection methods to electronic devices (McKenzie & van der Mars, 2015). Two tools described here have innovative apps for iPads (i.e., iSOFIT and iSOPARC, both available free on iTunes) that facilitate entering, storing, summarizing, and exporting data. These apps are especially attractive for use in larger-scale research or evaluation projects (e.g., multisite investigations).

SOFIT

SOFIT is used primarily during instructional sessions (e.g., physical education, dance, and sport) to simultaneously assess: participant PA levels (i.e., lying down, sitting, standing, walking/moderate and vigorous PA; lesson and session context (i.e., how lesson or session content is delivered, including time allocated for physical fitness, motor skill development, game play, knowledge, and session management); and teacher or coach behavior relative to the promotion of physical activity, skills, and fitness (McKenzie et al., 1991). Instructor gender, class location and gender composition, and number of participants in class are also typically recorded. The main focus of SOFIT is on individual students, and observers are paced by a visual or audible signal using an interval-recording format (e.g., 10 seconds observing and 10 seconds recording).

Typical SOFIT outcome data includes the number of minutes and proportion of session time that participants spend in various postures (i.e., lying down, sitting, and standing) and in walking/moderate and vigorous PA. Time in walking/moderate and vigorous PA are frequently summed to create moderate-to-vigorous PA (MVPA). Time in (MVPA) , lesson energy expenditure (kilocalories per kilogram), and energy expenditure rate (kilocalories per kilogram per minute) can be estimated from the observed data. SOFIT also provides important information on the physical education schedule (e.g., frequency of lessons, adherence to schedule, duration of scheduled and actual lesson length, and number of students participating), lesson context (i.e., minutes and percentage of lesson time spent in management, instruction, fitness, skill drills, gameplay, and free play), and instructor behavior (e.g., number and proportion of intervals instructors spend promoting PA, fitness, and skill engagement).

SOFIT (and its adaptations) has been used nationally and internationally in a variety of settings (e.g., preschools, sport instruction, special needs classrooms, and after-school programs) for over 25 years and has been part of more than 250 papers and theses (McKenzie & Smith, 2017). Examples include a nine-year longitudinal intervention study involving 76 elementary schools in four states (McKenzie et al., 2003); a cross-sectional study comparing PA and lesson contexts in high school physical education classes to Junior Reserve Officer Training Corps sessions, a common substitute for physical education in the United States (Lounsbery et al., 2014); an investigation of PA during extracurricular sports (Curtner-Smith et al., 2007); and a comparison of youth sport practice models (Kanters et al., 2015).

In addition to facilitating data collection, our recently developed iSOFIT app can provide a summary score (including bar charts) for participant PA levels, lesson context, and instructor behavior within five seconds of entering data. This feature, along with the capacity for storing data in Excel files and sending them immediately to others from remote locations (via iPads and Wi-Fi), makes the app ideal for providing feedback to preservice and beginning teachers and others.

System for Observing Children's Activity and Relationships During Play (SOCARP)

SOCARP is used primarily to obtain objective data on student PA levels on playgrounds while assessing the contextual variables of social group size, activity type, and pro- and antisocial interactions (Ridgers et al., 2010, 2011). While the PA codes and interval sampling protocols are similar to SOFIT, SOCARP does not focus on opportunities to learn physical skills but rather on an examination of social structures, especially during leisure-time PA periods. These variables include group size, PA type (competitive vs. noncompetitive), and child and supervisor interactions related to PA and social engagement (e.g., bullying).

Typical SOCARP outcome data includes the proportion of intervals (and session time) children spend in different activity levels, group sizes, and activity types. For social interactions, the percentage of occurrence of the different types of observed interactions (i.e., prosocial physical and verbal behaviors and antisocial physical and verbal behaviors) is most often used in analyses. Sample SOCARP studies include assessing children's PA and social behaviors at school to determine gender differences (Woods et al., 2012), differences among children with special needs (Bingham et al., 2015), changes over time (Ridgers et al., 2011), and the effects of a playground intervention (Mayfield et al., 2017).

SOPLAY

SOPLAY is used primarily to obtain objective data on the number of participants and their PA levels during play and leisure opportunities in predetermined targeted areas. In contrast to SOFIT and SOCARP, SOPLAY uses a group momentary time-sampling format (i.e., series of observation snapshots) to record the PA level (i.e., sedentary, walking, and MVPA) and additional characteristics of each individual (e.g., gender) and the target area using systematic scanning techniques (McKenzie, 2016; McKenzie et al., 2000). Separate scans are usually made for males and females, and simultaneous entries are made for area contextual characteristics, including their accessibility and usability and whether supervision, organized activities, and loose equipment are available. These five contextual characteristics are targeted for observation because they affect the number of students and their PA levels within a space and are predisposed to modification via policy, programming, and environmental changes. In addition, the predominant type of PA that area users are engaged in (e.g., basketball and dance) is recorded, as is other relevant information, such as time of day and temperature.

An enhanced version of SOPLAY (System for Observing Play and Recreation in Communities [SOPARC]) includes the recording of the age (i.e., child, teen, adult, and senior) and race or ethnicity (e.g., White, Black, Latino, and other) groupings of area users (McKenzie et al., 2006). SOPARC, most often employed to investigate park and recreation area usage, is also useful in school settings, especially to assess community and school shared use of facilities (Evenson et al., 2016; McKenzie, 2016; McKenzie & van der Mars, 2015). The iSOPARC app, for iPads, functions with both SOPLAY and SOPARC. It not only enhances the collection of area user and facility information, but it also permits the collection and exportation of photos and enables the identification, mapping, and spatial area calculations of target areas via the iPad's GPS technology.

Typical SOPLAY and SOPARC outcome data includes the number and proportion of participants in an activity area overall and by variable of interest (e.g., gender and age grouping) as well as the frequency and proportion of times during area observation visits that the facility was accessible, usable, and supervised and had organized activities and loose equipment available. Energy expenditure rates for areas (e.g., metabolic equivalent [MET] values) can also be calculated (using number of people present and their observed activity levels and previously validated energy constants for each activity level). In addition, an associated environmental inventory provides information on activity area characteristics, such as location, type, size, surface area, and structural enhancements. Examples of using SOPLAY and SOPARC in schools include the assessment of interventions during leisure time (e.g., recess and before- and after-school periods) in elementary (e.g., Huberty et al., 2014) and middle schools (e.g., Sallis et al., 2003), a study of shared use of facility agreements (Carleton et al., 2017), and comparisons of PA in schools that emphasized interscholastic versus intramural programs (Bocarro et al., 2012, 2014).

Self-Report Tools

This section summarizes three instruments that rely on the impressions of key informants (e.g., classroom teachers, physical education specialists, and school administrators), which can aid in the understanding of global school variables that relate to on-site PA. Compared to the instruments described earlier, the tools in this section have been used in research publications less frequently. Thus, supplementary resource information (e.g., instrumentation and protocol) is provided for them in this chapter.

School Physical Activity Policy Assessment (S-PAPA)

The S-PAPA tool assesses district- and school-level policy relative to environmental variables and PA at the individual school site. It targets policy related to physical education, recess, and other PA opportunities at elementary schools. S-PAPA uses open-ended, dichotomous, multichotomous, and checklist formatting and has seven background items and three modules: (1) physical education (40 items); (2) recess (27 items); and (3) other before-, during-, and after-school programs (15 items). In addition, background items provide a description of the respondent's professional role (e.g., position title and years in position), a brief profile of the school and student composition (e.g., grade levels, grades receiving physical education, number of enrolled students, and percentage of students eligible for free or reduced-cost meals), and facilities (e.g., gymnasium, multipurpose room, and fields) that are available for specific PA programs (e.g., physical education and after-school programs).

S-PAPA is designed to be completed by one or more key school personnel and can be done either face-to-face or online. The modules can be used alone or combined to include an assessment of all opportunities for PA at a school. The total administration time for background information and all three modules is approximately 23 minutes. Research studies have shown the S-PAPA items are reliable (Lounsbery, McKenzie, Morrow, Holt, et al., 2013) and useful in assessing PA policies at both elementary (Lounsbery, McKenzie, Morrow, Monnat, et al., 2013) and secondary (Kahan & McKenzie, 2017; Monnat et al., 2017) school levels. The S-PAPA instrument is available online at the Active Living Research website.

Physical Activity Record for Classes (PARC)

PARC provides information on the PA opportunities a school provides to students at the classroom unit level. It is usually completed by classroom teachers, who specify the opportunities for PA that their homeroom class receives during physical education lessons, recess, active lunch recess periods, and PA breaks during the school day.

Typical outcome variables for PARC are the frequency, duration, and total minutes of specific programs provided to the class per week. To reduce the burden on responding teachers, the weeks for recording PARC are often sampled (e.g., during four random weeks per semester or season), and respondents are permitted to complete the information either online (e.g., via school email) or in a paper format. PARC has been used in research studies in the assessment of school PA policies (Lounsbery, McKenzie, Morrow, Monnat, et al., 2013) and as a process measure during the Child and Adolescent Trial for Cardiovascular Health (CATCH) intervention in 96 elementary schools (McKenzie et al., 1994). Figure 17.1 presents an abbreviated PARC protocol and recording form.

Structured Physical Activity Survey (SPAS)

SPAS assesses participation in organized PA programs that are provided to students beyond physical education and free-play sessions (e.g., recess; Powers et al., 2002). Specific programs are identified (e.g., eighth-grade girls' basketball team practice) and classified into four mutually exclusive categories:

1. *Interscholastic activities.* Programs that provide competition for students at the school with those from other schools
2. *Intramural activities.* Programs that provide competition for students within the same school
3. *Club activities.* Competitive and noncompetitive PA groups that meet regularly (e.g., aerobics club)
4. *Other activities.* Sporadic or miscellaneous organized PA programs (e.g., judo workshop)

Participation in physical education classes and unorganized activities (e.g., unstructured pickup games at lunchtime) is typically recorded using SOFIT and SOPLAY rather than SPAS.

The school PA leader typically completes the SPAS daily by recording the frequency and duration of sessions, how many males and females participated, when programs were offered and who sponsored them, and whether there was a participation fee. Total weekly hours are calculated for each program (number of participants multiplied by time) as well as overall for the school.

The main outcome variables of SPAS are the number of minutes for structured PA programs (by type, gender, and overall) per week. Examples of SPAS in the research literature include a study of participation in extracurricular PA programs in 24 middle schools over several years (Powers et al., 2002) and investigations of the shared use of school facilities by community organizations during the school day, on weekends, and over the summer (Carlton et al., 2017; Kanters et al., 2014). Figure 17.2 provides a simplified SPAS weekly summary recording form.

Figure 17.1 PARC Protocol and Recording Form (Abbreviated).

I. General Procedures

The PARC form is completed by classroom or homeroom teachers during selected typical weeks in a semester. The weeks should represent normal or regular school programming and not include those with special events or holidays.

II. Protocol for Administration (Written Form Version)

a. The school liaison distributes PARC forms to classroom teachers by Monday morning of the data collection week. Teachers enter data by the end of each day.

b. On Friday afternoon, teachers put the weekly PARC form in the school liaison's mailbox.

III. Instructions to Classroom Teachers

a. Please take about one minute at the end of each day to identify opportunities children in your class had to be physically active.

b. For each day,

- record the *actual* number of minutes your class spent in recess, classroom physical activity breaks, and structured physical education lessons;

- enter the *actual* length of sessions, not necessarily their planned or scheduled length. The "class" is represented by the time the majority (over 50 percent) of your students spent there; and

- enter a number in each box. Write "0" for times when students did not have an opportunity to be physically active.

IV. Definitions

Recess refers to a scheduled break in the day for free play or leisure time and does not involve instruction. Include only recess periods when students have an opportunity to be physically active (e.g., outdoors or in a gym).

For *lunch recess periods*, record time allocated for physical activity opportunities only, not the entire lunch period. If students do not have an opportunity to be physically active (e.g., rain or no space), enter "0."

Classroom activity breaks refers to scheduled breaks in the school day when students are engaged in *directed* physical activity. This may or may not be a special program, such as TAKE10. *Physical education lessons* refers to instructional classes taught as part of the school curriculum. Circle "CT" for lessons taught by a classroom teacher and "PES" for lessons taught by a physical education specialist. Record "free play" time as recess, not physical education.

V. Recording Examples (Refer to corresponding letter in Monday column below.)

a. A scheduled 15-minute morning recess is canceled because of inclement weather.

   Enter "0" in the "AM recess" row for Monday.

b. After 13 minutes of a 30-minute lunch period, over one-half of the students go outside for free play.

   Enter "17" in the "Lunch recess" row for Monday.

c. For good behavior, the class is rewarded with a 15-minute free-play period held outside.

   Enter "15" in the "PM recess" row for Monday.

d. The classroom teacher conducts a 10-minute TAKE10 session in the morning.

(continued)

Figure 17.1 *(continued)*

Enter "10" in the "Classroom activity breaks" row for Monday.

e. A physical education class taught by the physical education specialist goes 6 minutes longer than the scheduled 30 minutes.

Enter "36" and circle "PES" in the "Physical education lessons" row for Monday.

	Monday	Tuesday	Wednesday	Thursday	Friday
AM recess actual # minutes	0 (A)	13	15	9	12
Lunch recess actual # minutes	17 (B)	18	11	18	22
PM recess actual # minutes	15 (C)	0	0	12	0
Classroom activity breaks actual # minutes	10 (D)	0	12	0	10
Physical education lessons actual # minutes	1. [PES] 2. CT 36 (E)	1. PES 2. CT 0	1. [PES] 2. CT 28	1. PES 2. CT 0	1. PES 2. [CT] 18

Figure 17.2 SPAS Summary Form (Simplified)

Structured programs during the week of _____

Program	When (circle)	Days per week	Duration (total minutes)	Mean # girls/boys
INTERSCHOLASTICS				
Example: Basketball grade 8	B L A D	2	90	0/14
1. 2. 3.	B L A D B L A D B L A D			
INTRAMURALS				
1. 2. 3.	B L A D B L A D B L A D			
CLUBS				
1. 2. 3.	B L A D B L A D B L A D			
OTHER				
1. 2. 3.	B L A D B L A D B L A D			

B = before school; L = lunchtime; A = after school; D = during school

A Summary Score and an Advocacy Tool

This section describes PAPOI, a tool that can be used with other instruments to summarize opportunities for PA (e.g., minutes per student per week) that a school provides within its various CSPAP programs. The section concludes with a description of PASS, a short web-based tool that enables users to assess opportunities for students to be physically active at their local site and to make comparisons to other schools. Because it provides feedback and increases user awareness of evidence-based PA practices, PASS can be used as an advocacy tool for school PA.

A Summary of the Core of PAPOI

PAPOI is based on the number of minutes a program operates and how many students participate in it; it serves as a summary measure for each CSPAP program and for the school overall. Data from other measures (e.g., SPAS and PARC) is combined to summarize the opportunities for PA that a school provides the average student during a week. As a result, PAPOI provides useful information for identifying areas of strength and weakness and can help in the prioritization of school-wide PA efforts.

The PAPOI score is calculated by summing the total minutes of program opportunities for PA from all school activity sources and then dividing the sum by the total student population (i.e., average daily attendance during the targeted week). It is important to remember that PAPOI provides information on *program opportunities for PA* and is not an actual PA engagement score. MVPA during program sessions, which can be assessed directly using SOFIT, SOPLAY, and other methods, is typically less than 40 percent of scheduled program time.

For illustrative purposes, table 17.2 compares two fictitious middle schools on the PA programs they provide. Muscle Middle School, which has required daily physical education for all students, a few class activity breaks, an extensive intramural program, and noncompetitive dance and martial arts clubs, provides the average student with 383.1 minutes of PA opportunities per week. On the other hand, Slug Secondary School schedules physical education classes only once a week and has a few classroom-based activity breaks and an interscholastic program but no intramural or club programs. Slug Secondary School provides the average student with only 138.5 activity program opportunity minutes per week, nearly one-third of the minutes provided by Muscle Middle School.

PASS: An Advocacy Tool

PASS is an eight-item web-based instrument designed to both assess and increase user awareness of evidence-based PA practices (e.g., physical education, recess, activity breaks, and active transport) at elementary schools (McKenzie & Lounsbery, 2014). The development and testing of PASS was commissioned by Active Living Research to create an advocacy tool that would help inform adults about the importance of school PA while enabling them to assess opportunities for children to be physically active at their local school.

Parents, teachers, school administrators, school board members, and others interested in learning about and assessing PA opportunities at an elementary school can use PASS to score the school on evidence-based items. Completing PASS takes about five minutes. After scoring each of the eight items, respondents receive numerical scores plus recommendations on how the school might improve relative to that item. Following question 8, an overall school score is provided along with a corresponding school grade (A-F). Respondents can subsequently compare their school's score to the scores of other schools both within and outside their state. PASS also provides links to relevant online PA information. PASS resources are available online for free.

Evidence-Based Recommendations and Applications

The quality indicator in *The 2018 U.S. Report Card on Physical Activity for Children and Youth* (National Physical Activity Plan Alliance [NPAPA], 2018) for schools was only a D-. That grade reflected the low prevalence of youth enrolled in physical education, gender and age disparities in physical education participation,

TABLE 17.2 Comparison of Physical Activity Opportunities at Two Fictional Middle Schools Using PAPOI

MUSCLE MIDDLE SCHOOL (600 STUDENTS)				
Source	**Students**	**Days per week**	**Minutes per day**	**Minutes per week**
Physical education classes	600	5	50	150,000
Recess (sixth grade)	200	5	20	20,000
Activity breaks	350	5	15	26,250
Intramurals	100	4	30	12,000
Interscholastics	40	5	60	12,000
Activity clubs	120	2	40	9,600
Total = 229,850 minutes per week				
PAPOI score = 383.1 physical activity opportunity minutes per student per week (229,850 minutes divided by 600 students)				
SLUG SECONDARY SCHOOL (600 STUDENTS)				
Source	**Students**	**Days per week**	**Minutes per day**	**Minutes per week**
Physical education classes	600	1	60	36,000
Recess	0	0	0	0
Activity breaks	50	5	30	7,500
Intramurals	0	0	0	0
Interscholastics	80	5	90	36,000
Activity clubs	60	1	60	3,600
Total = 83,100 minutes per week				
PAPOI score = 138.5 physical activity opportunity minutes per student per week (83,100 minutes divided by 600 students)				

and the low prevalence of CSPAP implementation (Katzmarzyk et al., 2016; NPAPA, 2018). While the whole-of-school approach to increasing on-campus PA has been supported for some time (Centers for Disease Control and Prevention, 2013; Institute of Medicine, 2013), the widespread adoption, feasibility, and effectiveness of CSPAP and its various components are not well known. Most of the research is based on snapshot surveillance studies that rely on self-reports, such as the *School Health Profiles 2014* (Demissie et al., 2015) and the *School Health Policies and Practices Study 2014* (U.S. Department of Health and Human Services & Centers for Disease Control and Prevention, 2015). Large surveillance studies of CSPAP programs conducted with on-site, ground-truthing, direct observations have yet to be conducted. Subsequently, it is important to build the capacity for assessing PA and associated CSPAP policies and practices. To best serve both researchers and practitioners in advancing professional practice, investigative tools need to be meaningful, easy to use, understandable, and generalizable.

This chapter provided an overview of eight selected tools that have been demonstrated to be useful in providing information about CSPAP programs. While diverse in focus and methodology, they are samples only, and other tools are available (McKenzie et al., 1991; McKenzie & van der Mars, 2015). CSPAP professionals (e.g., teachers, recreationists, and program directors) should conduct their programs based on scientific evidence, and there is need for them to be able to generate data within their own specific settings. Practitioners usually have substantial flexibility in the creation of instruments that will match their local, individual concerns. On the other hand, researchers typically strive to be influential beyond the local setting; thus, there is the need for them to be particularly concerned about the external validity of their work. There is currently no objective database using on-site observations of the conduct of CSPAP programs in the United States, and one is needed. For best value, CSPAP researchers should ensure their methods follow established protocols consistently and that they report their work in a uniform manner so that comparisons can be made to other studies and to state and national policy standards (McKenzie & Smith, 2017).

In terms of generalizability, there is also the need for both practitioners and researchers to consider how much data (e.g., number of observation days or questionnaire respondents) is necessary to ensure accuracy, diversity, and believability—all without exhausting available resources. There are limitations on how much information an observer can process and code; therefore, questionnaires need to be short enough so that respondents are willing to answer them in a reliable manner. It is also imperative to realize that obtaining solutions to important questions requires time and involves multiple factors. No single tool can provide all the information that may be of interest in assessing a program, which often makes triangulation among different methods necessary.

SUMMARY

CSPAP practitioners and researchers need to be able to generate data to assess, evaluate, and promote programs; thus, they need to be able to select from available tools or create their own. This chapter provides an overview of eight instruments that have previously been used to assess school physical education and PA policies and practices. The instruments range from sophisticated direct observation strategies for use by trained observers to easy-to-use self-reports by practitioners. Some are designed specifically for making onsite decisions, while others are more suitable for research purposes. The chapter concludes with case examples of how two widely used direct observation instruments (SOFIT and SOPLAY) have been used to assess physical education and leisure-time interventions in schools.

QUESTIONS TO CONSIDER

1. What do you consider to be the main advantages and disadvantages of using systematic observation to assess CSPAP components?

2. What are the main differences between the SOFIT and SOPLAY observation systems? Under what conditions would you select one over the other?

3. Although the systematic observation tools identified in the chapter are more reliable and valid than the self-reported ones, why might it be wise to sometimes use the self-reported instruments?

4. How do PA opportunity minutes and PA minutes differ? What would be needed to convert PA opportunity minutes to PA minutes?

5. How can data from the tools identified in the chapter be used to create a summary score that permits valid comparisons overall within schools and among separate CSPAP components?

CASE EXAMPLES

Following are two case examples provided to illustrate the use of two very different systematic observation tools. Both tools were used to assess large-scale intervention studies in San Diego County, California, funded by the National Institutes of Health (NIH). Example 1 shows how SOFIT was used to assess physical education in elementary schools, and example 2 shows how SOPLAY was used to evaluate before-, during-, and after-school leisure-time activity periods in middle schools.

SOFIT and Sports, Play, and Active Recreation for Kids (SPARK)

While at San Diego State University, Jim Sallis and I (the author of this chapter) received funding ($2.4 million from 1989-1996) from the NIH to develop and evaluate SPARK, an evidence-based, health-related physical education program for grades 3 to 6 (McKenzie et al., 2016). The program we developed consisted of a physical education curriculum designed to provide ample amounts of PA in class, a behavioral self-management curriculum to promote PA outside of school, and extensive teacher training and support. Because physical education in U.S. elementary schools is frequently taught by classroom teachers, we designed the SPARK curriculum to be a practical resource for both classroom teachers and physical education specialists. We sequenced the instructional units and lesson plans and provided details for managing students and equipment. As well, we partially scripted lesson plans to aid inexperienced teachers in using appropriate instructional cues. The initial SPARK project included

- a year of funding that allowed both measurement and intervention strategies to be developed;
- schools being randomly assigned to intervention or control conditions;
- diverse measurement strategies to assess multiple formative, process, and outcome variables;
- separate intervention and measurement teams to reduce bias;
- collaborative research across disciplines and agencies (i.e., university, school, and community); and
- follow-up measures postintervention.

SOFIT (McKenzie et al., 1991), which simultaneously assesses student PA levels, lesson context, and teacher behavior, played a prominent assessment role throughout the study. For example, before moving to intervention schools, we used the instrument in both low– and high–socioeconomic status nonstudy schools to ensure the curriculum we were designing indeed promoted student MVPA and kept lesson management time to a minimum. SOFIT also permitted us to assess the intervention effects separately for classroom teachers and physical education specialists on motor skill development (McKenzie et al., 1998), physical fitness (Sallis et al., 1997), PA during class time (McKenzie et al., 1997), adiposity (Sallis et al., 1993), and student academic achievement (Sallis et al., 1999). Later, in one of the very few studies to assess the long-term effects of a physical education intervention, we used SOFIT to examine physical education in the schools after the SPARK intervention was completed (McKenzie et al., 1997). As a result of the findings relative to being a successful evidence-based program, SPARK became nationally and internationally known, and after 30 years, SPARK programs (which are updated regularly) remain available for widespread dissemination.

SOPLAY and Middle School Physical Activity and Nutrition (M-SPAN)

As a result of our successes with SPARK in elementary schools, Jim Sallis and I received an additional five-year grant (M-SPAN, 1996-2000) from the NIH to develop and assess expanded interventions for middle schools (Sallis et al., 2003). Our goals were to expand the intervention beyond physical education curriculum and staff development efforts to improve PA and eating behavior through environmental and policy approaches, the least evaluated components of school health interventions at the time. We tested this multi-component intervention in 24 middle schools in 9 school districts in San Diego County, California. The schools were diverse in size, facilities, and population characteristics. They had an average enrollment of 1,109 students, with 45 percent being non-White and 39 percent receiving free or reduced-cost meals. Following baseline measures, the schools were stratified by school district and then randomly assigned to receive two years of intervention ($N = 12$) or to be a measurement-only control school ($N = 12$). In addition to targeting physical education classes that were assessed using SOFIT, we designed an intervention that focused on increasing PA during leisure periods at school when students could make choices. A major component of this out-of-physical education program was the recruitment of adult volunteers (Strelow et al., 2002).

In addition to using SOFIT to assess physical education in M-SPAN, we used SOPLAY throughout the study to simultaneously assess the number of students and their PA levels during play and leisure opportunities in 151 targeted PA areas at the 24 schools (McKenzie et al., 2000). As indicated previously, SOPLAY is a place-based assessment tool (McKenzie, 2016), and we trained observers to made systematic scans of each target area during three measurement periods (i.e., before and after school and during lunchtime). Before-school observations were staggered so that the last area was observed 15 minutes prior to the start of school. Lunchtime observations began 15 minutes into the lunch period, and after-school observations were made at 15, 45, and 75 minutes after classes were dismissed for the day. We made separate scans to code the PA levels (sedentary, walking, and MVPA) of girls and boys and to simultaneously assess the contextual characteristics of the areas, including their accessibility and usability and whether supervision, organized activities, and equipment were provided. We also coded the predominant type of activity (e.g., basketball and dance) that area users were doing.

During baseline, we made SOPLAY observations at each school on three randomly selected days; during the intervention, we observed during two randomly selected days each semester. Baseline measures showed that few students used the school spaces to be physically active during leisure time; more students, however, used activity areas at lunchtime (19.5 percent of the daily attendance) than before (4.1 percent) or after (2.1 percent) school. There were also substantial gender differences, with more boys than girls using the areas and engaging in more vigorous PA. Target area environmental conditions explained 42 percent of the variance in the proportion of girls who were physically active and 59 percent of the variance for boys (Sallis et al., 2001). Both girls and boys were more physically active when the activity areas had received structural improvements and adult supervision was present. Overall, the out-of-physical education intervention was more successful with boys than with girls (Sallis et al., 2003).

CHAPTER 18

Evaluating CSPAPs: Measuring Implementation and Impact

Erin E. Centeio, PhD
Wayne State University

Nate McCaughtry, PhD
Wayne State University

There are many documented interventions that have been designed to increase the daily PA of youth in the school setting. Although many of these interventions have been successful at increasing minutes of PA and positively affecting the health of children, most of them are limited to specific parts of the school day (e.g., physical education, recess, or classroom time). More recently, agencies, such as the Centers for Disease Control and Prevention (2010) and the National Academies of Science, Health and Medicine (Institute of Medicine, 2013), have recommended that schools should play a key role in providing PA opportunities for children throughout the school day. Although the authors would assume that more PA opportunities during the school day would subsequently increase youth PA levels, little research has been done on the implementation of CSPAPs and their impact on PA and the health of children. This chapter will review the research focused on evaluation of CSPAPs, identify knowledge gaps, propose recommendations for future research and evaluation, suggest practical implications, and provide a case example of a CSPAP evaluation.

Review of Research

The following sections will review literature pertaining to school-based interventions. The first section will examine key school-based interventions that preceded the term "CSPAP," and the second section will specify evaluation studies performed on CSPAP interventions.

Pre-CSPAP Evaluation Studies

When thinking of seminal work regarding multicomponent school PA interventions, the Sports, Play, and Active Recreation for Kids (SPARK) project (Sallis et al., 1997) is at the top of the list. SPARK was a PA intervention designed to increase PA of elementary aged youth both in physical education class and at home. The intervention was based primarily in physical education. However, a self-management program that focused on increasing PA outside of school included newsletters and homework for youth and families. Results showed a significant increase in PA for those youth who participated in the SPARK intervention, with youth who were taught by a certified physical education teacher experiencing the most gains. Girls also experienced significant gains in abdominal strength and cardiovascular endurance.

The Coordinated Approach to Child Health (CATCH) program has shown numerous benefits to youth over the past decade with early results focusing on significant changes in cardiovascular risk factors (Luepker et al., 1996). A total of 56 intervention schools (40 control schools; $N = 5,106$) participated in the CATCH program, which included food service modifications, enhanced physical education, and classroom health curricula, and half received additional family education components. The randomized controlled trial that took place across four states showed increases in moderate-to-vigorous PA (MVPA) and a decrease in fat content served at lunch (Luepker et al., 1996). A follow-up to the original CATCH study showed behavioral changes were still present after a three-year period following the intervention (Nader et al., 1999).

In 2003, Caballero and colleagues examined a three-year healthy eating and PA intervention among American Indian youth. The purpose of their study was to examine a multicomponent

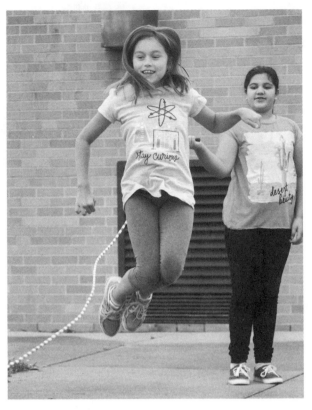

Students in the Building Healthy Communities program participating in active recess.

Photo provided by the Building Healthy Communities Program.

intervention that included both nutrition and PA components. The PA components included classroom PA breaks; increased energy expenditure during physical education; guided play during recess; and family and community engagement in the form of family fun nights, workshops, and family packs linked to the classroom curriculum. A total of 1,704 youth across 41 schools participated in the study. A decrease in total fat intake but not a reduction in body mass index (BMI) were found.

The Lifestyle Education for Activity Program (LEAP) was designed to increase the PA levels of high school girls through a comprehensive school-based intervention (Pate et al., 2005). The LEAP program was designed after the CATCH program and focused on physical education, health education, school environment, school health services, faculty and staff health promotion, and family and community involvement. This program was unique because it targeted high school girls and increasing behaviors and attitudes toward PA. After one year of intervention, girls in the intervention schools significantly increased vigorous PA compared to those in comparison schools. It is important to note that this program was based on self-reported, three-day PA recall and PA was not objectively measured.

Lubans and colleagues (2011) designed a comprehensive intervention for adolescent boys, which took place in secondary schools in Australia. The primary outcome of the intervention was decreased BMI; secondary outcomes included decreased percent body fat and waist circumference and increased muscular fitness and PA. The duration of the program was six months; the program consisted of school sport sessions, interactive seminars, lunchtime activities, PA and nutrition handbooks, leadership sessions, and pedometers for self-monitoring. Significant reductions were found for BMI and percent body fat, but no change was found for waist circumference, muscular fitness, and PA.

Also, in 2011, Puder and colleagues worked with preschool children to determine if a multicomponent preschool intervention that was culturally relevant for migrant children would decrease BMI and body fat while increasing aerobic fitness. The intervention consisted of structured PA lessons during the week, nutrition lessons, family communication about PA, sleep and screen time, and built environment changes within the preschool classroom. Although BMI did not significantly decrease, there were positive effects on aerobic fitness, waist circumference, percent body fat, PA, media use, and eating habits.

Finally, the Healthy, Energetic, Ready, Outstanding, Enthusiastic, Schools (HEROES) program (Seo et al., 2013) included 1,091 students who participated in a comprehensive intervention with a goal to increase PA of students. Schools made changes in their environment based on individual situations, but all intervention activities were led by a school wellness coordinator. Students significantly increased vigorous PA over the 18-month period but did not significantly improve moderate PA. School-level implementation, however, was a significant predictor of vigorous PA, and small school size predicted moderate PA.

CSPAP Evaluation Studies

Given that the term CSPAP is new, there are fewer studies that identify themselves as evaluating a CSPAP, although some would argue that many studies mentioned previously would qualify as CSPAP interventions. Literature detailing specific CSPAP interventions most often refers to outcomes in metrics, such as increased PA and aerobic capacity, decreased sedentary time, and the prevalence of obesity. Some literature apply more of a whole-of-school approach, which also include nutrition, to study more distal outcomes, such as classroom behavior and academic achievement.

In 2014, the *Journal of Teaching in Physical Education* released a monograph that included the first set of published research articles that were identified as CSPAPs. In this issue, Centeio and colleagues (2014) described a CSPAP that was implemented with urban students that affected PA levels of both students and parents. Specifically, an intervention that included quality physical education, classroom PA, and after-school PA clubs was implemented across one school year. The primary outcome measure was PA, which was objectively measured with students and subjectively measured with adults. After eight months, Centeio and colleagues (2014) reported that students had increased their MVPA by 4.5 minutes a day, and parents also reported an increase of PA.

Also in 2014, Carson, Castelli, and colleagues trained teachers to become PA leaders. Teachers were then expected to implement CSPAPs in their respective districts in the upcoming school year. Carson, Castelli, and colleagues measured the number of PA opportunities offered by teachers as well as students' PA levels and sedentary behavior using a wearable device. They found that teachers implemented significantly more opportunities for students to be physically active but the effect on students' actual behaviors over eight months was small. All students decreased their time spent in MVPA and increased time spent in sedentary behaviors, with students of trained teachers recording slightly better levels at postintervention (e.g., spent more time in MVPA and less time being sedentary than comparison students).

Step counts were targeted for a CSPAP intervention that was conducted by Burns and colleagues (2015), which focused on quality physical education and having students spend 50 percent or more of physical education classes in MVPA. Additionally, schools promoted active recess and integrated classroom PA breaks. Results showed that intervention students increased their steps from pre- to postintervention by approximately 1,126 steps per day (Burns et al., 2015).

In a related CSPAP study conducted by similar authors with at-risk elementary aged youth ($N = 1,460$), Brusseau et al. (2016) reported that the three-month CSPAP intervention significantly increased students' steps (an increase of ~603 steps per day) and time spent in MVPA (~5 minutes per day) as well as health-related fitness measures (Progressive Aerobic Cardiovascular Endurance Run [PACER] laps, push-ups, and curl-ups; Brusseau et al., 2016). A significant decrease in BMI (small effect size) was also found at the end of 12 weeks. This intervention consisted of three CSPAP components: quality physical education, PA during the school day (classroom and recess), and PA before and after school. These results are consistent with the results found by Centeio and colleagues (2014), who reported an increase of MVPA of approximately 4.5 minutes a day.

In 2016, Burns and colleagues (2016) examined change in elementary children's ($N = 1,460$) classroom behavior while a CSPAP was being implemented. Although there was no control group, they saw a significant increase in on-task behavior after CSPAP implementation in 70 classrooms over 6- and 12-week periods.

In 2017, Centeio and colleagues reported the impact of an eight-month CSPAP program on youth rate of improvement in reading and math achievement. They found that levels of PA (measured in steps) had a direct impact on youth rate of improvement in math and the level of school implementation of the CSPAP had a direct impact on rate of improvement in reading (Centeio, Somers, et al., 2018). Although there was no control group, this study is one of a few studies that examined a full CSPAP in relation to academic achievement of youth.

Also in 2017, Burns and colleagues used cardiometabolic health markers as an outcome measure of a nine-month CSPAP performed in five low-income schools. In this study, the schools hired a physical activity leader to assist in implementing PA experiences throughout the school day. The physical activity leader was responsible for helping the physical education teacher implement quality curriculum, provide semistructured recess for students, instruct classroom teachers on how to implement activity breaks, and provide opportunities for drop-in PA events. Improvements were made among third- through sixth-graders in high-density lipoprotein cholesterol, triglycerides, and mean arterial pressure, and sixth-graders also showed improvements in low-density lipoprotein cholesterol (Burns et al., 2017). Although this study did not employ a control group, it is the first of its kind to measure the effects of a CSPAP on the cardiometabolic health markers of youth.

Centeio, McCaughtry, and colleagues (2018) found that the Building Healthy Communities (BHC) program led to a decrease in obesity and central adiposity of fifth-grade students. The program was a whole-of-school approach (including a CSPAP) that targeted both PA and healthy eating, with a central focus on PA. The program consisted of six components: quality physical education, principal engagement, classroom education and activity, active recess, student leadership teams, and an after-school PA club. The program was evaluated using a quasi-experimental design with four treatment and two comparison schools. Students in the treatment schools significantly decreased their central adiposity (measured by waist-to-height ratio) and BMI compared to students in the comparison schools, who slightly increased their central adiposity (Centeio, McCaughtry, et al., 2018).

The previously discussed examples measure CSPAPs with different outcome measures. However, the most common measure used has been the PA behavior of students. Few articles examine the impact outside of student outcomes. The study conducted by Centeio and colleagues (2014) assessed the impact of CSPAPs on teachers' and parents' PA levels, and Pulling Kuhn and colleagues (2015) found that the work engagement of CSPAP-trained teachers significantly increased when compared to a control group.

Knowledge Claims

Given the information previously provided, following are the knowledge claims that we know about CSPAPs.

- Many multicomponent school intervention programs have been successful at increasing PA behaviors of youth, irrespective of gender. Most programs measure physical activity or MVPA, but some of them have shown success in decreasing BMI.
- Most outcome measures of the evaluations conducted focus on youth PA levels and overweight and obesity. Although not a focus of this chapter, many of the successful interventions also include nutrition programming in addition to the PA programming.
- Few studies saw a decrease in BMI or obesity-related measures.
- Among the few studies that have examined the extended impact of multicomponent school programming in adults (parents and teachers), the effects are promising.
- Common components include classroom PA breaks and quality physical education as the two components mostly present in the current CSPAP interventions.

Knowledge Gaps and Directions for Future Research

Understanding where the field has been and where it should be headed regarding the evaluation of CSPAPs is important. After reviewing the evaluation literature in relation to CSPAPs, the authors have outlined where they believe knowledge gaps exist and some suggestions for future research. To begin, little if any CSPAP research has been conducted with randomized controlled groups or using a randomized controlled trial (Centeio, McCaughtry, et al., 2018). Future research should include randomized controlled groups in order to fully understand the impact of such interventions. Additionally, little research has examined the effect that CSPAPs have on the collective school environment (e.g., policies) and longitudinally how these cultural shifts might affect youth health and

behaviors post-CSPAP intervention. Furthermore, few CSPAP studies have focused on outcome measures beyond physical health indicators (e.g., academic achievement and on-task behavior). Understanding the collective effects of CSPAPs on academic achievement could be one way to advocate for CSPAPs among principals and school personnel who value academic classroom time.

In addition to the previous suggestions, among the literature that was reviewed, most programs are designed for elementary aged students, and few of the interventions previously mentioned are specifically designed for preschool or secondary education settings. Although there have been successful interventions at the elementary level, future research should be conducted to better examine preschool- and secondary level interventions to evaluate the effectiveness of these programs. In addition, few if any publications discuss process evaluation of CSPAP programming. Carson, Pulling, and colleagues (2014) presented a mixed-methods evaluation of the delivery of national CSPAP trainings, but published manuscripts have yet to examine the process that it takes to implement the resultant comprehensive programs. Additionally, there is no known literature that discusses the cost effectiveness of implementing CSPAPs into the school setting and the amount of money they are saving long term. Finally, to date, there is no longitudinal data about the impact that participation in CSPAPs during youth has on adult PA and beyond the K-12 environment. Given the amount of time and money that it takes to implement CSPAPs into the school setting, understanding beyond the short-term effects is important because it influences the health benefits tracking into adulthood.

Evidence-Based Recommendations and Applications

Based on the existing literature around CSPAPs and other similar school-based PA interventions and the authors' experience in conducting research on these types of programs over the past 15 years, the authors have found that evaluating healthy school interventions is both essential and complicated. Implementing CSPAPs is a costly, labor-intensive process that often requires significant changes in the operational and political culture of schools. Hence, knowing that such initiatives have meaningful impacts on student health and learning is paramount. Without sound evaluation, schools and project leaders are left devoid of evidence as to whether any real change happened other than word-of-mouth and opinion-informed evidence. However, evaluating CSPAPs is also a complicated process and one that needs to be conceptualized at every turn of the program's implementation as the program develops from the initial design of the PA programming and throughout its implementation.

Given the importance and complexities involved in evaluating CSPAPs, in this section, the authors advocate for a four-part strategy that works in unison to fully understand the CSPAP experience in schools. It is understood that this strategy represents a fairly comprehensive approach that could be undertaken under ideal circumstances. However, the authors recognize that evaluation is often bound by budgets, evaluator skills and capacities, perceived disruptions to school operations, and the kinds of things that different stakeholders hope to learn about their new programs. Nevertheless, their recommendations will be global and hopefully allow future CSPAP leaders to understand the possibilities in evaluation so they are able to make informed decisions about the design and implementation of CSPAP evaluations that are tailored to each unique context.

Understanding School Context as a Starting Point

Often, evaluators commence their work when the programs begin, perhaps when they collect baseline data on the built environment of the school and various student-related variables. We contend that to fully understand the CSPAP experience, evaluation should begin at the inception of the process, when schools and other stakeholders decide that change should occur. The reality is that CSPAPs emerge for a range of reasons and those reasons set in motion the context in which CSPAPs will either flourish or fail. Here are three examples to make this point. First, a CSPAP may emerge as an initiative by university researchers

who have some degree of funding and wish to recruit schools willing to embark on a journey. Second, schools might apply to a CSPAP-oriented program offered by an outside organization because a key stakeholder at the school hopes to change a school's PA culture. Third, school personnel might recognize the importance of PA in their schools in the areas of student health and potentially academic achievement, and they set about developing their own CSPAP. The point is that the reasons and culture that give rise to the origination of CSPAPs matter to the overall story and learnings about programs and outcomes. For instance, who launched the idea (e.g., district administrator, principal, teacher, or parent)? How supportive are all of the other stakeholders? What kinds of cultural issues might facilitate or constrain a CSPAP program (e.g., equipment, facilities, curricular mandates, standardized testing, and weather)? How are programs designed? How much institutional change will they require? Which curriculum will be used and why? How much funding is available to support that change? The list of questions can go on indefinitely. However, knowing the genesis of programs from a multitude of perspectives is vital for evaluators to tell a complete story about a CSPAP experience. Moreover, evaluators may often play a role in many of the issues just described, and documentation of their involvement is yet another important piece in the evaluation puzzle.

Tracking Implementation and Environmental Change

The second step in a comprehensive CSPAP evaluation involves tracking implementation and environmental change. The authors have found that the tracking process itself involves three steps: establishing a baseline of past school norms for PA and nutrition, designing and implementing a tracking system, and developing implementation metrics.

Establishing a Baseline

First, it seems likely that an end goal of a CSPAP evaluation would be to report ways in which the school environment changed over time. The evaluators will also likely want to report changes in a range of student; school personnel; and, poten-

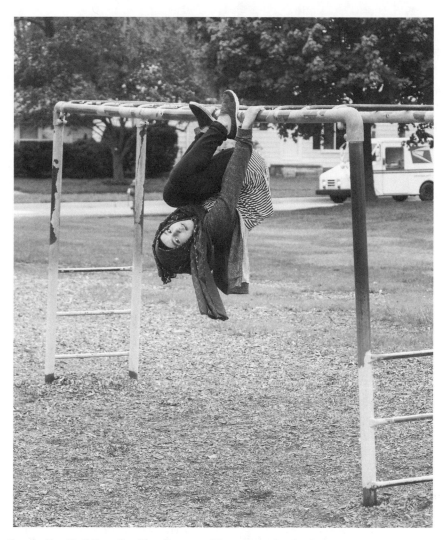

Student participating in the Building Healthy Communities program playing at recess.

Photo provided by the Building Healthy Communities Program.

tially, parent variables (discussed in the following section) stemming from new programs. The key is that none of this evaluation is possible without an accurate understanding of what happens in schools before CSPAPs begin. To have an accurate understanding, one might consider the following questions pertaining to integrating classroom PA in schools:

- How often are classroom PA opportunities offered?
- What curriculum is taught when integrating PA in the classroom?
- How active are students during classes?
- How long do classes last?

- What PA equipment do classroom teachers have to use in their teaching?

Similar questions might apply to recess, especially if it is one of the components in the CSPAP reform:

- How often do students get recess and for how long?
- What equipment do students have to use at recess?
- What are the norms for PA during recess?

The point here is that an evaluator must fully understand the norms of the school environment, especially related to PA, if he or she is going to eventually make claims about the ways in which

CSPAPs affected the school environment or led to changes in student and other stakeholder variables. Of course, as with measuring anything, there is a range of options an evaluator could use. For instance, an evaluator might employ ethnographic methods through school observations, interviews, document collection, or design tailored surveys for various school personnel to report their schools' norms. Regardless of the strategy, the evaluator must understand the point where CSPAP implementation began to fully understand and report where CSPAP implementation eventually ends up.

Designing and Implementing a Tracking System

Once a baseline of school culture is established and intervention programs ensue, evaluators must develop a system for tracking what happens. Inevitably, for various reasons, an evaluator needs to report the specifics about the intervention or program that took place. It is well known that schools rarely implement health-related programs the same way. On one end of the spectrum, some schools face challenges that prevent ideal or even minimal implementation (e.g., teacher resistance, political pressure not to decrease instructional time, and lack of resources). On the other end of the spectrum, some schools find immediate success, have strong stakeholder support, and end up implementing far more than they originally anticipated. Of course, other schools fall somewhere within this spectrum. It is important that evaluators acknowledge where schools fall on the spectrum when analyzing a school's implementation process and contributing outcomes.

Logically, however the evaluator designs the system of implementation tracking (otherwise known as intervention fidelity or ground truthing), it must have correspondence with the baseline data that was initially collected about school norms. It also should follow the simple strategy of reporting who, what, when, where, and how. Think back to the physical education example. The evaluator must design an approach that captures information such as who taught the lessons, which lessons were taught, did the lessons follow the same schedule as before the intervention, how active were the students, was the curriculum new,

was the teacher given new equipment or facilities to use, and was there professional development? To make claims about what changed in physical education and the impact it may have had on student outcomes, the evaluator needs to know exactly what happened. Of course, similar types of questions and corresponding tracking need to be included in all components of the overall CSPAP program, whether it includes, for example, interventions at recess, in classroom PA breaks, or in after-school programs.

There are many methods of tracking the who, what, when, where, and how of intervention implementation. An evaluator might design tracking logs on Survey Monkey or in paper format for teachers to report their activities. To add rigor, the evaluator could conduct site visits to verify the accuracy of the information being reported by teachers. If there are sufficient resources, an evaluator might place research staff at schools daily to observe and record the information that is required. Regardless of the approach, the importance of having detailed and accurate information about the who, what, when, where, and how of the program implementation is the foundation to understanding what changed at a school and whether those changes affected students. Evaluators should appreciate at the outset the volume of data that will be absorbed through this process and the kinds of resources and efficiency processes that will be needed to keep pace.

Developing Implementation Metrics

Once baseline data has been collected before any intervention activities take place and an accurate and comprehensive system of intervention tracking has occurred, the evaluator is now in a position to develop evaluation metrics. This is especially the case when interventions take place at more than one school. Mentioned earlier, schools often implement CSPAP programs in different ways and at different rates. Some do the minimum (or even less), and others outperform and make an extra effort to excel. Each school has a unique story to tell about what worked, what did not, and why. Furthermore, when an evaluator has outcome or impact data to explain how an intervention affected the school environment, or students, or teachers (see the following section), that outcome or impact data can fully be understood only in relation to the who, what, when, where, and how of the program implementation. For example, if two schools implemented CSPAP programs intending to increase student MVPA, one school could implement the bare minimum of the program, and the other school could implement far more than intended. This difference in intervention implementation may very well play an important role in explaining why, for instance, one school's students increased their MVPA far more than another's students. Both implemented CSPAPs but did so differently; hence, differences in the impact of those programs resulted. The point here is that an evaluator cannot assume that all schools implement programs identically. In fact, implementation needs to be tracked through baseline measurement, implementation tracking systems, and composite scoring so that how a CSPAP was actually rolled out in schools can be factored into the understanding of how implementation led to various types of culminating effects.

Identifying and Measuring Outcomes and Impact

Clearly, stakeholders design and implement CSPAPs to accomplish something and for some anticipated reason. For example, schools might embark on labor-intensive CSPAPs because they value the health of their students or they want students to adopt healthy life habits. They might even seek improved academic results because they recognize the connections between PA and learning. Whatever the reason, evaluators need to understand from the outset what stakeholders eventually hope to accomplish and factor that into their evaluation design. While the implementation tracking described in the previous section is able to capture how the school environment did or did not change, which is in itself important, a comprehensive evaluation system must also seek to understand how stakeholders were affected. In a perfect world, CSPAPs have the ability to produce desired effects on students, school personnel, and parents. Of course, the primary point of CSPAP impact should be with students. However, schools, like any place of employment, want healthy and happy workers for both altruistic and workplace performance reasons. In addition, it seems reason-

able that CSPAPs have the ability to influence student outcomes through interventions at schools but also the activities that take place at school are ideally transitioned to the home environment and have an effect on home environments and broader family health. This is especially the case when programs are designed with activities to specifically bridge school initiatives to students' home lives. Therefore, measuring the effect of CSPAPs on students, school personnel, and parents can provide the fullest and most wide-ranging explanation of a program's success.

Effect on students is typically the primary reason schools implement CSPAPs. The authors suggest that CSPAPs have the ability to affect students in eight areas, all of which an evaluator might consider to be necessary components to measure the comprehensive evaluation system that is developed. See the sidebar titled "Measuring Impact."

Mode of Evaluation (How)

Measuring the effect of CSPAP programs on students is clearly a wide-ranging enterprise. There are many options to consider, and within each variable, there are many data collection techniques ranging from highly to less rigorous. For instance, when measuring PA behaviors, evaluators can choose from a range of options, each option having its own level of scientific rigor, labor requirement, and cost. PA could be measured using state-of-the-art accelerometers or less costly pedometers, which capture step counts or MVPA, or research staff can systematically observe students and do time-interval recordings. The least costly option would be to use valid and reliable self-report scales, where students report their activity levels. Of course, there are even more fine-grained details to consider, such as whether evaluators want to track activity levels throughout the school day so they can report where in the school environment activity takes place or whether they want to obtain measures of student PA both at school and outside of school so they have an understanding as to how school programs affect behaviors in both places. In the end, there are a great many things to consider when designing an evaluation plan to measure the impact of CSPAPs on students. All of these areas are worth including in a comprehensive strategy,

Measuring Impact

Before discussing the many variables that an evaluator might measure to determine the impact of CSPAPs on students, all measures must be collected in a pre- and postintervention format so that change over time can be understood. Even more important, because evaluators typically hope to attribute eventual outcomes to the CSPAP intervention, both a control and a comparison group should be measured. In other words, the evaluator collects data with two groups of students: those who participate in a CSPAP program at their school and those who attend a school not implementing a CSPAP program (ideally a school without an extensive PA focus). Therefore, when combined into an experimental design, if the evaluator finds that student variables at the CSPAP school changed but those same student variables at the non-CSPAP school did not, then the evaluator can attribute those changes in student variables to the CSPAP intervention with more confidence. This results in the changes in student variables being attributed to CSPAP intervention activities and not to coincidence or some other mediating reason.

The eight areas of student impact that should be considered by evaluators for inclusion into the overall evaluation design range from direct health and behavioral measures to more psychological and distal variables.

1. When the intervention is designed to improve student health, saliva and blood tests that are capable of measuring a range of biomarkers (e.g., cholesterol, immune functioning, cortisol, and diabetes) might be considered.

2. To measure effects to obesity or body composition, evaluators would collect anthropometric measurements, such as weight-to-height ratio or BMI.

3. To understand the effect of programming on students' fitness levels, evaluators could measure aerobic capacity, muscle strength and endurance, and flexibility.

4. Given the overall goal to meet national PA guidelines, evaluators might measure the amount of time students engage in light PA or MVPA or the amount of time they are sedentary.

5. To teach students how to lead healthy and active lives, evaluators could develop PA knowledge scales that measure how much of the PA and healthy living knowledge students have learned through programming.

6. Measuring psychosocial variables is important because they are often used as proxy measures of program impact. These variables have origins in a range of theories (e.g., social cognitive theory, ecological theory, theory of planned behavior, self-determination theory, and expectancy-value theory). Some of the variables that can be measured include attitudes toward PA, PA enjoyment, social support, competence, autonomy, and values.

7. PA can have important influences on non-PA areas in life. As a result, a seventh evaluation measure that could be used might focus on issues regarding quality of life (e.g., social connectedness, depression, and feelings of well-being).

8. A measurement area gaining increased popularity is academic performance. This is especially the case given the vast research emerging that shows the connections between PA and cognition, learning, creativity, academic achievement, school attendance, and pro-social behavior. School performance measures might include attendance and disciplinary data, cognitive function tests, curriculum-based assessments, grades, and standardized test scores.

but evaluators are often bound by funding, staff, school permissions, and stakeholder outcome requests, which force them to make difficult decisions about which variables to measure and how to measure them.

Target of Evaluation (Who)

Beyond student variables, evaluators should also consider whether to include school personnel and parent measures. The reality is that teachers and school administrators who adopt CSPAPs are at least partially committed to issues of health and wellness. They also operate in a health-enhancing climate for an academic year. Measuring variables related to school staff PA, healthy living knowledge, and various psychosocial constructs (e.g., social support, PA enjoyment, competence, relatedness, and autonomy) might have two upsides. For one, knowing that an initiative has positive benefits for students is important, but knowing that it also has positive influences on school personnel provides even more justification for the importance and viability of school-wide PA. Further, from an analytical perspective, such measurement allows evaluators to adopt nested research designs where changes in student variables can be examined in relation to principal and teacher variables. From a slightly different perspective, part of the rationale for adopting CSPAPs is the hope that behaviors learned at school will have some carryover to students' home lives. Therefore, to fully measure the impact of CSPAPs, evaluators should consider whether to extend their evaluation approaches to students' parents and home contexts. Evaluators might elect to pursue measuring parent PA, healthy living knowledge, and psychosocial constructs and the built environment that parents provide for their children around PA.

Understanding the Context of Change

The fourth part of an overall strategy for evaluating CSPAPs focuses on understanding the process whereby change took place. As mentioned earlier, every school has its own political, cultural, economic, and social dimensions. No two schools are alike. Whereas one school might have strong consensus to pursue CSPAP initiatives, another school might have administrative support but teachers who are not willing to change routines and implement changes. One school might have abundant resources to support a change effort, and another school might be facing budget cuts and be located in an economically disadvantaged community with fewer resources. Evaluating what happened (implementation tracking) and what resulted (student, school personnel, and parent impact) is not entirely sufficient to fully understand a school's CSPAP experience. Missing in the current literature is *how* change actually happened in the school. For example, how did teachers react? Were they willing, or were they forced to operate differently or learn new things? What kinds of barriers or challenges did principals face in leading a CSPAP, or were they the ones being forced to embrace implementation? How did original plans change and get modified as the program progressed? With the complexity of CSPAPs and their many variations, the complexities of schools, and the time during which real change happens in schools, there are infinite important stories to be told about the process of change. It is important that these stories be captured as part of the evaluation not simply to chronicle an individual school's journey but also to contribute to growing a national movement around school PA. Schools inevitably must learn from each other's journeys to avoid common errors and pitfalls, anticipate challenges, and have a repertoire of strategies available to move forward. Research has shown how extraordinarily emotional and complex school reform and change can be. Implementing CSPAPs is no different.

A concluding recommendation is that evaluators employ a range of qualitative methods to understand how CSPAPs play out. Regularly interviewing students, teachers, administrators, and parents; observing change in action; and developing an archive of change-related documents can help the evaluator to tell the story of how change occurred. For example, schools, researchers, and evaluators should develop more case studies that describe how CSPAPs began. Within these stories should be information about what happened along the way, the outcomes that occurred, and the story of how it all took place. These case studies could then serve as blueprints for other schools.

SUMMARY

This chapter focused on how to evaluate CSPAP programming. A review of literature was conducted, and knowledge gaps were identified, including lack of programming within the early elementary setting and within high schools. Additionally, little program evaluation has been conducted on CSPAPs with rigorous methodologies (i.e., a randomized controlled design). The authors suggested that evaluating CSPAPs is complicated and there is no one-size-fits-all formula for evaluation. Therefore, it is imperative that evaluators tailor evaluations within the unique context of the CSPAP. A four-step process was suggested for evaluation: (1) understand the unique context, (2) track implementation and environmental change, (3) identify and measure outcomes and impact, and (4) understand the context of change.

QUESTIONS TO CONSIDER

1. What are the major contextual factors in your school or the school you are partnering with that should be examined when thinking about designing a context-relevant CSPAP?

2. Based on the overall goals and design of your CSPAP program, what are the most important outcomes that ought to be measured?

3. What kinds of impact assessments will stakeholders require to evaluate the success of the CSPAP program, and how many resources are available to support the evaluation program?

4. What social theories will serve as a framework for the CSPAP design, and how should that influence the evaluation design?

5. How will the CSPAP program be tracked during implementation as a basis for understanding how the programming resulted in measurable outcomes and impact?

CASE EXAMPLE: BUILDING HEALTHY COMMUNITIES (BHC)

The Building Healthy Communities program is a comprehensive nutrition and PA intervention that takes place in elementary schools across the state of Michigan. The program was created in 2009 by Blue Cross Blue Shield of Michigan. It was transformed in 2012 when Wayne State University joined Blue Cross Blue Shield of Michigan to create Building Healthy Communities: Engaging Elementary Schools Through Partnership (BHC). The partnership and dedication of like-minded people and organizations has led to the program's being delivered in over 228 schools and reaching more than 85,000 students.

The BHC program is now a partnership between Blue Cross Blue Shield of Michigan, Wayne State University's Center for Health and Community Impact (WSU-CHCI), Michigan Department of Health and Human Services, United Dairy Industry of Michigan, and Michigan Fitness Foundation. WSU-CHCI is the implementing agency for the BHC program and is responsible for overseeing all of the program implementation and evaluation. As a partner, the United Dairy Industry of Michigan supports the Fuel Up to Play 60 program with Blue Cross Blue Shield and the Michigan Department of Health and Human Services by supporting the partnership with generous funding, program oversight, as well as media and marketing support.

The BHC program is designed to improve the health of young people and the health of their families and communities by creating a comprehensive, school-wide network of PA and healthy eating opportunities and education. The program consists of six main components that address both PA and nutrition: principal engagement, classroom education on PA and healthy eating, quality physical education, active recess, student leadership team, and Healthy Kids Club (see figure 18.1). For the purpose of this case example, the authors will address all components of the program given that the CSPAP is strategically intertwined throughout each component.

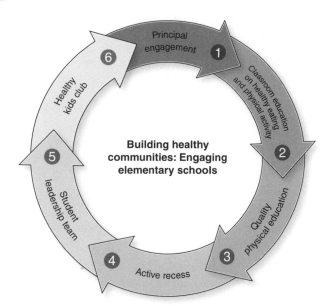

Figure 18.1 BHC six-component model.

Reprinted by permission from Blue Cross Blue Shield of Michigan.

Principal Engagement

For school-based health initiatives to be successful, school principals must be fully engaged. Research shows that schools are most successful in implementing comprehensive health programming when principals are supportive and engaged in the process (Centeio et al., 2016; Kulik et al., under review). As part of the BHC program, principals

- attend the BHC kickoff at the beginning of the year with their staff,
- read the Healthy Tip of the Day each morning,
- display health promotion messaging throughout the school,
- send healthy eating and PA messaging home to parents and caregivers through school communications (e.g., newsletters, emails, and social media),
- support publicly all school personnel in their individual program roles, and
- complete the Healthy School Action Tool.

Classroom Education on PA and Healthy Eating

Academic classrooms provide an ideal location to promote healthy eating and PA. Students spend most of their time in the homeroom, especially at the elementary level. The classroom-level contact also provides a way for families to receive educational materials about healthy living. As part of the BHC program, classroom teachers

- teach healthy eating lessons;
- implement PA breaks; and
- share healthy living resources, healthy homework, and tip sheets with parents.

Quality Physical Education

Quality physical education lays the foundation for a lifetime of PA (Sallis & McKenzie, 1991). The Exemplary Physical Education Curriculum, or EPEC, is an award-winning, evidence-based curriculum developed by the Michigan Fitness Foundation that also reinforces healthy eating. As part of the BHC program, physical education teachers

- receive a full set of age-appropriate physical education curriculum and the equipment,
- participate in one EPEC and physical education best practices professional development,
- implement EPEC at all grade levels and carry out best practices in physical education, and
- share physical education materials and messaging with parents.

Active Recess

PA equipment and play guidance at recess increase students' PA levels and learning readiness (Murray et al., 2013). To support active recess,

- schools receive a mobile recess cart fully stocked with PA equipment, and
- the physical education teacher and recess monitors receive training to promote high-activity recess games outside as well as active recess inside.

Student Leadership Team

Getting students engaged in the school transformation process is an excellent way to help schools make and sustain change (Wallerstein & Berstein, 1988). Through Fuel Up to Play 60, students

- form a leadership team,
- evaluate the PA and nutrition environment of the school,
- design and implement PA and nutrition reforms ("plays"), and
- advertise and celebrate success.

Healthy Kids Club

After-school programs can significantly increase students' PA and healthy eating behaviors to help meet national activity and eating guidelines (Demetriou et al., 2017). As part of the Healthy Kids Club, schools

- implement fun and culturally relevant MVPA clubs,
- provide healthy snacks,
- design walking or running sessions that include record keeping and goal setting, and
- share PA and healthy eating materials and resources with families.

Understanding Context

Each January, the BHC partnership releases a statewide announcement that invites schools to apply for the program the following year. Schools then complete a comprehensive application. Once the applications are reviewed and scored, applicants are interviewed to learn more about their school context, capacity, and readiness to undertake a culture change around PA and nutrition.

After schools are awarded the program, they are assigned a healthy school coordinator who works with the school to understand its needs and perceived barriers and then helps determine how to effectively implement all components of the program within each individual context. During the process of applying, being interviewed, and working with the healthy school coordinator, understanding the context of each school takes place.

Tracking Implementation and Environmental Change

As part of implementation tracking, three steps outlined in this chapter are followed: establishing a baseline, designing and implementing a tracking system, and developing implementation metrics.

Establishing a Baseline

During the application process, applicants are asked to provide a substantial amount of data about their schools. For example, they are asked to provide general information about the number of students, student-to-teacher ratio, number of physical education teachers in the building, information about a school wellness committee, what other healthy eating and PA programming is occurring, and who the food service director is. Then, beginning yearly in September, the healthy school coordinator follows up with the principal and other key personnel to begin collecting baseline data regarding the BHC-specific components as well as current policies in the school. Through these interviews, which provide baseline data for tracking implementation and environmental changes, healthy school coordinators gather information such as what free opportunities there are for students to be active before and after school, how recess is organized and monitored, and the number of minutes of physical education and PA. This initial interview helps create a baseline of each component for evaluation purposes and helps the healthy school coordinator understand each school context independently in order to help with future implementation of the CSPAP in each school.

Designing and Implementing a Tracking System

As the program unfolds in each school, the healthy school coordinator and school personnel complete monthly reports. The healthy school coordinator regularly visits each school to help implement each component of the program and ensure that the activities being reported are actually taking place. For example, a physical education teacher might report that he or she taught four different EPEC lessons a day for the entire month. The job of the coordinator is to drop in on the physical education teacher to observe a lesson in physical education and document whether the teacher is teaching part of the EPEC curriculum. Furthermore, the healthy school coordinator will follow up with the physical education teacher and ask specific questions about what the teacher had written on his or her monthly log. He or she might say, "I saw that you taught basketball dribbling last week with fourth grade. What was the EPEC lesson that you taught? Did the students enjoy it?"

Developing Implementation Metrics

Healthy school coordinators are given a checklist and follow-up questions to ask when visiting schools and observing the components of the program. By following this checklist, the coordinator is able to gather information and then report detailed information back to the program evaluation team on a regular basis. Figure 18.2 outlines the type of tracking documents and procedures that are collected to ground truth and tell a complete implementation story.

Understanding Outcomes and Impact

As part of the BHC program, the evaluators measure student, parent, and staff outcomes as well as policy, systems, and environmental change. Each year, a team of researchers meets and discusses the focus for the current year of outcome measures. Figure 18.3 is a culmination of outcomes that we have collected from schools that have participated in the BHC program. Of the data that is presented, some of it is collected every year, and some of

Observations	Tracking documents internally	Tracking documents for school personnel

• Physical education
• Classroom lessons and PA breaks
• Active recess
• Student leadership teams
• Healthy kids club
• General school environment
	• **Monthly**
	  • Healthy school coordinator report
	
	• **End of year**
	  • Final report on key changes throughout the year
	  • Master spreadsheet created with monthly implementation documents
		• **Monthly**
		  • Surveys filled out by classroom teacher, physical education teacher, student leadership team advisor, and after-school club advisor
		
		• **End of year**
		  • Final surveys filled out by each key personnel
		  • Healthy school action tool action plan

Figure 18.2   BHC implementation tracking.

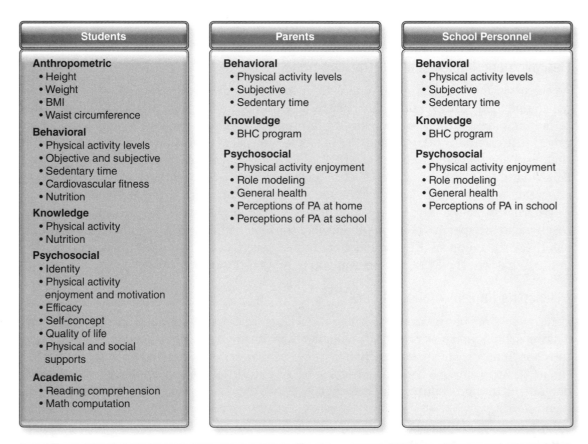

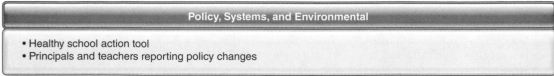

Students	Parents	School Personnel
Anthropometric • Height • Weight • BMI • Waist circumference **Behavioral** • Physical activity levels • Objective and subjective • Sedentary time • Cardiovascular fitness • Nutrition **Knowledge** • Physical activity • Nutrition **Psychosocial** • Identity • Physical activity enjoyment and motivation • Efficacy • Self-concept • Quality of life • Physical and social supports **Academic** • Reading comprehension • Math computation	**Behavioral** • Physical activity levels • Subjective • Sedentary time **Knowledge** • BHC program **Psychosocial** • Physical activity enjoyment • Role modeling • General health • Perceptions of PA at home • Perceptions of PA at school	**Behavioral** • Physical activity levels • Subjective • Sedentary time **Knowledge** • BHC program **Psychosocial** • Physical activity enjoyment • Role modeling • General health • Perceptions of PA in school

Policy, Systems, and Environmental
• Healthy school action tool • Principals and teachers reporting policy changes

Figure 18.3   Outcome variables measured during BHC program evaluation.

it is collected on designated years. Some of the data has also been collected in comparison schools in order to get a better understanding of the impact on the program compared to schools that are not enacting a comprehensive healthy school initiative.

The BHC program has a team of data collectors who are trained on each protocol before going out into the school setting. Once trained, data collectors spend one week in a designated school to collect all measures. During this week, surveys are distributed to parents and school personnel, and multiple efforts are made to encourage completion.

Understanding the Context of Change

To understand the context of change, the BHC evaluators utilize a variety of methods to capture a complete story of change within each school. The healthy school coordinator is constantly engaging in informal interviews with key school personnel (e.g., principals, secretaries, and team leaders) to document changes in the school environment. The healthy school coordinator makes sure to document these conversations in a journal and then reflect them on his or her monthly reports. In addition to informal interviews, at the end of each school year, key school personnel as well as parents and students are asked open-ended questions to capture changes, successes, and challenges that have taken place throughout the year. Another document that is collected at the end of the year is the Healthy School Action Tool (HSAT) action plan. This document is created once schools have completed the HSAT online. It is a documented action plan that tells them where improvement needs to happen in relation to PA, nutrition, and health. Through these surveys, we are better able to understand the change that schools have gone through over the past year and determine key areas that they are looking to improve next. Using a combination of all the data collected allows us to build case studies that describe how CSPAPs began, what happened along the way, and what outcomes occurred and helps us tell the story of how each school was successful in its own way.

CHAPTER 19

Advocating for CSPAPs

Heather E. Erwin, PhD
University of Kentucky

Erin E. Centeio, PhD
Wayne State University

*A*dvocacy is the "act or process of support-ing a cause or proposal" (Advocacy, n.d.). The World Health Organization (1995) better defined it as a combination of individual and social actions with the intent of advancing political promise, policy aid, social tolerance and approval, and backing for a particular health goal or program. In the world of education, advocacy for PA and physical education for youth is immi-nent because of negative stigma surrounding physical education, the looming pressure placed on teachers for students to perform academically at high levels, and the stress surrounding college and career readiness and high school graduates' abilities to succeed in our society. Additionally, youth are not accruing adequate PA levels, which leads to obesity. And physical education is the only subject in the school system that adequately teaches the whole child by addressing psycho-motor, cognitive, and affective learning domains (Darst et al., 2014). From a health standpoint, PA has numerous benefits, including building healthy bones and muscles, reducing the risk of developing chronic disease risk factors, improving muscular strength and endurance, and reducing stress and anxiety (Physical Activity Guidelines Advisory Committee, 2008). Therefore, advocacy for PA and physical education is imperative not only because of the multiple related health benefits but also for the cognitive and affective benefits (Centers for Disease Control and Prevention [CDC], 2010). Physical activity provided within and outside of school contributes to the success of the whole child. In this chapter, we review the research on advocacy for CSPAPs, summarize the existing research, identify holes and possible directions in the literature, recommend strategies for advocat-ing for CSPAPs in the future, and share two case examples of successful advocacy efforts by CSPAP champions. Because of the focus on advocacy in this chapter, we attempt to pull from advocacy techniques and strategies in other health promo-tion areas to make broad suggestions for advocacy in CSPAPs.

Review of Research

To date, very little has been published on the advocacy of PA and physical education for youth, yet advocacy is one of the standards for national board certification for physical education teachers (National Board for Professional Teaching Standards, 2014). It is expected that accomplished physical education teachers will "advance their work through advocacy by actively promoting outcomes that benefit students" (p. 62). This can be done through the promotion of school programs; collaborating with community partners; and working with parents, community members, and professional organizations to write grant proposals, raise money, and form coalitions with groups to enhance PA opportunities.

Shilton (2008) indicated that while advocacy for the field of PA has made progress overall, it has still not reached its potential. Much of the related literature encourages people to advocate for both quality physical education and PA in schools. SHAPE America offers a multitude of resources for advocating for physical education and PA on its website, which provides statistics on a number of items, related legislation and policy, and steps to take action. The CDC (2011) also specified schools as avenues for promoting PA within the community. One might ask why advocate for PA and physical education? Loland (2006) argued that three justifications for physical education were moralism, health, and meaning. *Moralism* is the mix of morality and ethics held by an individual, group, or society and defines what is good or bad for them. *Health* is a rationale for physical education because of the scientific evidence available to support the positive outcomes of regular engagement in exercise or PA. Finally, physical education or PA should be *meaningful* to the users so they can realize their human potential.

Most of the published literature details advocacy and campaigning strategies in larger contexts within the realm of health promotion; however, there are essentially no known publications that research the effectiveness of advocacy for PA or physical education specifically. Nearly 20 years ago, Bauman and colleagues (2001) published information on a mass media campaign in Australia that targeted PA. This campaign was a statewide effort that included television and print media advertising, mailings, and support programs at the community level. Based on telephone surveys, they found substantial changes in adult recall of activity messages and awareness in the campaign state compared to others within Australia. Participants in the campaign state were 2.08 times more likely to increase their PA by one hour per week than those not targeted in the campaign (Bauman et al., 2001). Another research publication describing the effects of the mass media was from Huhman and colleagues (2005). The subject of this publication was the VERB campaign, which was conducted by the CDC to increase PA among youth and comprised advertisements within schools and communities and Internet activities. They found that three-fourths of children surveyed were aware of the campaign. The average 9- to 10-year-old children who were aware of the campaign engaged in 34 percent more free-time PA than those who were not aware of the campaign. The researchers suggested utilizing commercial advertising to promote youth PA. Strategies and principles similar to these two examples may be valuable for physical education teachers and school champions to advocate for CSPAPs and could possibly result in more PA for students, staff, and community members.

In 2010, two major campaigns were launched in the United States to promote PA among youth: Nike's Designed to Move campaign and former First Lady Michelle Obama's *Let's Move!* campaign. Nike, in conjunction with the American College of Sports Medicine and the International Council of Sport Science and Physical Education, was a leader in the campaign, with 70 other public-, private-, and civil-sector organizations. The purpose of the Designed to Move (2015) campaign was to inspire a unified approach to end the growing epidemic of physical inactivity and coordinating aligned action forward. As a result of the movement, a series of tangible items for consumers to use to promote and implement PA were published. The playbook is a comprehensive document that organizes research, case studies, and benefits of getting kids moving as well as suggestions on how to make change happen. An executive summary was created to give a brief version of the report, and an infographic was created to tell the story and spread the word in an easy-to-read manner. To date, there are no known results as to the impact of the campaign on physical inactivity of youth.

Let's Move! was also launched with the intent to help kids and their families lead healthier lifestyles. This campaign by the former First Lady led to the first-ever task force on childhood obesity and to the development of a national action plan that encouraged public and private sectors to come together to help engage families and communities in improving the health of children. As part of the overall *Let's Move!* campaign, many changes were made across the nation regarding children's health. School meal nutrition programs were updated through the Healthy, Hunger-Free Kids Act of 2010 (Public Law 111-296), and the Food and Drug Administration modernized food labels. The U.S. Department of Agriculture launched its own campaign of MyPlate and MiPlato, which sought to educate youth and adults about the five food groups to help Americans make healthy choices. These efforts also influenced the updating of the President's Challenge Youth Fitness Test and expanded the mission of the President's Council on Fitness, Sports & Nutrition. Finally, as part of *Let's Move!*, many subsidiary campaigns developed to target specific areas of childhood obesity, including *Let's Move!* Salad Bars to Schools; *Let's Move!* Active Schools; *Let's Move!* Outside; Every Kid in a Park; Eat Brighter; Drink Up; FNV (Fruits and Vegetables); *Let's Move!* Cities, Towns, and Countries; and *Let's Move!* Child Care.

Of most importance to this chapter is the *Let's Move!* Active Schools campaign, which was launched in 2013. *Let's Move!* Active Schools promotes using a CSPAP to ensure that all K-12 students are receiving 60 minutes a day of PA. Using the slogan "Active Kids Do Better," the *Let's Move!* Active Schools campaign helps schools understand the benefits of PA in the school setting and promote integrating opportunities to be physically active before, during, and after school. In its infancy, the campaign was backed by a large variety of public, private, and civil organizations, including SHAPE America, Alliance for a Healthier Generation, Nike, and the President's Council on Fitness, Sport & Nutrition. In 2016 in schools, *Let's Move!* transitioned to Active Schools during the former First Lady's transition out of

office. Active Schools continues to be run by the Partnership for a Healthier America. Its mission remains the same, to influence schools directly by encouraging children to be active 60 minutes a day, but it also seeks to influence systems and policy changes that will enable schools to educate the whole child. The impact of the *Let's Move!* campaign and its subsidiaries is not yet known because it will take many more years to understand the impact this campaign had on childhood obesity and physical inactivity of youth.

Social marketing is also important in advocating and promoting PA programming (Tannehill et al., 2015). Its purpose is to benefit the people who engage in the behavior. Similar to business marketing models, the four keys to marketing physical education and PA are product, price, place, and promotion. *Product* is the PA itself. For youth, this product should provide for success; offer choices; and be fun, inclusive, and developmentally appropriate. The idea of being physically active should be as enticing as possible for the user. *Price* concerns costs and barriers to partaking in PA; the cost–benefit ratio should be low. Selecting school times to offer PA can help with costs because students are typically on campus before school and during the day and additional transportation would not be required. Communicating with local businesses, contacting individuals who are willing to provide free PA services or resources, and hosting fund-raisers to lower the overall costs are recommended. *Place* is another key to marketing. The locations for PA opportunities should be visible, usable, and accessible to all those involved. Ideally, PA opportunities offered beyond the school hours would take place at the school to lower costs, and the school would serve as a familiar location. *Promotion* serves to inform students, families, and faculty and staff of all the opportunities available to them. A number of promotion strategies are suggested, such as visual prompts (e.g., point-of-decision prompts or advertisements through social media), branding the CSPAP and creating a logo, auditory prompts via daily announcements, or special events (e.g., school assemblies or family nights).

One form of social marketing is point-of-decision prompts, which are motivational signs designed to influence individuals to make certain behavioral choices. Kahn and colleagues

(2002) found sufficient evidence in their review that point-of-decision prompts were effective in a variety of settings for increasing levels of PA. However, no point-of-decision prompt studies have been conducted with youth or in a CSPAP environment. The authors suggest that tailoring prompts to specify the benefits may increase the effectiveness of the intervention or advocacy. For example, on the playground, a point-of-decision prompt may read, "Walking four full laps around the playground is the same as a half mile!" Another example of a point-of-decision prompt may be a sign located in the hallway of a high school that reads, "Drop in for some activity after lunch to burn off some calories and energize your brain!"

In summary, advocacy is a fairly new field of study in PA and physical education. A number of national and regional campaigns have been instigated to push for PA for youth, yet to date, their impact is unknown. Many of them use social marketing campaign strategies to advocate for PA programming. It is anticipated that product, price, place, and promotion may be utilized as strategies to successfully increase PA for youth. Point-of-decision prompts are also a potential means for influencing youth to be active.

Knowledge Claims

The following evidence-based claims can be made about CSPAP advocacy based on the available research reviewed in previous section.

- Research supports the four keys to marketing to advocate for a CSPAP: product, price, place, and promotion. The product (PA) should be fun and enticing for the user. The price (costs and barriers) must be affordable and appropriate, with the benefits outweighing the barriers. The place (location) should be noticeable, practical, and available to anyone taking part. The promotion (advocacy) is meant to make students, families, and staff aware of and welcome to participate in all the opportunities available (Tannehill et al., 2015).

- To the best extent possible, television and print media should be utilized for advertising, social media, mailings, and support programs at the community level to promote CSPAP events (Bauman et al., 2001). For a

teacher, this may include advertisements played during morning announcements over the public announcement system, reminders via social media (e.g., Twitter, Instagram, and Facebook), notes home in student folders, and advertisements throughout the community (e.g., signs in yards and at local grocery and department stores and displays at the local community center or churches).

- The VERB campaign encourages PA every day and provides a good foundation for targeting tweens. Teachers or CSPAP champions should offer advertisements within schools and communities to advocate for PA. Additionally, utilizing the Internet to improve personal and social welfare has been shown to be effective with youth (Huhman et al., 2005).

- Commercial advertising may be a promising way to advocate for a CSPAP. It was found to be effective with a nationwide campaign effort for adult PA (Bauman et al., 2001).

- There is much synergy around increasing PA during the school day in the United States, although the campaigns are relatively new and it is impossible to understand the overall impact they are having to date.

- Point-of-decision prompts may be an untapped resource for advocating for CSPAPs, specifically to encourage youth to be more active. They have been shown to be effective in increasing stair use with adults (Soler et al., 2010), yet research is warranted regarding their influence for youth PA.

Knowledge Gaps and Directions for Future Research

Shilton (2006) described a three-step model for advocating for PA that includes the why, what, and how of advocacy. Step 1 is gathering and translating PA evidence. The evidence indicates why it is important to advocate for PA. Step 2 is the message or the agenda. What should be advocated? Step 3 includes the strategy to influence support. The strategy involves political advocacy, media advocacy, professional mobilization, advocacy from within the organization (or school), and community mobilization. Presently, there are no known data-based publications focused on advocacy specific to CSPAP and PA outcomes.

Future research should be conducted around the impact of advocacy in relationship to CSPAPs. Specifically, what types of advocacy are occurring in relation to CSPAPs, and what impact has they had on increasing PA opportunities and the PA participation level of youth? Research should also begin to examine the level of effectiveness of different types of advocacy in producing change.

Evidence-Based Recommendations and Applications

In this section, we provide evidence-based recommendations for teachers, administrators, and school champions to consider when advocating for their CSPAP. First, advocacy is framed within the nested ecology of advocacy, which blends nicely within the CSPAP conceptual framework as outlined by Carson and colleagues (2014). Next, messaging strategies are provided in preparation for asking for resources. Finally, professional development suggestions are offered as a means of closing the gap between transitioning from preservice physical education teacher candidates to in-service teachers to fulfill the role of CSPAP champions.

Nested Ecology of Advocacy Framework

The social-ecological framework as described by Sallis and colleagues (2008) suggests that multiple levels of factors work together to influence health change. The CSPAP conceptual framework (Carson et al., 2014), which was built on the social-ecological framework, suggests that daily PA is the epicenter of the framework, but it adds four additional levels of influence (components, facilitators, leaders, and culture). To advocate for health change among youth, specifically through CSPAP programming, targeting different levels within the CSPAP conceptual framework is key. These levels can be thought of as a nested ecology of advocacy (see figure 19.1). As in many promotional efforts, there are several levels that should be targeted when advocating for CSPAPs, stemming from the epicenter, where the student is engaging in 60 minutes a day of PA, to culture and policy. Advocacy will look different depending on what is being advocated and to whom. It is important that when advocating for something begins, a specific level within the framework is targeted. The CSPAP conceptual framework lays the foundation for the practical initiatives, which are informed by best practices within the field. However, to advocate for mainstream use of such models, researchers also must take a nested

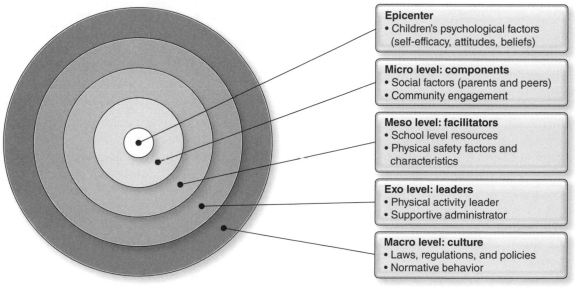

Figure 19.1   Nested ecology of advocacy.

approach; they need to embed the CSPAP with the implications of the social-ecological model in order to consider the far-reaching determinants that affect the implementation, dissemination, and sustainability of CSPAPs in schools.

The nested ecology of advocacy indicates that the target audience for each layer is different depending on the goal. To help visualize these layers, a discussion follows of each layer with examples of how to prepare for and target that layer within the nested ecology to advocate for CSPAPs.

Epicenter

When advocating at the epicenter, increasing the amount of daily PA in which students are participating should be targeted with a goal of 60 minutes per day. Similar to the social-ecological framework's intrapersonal levels of influence, the CSPAP's framework asserts that the epicenter of the individual student's daily PA is influenced by social and emotional factors toward PA participation (e.g., self-efficacy, attitudes, and intentions to be active).

Advertising and promoting activities that are fun and engaging for all students, culturally relevant, and convenient fall within this level. When encouraging youth to be active, consider how youth might perceive the activity, whether they have intentions to participate, and how to entice them to *want* to take part.

Microlevel: Components

The microlevel sheds light on the interactions between the individual child's daily PA and the sociocultural school environment. When placed into the context of the CSPAP model, there are five components offered across the school day that influence the individual child's daily PA behaviors. Social factors can influence behavior. For example, social interactions with family and friends would be a point of target within the microlevel. At this level, one would advocate for activities that are social in nature. Designing activities around social experiences, such as a neighborhood walking club or a family fitness night, is a way to incorporate PA at the microlevel. When looking for sponsors, people and organizations that have experience with designing or offering activity

within the intrapersonal level should be targeted. Such targets may include group fitness classes or Zumbini (Zumba for families).

Mesolevel: Facilitators

This organizational level, conceptualized within the social-ecological framework as the mesolevel, comprises the structural inputs and resources that facilitate the CSPAP model as a whole. Without health-based resources and surveillance of best practices to ensure the dissemination of knowledge and resources as well as opportunities for skill enhancement, a healthy environment cannot be sustained. School–community facilitators would include physical characteristics of spaces, such as access to recreational facilities and parks and well-maintained bike paths and walking paths. They can also include perceived safety and attractiveness of those spaces. Advocating within this level might include discussing the importance of safe places to walk to facilitate walking clubs or talking with the city board about having lights installed on local recreational facilities.

Exolevel: Leaders

The social-ecological framework considers the impact of strong community stakeholders, which align with CSPAP champions. A strong community champion utilizes facilitators to advocate for the core components—access to quality physical education and PA as well as the space to engage through facilitators. Advocating for classroom- and school-level policies around recess and PA time or targeting principal support for an after-school club would fall into this nested level. For instance, a physical education teacher may have a desire for his colleagues to offer PA breaks during classroom time, but this will not just happen. First, he needs to advocate to his principal and classroom teachers to get them on board by telling them the benefits of PA. Not only should the physical benefits for students be described but also how PA is likely to improve academic achievement, time on task, and student behavior issues. Another example would be advocating to the principal to offer multiple PA opportunities throughout the day. Although it may not seem like implementing these changes would take much effort, it would require juggling the school schedule and organizing to make sure that time offered was equal across grade levels.

Macrolevel: Culture

The macrolevel of the social-ecological model highlights the need for public–private partnerships whereby implementation of health-based initiatives, such as a CSPAP, is advocated for and supported at the state and national levels. Once policies of this magnitude are adopted, the normative behaviors and beliefs of the surrounding culture make the CSPAP model the status quo. The public policy level includes policies at both the state and national levels. This level is probably the most difficult in which to advocate and create meaningful change. It often takes an enormous amount of time and effort. However, if small changes in policies can be made at this level, often, big cultural changes can be seen within other layers of the system.

Messaging Strategies

There are three important components to multilayered messaging:

- *Strategy.* Know the audience and tailor the message to that audience.
- *Content.* Create a comprehensive message.
- *Vehicle.* Create the package for delivering the content.

These components should be considered in preparation for advocating for a CSPAP. First, each ask is different. What the prepared message is will depend on the ask and the audience. When advocating, have a plan and a strategy. Be very specific about the ask, and consider how it can be mutually beneficial. The second strategy is about content. Be prepared, do the homework, and create a comprehensive message about the ask. When creating comprehensive messaging, there should be no room for error. Think it through, conduct preassessments, and prepare for the implementation of the ask. Using data-based advocacy is extremely important in crafting the argument for the ask. Finally, how to package the ask, or creating the vehicle in which it is delivered, is paramount. If a 30-second stairwell speech is prepared to advocate about a certain topic, the ask is going to come across better than rambling on about the desire to create more time for PA. Being prepared and succinct while giving detailed information is an art.

Suggestions for Professional Development

A huge gap in the literature and in everyday practice involves preparing preservice and inservice physical education teachers to advocate for CSPAPs. In 2013, the CDC (2013b) published a resource titled *Make a Difference at Your School,* which provides strategies for promoting PA and healthy eating in the school environment. It is free and can be accessed on the CDC website. The strategies are based on scientific evidence reviewed by researchers. The CDC suggests building the foundation at a school by implementing a coordinated school health program, maintaining an active school health council, designating a school health coordinator, and conducting a self-assessment of school health policies and programs and using that data to strengthen the policies. Next, the CDC suggests taking action by including a high-quality health promotion program for school staff, implementing K-12 quality physical education, and increasing opportunities for students to participate in PA. This publication may be a foundation for school administrators or professional development providers to refer to when helping teachers advocate for their programs. Additionally, some physical education teacher education programs are beginning the process of preparing their teacher candidates to implement quality CSPAPs (Carson et al., 2017). A two-part special feature of the *Journal of Physical Education, Recreation & Dance* emphasized coursework, learning objectives, field experiences, certification and trainings, research initiatives, and future strategies that these particular programs will take to prepare physical educators for what lies ahead regarding CSPAPs.

When available, partnerships between a nearby university and K-12 schools can be valuable and impactful. Bryan and Sims (2011) have suggested a number of ideas for K-12 physical educators and university faculty to consider in advocating for their programs. For example, physical education teachers can meet with physical education teacher educators to plan activities that will mutually benefit preservice teachers and K-12 students and inform the media of special events occurring at the time. University faculty members can seek out physical education teachers who desire to promote PA and inform the university public relations office to let them know of partnerships in which university and K-12 students are engaged. University faculty members can also provide professional development for local and regional physical educators regarding CSPAPs and how to advocate for them.

SUMMARY

Advocacy for physical education is imminent because of the negative stigma surrounding it. Little has been published on the advocacy of PA and physical education for youth; however, there are a multitude of resources available for helping individuals gain support for their programs. The VERB campaign was one of the first to advocate for PA for youth, followed by Nike's Designed to Move and former First Lady Michelle Obama's *Let's Move!* campaigns. One approach to advocating is social marketing, in which product, price, place, and promotion are the focus. Point-of-decision prompts have also been found to be effective for influencing behavior; utilizing this type of advocacy with youth is needed to determine its usefulness on children and adolescent behavior. The nested ecology of advocacy framework is suggested for targeting CSPAP promotional efforts. Professional development that highlights how to advocate and promote PA and physical education is warranted.

QUESTIONS TO CONSIDER

1. What types of research have been conducted for advocacy in physical education and PA? What roles did Designed to Move and *Let's Move!* play in advancing the field?

2. What is the best approach for a physical education teacher to advocate for PA and CSPAPs?

3. How can product, price, place, and promotion be applied to physical education marketing in your school? Describe each of these components and how they can be advocated within your particular program.

4. What four layers are within the nested ecology of advocacy, and how does PA fit within each one?

5. Using the message strategies described, how could you develop a 30-second stairwell speech to support the addition of one extra CSPAP component within your school? Prepare this message as if you were presenting it to your principal or assistant principal.

CASE EXAMPLES

Following are two case examples of advocacy for CSPAPs. In the first example, Emily Elizabeth, physical education teacher at Apple Orchard Elementary, shares how she made the case for more PA at her school via the number of minutes devoted to recess. In the second example, Forest Public Schools district physical education coordinator, Jane Doe, describes how she revitalized her program to train physical education teachers and other champions to lead the CSPAP efforts across the country. Pseudonyms are used throughout the case study examples, but the case studies are representative of real-life stories.

Emily Elizabeth, Physical Education Teacher at Apple Orchard Elementary

In 2015, I learned that several of my students were losing their recess time because they had not completed their homework and that students were losing recess minutes on a daily basis for discipline purposes. To find out more, I decided to administer a questionnaire to my teachers to determine how often recess was being offered, the rules teachers were using regarding using recess for disciplinary purposes, and the frequency in which these offenses were occurring. I found that over half of the 25 teachers who responded offered 20 minutes or less of PA to their class each day and the other half offered more than 20 minutes. All 25 teachers believed their students benefited in the classroom after PA. Sixteen out of 25 teachers indicated that one or more students were walking laps as punishment or sitting out at recess at least two or three times per week. Fifteen out of 20 thought walking laps at recess helped reduce the problem behaviors in class throughout the year, yet 19 out of 21 respondents indicated that it was usually the same misbehaving students who walked laps at recess. Overwhelmingly, the teachers indicated there was a need for alternative behavior consequences at our school.

Simultaneously, our principal was a participant in a 21st-century learning academy through the local university in which the focus was student voice. Based on what the principal learned in the workshop, she had students complete a questionnaire in which they were asked what types of things they desired in their school. They were also involved in focus group interviews to find out more details on their replies. Overwhelmingly, the students' responses included more PA. She checked with the state department of education to determine how many instructional minutes could be devoted to recess (not including physical education); 150 minutes per week were allowed. Any additional minutes offered as recess time would not be counted as instructional time, but they were allowed because of the number of minutes the students were at school each day.

I approached the principal with my concerns because I felt strongly that PA was so important for the students and I wanted to help enforce a policy regarding protecting recess minutes. She was 100 percent on board given the students' responses. She told me to contact the site-based decision-making council at our school to see if they would consider adding more PA opportunities during the school day.

Because I had support from the principal, a quality physical education program, and baseline data to support my request to enforce a PA policy, the council members not only approved a protected 20-minute period of recess, but they also voted to implement a second recess of 10 to 15 minutes each day. The morning recess time is protected; the afternoon recess time can be used to take away minutes for behavior issues or for students to walk for punishment. While I am not supportive of using or taking away PA as punishment, I am pleased that there is an automatic 20-minute recess per day and they have up to 35 minutes per day they can earn.

Overall, the teaching staff is supportive of the policy, based on the questionnaire teachers completed postimplementation. They raved about how much time they "get back" because the students are able to be active and get their "wiggles" out. Some of the teachers use the morning recess period for having students simply run around in an open field, and other teachers use it to allow students to do an indoor activity, such as GoNoodle. Another outcome the teachers discussed is the positive socialization they notice as a result of the PA. Their students interact so much better with one another now that they have two times during the day to be active and a kid.

Jane Doe, Forest Public Schools District Physical Education Coordinator

Advocating for a CSPAP within an individual school is a hard task, but changing the environment of an entire district is monumental. This is a case study example of a large urban district in the northwest part of the United States and the district's journey over the past eight years in advocating for and implementing a CSPAP into the everyday lives of school-aged youth.

In 2007, the superintendent of Forest Public Schools had a vision. She saw the "whole child" and wanted to make sure that the whole child was being serviced in all the Forest Public Schools. One of the missing factors at that time was the lack of leadership within the physical education department of the district. To fill this void, the superintendent set out to recruit an advocate for physical education. This person would have to be someone who understood the importance of the whole child, had a vision for what the department could become, and understood how physical education fit into the overall mission of the district.

I was brought to Forest Public Schools in 2007 as a past SHAPE America Teacher of the Year. I had previously led what I believe was a high-quality high school physical education program of my own and recently been given the opportunity to travel and share my skills around the United States. I also had experience in CSPAPs because I had been part of the initial group to help give context to the CDC document titled *Comprehensive School Physical Activity Programs: A Guide for Schools* (2013a). Most importantly, I had a vision. I knew that I wanted Forest Public Schools to have the best physical education programs in the nation; I just didn't quite know how to manifest that vision.

When I first arrived in Forest, I decided to conduct some initial assessments of the schools. I was looking for what was and wasn't going well regarding physical education. I personally visited every school over the first year. I made sure that my visits were unannounced so that I could get an accurate picture of how physical education was perceived and delivered in each school. Over the year, I realized that there was no set curriculum for physical education and no consistency across buildings. Once I had made my initial assessment, I reached out to teachers in the district who were like-minded, and together we created a vision for the district. This vision included messaging and key points that were pushed by the superintendent, including equity and access, sustainable systems, and community partnerships, but that also featured quality physical education that was sequential in nature and standards based.

A key to the transformation of physical education in Forest Public Schools was building a platform for sustainability. We realized that changing a culture started from the ground up; based on this premise, we decided to implement a train-the-trainer model within our own district. We taught teachers how to be thoughtful about quality physical education and how to implement quality lessons; then, we had those teachers practice and share their passion with others through a self-created mentor program. Simultaneously, I began looking for funding. I knew, as with anything, if real change were going to happen, monetary support would need to be present to get the ball rolling. The district began applying for grants; the first bit of funding came from national funds at the county level through a public health funding stream. It funded 32 Title I schools in the district to improve physical education programming. Receipt of these funds started the momentum rolling with funding. I was able to use data we collected from the initial funding to document change and keep advocating for more funding to help support our core vision. I knew that if I weren't out telling our story, then we would never make CSPAPs a reality. In 2011, another grant was given to Forest Public Schools. This time it was a three-year Carol M. White Physical Education Program (PEP) grant. The PEP grant was designed not only to provide quality physical education for the district, but it also helped to establish a district physical education policy, which in turn, led to a district wellness policy that incorporated CSPAPs into the school day. Additionally, advocating within the district to classroom teachers and union representatives resulted in mandatory recess for the elementary students. Although there were other reasons for recess being mandated (mainly mandatory break time for teachers), mandatory recess met the vision of increasing opportunities for students to be physically active during the school day. Through the district policies that were put into place that coincided with the PEP grant, professional development for teachers was also supported to help create a platform to sustain the changes that were taking place across the district.

Once the policies were in place, schools started to implement not only quality physical education but also CSPAPs into their school buildings. As a large school district, oftentimes, community organizations reached out because they wanted access to the student population. One of the key advocating pieces that has helped create CSPAPs in schools in Forest is the ability to hold community partners accountable. Yes, we would like free programming to offer our students, but our overall vision should not be compromised. Hold community partners accountable. Have them create quality lesson plans for programming, and express the need that equity is important. If they would like to offer programming in one school, then it needs to be available for all schools. Then, work with the community partners to figure out how to make that happen. It is also important that you give back to that community partner, remembering that it is a give-and-take relationship. Ask them what their needs are, and try to work together to meet them.

Work is never complete. There is always more to do and ways to improve programming. Understand that you are always advocating for what you want and what you believe is important. Although Forest Public Schools has made tremendous changes over the past eight years, there is always more that can be done to improve the physical education and PA environments within the school setting.

A leader with a clear vision was key for Forest Public Schools in changing the culture around physical education and PA within their district. Advocating started with one leader and was continued by a passionate teacher with a vision. Although barriers pop up, keeping a positive attitude and addressing roadblocks as they come is essential along with keeping a clear overall vision. Jane says, "Without vision and a clear goal, nothing can happen." She goes on to say that "the most important part of advocating for change is knowing what you have to do. You must first gather all the information and then backward plan; then, look at the map you created and figure out exactly how you are going to get there."

PART VI

Looking to the Future

Preparing Preservice Physical Education Teacher Educators for CSPAP Implementation

Grace Goc Karp, PhD
University of Idaho

Helen Brown, MPH, RDN
University of Idaho

Ja Youn Kwon, PhD
Arizona State University

Pamela Hodges Kulinna, PhD
Arizona State University

Researchers suggest that it is essential for physical education teachers to take the lead in promoting youth PA via CSPAPs (Beighle et al., 2009; Castelli & Beighle, 2007; Erwin et al., 2013; Scruggs et al., 2010). Others argue that the expansion into CSPAPs broadens and weakens the curricular offerings in physical education teacher education (PETE) and sufficient time is not available to adequately prepare preservice students for both the roles of a physical education teacher and a PA leader (PAL; Webster et al., 2014). The success of a CSPAP is largely dependent on the ability of PETE programs to successfully train preservice teachers to become confident and capable PALs while meeting state physical education standards in teaching physical education (Carson, 2012). Teaching physical education in K-12 schools is challenging, and the goal of PETE is to graduate highly competent students with the skills and knowledge to become effective teachers. If physical education is expected to align itself to meet broader public health goals to improve the nation's health, then it is necessary to know how to train preservice physical education teachers to meet this expanded expectation.

This chapter will review the research, propose knowledge claims based on this research, identify knowledge gaps and propose recommendations for future research on PETE, suggest practical implications from the existing research on PETE, and provide a case example of a successful PETE program.

Review of Research

This section includes a discussion of three frameworks for consideration when preparing physical education teacher educators to be PALs for CSPAPs: the public health model, the CSPAP model, and a leadership model. Each framework provides structure and a foundation for designing CSPAP learning and experiences for PETE students.

Public Health Alignment

In its 1988 and 2003 reports, the Institute of Medicine (IOM) posited the idea of a "public health system" as being a complex network of individuals and organizations working together to represent "what we as a society do collectively to assure the conditions in which people can be healthy" (1988, p. 1). In view of the multiple factors that shape the public's health, the committee recommended participation across many sectors, including schools, as key partners in meeting public health goals. A CSPAP approach to increasing PA aligns well with several suggested actions, particularly the recommendations to build a new generation of intersectoral partnerships. CSPAP development efforts can be informed by public health colleagues' interdisciplinary approaches and methods that address health issues primarily through prevention strategies (IOM, 1988, 2003).

Physical education is slowly providing evidence of alignment with public health goals and prevention strategies (Office of Disease Prevention and Health Promotion, n.d.; Pate, 2014). Sallis and McKenzie (1991) proposed that physical education should prepare youth for PA and provide opportunities to help establish PA habits to improve and sustain health. The National Association for Sport and Physical Education (2004) supported the goal of preparing youth for a lifetime of PA, and federal and state organizations have advocated for daily

PA and moderate-to-vigorous PA (MVPA) during physical education. More recently, CSPAP proponents (SHAPE America, 2013) and the Centers for Disease Control and Prevention (CDC, 2013) advocate for school and community-wide PA promotion. The National Standards for Initial Physical Education Teacher Education (SHAPE America, 2017) provide guidance to train PETE students to meet some of these goals. Current standards primarily provide knowledge-based standards (SHAPE America, 2017) but do little to ensure competency in the skills needed to promote school and community PA. There are pockets of change occurring, though. Sixteen states identify expectations for measuring PA levels in their teacher standards, and recently, in some states, such as Idaho, PETE standards include expectations for promoting school-wide PA and working with community partners to foster PA opportunities.

The three core functions of public health are assessment, policy development, and assurance, and the attendant 10 essential public health services provide PETE educators and students with a framework for undertaking impactful CSPAP leadership. Sharing public health practice models, such as MAP-IT (mobilize, assess, plan, implement, and track), provides a framework for public health interventions (Office of Disease Prevention and Health Promotion, n.d.) that are translatable to CSPAPs.

The long history of public health practice and research provides scaffolding for CSPAP approaches. PETE students can learn to assess PA needs and strengths through data collection, monitoring, and surveillance, all of which provide baseline data for evaluative purposes, build data-driven support for increasing PA, and enhance PETE student research and evaluation skills. Investigating the causes and identifying those at risk for insufficient PA will build PETE students' skills in primary and secondary data collection, enhance competency reading and extrapolating from scientific literature, and prepare students to identify and use defensible assessment tools. Public health professionals stress the unitization of evidence-based interventions to improve health conditions. A CSPAP approach allows PETE students to gain a rich understanding of research-based practices and methodology for planning effective PA interventions. In addition, integration of public health models may enhance PETE students' self-efficacy and self-respect because these models employ effective evidence-based interventions and demonstrate and disseminate successful outcomes via robust evaluation.

CSPAP Conceptual Framework

Public health–aligned recommendations are consistent with CSPAP recommendations to expand the physical education teacher's role to include leadership skills necessary to be a PAL. Carson and colleagues (2014) created a framework for school-based PA promotion, based on the social-ecological model, including interpersonal, organizational, community, policy, and environmental systems to support and maintain healthy behaviors (McLeroy et al., 1988; see figure 3.1 in chapter 3 for a visual depiction of the model).

Carson and colleagues' (2014) conceptual framework offers an important starting point for developing a PETE–CSPAP curriculum to address the interplay of complex and interrelated social, behavioral, environmental, and biological factors that interact and contribute to improved individual and community-wide PA and health outcomes. To carry out a CSPAP, PETE students need to attain the knowledge and skills necessary to address PA at each level of the conceptual model and understand the relational aspects of the layers of the model. For example, family and community engagement is more likely realized and sustained when students are well versed in the knowledge of engagement principles, skilled at forming and maintaining collaborative partnerships, and have favorable attitudes toward engagement and the opportunity to plan and implement engagement activities that require them to identify and engage with stakeholders.

Students need a clear understanding of the role CSPAP leaders play in the vision, support, and decision making for successful parent and community engagement. Exploring leadership development models, principles and practices, committee formation and function, and volunteer development and engagement is essential for all CSPAP components. Finally, understanding the critical importance of policy, culture, and normative behaviors and beliefs is essential for PETE–CSPAP curricula. Integrating school policy, culture, and

climate assessment into the curricula introduces students to these more ephemeral domains of the framework (CDC, 2014, 2015). Exploring examples of policy adoption and adherence that challenge normative practices is crucial for PETE students, to grasp the interactions and synergies inherent in the CSPAP framework to support PA.

Leadership Framework

Many leadership skills and competencies developed for public health practice fit well with the CSPAP framework. Rowitz (2013) offered a model of public health leadership with three intersecting leadership competency areas: human, analytical, and execution. Considering the CSPAP framework (CDC, 2017), the teacher leadership skills framework (Center for Strengthening the Teaching Profession, 2009), teacher leadership competencies (Jackson et al., 2010), and Dweck's (2006) work regarding a growth mindset, a possible CSPAP leadership framework might include these three intersecting areas: people, growth, and process mindsets (see figure 20.1). Each of the three leadership competencies requires sufficient knowledge and skill acquisition, disposition growth, and attainment through supportive experiences and opportunities. This framework of desired CSPAP leadership competencies is not exhaustive; it is meant to be a frame for discussion around the formation of PETE–CSPAP student leadership development.

A people mindset is needed for personal leadership development and working with interdisciplinary teams across disciplines and with community partners. Self-reflection and evaluation of learning and skill attainment is critical for continued growth. A growth mindset speaks to the expansion of the thinking and abilities needed for adopting interdisciplinary approaches and considering social justice, cultural competence, and the importance of advocacy. A process mindset includes the functional and mechanistic skills and abilities needed to operationalize CSPAPs within schools and into the community (York-Barr & Duke, 2004). Traditional PETE faculty and students may find these modes of thinking out of their comfort zones. In one exploratory study (Webster, Russ, et al., 2016) examining faculty perceptions about the preparation of preservice

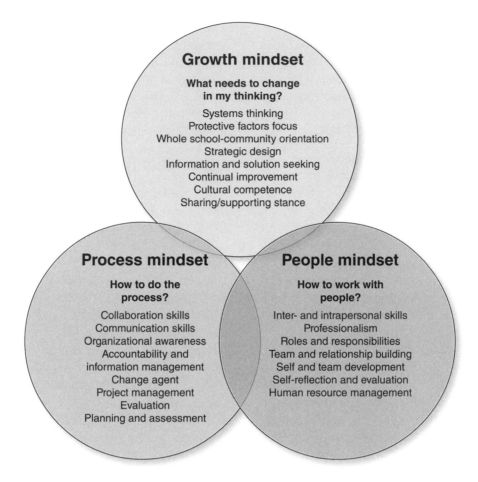

Figure 20.1   Framework for CSPAP leadership mindsets.

Data from Rowitz (2013); Center for Strengthening the Teaching Profession (2009); Jackson et al. (2010).

teachers for CSPAP roles, participants indicated the least agreement on whether programs should prepare majors for leadership roles, specifically those related to school employee wellness and PA promotion. Applying a growth or process mindset provides direction for identifying essential skills needed for CSPAP education (McTighe & Wiggins, 2012). Several PETE programs are now starting to develop and examine CSPAP skills (Carson et al., 2017; Erwin et al., 2015).

Knowledge Claims

This section identifies claims related to CSPAP types of knowledge, skills, and experiences; the PETE–CSPAP profile; PETE–CSPAP desired results, assessment, and experiences; training classroom teachers; qualifications, practice, and

professional development for mentor teachers and PETE faculty; and the PETE researcher.

CSPAP Knowledge, Skills, and Experiences

- The sequence of and amount of time allocated to developing knowledge, skills, and experiences are often determined or influenced by state, institutional, and departmental requirements and priorities. PETE programs must generally meet state and national requirements for teacher education. As mentioned earlier, currently, few states have modified their requirements to include public health–aligned standards and CSPAP components and experiences.

- Candidate competency should include knowledge that is specific to school- and community-wide PA promotion, culturally relevant for local settings, and based on behavior change theory. It is recommended that candidates gain skills in collaborating and advocating for physical education programs as well as promoting school and community PA (Webster, Stodden, et al., 2016).

- Gaining leadership skills for school and community PA promotion is an identified need (Beighle et al., 2009; Carson, 2012; Centeio & McCaughtry, 2017; Heidorn & Centeio, 2012; see table 20.1 for the proposed skills for this curriculum).

- Engaging stakeholders (e.g., students, parents, and policy makers) requires pedagogical content knowledge related to how to structure and represent CSPAP content for stakeholders; common conceptions, misconceptions, and difficulties that stakeholders encounter when learning about CSPAPs; and specific teaching and leadership strategies that can be used to address CSPAPs in particular circumstances (Centeio, Erwin, et al., 2014; Ciotto & Fede, 2017; Mosier & Heidorn, 2013; Russ et al., 2015; Webster et al., 2015).

PETE–CSPAP Profile

Both student and faculty perceptions about the role of the physical educator are mostly traditional and conflict with the role of a PAL (Berei et al., 2018; McMullen, van der Mars, et al., 2014; Wester & Nesbitt, 2017; Webster, Russ, et al., 2016). Identifying prospective students and mentor teachers predisposed to a CSPAP role for physical education teachers along with the traditional role (background and skills in PA and sports) may be a critical consideration. PETE programs can provide opportunities for prospective students and faculty to explore existing beliefs about the role and reality of the traditional physical educator and a PAL.

PETE–CSPAP Desired Results, Assessment, and Experiences

- Kwon (2016) reported that many PETE programs do not offer separate learning experiences for CSPAPs. PETE programs most often integrate CSPAP knowledge and skills into existing coursework, practica, and internships

for PETE student CSPAP skill development (Carson et al., 2015).

- Using a backward design, programs could decide what results are desired (the big ideas), what performances and assessments will provide evidence for achieving the results, and what activities and experiences will lead to the desired results and success in the assessments (McTighe & Wiggins, 2012). Table 20.1 provides a proposed backward design for a CSPAP curriculum.

- There is more faculty consensus and support for the effectiveness of current programs in preparing physical education teachers for quality physical education (McKenzie, 2007; Webster et al., 2014; Webster et al., 2015) than for the other four components of a CSPAP (Webster, Russ, et al., 2016). Some faculty members believe that preparing majors for a leadership role in staff wellness, staff involvement in PA promotion, and before- and after-school PA is peripheral and beyond professional responsibilities (Webster, Russ, et al., 2016). Given this attitude, CSPAP components beyond physical education are often limited. Some programs do include opportunities for majors to organize school PA clubs, before- and after-school PA experiences, staff pedometer challenges, and PA family night events.

- Foundational aspects of a CSPAP, such as developmental responses to exercise (McKenzie & Kahan, 2004), social-ecological models of PA behavior, behavior change theory, PA-related public health practices, and health promotion, are critical areas of knowledge. It is possible to infuse this content into foundation coursework, such as wellness and introduction to physical education, sport sociology, health education, and health psychology courses, or as separate courses (CDC, 2013; Centeio, Castelli, et al., 2014; van der Mars et al., 2017).

- Little is known about assessing PETE students' CSPAP skills. Some PETE programs report determining effectiveness through the use of portfolio-type artifacts that are generally limited to one CSPAP component (Carson et al., 2017; Heidorn & Mosier, 2017). Other assessments include examining K-12 students' PA across the school day (Webster, 2017)

TABLE 20.1 CSPAP Curriculum Map Using a Backward Design

DESIRED RESULTS	
ESTABLISHED GOALS	
Demonstrate knowledge and skills in delivering the five components of a CSPAP	
Understandings	**Essential questions**
PETE students will understand that	
• CSPAP components provide a variety of school-based activities to enable students to participate in 60 minutes of MVPA each day; • CSPAPs require coordination between components and stakeholders to create a culture of PA; and • the physical education teacher is ideally situated to lead, develop, and implement CSPAPs with the support of others.	• How can CSPAP components enable K-12 students to achieve 60 minutes of MVPA each day? • What is your role in developing a culture of PA in a school through a CSPAP?
PETE students will know	PETE students will be able to
• the goals of a CSPAP; • their role in a CSPAP and the roles of others in establishing a culture of PA in the school environment; • key aspects of each of the five CSPAP components; • how to deliver, advocate, and promote the five CSPAP components with a variety of stakeholders; • how to lead, coordinate, and train others, using effective motivation and communication strategies; and • steps and strategies for planning and evaluating a CSPAP.	• identify their perspectives about being a PAL, • develop a plan to establish a culture of PA in a school setting, • demonstrate skills related to each component of a CSPAP, • demonstrate skills in coordinating one or more components of a CSPAP within a school setting and with stakeholders, • demonstrate skills in training others to lead a CSPAP component, • develop a plan to lead and sequentially implement a CSPAP with the support of stakeholders, • use a variety of promotional strategies to promote PA and a CSPAP, and • use assessment to examine and promote PA in a school.
ASSESSMENT EVIDENCE	
Sample performance tasks	**Other evidence**
• Achieve competency in delivering one strategy for each of the five CSPAP components in a school setting. • Demonstrate effective leadership in coordinating with stakeholders in one or more components of a CSPAP. • Provide assessment data of impact on one or more CSPAP components. • Develop a plan for fostering a culture for CSPAP implementation.	• Examination of PAL role experience, frustrations, and opportunities • Use of promotional strategies (including technology) to develop a culture of PA

LEARNING PLAN
SAMPLE LEARNING ACTIVITIES
• Conduct a needs assessment using the School Health Index (CDC, 2015), School Physical Activity Policy Assessment (Lounsbery et al., 2013), and Physical Education Curriculum Analysis Tool (PECAT) (2006). \ • Interview a physical education teacher who is using a CSPAP about his or her role, daily activities, and progress in establishing a CSPAP at the school. • Engage and monitor students in MVPA, and use LET US Play (Brazendale et al., 2015; Weaver et al., 2013) principles. • Create and implement point-of-decision prompts and activity zones for gymnasiums, school places, and playgrounds. • Promote PA during breaks and free periods (e.g., PA drop-in programs). • Implement recess activities and activity zones, and assess success. • Create integrated PAs for classroom teachers (Erwin, H.E.; n.d.), and use existing resources, such as Energizers (Mahar et al., 2006), TAKE10! (Kibbe et al., 2011), and HOPSports. (n.d). Create PA videos for classroom. • Teach classroom teachers how to use activity breaks. • Engage in active transportation before and after school (e.g., Safe Routes to School (National Center for Safe Routes to School, (n.d.). • Evaluate the impact of a district's wellness policies, compare and contrast policies, interview stakeholders, and observe settings to report on implementation. • Organize and report on a staff wellness program (e.g., pedometer challenge). • Develop social marketing strategies for promotion of PA for stakeholders. • Implement strategies to communicate with parents (e.g., parent–teacher association, newsletters, parent nights, and website). • Develop, market, and evaluate events that include parents (e.g., Kids Heart Challenge, American Heart Association, n.d.). • Develop a list of PAs that require little or no equipment for recess and at home. • Implement strategies for community collaboration (e.g., after-school programs, coaching, and Special Olympics).

Data for some examples from CSPAP: A Guide for Schools (2014), Beighle et al. (2009), Carson et al. (2017); Webster and Nesbitt (2017).

or preservice teacher growth in leadership and collaborative skills (Carson et al., 2015). Further discussion is needed to clarify what measures are truly indicative of successful CSPAP preparation.

- CSPAP service learning opportunities provide occasions to assess PETE students' knowledge; changes in attitudes, values, and belief systems; and teaching and promotional behaviors resulting from their participation in such programs (Carson & Raguse, 2014; Carson et al., 2015; Dauenhauer et al., 2015; Doolittle & Virgilio, 2017; Webster et al., 2017).

- Students' perceived confidence and self-efficacy could provide evidence for CSPAP training needs. Compared to high-perceived confidence in teaching physical education, PETE students reported they were the least confident in implementing family and community engagement (Kwon et al., in press) because of lack of practical learning experiences in school settings.

- Programs that have collaborative school partnerships with existing CSPAP components are able to provide experiences for students to observe, apply skills, and collect data (Erwin et al., 2015; Goc Karp et al., 2017; Kwon, 2016).

Training Classroom Teachers

- CSPAP encompasses multiple school contexts, and classroom teachers play an important role in providing opportunities for PA and promoting healthy behavior among students. Evidence from the research indicates that classroom teachers need training in providing successful PA opportunities (Cothran et al., 2010; Goh et al., 2013). As a PAL, preservice teachers should be made aware of this research and how to address training classroom teachers as subsequently described.

- By shifting the mindset toward PA opportunities and barriers and identifying personal benefits of a physically active lifestyle, classroom teachers can change their beliefs and practices regarding their role as PA advocates (Goh et al., 2013; Webster et al., 2013), particularly if being a PA advocate aligns with their own personal wellness priorities and they

care about their students' health (Cothran et al., 2010).

- McMullen, Kulinna and colleagues (2014) recommended teaching classroom teachers sample classroom PA breaks (content knowledge) and space and movement management knowledge (e.g., demonstrating how to quickly and efficiently organize students into pairs or teams [pedagogical content knowledge]). For example, teaching about short bouts of instruction time, freezing students, and dispersing and retrieving equipment can increase successful implementation and thus adoption of classroom PA (McMullen, Kulinna, et al., 2014). The more classroom teachers are engaged in practical and enjoyable experiences, the more their competence, acceptance, and attitudes to this role improve (Webster et al., 2010).

Qualifications, Practice, and Professional Development for Mentor Teachers and PETE Faculty

- Mentor teachers and PETE faculty with strong content knowledge and teaching experience are able to provide expertise for the pedagogical and clinical parts of a program. Most mentor teachers focus on only one or two CSPAP components; very few (perhaps successful Carol M. White Physical Education Program [PEP] grant awardees) have engaged in a system-wide approach using all five components (Berei et al., 2017; Jones et al., 2014).

- Most faculty members agree that their programs effectively prepare majors for one component of a CSPAP, quality physical education. Faculty are not in consensus that PETE students should be prepared for roles related to staff wellness and their involvement in school-wide PA promotion (Webster, Russ, et al., 2016).

- Faculty knowledge and program constraints may influence the lack of CSPAP training in PETE programs. CSPAP implementation enables faculty and mentor teachers to learn the language and requisite skills for implementing the public health approach to the training mentioned earlier (Erwin et al., 2015; Goc Karp & Scruggs, 2012).

- Learning communities can foster support for organizational improvement, including professional development, innovation, and enhanced practice (MacPhail et al., 2014; Talbert & McLaughlin, 1994); breaking up academic isolation; and developing professional capital (Hargreaves & Fullan, 2012). PETE programs can engage students, mentor teachers, and faculty members in learning communities related to fostering individual and collective research and praxis capacity for CSPAP education (Tannehill et al., 2015).

PETE Researchers

- Faculty members with positive dispositions for CSPAPs could train PETE doctoral students to embrace CSPAPs in research and teacher training education.

- Detailed examples of doctoral programs with a CSPAP focus are available (e.g., Brusseau, 2017; Webster, 2017). The University of Utah includes content and experiences for CSPAPs integrated into its four core courses and offers additional interdisciplinary experiences (particularly related to public health) and research campus wide. At the University of South Carolina, CSPAP content and experiences are integrated across the doctoral program, including three-semester research practicum, peer reviews, teaching at the university, a grant-writing class, and the dissertation.

Knowledge Gaps and Directions for Future Research

The research regarding the preparation of PETE students for CSPAPs is in its infancy and generally focuses on program, student, or school and child outcomes (Carson et al., 2017). Although there are many programs for implementing CSPAPs using a variety of approaches, more research is needed to evaluate the most efficacious practices. Likewise, more evidence is needed to ensure that the content and skills espoused for implementing CSPAPs actually do prepare students and teachers to affect PA and health outcomes. Another key area of needed understanding surrounds the issue of

resistance and conflict around the depth of CSPAP implementation. We have many questions left to answer; here are a few: Does a PETE student and faculty profile affect how CSPAP is implemented? If so, to what extent? What barriers and conflicts have PETE programs overcome to successfully integrate CSPAPs into their programs? Are CSPAP components subjected to differential implementation in PETE programs? If so, how and why? How do we know when programs have successfully implemented CSPAPs? How do we assess successful achievement of CSPAP-related skills? How well do physical education teacher educators successfully implement and sustain CSPAPs once in the field? Has CSPAP training affected physical education instruction and the PA of students? Do CSPAP efforts extend beyond students to staff, families, and the community?

With the success of CSPAPs partially dependent on effective outside engagement with stakeholders, questions emerge related to effective preservice preparation for teamwork with stakeholders and community partners, such as what leadership skills are required for effective engagement, and how are preservice teachers best trained to effectively engage with community partners? Answers to these and many more questions will help inform PETE programs.

Evidenced-Based Recommendations and Applications

Currently, our knowledge about the successful integration of CSPAP knowledge into PETE programs is limited. Program implementation runs the gamut from contributions or additive approaches (DePauw & Goc Karp, 1994), where students develop CSPAP implementation awareness, knowledge, and skills, to transformative approaches, where all stakeholders examine and support CSPAPs and PETE students develop leadership skills that enable them to increase school PA through CSPAP policies, programs, and environmental modifications. Faculty members in PETE programs have conflicts as to the role of the physical education teacher and whether the curriculum can and should be expanded to include a PAL role. It is important for researchers to study PETE programs that are successfully training preservice students for these roles. Identifying barriers and facilitators for including CSPAP knowledge and experiences in PETE programs and the processes, training, and methods used to introduce and implement changes that embrace CSPAPs would provide valuable information to assuage these conflicts.

Current practitioners also need training opportunities to expand and transform their current quality physical education programs to CSPAPs. SHAPE America supports CSPAPs in many states. Local chapters of SHAPE America give teachers the opportunity to participate in PAL training at little or no cost to teachers. Initiatives such as the University of Kentucky's Physical Activity and Wellness in Schools (PAWS; Erwin et al., 2017) and Creating Physically Active School Systems

(PASS; Ciotto & Fede, 2017) provide opportunities to infuse CSPAPs into current physical educators' roles and thus ensure quality field experiences for CSPAPs. Finally, PETE graduate programs that support CSPAPs also need to consider how to train future faculty to expand the role of physical education teachers to include CSPAP programming. The University of Utah provides an example of a doctoral program in training future faculty as teacher educators who will then train teachers for this expanded role.

The PETE field is making progress in training PETE students to take on the CSPAP role, and more training is needed at all levels to prepare school and university personnel for these role changes. Studies of these changes, stakeholders' perceptions of these changes, and student outcomes from program transformations are needed for the field to continue to move schools and communities forward in these efforts.

SUMMARY

There are many issues that surround the integration of CSPAPs in the training of preservice physical education teachers (Carson et al., 2017). PETE faculty members have conflicts as to the true purpose of physical education (skill based vs. public health) and whether the role of the physical educator should be expanded. PETE programs face increasing scrutiny regarding accreditation requirements and beginning teaching standards that leave little room or need for expanding or infusing CSPAP-related skills and experiences. Pioneering PETE programs that integrate CSPAPs in their curriculum and experiences demonstrate the feasibility of preparing preservice teachers for their expanded roles as PALs. Yet PETE students' assessment of their perceived effectiveness in the PAL role is limited.

QUESTIONS TO CONSIDER

1. To what extent can or should PETE programs integrate CSPAP content into the curriculum? What are some of the barriers and facilitators to this integration?

2. How do we add the necessary skills and knowledge related to CSPAPs to enable future teachers to master into the national and state standards for physical education as well as into the SHAPE America guidelines for beginning teachers?

3. How are experiences for all CSPAP components provided and assessed?

4. How do we (or even should we) increase expertise related to CSPAPs across faculty members, graduate students, and mentor teachers within a program?

5. How do we address challenges in providing opportunities in partnership schools that model CSPAPs?

CASE EXAMPLE

Julia Werner wants to become a physical education teacher and seeks opportunities to be involved in various PA programs. In 2010, she enrolled as a PETE major at Highland Park University. Also in 2010, the PETE program at Highland Park University expanded its teacher preparation to teach its preservice physical education teachers not only how to teach a quality physical education program but also how to promote PA in schools and communities. In partnership with a local school district, which received a PEP grant to implement CSPAPs, Highland Park University broadened its curriculum to provide more authentic CSPAP preparation for preservice physical education teachers. The newly revised curriculum develops preservice physical education teachers' planning, communication, collaboration, and assessment skills along with content knowledge through coursework and class projects. Students have the opportunity to expand their perspective and beliefs about the role of physical educators within the CSPAP framework.

In the first two years, Julia and her cohort members are required to take several departmental core courses to develop basic CSPAP knowledge and skills for teaching physical education. The training focuses on implementing components of a CSPAP program along with principles of physical activities, health and wellness, movement integration, fitness and nutrition, and PA pedagogy. These courses were revised to include the basic ideas of CSPAPs via lectures, discussions, and assignments. During these two years, Julia evaluates the school district's wellness policies, interviews physical education teachers about their roles in establishing CSPAPs at the schools, and assesses PA opportunities and resources in the local community. She and her cohort members as a team are required to develop CSPAP promotional skills and marketing strategies, such as creating a newsletter for parents for informing them of CSPAP programming and activities and developing wellness bulletin boards for students and school staff.

In the next two years, Julia and her cohort members have ample opportunities to implement CSPAPs in various ways. First, in two methods courses, Julia learns how to teach specific content areas (e.g., lifetime activities, team sport, group exercise, and strength and conditioning for health) as part of an effective physical education program and how to apply the instructional strategies to other PA programs in schools. She leads short PA breaks for her cohort members during methods courses. With her peers, she develops age-appropriate PA break plans and trains classroom teachers to implement them. Fortunately, Julia has an opportunity to be involved in a local community PA event as a volunteer. A PETE professor arranges this event and provides Julia an opportunity to develop leadership skills and learn community collaboration strategies.

Following two consecutive internships over two semesters, Julia and her cohort members complete focused observations of physical education lessons and PA programs in schools and teach mini and full lessons. During observations, she and her teammates are required to evaluate CSPAP implementation in schools and develop PA promotion plans to improve their CSPAPs. The improvement plans are specific and realistic to each school in all components of a CSPAP. In addition to the instructional aspect of the physical education program, Julia and her peers plan for before- and after-school PA programming, including a running program and a Safe Routes to School event. Across all of these PA opportunities, a plan for using pedometers and tracking PA patterns is included. The component of PA during school includes PA breaks in the classroom and structured recess activities along with point-of-decision prompts posted around the school. To disseminate useful information to parents and school staff about the CSPAP programming, Julia and her team prepare several marketing strategies, including a website, newsletters, bulletin boards, prompts, and presentations. Julia and her cohort members have had regular meetings with a mentor teacher and a supervising professor from Highland Park University to discuss their progress

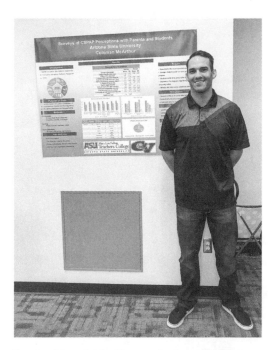

Coleman McArthur standing by his culminating project on CSPAP to complete his MPE degree with teacher certification at Arizona State University, May 2018.

© Pamela Kulinna

and the CSPAP improvement plans, and now, all of the plans are ready to be reviewed and approved by the mentor teacher and supervising professor.

Following the internships, during the two student teaching semesters, Julia and her cohort members are expected to implement their CSPAP plans in their placement schools. They organize recess and lunch programs; teach classroom teachers PA breaks; and create PA prompts, which are posted around the school. Julia and her team send out staff newsletters, plan an event (e.g., district staff pedometer challenge), and organize school wellness activities. They promote Safe Routes to School; provide a website for parents and guardians; and organize several events for families, such as Special Olympics and a health fair. They update the website biweekly with relevant information. Reflection is an important aspect of this work. At each weekly meeting with her mentor teacher and supervising professor, Julia discusses her experiences and reflects on what went well, what needed improvement, what she learned, what she expected, and what surprised her. Julia documents this discussion and submits the piece as a student teaching assignment.

Last, Julia is required to complete a teaching portfolio as a CSPAP-specific culminating assignment at the end of the second student teaching semester. The teaching portfolio includes her assessment of each CSPAP component used in her placement school, plans for improvement for each component, a short summary of the reflections for actual application, and photo and video evidence of CSPAP programs in action.

When asked for program feedback, Julia and her peers suggest that the program faces some challenges. Most notably, students offer that it takes time for PETE students to develop CSPAP roles, they find the group work demanding, and more time is needed for preservice teachers to develop advocacy skills and engage in bringing about change. In addition, faculty members provide input that the program faces challenges that hinder expanding authentic CSPAP preparation for teacher candidates, such as already arduous state requirements for licensure in physical education, packed course schedules, university education requirements, and burdens related to finances and staffing.

CHAPTER 21

Progress and Possibilities for Technology Integration in CSPAPs

Zan Gao, PhD
University of Minnesota–
Twin Cities

Zachary Pope, PhD
University of Minnesota–
Twin Cities

Nan Zeng
Colorado State University

Daniel McDonough
University of Minnesota–
Twin Cities

Jung Eun Lee, PhD
University of Minnesota–Duluth

School-based PA programs (e.g., physical education) have taken an approach more aligned with public health in recent years (Kohl & Murray, 2012). With this public health emphasis has come the search for activity modalities that can affect children's lifelong PA behaviors and positively influence children's PA antecedents (e.g., self-efficacy and motivation). As technology continues to become ever more pervasive in our daily lives and remains of great interest to this generation of children (see Gao & Chen, 2014), educators have begun to integrate innovative and emerging technology into not only CSPAPs but also into assessment methods of children's PA and fitness and motor skills. In this chapter, the authors review literature concerning emerging technologies in PA, propose knowledge claims based upon the literature; offer evidence-based recommendations and applications for practice for all stakeholders in CSPAPs, identify knowledge gaps and propose recommendations for future research on technology integration in CSPAPs, and provide a case example of successful implementation of emerging technology in CSPAPs.

Review of Research

Early integration of technology within CSPAPs involved video cameras and audio players but has since progressed to the integration of pedometers, active video gaming (AVG, or exergaming—e.g., Wii, Xbox), smartphone and tablet applications (apps), global positioning systems (GPS), and high-tech heart rate monitoring devices (Gao, 2017b). For instance, AVGs have seen a rapid growth rate within physical education and other extracurricular settings over the past decade (Gao, 2017b; Gao & Chen, 2014). More recently, however, technology, such as mobile device apps, have been posited as a means to engage children in more PA as well as educate and assess health and motor skills among youth (Martin et al., 2015).

Despite the new interest in the integration of smartphone apps, GPS and motion sensors, and high-tech heart rate monitors within CSPAPs, little to no research has been conducted within this context, which represents a knowledge gap in the literature. Martin and colleagues (2015) have provided a brief overview of how to integrate technology—namely, AVGs and smartphone apps—into school-based PA programs. Yet no thorough review of literature related to the use of smartphone apps, GPS and motion sensors, and high-tech heart rate monitors, with further emphasis on how researchers and educators can apply this technology within CSPAPs, has been conducted. Therefore, the purpose of this section is to review research on the use of emerging technologies in CSPAPs and the effectiveness of these technologies.

Technology has become relevant in all aspects of our lives, which has had both positive and negative implications on population health (Gao, 2017b). Technologies such as television and video games have long been demonized for decreasing children's levels of PA and consequently, negatively affecting their health and resulting in conditions such as obesity and type 2 diabetes (Gao, 2017a). Luckily, as the prominent Chinese expression "fight fire with fire" suggests, today's health professionals are on the forefront because they are purposefully integrating novel technologies, such as AVGs, into community-based settings with the intent of promoting PA. Presently, children and adolescents have become attracted to these emerging technologies for PA promotion as they continue to be integrated into our schools and other institutions. Because traditional technologies (e.g., telephone, mass media, computer and Internet, electronic devices) have been reviewed extensively in two relevant textbooks (see Castelli & Fiorentino, 2008; Leight, 2014), we will not reiterate these technologies in this chapter. Rather, we will focus primarily on the application and effectiveness of emerging technologies in CSPAPs.

AVGs

Exceedingly high rates of overweight and obesity and associated conditions have led to the condemnation of sedentary video games (Gao & Chen, 2014; Gao et al., 2012). Contrastingly, AVGs may spark physically active lifestyles (Gao & Chen, 2014; Gao et al., 2015). In brief, AVGs are video games that require gross motor activity to play. CSPAPs have benefited from AVGs (e.g., Dance Dance Revolution [DDR], Wii Sports/Fit, Xbox Sports) and their interactive modes of play (Gao, 2012; Gao et al., 2012; Hansen & Sanders, 2012). Apparent increases in PA and decreased sedentary time have been observed among individuals with interest in computer- and video-based interactions following the addition of product-specific PA equipment (Mears & Hansen, 2009). Thus, as the popularity of AVGs continues to increase, school staff and community partners should be informed of their up-to-date, practical applications derived from a synthesis of in-school research findings. Such efforts may improve the effective delivery of AVGs at schools.

Over the past several years, research has popularized investigating the efficacy of AVGs among children and adolescent populations (Christison & Khan, 2012; Gao, 2012; Gao & Podlog, 2012). While the majority of the current literature regarding AVG integration in community-based settings indicates significantly positive health effects, the effectiveness of AVG interventions in schools is mixed (Gao, Hannan, et al., 2013; Gao et al., 2012; Gao & Xiang, 2014; Sheehan & Katz, 2013). In detail, some CSPAP studies have reported modest effects of AVG (Duncan & Staples, 2010; Gao, 2012; Gao et al., 2011). Two studies in particular favored AVG interventions over traditional physical education curricula because findings suggested that the AVG group had increased PA and balancing ability following the intervention than what was observed in the control group (Fogel et al., 2010; Sheehan & Katz, 2013). Further, positive trends were reported for cardiorespiratory fitness in addition to PA in three other CSPAP intervention studies (Gao, Hannan, et al., 2013; Gao et al., 2012; Gao & Xiang, 2014).

Notably, traditional sport still outperforms AVG gameplay for PA promotion, particularly among adolescents. Indeed, while Whittman (2010) observed AVG participation resulted in significantly more PA among children compared to two common after-school activities, Gao et al. (2011) observed adolescents to have significantly increased percentages of moderate-to-vigorous PA participation during fitness and football compared to DDR gameplay. Further, when compared to AVG gameplay, PA has been observed to be significantly higher during fitness and aerobic dance curricula within physical education (Gao, Zhang, et al., 2013; Sun, 2012). Finally, Miller and colleagues (2013) demonstrated that, compared to the AVG stand-alone classes, the physical education class with traditional sports and fitness resulted in significantly higher energy expenditure among children. These inconclusive findings may be ascribed to the nature of AVGs (e.g., some games require more movement), the research design (e.g., randomized design versus convenience sampling), instruments (e.g., measuring PA subjectively or objectively), and other confounding factors (e.g., familiarity with AVG units, participant age, and program consistency). Therefore, these research findings must be thoroughly evaluated.

There also appears to be consensus among the literature that AVGs are enjoyable (Gao, 2012; Sun, 2013). Undoubtedly, AVGs are an attractive means of complementing traditional physical education classes. As such, public health promotion and educational institutions may directly benefit from AVG use. However, longitudinal effectiveness of AVG implementation in CSPAPs has been noted in only two studies to date (Gao et al., 2012; Gao et al., 2017). Indeed, two other studies observed elementary school–aged children to demonstrate a significant loss in situational interest during AVG curricula from the start to the end of instruction (Sun, 2012, 2013)—congruent with findings

from other studies (see Gao & Podlog, 2012) and introducing uncertainty as to the sustainability of AVGs in CSPAPs. Consequently, some researchers propose that AVGs may promote only acute PA participation (Duncan & Staples, 2010). In fact, because AVGs require gross motor activity to play and achieve health benefits, they have been widely accepted as practical alternatives to uneventful, sedentary video games. That is, AVGs may serve as a substitute for sedentary technologies (e.g., computer games and television), though traditional PA remains unrivaled. As such, it is imperative that AVGs do not steer children away from traditional PA.

The study of the integration of emerging technologies in CSPAPs is still in its infancy with current literature largely concerned with the implementation of AVGs within physical education curriculum. While reviews of school-based AVGs indicate this activity modality to show promise in the promotion of children's PA engagement (Gao & Chen, 2014; Gao et al., 2015), new technologies, such as smartphone apps, health wearables, virtual reality, and GPS and motion sensors, have also gained the attention of researchers and physical educators. Today, fourth-screen technologies (e.g., tablets and smartphones) preoccupy much of our daily lives and have altered the way in which we communicate with each other. Notably, numerous social media platforms have become widely available and capable of being accessed via smartphones and tablets. Finally, wearable technologies have also increased in popularity as a manner by which to self-regulate health behaviors. The following is a review of these technologies and their applications.

Online Social Media

Computers have rapidly evolved with time, moving from vast, in-home units to micro-computers that function in the palm of our hands. Since the early 21st century, computers and Internet services have transformed from simple, text-based media to elaborate communication platforms for music, video streaming, and instantaneous communication. In 2003, Myspace was the first social media platform to launch, followed soon by the release of Facebook and Twitter in 2005 (Terrel, 2015). These social media pioneers were the first to allow users to post text, video, and music media; read world news; and socialize with friends via embedded messaging services. Recently, more and more researchers and practitioners are using Twitter and Facebook as an intervention channel in PA and health promotion in communities, including schools.

Other interactive Internet media, such as online diaries, have since emerged, allowing users to reflect on specific topics. Further, wikis, which are server software, were created to enable an individual to freely construct and edit web content. As the desire to share, edit, and construct web content increased, Google developed Google Drive (Google Docs, Sheets, and Slides), which serves to store and synchronize files in the cloud and collaborate with other users to share and edit files (Mossberg, 2012). The development of Google Drive led to the development of Google Hangouts, a communication platform that includes video chat, instant messaging, and Voice over Internet Protocol (VoIP) capabilities. Collectively, these services allow for complete communication via the Internet and have great potential in PA promotion in CSPAPs.

Computers, along with the Internet and social media, have undoubtedly changed our lives. In effect, researchers have since been perusing methodologies to increase PA and health interventions using such technologies (Gao, 2017b). Specifically, studies relative to social media–based PA interventions have been conducted primarily on healthy, inactive individuals, mostly among adults, with a paucity of research in youth populations. To our knowledge, the efficacy of social media–based PA interventions has been examined among children and adolescents in only two studies. A 12-week Facebook-based intervention on PA and body mass index was conducted on overweight and obese Finnish teenagers (Ruotsalainen et al., 2015). Findings indicated no significant differences for body mass index or PA levels between the intervention group receiving healthy lifestyle and self-monitoring assistance and the control group. Teenage girls' perceptions of PA and social media–based PA interventions, primarily on Facebook, were examined in the other study (van Kessel et al., 2016). Nineteen Australian female adolescents (aged 13-18 years) with differing PA levels and socioeconomic statuses were participants within six focus groups.

Humorous animated imageries and walking protocols proved undesirable by the girls, with the ability to socialize and compete with friends during social media–based PA interventions most desired among this population. That said, parents were found supportive of such social media–based PA promotion strategies, particularly when the protocol was not advertised for weight loss (van Kessel et al., 2016). Taken together, the Internet and online social media can serve as a valuable resource for PA promotion among youth and adults alike. Future endeavors should continue using these resources for behavior change and health promotion at a larger scale in CSPAPs.

Mobile Devices and Apps

Mobile phones are now deemed "smartphones," owing to capabilities such as sending and receiving text messages, photography, and connectivity to 4G and Wi-Fi networks. Today, smartphones are in the hands of 64 percent of adults, with this trend growing annually (Smith, 2015). Tablet computers are another common mobile device initially popularized with Apple's release of the iPad, with comparable features of a laptop but smaller in size. Like smartphone use, tablet popularity continues to see exponential growth, with 40-80 million tablets shipped annually (Statista, 2016). Regardless of whether a smartphone or tablet is being used, mobile devices allow educators and researchers the ability to apply mobile device apps for health promotion in CSPAPs.

Because children do not typically own smartphones, literature on mobile device health apps (mHealth apps) for PA promotion is sparse and has primarily focused on adolescent populations. For example, two randomized controlled trials from Smith and colleagues (2014) and Lubans and colleagues (2014) used ATLAS (a multicomponent, theoretically driven, app-based intervention), which resulted in reduced sugar-sweetened beverage consumption, increased PA, and lower screen time among adolescents in low-income schools. The latter of the two trials yielded the ATLAS 2.0 protocol's (Lubans et al., 2016) current implementation. Successful school-based mHealth interventions have been noted in other studies (e.g., Watterson, 2012), though young children remain an understudied population. Because childhood is so critical to one's development and health habits, we outline potential mHealth PA interventions for future research.

Interventions utilizing mHealth apps among children should take place at the classroom level, placing the responsibility on school administrators and teachers given children's sparse smartphone or tablet ownership. Within physical education and classroom settings, one study indicated 40 percent of K-12 teachers currently use apps related to their instruction on mobile devices (Kervin et al., 2013). In physical education classes, facilitation of motor skill development and PA excitement has been introduced by apps, such as Iron Kids, though no known intervention literature has utilized this or other apps for such purposes (Martin et al., 2015). Nonetheless, mHealth apps allow for endless possibilities in the synchronization of educational curricula, such as math, with PA opportunities. For example, a student may complete the math equation "5 + 6" on an mHealth app, after which the student and his or her peers might be asked to do 11 jumping jacks (i.e., the sum of the math equation). Notably, this type of PA-based learning may improve students' in-class behavior and performance, as noted by Mahar (2011). More detail regarding such PA programs can be found in chapter 7 of this book. Through their work, researchers may educate PA leaders (PALs), administrators, and community partners regarding the effectiveness of these interventions to not only increase PA participation but also to improve in-class behavior.

Health Wearables

Quantifiable data on movement of the human body and PA patterns has been tracked by wearable electronic devices (e.g., heart rate monitors, accelerometers, and pedometers). Pedometers track and count steps taken during PA. In detail, an internal lever arm electrically, mechanically, or via a piezoelectric strain gauge (e.g., New Lifestyles NL-1000) registers steps. Similarly, accelerometers track minute-to-minute patterns of frequency, intensity, and duration of bodily movement. Specifically, accelerometers estimate energy expenditure by assessing ambulatory activity (total) levels by way of triaxial accelerations. Heart rate monitors measure intensity of

individuals' PA and can approximate their individual energy expenditures. These devices are optimized to estimate burned calories during steady-state PA because of the linear relationship between energy expenditure and heart rate.

Though these devices have been widely available for decades, they have long possessed inadequate capabilities to track multiple modes of PA (e.g., pedometers track only walking or running) or, like accelerometers, were historically too expensive for average consumers and, therefore, used only in research settings. Today, PA monitoring devices (i.e., health wearables) have flourished because they are widely available to and affordable for the general public. Health wearables are the most novel forms of PA-tracking technology currently used in the promotion of PA and health. Indeed, heart rate monitors as a traditional health wearable have been extensively used by PALs and physical educators in CSPAPs in the past decades, and studies with this device have been widely reported in the scientific community. Therefore, purchasing sets of health wearables for school use is feasible. Yet very few newly developed health wearables have been used in CSPAPs so far, and few studies have examined the use of innovative health wearables, such as Fitbit and other fitness bands, in CSPAPs.

Health wearables (e.g., Fitbit) utilize sensors to assist users in automatically setting and tracking goals (e.g., burned calories and steps taken), diet, and sleep to optimize health patterns (Almalki et al., 2015). Outcomes, such as heart rate, number of stairs climbed, and active time, can be tracked on health wearables and subsequently transferred wirelessly to free mobile apps for immediate PA feedback and long-term data storage (Cadmus-Bertram et al., 2015; Lyons et al., 2014). Interventions using health wearables (e.g., Fitbit, Microsoft Band, Apple Watch) have been employed for self-evaluation, monitoring and reinforcement, and goal setting to enhance PA and wellness among all age groups (Cadmus-Bertram et al., 2015; Michie et al., 2011; Wang et al., 2015). Most wearers report that health wearables have changed their lives because of their unmatched capabilities to provide specific PA feedback (Michie et al., 2011). For example, Fitbit, one of the most popular health wearables on the market, is user friendly and has been utilized for behavioral change and health promotion in youth and adults alike. It is possible that if CSPAP leaders, PALs, and physical educators implement Fitbit into the daily lives of the school staff and students, the health benefits would prove tremendous.

Virtual Reality and Augmented Virtual Reality

Virtual reality (VR) and augmented VR (simulation technology) are among the newest and possibly most compelling technologies available to aid in PA promotion. VR allows for user interaction via digital technology that reproduces an authentic or imagined environment, which simulates one's physical presence within this environment. The PlayStation VR, HTC Vive, Oculus Rift, and Samsung Gear VR are the latest commercially available technologies in the VR market, all of which artificially trigger interactive sensory experiences with auditory, tactile, and visual stimuli (Isaac, 2016).Augmented VR is slightly different because this technology offers a depiction of live, real-life environments where computer-created sensory inputs (e.g., sounds and visuals) are integrated with GPS location and graphics (Graham et al., 2013). Indeed, augmented VR games, such as Pokémon Go, are distinct in that they synchronize real and animated worlds into a single experience.

Though considered cutting edge, the use of this technology to effectively promote PA at schools is still in its infancy (Pasco, 2013). Nonetheless, thanks to organizational support from SHAPE America and other major health organizations, VR is quickly becoming a player in the mission of increasing youth PA (Hansen & Sanders, 2012). Nationwide, physical educators have increasingly implemented both forms of VR into their curricula—VR exercise bikes, sporting games, rhythmic dance machines, balance boards, and other VR-based equipment—to increase PA appeal and motivation (Hansen & Sanders, 2012; Zeng et al., 2017).

VR in schools also has the potential to prevent injuries, enhance students' self-training awareness, and bypass gym-space limitations. Students (K-12) in Florida's Polk County Public Schools and San Francisco's Unified School District were some of the first to use Nearpod VR in their lesson

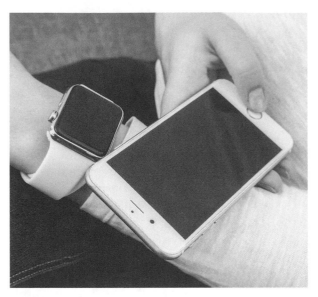

Smart sports tracker is used to capture physical activity behavior.

Photo from Pixabay.

plans. Further, Google Cardboards allow teachers to send classes on over 25 VR field-trip lessons in various curricular areas (e.g., math and science; Liao, 2015). Yet VR research is still lacking in its effectiveness in CSPAPs, meaning this technology's effect on PA and health in youth remains unclear. Though initial studies showed promise, schools still hesitate to embark on VR lessons because funding, space limitations, and curricular restraints as well as the maturity of VR equipment remain issues (Liao, 2015), thus explaining the scarcity in research.

Finally, because the environment in which individuals desire to engage in VR gameplay has changed, researchers have become interested in the accompanying health benefits (Baranowski, 2016). For example, Pokémon Go encourages PA and promotes geographic learning as users maneuver through their respective locations. Notably, Pokémon Go might also enhance social interactions as nearby users compete with one another, which might explain the positive effects on emotion and mood observed after engaging in Pokémon Go play (Serino et al., 2016). Thus, CSPAPs may benefit from this type of augmented VR game within after-school and staff wellness programs.

GPS and Geographic Information Systems (GIS)

Among the most advanced modern technologies utilized in PA and health promotion, GPS and GIS—two complementary technologies now used for health promotion—show great potential in CSPAPs. Briefly, GPS records activity utilizing geographic reference points determined by up to 24 satellites and ground stations, which accurately calculates the geographic location. When combined with accelerometry, GPS can monitor and assess PA markers, such as PA time and distance, average velocity, and altitude (Rodriguez et al., 2005; Troped et al., 2008). GIS is a computer-based system that stores information relative to location and the local environment. As such, GPS data on PA can be examined by GIS relative to PA location, allowing researchers to establish associations between environmental features and exact locations (e.g., street construction, land occupancy, and rail systems), which may deter or promote PA participation (Troped et al., 2001).

As GPS and GIS technologies have improved over the past several years, research has transitioned from a concentration on validity and reliability of this technology during PA assessment to the implementation of GPS-based PA and health promotion interventions. Specifically, investigators in this field are researching how modifications to the built environment can mold behaviors in youth and adults to improve health promotion (Gao, 2017b). Exclusive to research among youth populations, multiple large-scale studies have been conducted using GPS and GIS, in addition to accelerometry, to examine the PA location and associated PA levels at these locations among youth. Presently, GPS and GIS devices show promise in linking environmental attributes with PA tendencies despite the lack of literature utilizing such technologies in PA interventions within school- or community-based settings. Finally, geocaching, a sport similar to treasure hunting, requires GPS-enabled participants to bike, walk, climb, and hike their ways to specific locations marked by GPS coordinates (Groundspeak, 2016). Per geocaching rules, players must leave an item of equal value to the item they took and note their finds within the provided logbook (Groundspeak, 2016). Geocaching might be a promising addition to promote PA within after-school programs among youth.

Overall, emerging technologies are continually evolving and changing our lives. On the horizon are novel and exciting, cutting-edge technologies that have great potential for PA promotion in CSPAPs. In fact, school staff and community partners have applied technology in promoting PA at schools and communities for years. Yet in this rapidly changing era, emerging technologies are providing us with more exciting opportunities to promote PA and foster healthy lifestyles on a larger scale.

Knowledge Claims

The major knowledge claims based on the preceding sections follow.

- AVGs can be a substitute for less active forms of screen entertainment (e.g., computer games, sedentary video games, and TV), but they are not a stand-alone replacement for traditional PA in CSPAPs.

- The Internet and social media have advantages over traditional, face-to-face interventions because interventionists can reach a large and more diverse sample of individuals while also reducing the burdens that might arise during typical face-to-face interventions. Likely, they will play a part in PA intervention delivery in CSPAPs for many years to come.

- Research evidence has shown positive effects of mobile- and smartphone-based app PA interventions among youth. More studies are needed, however, to explore the long-term impact of mobile- and smartphone-based app interventions on PA and health in CSPAPs.

- Evidence regarding the effectiveness of health wearables in promoting PA and health in CSPAPs is inconclusive, yet studies have demonstrated that these devices hold great promise for promoting healthier lifestyles in youth and adults. The market for health wearables continues to grow in popularity, and the potential utility of using these devices to promote health is considerable.

- VR technologies have been applied in physical education and sport settings to promote

PA and athletic performance. However, few large-scale, methodologically rigorous studies have been conducted, with no high-quality studies completed in a physical education setting. Therefore, researchers and educators should continue to explore the benefits of VR and augmented VR games as well as harness their potential in the promotion of PA and health in CSPAPs.

- GPS and GIS systems show promise as modalities for improving our understanding of the relationship between environmental attributes and PA behavior at the population level, despite the relative paucity of literature using these technologies in CSPAPs.

Knowledge Gaps and Directions for Future Research

Technology has played a paramount role in shaping the lifestyles and health status in youth. Emerging technologies bring exciting opportunities for the promotion of PA and health in CSPAPs. This section provides the limitations inherent in the empirical studies regarding the use of emerging technologies in PA interventions and the directions for future research discussed in each technology's individual section. It is important to note that careful consideration of knowledge gaps, challenges, and opportunities sets the stage for transformative approaches to scientific discovery and effective PA intervention implementation in CSPAPs. The rapid growth of technology, coupled with the emerging CSPAP field, has created both obstacles and opportunities that require further attention from researchers.

Emerging Technology for PA Assessment

Fifteen years ago, PA questionnaires were replaced with health wearables (e.g., pedometers, heart rate monitors, and accelerometers), which measured PA and tracked and calculated human movement patterns for analyses. Further, they may motivate youth by providing feedback for them to build upon. Accelerometers are now appearing in smartphone and GPS units and are capable of measuring PA intensity. Innovative technologies, such

as apps, GPS and GIS, and health wearables, now create seamless interactions (e.g., integrated data from multiple devices), making them attractive assets to health professionals. With this information, knowing where, when, and how PA occurs allows for greater understanding of PA patterns and more effective PA behavioral changes.

Multisensor systems now exist that identify previously unidentifiable PA (e.g., stair climbing and bench pressing) using accelerometers or pedometers by themselves. Presently, the vast majority of apps (e.g., MapMyFitness), devices (e.g., Polar M430 sports watch), and monitors (e.g., ActiGraph) are capable of sending data to one's personal account or to the associated communities.

Though it is necessary to test the validity of technologies when used in PA interventions, researchers must also consider the following: (1) New technologies may seamlessly elevate our abilities to analyze PA patterns. (2) Data from large populations can easily be transferred from a longitudinal perspective. (3) Developing technologies with the live data-sharing abilities can advance the enduring, methodical process appraisal of any interventional PA program. (4) Big data can be data or text mined (e.g., PA data and online posts). PA data will be better accessed with improved algorithms and mathematical models. (5) The traditional scientific model may be outdated for these technology-based PA interventions (e.g., self-tracking PA; Graham & Hipp, 2014).

Emerging Technologies in PA Promotion

School-based interventions that employ emerging technologies to promote PA have attempted to fill the curricular gaps where the behavioral aspects of PA have suffered. This has been achieved through the implementation of persuasive technologies (e.g., computers, mobile devices, and the Internet), which leverage readily accessed social influences and encourage the students to play without being coercive as some traditional physical educational practices have been perceived (Fogg, 2003). Literature examining these persuasive technologies have been computationally and interactively based, though the use of human–computer interactions and behavioral theories has become more prevalent (Dominic et al., 2013). The emergence of such technologies has shown great promise for reshaping PA behavior in predefined methodologies in noncommercialized domains.

Specifically, some emerging technologies have proven effective in the promotion of PA in that (1) they act as tools (e.g., record heart rate), (2) they link to social media (e.g., transfer exercise data from app to social media), and (3) they allow for social interaction. The implementation of such technologies increasingly appears in our daily lives. DDR, for example, is an AVG utilizing dance movement that gives scores and instantaneous feedback to users relative to each of their movements and allows them to exercise in an enjoyable environment.

Per Dominic et al. (2013), emerging technologies are seen as tools, and simply using the technologies by themselves will not produce the expected behavior changes or health outcomes. Changing behavior through PA intervention is a fundamental by-product of changing behavior through behavioral theories. Theories, such as the social cognitive theory, have been openly used in behavior-altering PA interventions. Lastly, it is important to recall that multiple technologies have now been integrated into singular apps. By utilizing the power of each technology and combining the technological units, incredible power for users is provided. Now, PA assessments and delivery of interventions are available on singular apps.

In all, technology is ever changing and will forever have dramatic effects on our lives. New and exciting technologies are being produced continually, and all of them have amazing potential for PA promotion. Larger-scale PA promotion has been made possible with these technologies when combined with relevant behavioral theories—especially with VR and AVGs. Distinctly, the technology age is the perfect time for researchers to apply new technologies for health promotion in CSPAPs.

Directions for Future Research

Given the limitations inherent in the empirical studies with AVGs, researchers and educators have several questions to answer before successfully and effectively promoting PA and health in fun and innovative ways through AVGs in CSPAPs.

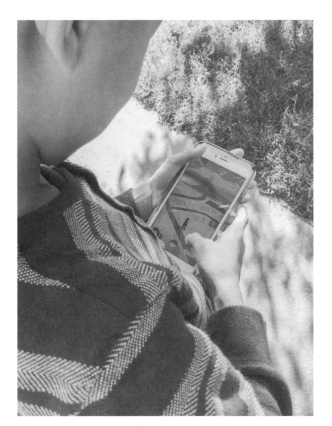

A child is playing Pokémon Go.

© Zan Gao

Some recommendations for future research across different contexts follow (Gao, 2017a):

- Investigate the extent to which AVGs can promote players' learning and maintenance of new movement and cognitive skills (e.g., concentration), and improve the understanding of the impact of exercise on their bodies.

- Examine the long-term efficacy of AVG use in CSPAPs using group randomized controlled trials and the potential benefits of group play and potential barriers in such settings.

- Ascertain the effectiveness of using a multi-player mode in comparison to a single-player mode in CSPAPs.

- Explore AVGs in early childhood and their subsequent effectiveness.

- Determine whether youth with access to AVGs actually replace their screen time with AVGs as opposed to traditional sports or PA.

- Quantify the role of AVGs in contributing to youth daily PA levels.

- Examine the long-term effectiveness of playing AVGs in unstructured and structured settings.
- Develop and implement serious games or storytelling games that promote PA behaviors.
- Conduct process evaluation for AVGs to ensure intervention fidelity.
- Investigate the effects of multiple sports-based AVG types (requiring whole-body versus lower or upper body movement) and different AVG consoles on specific motor skills.

Online social media is promising in the promotion of PA and health given that this technology allows educators to reach large numbers of participants while eliminating more bothersome tasks associated with face-to-face interventions (e.g., transportation needs and time off work). However, it also has knowledge gaps that need to be filled. Specific to CSPAPs, popular quasi- and nonexperimental study designs disregard a control group, which results in the inability to discern causal (direct) effects of CSPAP interventions on health outcomes. Further, because social media–based PA interventions are in their infancy, small sample sizes and low study power make it difficult to establish between-group differences. Moreover, some studies lacked objective PA measures, which has limited the validity of the assessed PA outcomes (Valle et al., 2013). Hence, future research should implement true experimental designs that objectively measure PA with larger sample sizes and further examine the long-term health effects of short-term interventions—interventions that might be utilized among older youth populations using mHealth apps.

Research utilizing mHealth app interventions within CSPAPs to improve the health of youth is one manner by which researchers can recommend changes in recent policies and regulations that limit students' PA. To achieve this objective, however, the validity and reliability of mHealth apps that can track PA and physiological variables must be further evaluated (Charara, 2016).

Health wearables—many of which also have dedicated mHealth apps akin to those discussed previously—have had a positive effect on health promotion. By providing users valuable feedback (e.g., energy expenditure and steps taken), these devices encourage health and well-being by allowing individuals to self-regulate behaviors toward greater alignment with improved health. Additionally, the feedback also provides researchers raw data for analysis, which can be utilized for subsequent behavior intervention development.

Nonetheless, challenges to the implementation of health wearable technology for CSPAPs do exist. To begin, sparse literature exists confirming the efficacy of health wearables in free-living conditions, with more research needed comparing the health metric information of commercially available health wearables to research-grade health wearables (e.g., ActiGraph and Actical; Powell et al., 2014). Noteworthy is the fact that ActiGraph has produced a watch similar to its popular ActiGraph Link. The ActiGraph Link has an associated mobile device app, which might prove valuable for research and daily use while also being more accurate given the high-quality reputation of the ActiGraph Corporation.

Second, convincing previously sedentary individuals to track their PA is another challenge, particularly, as the initial novelty of such technologies wanes. Thus, PALs and administrators need to expect and prepare for students' potentially decreasing interest in this technology.

Finally, health wearables must be affordable for everyone so that PA can be tracked by a desired population, with this PA information subsequently shared with a PAL and used in the development and implementation of the health promotion plan. Yet because consumer-based products, such as the Apple Watch #3 and Fitbit Surge, sell for $300 to $400 (Wang et al., 2015), assisting populations, such as the socioeconomically disadvantaged, remains difficult and unsustainable long term—an unfortunate fact because individuals of lower socioeconomic status are those most likely to suffer from sedentary behavior–related health issues (Patel et al., 2015).

Therefore, in the years to come, a collaborative effort must be made among PALs, administrators, and community partners if health wearables are to facilitate PA and health promotion in CSPAPs. For example, school staff and community partners can use health wearables to regulate PA and sedentary behaviors and adopt healthy and active lifestyles, which set a good example for the youth.

Population-level health promotion might also be possible when utilizing certain types of VR technology, particularly when considering augmented VR games, such as Pokémon Go. Despite the positive initial findings of VR investigations, no large-scale, methodologically rigorous studies have been completed, with little to no study of this technology within CSPAPs. Because of its infancy, VR in CSPAPs requires more research to prove its efficacy in promoting PA and athletic performance. Thus, the following research questions should be considered in the future:

- How might PALs get administrators to understand the potential of VR on health and educational outcomes given the costliness of in-school VR programs?

- Once implemented, how might VR serve as a teaching tool to optimize teaching content?

- Using VR-based teaching methodologies and provisional content, how effective is VR in aiding physical educators in facilitating youth attainment of national PA standards (e.g., development of physical literacy and preparing youth to become lifelong movers; Pasco, 2013).

As the technology progresses, games, such as Pokémon Go, also deserve further investigation among the youth population. Baranowski (2016) has provided a series of questions for future research and directions to follow in this emerging field, including the following: "Was playing it with friends (cooperators or competitors) critical to the experience?" and "Were some aspects of the game more played or more effective, or did different aspects (e.g., different characters, different locations) motivate different people?" It may, therefore, be expected that emerging empirical studies will compile within this field over the next five years.

Finally, literature is inadequate at present connecting GPS and GIS to PA and health promotion strategies. While GPS- and GIS-based games, such as geocaching, may be effective for changing PA behaviors, the safety of this game will turn off users—particularly parents of children (Flett et al., 2010)—a fact that should be accounted for by researchers. Other research questions concerning use of GPS and GIS for PA and health promotion include (1) What is done if the participant loses the GPS signal for prolonged periods of time? (2) How can GPS and GIS produce reproducible

results for PA intensity and type? (3) Can this technology seamlessly integrate into one's daily life? Distinctly, further research is needed for GPS and GIS in CSPAP settings.

Evidence-Based Recommendations and Applications

PALs and community partners can play a valuable role in the selection and integration of emerging technologies in CSPAPs. This section will provide the requisite knowledge base concerning evidence-based applications and recommendations for practice (Gao, 2017a; King et al., 2015). It is hoped that this information will promote further integration of emerging technology in CSPAPs by researchers and educators alike.

For School Staff

Within health care, the most persistent issue has been stakeholder buy-in regarding the incorporation of technology within primary care clinics and hospitals for PA and health promotion, resulting from worries about the security measures for clients' electronic health data (e.g., the total PA an individual participates in; see West, 2012). Schools, which have a large population of youth who could benefit from technology integration, also suffer from stakeholder buy-in. To incorporate health-promoting technologies into schools, administration and teachers could require proof of effectiveness when using technologies, such as AVGs and mHealth apps, for promotion of PA and health within classroom and physical education settings. Regardless, implementing PA and health interventions in school settings is important for challenging the existing stigma linking technology to poor youth health.

Although the use of technology to improve health and well-being can be researched in CSPAPs, most schools need funding, space, and other resources to embrace efficacious technologies. To change this, it is critical that grant monies or other funds reward proposed CSPAP studies, which detail how emerging technology will be disseminated into schools. In addition, while the use of emerging technologies in health promotion in CSPAPs will always face challenges, the way educators teach and train their students in the use of technology for these purposes will affect the level of integration of these technologies seen in CSPAPs. As such, it is important for educators to take note of the potential challenges mentioned in this chapter.

For Community Partners

Researchers face numerous challenges in reducing the gap between the development of health-promoting technologies and their implementation in the real world. First, experts from various disciplines are required to develop and apply technology with the purpose of improving health in school settings. For example, computer scientists have developed many well-functioning mobile device health applications that did not meet the needs of clients and led to slight or no PA intervention effectiveness. Consequently, it is crucial to recruit educators and researchers from varied disciplines, such as PALs, health practitioners, and computer scientists, whose combined knowledge can be used to develop and execute efficient PA promotion strategies utilizing technology. Second, to effectively implement technology-based PA promotion, it is imperative to understand stakeholders' interests and needs as well as the community and organizational systems. For example, students can be offered more choices in school-based PA programs when a technology such as AVGs is integrated within this setting because children can choose from different games (e.g., Kinect Just Dance, Wii Fit, and DDR) most appealing to these interests and, therefore, most likely to stimulate increased PA. Further, the increased independence facilitated during the aforementioned situation might also serve as a motivational tool to improve children's PA and increase class involvement. That said, lack of support from school administration makes it difficult to implement these types of school-based programs, with budget deficiencies, space limitations, and curricular clashes being notable barriers. As such, King and colleagues (2015) have suggested collaborating with organizational workers from diverse community areas and within industry to increase the appeal of technology-based health promotion strategies within schools.

In addition, many concerns are present when it comes to the digital realm and its history with the undermining of anonymity. The largest undesirable feature for the use of emerging technologies in PA promotion is the confidentiality of health information while using these new technologies (Lobelo et al., 2016; Richardson & Ancker, 2015). It is critical that all parties, including community partners, remain ethically concerned about the issues of privacy, participant consent, and anonymity as they pertain to emerging technologies that are constantly collecting statistics on behavioral as well as environmental and social characteristics. Researchers are tasked with the responsibility of finding solutions in CSPAPs to collect data for health-promotion purposes while continuing to protect the participants' information.

SUMMARY

Throughout this chapter, we have illustrated the reality of today, that emerging technologies have changed our lives and are continually upgrading the intervention channels in CSPAPs. Indeed, technologies have gained entry into most PA and behavioral change programs in schools. Where technology was once demonized for its role in contributing to the diminishing levels of PA and overall health, researchers and educators have fought fire with fire and leveraged society's vast interest in technology to *promote* PA and health in youth and adults. Thus, the paradigm has shifted, and the emergence of such technologies has opened up new windows of opportunity to promote PA and health at scale and in an enjoyable manner. To effectively promote PA through emerging technologies, we should consider the feasibility, cost, and behavioral theories as well as build partnerships between PALs, administrators, community partners, and other stakeholders within CSPAPs. As such, the promise of using emerging technology in fostering a healthy and physically active lifestyle through CSPAPs can be realized more fully.

QUESTIONS TO CONSIDER

1. What makes emerging technologies important tools for promoting PA in CSPAPs? Can they also do the opposite?
2. What features are important in an AVG to make it a healthy and sustainable exercise option at schools?
3. How can the VR exercise programs in a CSPAP provide incentive for further play once the novelty wears off?
4. How can long-term use of health wearables among school staff, students, and community partners help prevent lifestyle diseases?
5. What are the directions for future studies with emerging technologies in CSPAPs?

CASE EXAMPLE

Mr. Smith, the only physical education teacher at the Jefferson Elementary School in Blaine, a town in a midwestern state, describes his plan to integrate emerging technology at the school.

He decided to implement a 50-minute AVG session in his physical education class in addition to two other physical education lessons every week for 12 weeks. He chose DDR, which requires fast foot movements synchronized to energetic music and visuals, a very popular AVG among youth. To successfully initiate the program, he purchased a set of DDR systems and relevant accessories with his annual allotted physical education budget ($500). Fortunately, he also had learned how to play and organize DDR during a workshop at the SHAPE America National Convention this past year, making designing this program much easier.

The DDR program has proven to be a great way to get the students moving. Specifically, during gameplay, students move their feet to a set pattern and step in time to the general rhythm or beat of a song. Arrows are divided into quarter notes, eighth notes, and so on, up to about thirty-second notes. Arrows scroll upward from the bottom of the screen and pass over stationary, transparent arrows near the top. The students must step on the corresponding arrows on the dance pad when the scrolling arrows overlap the stationary arrows. For the longer green and yellow arrows, arrows that freeze movement, the students must hold them down for the entire count. If students fail a song three times, the game is over. Otherwise, students can see the results on the screen, which include a rating of their performance with a letter grade and a numerical score as well as other statistics. Depending on the version of the game, dance steps can be categorized into varying levels of difficulty. As the steps increase in difficulty, the challenge begins to resemble real dancing.

To begin the DDR program in the physical education classes, he adopted the following processes according to the practices employed in a related DDR field experience, which he learned in the SHAPE America workshop. First, he instructed students to master the basic knowledge of rhythm and beat by clapping, stepping, snapping, or using percussive instruments on specific counts of a basic 4/4 beat. Second, he asked the students to follow the easy on-screen instructions in lesson mode. This mode is great for learning how to play DDR. It starts off with the basics and gradually works up to combination moves and jumps. Third, he let four students stand in the middle of the interactive dance pad and stomp the arrows with their feet on the mat to play DDR while the rest of the students practiced on the rubber dance pads, which are not connected to the game consoles. This drill allows students to familiarize themselves with the DDR process and timing. Additionally, students practiced stepping in the four directions required by the game (right, left, up, and down). Finally, as students mastered basic concepts, such as the 4/4 beat and stepping in all four directions, variations and new challenges were introduced to make these dances more realistic. This drill also allowed students to assess their progress and success during gameplay in physical education.

It should be noted, however, that there were limited interactive dance pads for DDR gameplay during these physical education sessions, with only four children able to play on an interactive DDR pad (i.e., pads that provided live feedback). Therefore, Mr. Smith developed methods of "dry play" for the remaining students, such as imaginary dance pads, rubber practice pads, poly spots, and marking arrows on the floor to mimic the actual DDR pads and allowing the students to engage in the same body movements. Notably, he was also able to borrow a large projection system (to project the screen onto the gym wall) so that dozens of students could follow along with the motions at the same time. Technically, students still get the full activity benefits, minus the live accuracy feedback. After each song, Mr. Smith had students take turns rotating on and off the interactive dance pads. His advice is that whatever rotation system works best for the activity in physical education can and should be employed.

CHAPTER 22

A Synergized Strategy Guide for Advancing the Field

Russell L. Carson, PhD
University of Northern Colorado

Collin A. Webster, PhD
University of South Carolina

The CSPAP is a unifying model that can bring together a range of supporters—those affiliated with schools and anyone genuinely interested in promoting lifetime PA behaviors for youth. CSPAPs are uniquely inclusive of all possible philosophical and curricular positions and adaptable to varying school contexts (see chapter 1). Since the conception of CSPAPs in 2008, we have witnessed an explosion of dedicated professionals researching and implementing school-wide PA initiatives with CSPAPs in mind. National groups and guiding documents have surfaced in dramatic fashion and mobilized CSPAP fields of research and practice (Centers for Disease Control and Prevention [CDC], 2017; CDC, 2018; National Physical Activity Plan Alliance [NPAPA], 2016). The timely publication of this book offers an organized, up-to-date resource to the growing body of science and practice in the rapidly progressing CSPAP field. This book intends to accelerate cross-disciplinary inquiry and practice around CSPAPs for the coming years.

To jump-start this work, this chapter will address the guiding questions posed in the preface, using bulleted summary points of the overlapping knowledge claims, gaps, and directions presented across the chapters. The goal is to provide quick takeaways to facilitate action for research and practice. The pertinent chapters will be referenced throughout these summaries along with complementary sources for consideration. The chapter will conclude with the top 10 at-a-glance strategies to advance CSPAP research and practice. The goal is to leave readers with a path for what CSPAP research and practice can become.

How Does the Policy Landscape Reflect the Evolving Values and Traditions of the CSPAP Model?

The bulleted response material in this section comes from part I, Foundations and Contemporary Perspectives; and part V, Developing, Measuring, and Promoting CSPAPs.

- Public policies related to CSPAPs aim to promote one of their overarching goals: PA behaviors among youth. Most CSPAP-related policies are implemented at the state level ("big P" policy) rather than at the school or district level ("little p" policy), with main focuses on either the foundational component of CSPAPs—physical education and the time mandates for physical education—or the allotted time for PA at school. Public policies have yet to reflect the multicomponent principles of CSPAPs (chapter 2).

- Studies suggest that state policies correspond to greater time requirements for physical education and more time spent being active during physical education classes, despite policies on the actual amount of time devoted to moving in physical education existing at more district than state levels. Regardless of the mandates at the state level, all districts should clearly articulate general physical education and PA requirements (separately) in their local policy statements (chapter 2).

- CSPAP-related policies have the utility to increase youth PA levels if they are imple-

mented at the local level using enforceable wording that is inclusive of the opportunities for movement throughout the entire school setting (chapter 2). Involvement of and, ideally, leadership from school-level administrators is paramount to local-level policy adoption and implementation (Greenberg & LoBianco, in press). Limited research has examined the effect that CSPAPs have on the collective school environment (e.g., school-level policies) or, longitudinally, how these cultural shifts might affect youth health and behaviors (chapter 16).

- Despite there having been no federal mandates on PA and physical education in schools in the past, there are now opportunities for researchers and practitioners to explore the relationships between new national policies, such as the Every Student Succeeds Act (ESSA), and youth PA levels (chapters 1 and 2).

What Conceptual and Theoretical Approaches Could Guide CSPAP Practice and Collaboration?

The bulleted response material in this section comes from part II, Conceptual Models for CSPAP Implementation; and part V, Developing, Measuring, and Promoting CSPAPs.

Conceptual Guides

- Although many view the CSPAP concept as new, its multicomponent principles are rooted in a conceptualization of the promotion of school health, initially and more broadly known as the Coordinated School Health (CSH) model (Allensworth & Kolbe, 1987) and, since 2014, the Whole School, Whole Community, Whole Child (WSCC) model (Association for Supervision and Curriculum Development [ASCD], 2018). The ways both the CSPAP and WSCC models inform one another are worthy avenues of research exploration and meaningful practice.

- Carson and colleagues (2014) proposed a conceptual framework to guide CSPAP research and practice. The framework highlights the importance and interconnectedness of CSPAP facilitators (i.e., knowledge, skills, disposition, safety, and resources), leaders (i.e., champion, administrator, and committee), and culture (i.e., policy, norms, and beliefs) to reach the goal of increasing youth PA at school (chapter 3). This conceptual framework has been included to guide many research studies or interventions implemented at many different levels (e.g., student, teacher, school, and community; chapter 4). The framework can also be used as a template for the several layers of advocacy efforts and targets, referred to as the nested ecology of advocacy (chapter 19).

- While the available evidence does support the idea that implementing more CSPAP components provides more desired PA outcomes for youth, it is also clear that various iterations and alternatives to the five-component model can work well for different schools. Perhaps conceptualizations of CSPAPs should be geared less toward the number of components and more toward any combination of enhanced, extended, or expanded opportunities for youth PA promotion (Beets et al., 2016).

Theoretical Guides

- Twenty CSPAP studies were guided by a theoretical foundation (chapter 5), suggesting that the majority of published CSPAP studies have theoretical underpinnings.

- The main theoretical foundation applied to CSPAP studies is social cognitive theory (Bandura, 1986), an interpersonal-level theory that emphasizes the dynamic interaction between *people* (personal factors) and their *environments* (social and physical contexts) and *behavior* (chapter 6). The diffusion of innovations theory (Rogers, 1995) adoption factors (e.g., perceived attributes that influence adoption of an innovation) provide helpful guideposts when planning for CSPAP sustainability (chapter 4).

- *Youth PA behavior* is the primary behavioral focus of theoretically applied CSPAP studies, followed by body mass index, fitness levels, and motor skill competency (chapter 5).

- The foremost theoretically driven approach to changing youth PA behavior was through

personal factors of either self-efficacy or perceived competence, followed by youth enjoyment for PA and youth satisfaction of autonomy needs, a main underpinning of the self-determination theory (Deci & Ryan, 1985), which represents feeling in control of one's behavior (chapters 5 and 6).

- Salient theory–based *environmental factors* guiding CSPAP studies are social influences (e.g., teachers, parents, peers, administrators, paraprofessionals, and recess monitors) and physical environmental features that facilitate autonomy-supportive (e.g., activity zones and stations with various points of entry and challenges) rather than controlling school PA contexts (e.g., only one PA option, chosen by the teacher, is provided at recess or during classroom movement opportunities; chapter 5).

- Research findings from theoretically based CSPAP studies can inform factors for consideration in CSPAP practice. Collectively, to date, when youth PA behavior is the goal, CSPAP implementers and stakeholders should integrate theoretically derived personal factors that facilitate youth self-efficacy, perceived competence and ability, and enjoyment along with supportive environmental factors of PA encouragement and autonomy-driven PA contexts (chapter 5).

Approaches to Guide CSPAP Practice

Beyond CSPAP or WSCC conceptual guides or social cognitive theory or diffusion of innovation theory theoretical guides, in the end, sustainable CSPAP practice relies on the guidance from having a three-way personnel structure in place, known as the CSPAP leadership triad (chapter 3).

- *PA champion* (preferably, a physical education teacher): Support by physical education teachers is commonly identified as another crucial lever for implementing a CSPAP. However, there is a scarcity of research examining physical education teachers' CSPAP-related perceptions. While physical education teachers often are called upon to be the central protagonists in the CSPAP movement, it is unclear whether most physical education teachers wish to serve in this capacity or view a CSPAP as a realistic goal for their schools (chapter 3).

- *Supportive school administrator*: Administrative support for the program is vital to successful CSPAP initiatives. Garnering and securing administration support is an early CSPAP implementation step (CDC, 2013). The lack of research on school principals' perceptions of CSPAPs leaves a gaping hole in the knowledge needed to recruit this key stakeholder group as activists in the CSPAP movement (chapter 3).

- *CSPAP committee*: Advisement and assistance with CSPAP coordination and implementation should come from a three-member committee, consisting of the PA champion, the building administrator, and one more influential leader in or around the school. Including or engaging a district-level person in the committee work can expand CSPAP participation, reach, and partnerships within and beyond the community (chapter 3).

Approaches to Guide CSPAP Collaboration

- School practitioners and researchers may struggle to maximize the effectiveness and sustainability of a CSPAP without collaborative support from varied entities and the extra resources they can provide (chapter 3). Practitioners might apply a *community-organizing approach*, based on the notion that the most successful CSPAPs are those that are initiated, implemented, and cultivated by the members of the school community (within and outside of school grounds; chapter 4). Researchers might apply *community-based participatory research (CBPR) strategies* to form community partnerships through the integration and understanding of local opinions, strengths, and barriers in the research process (chapters 3 and 4).

- Webster and colleague's (2015) partnership model highlights three approaches, CBPR, communities of practice, and service learning, which collectively bridge *internal supports* (existing within the school) and *external supports* (existing outside of the school) to build community will, relationships, and capacities for CSPAPs (chapter 4).

- *External supports* can come from a myriad of community partners, such as university faculty, service providers, and professional networks (chapters 4 and 12). External support strategies may include personnel trainings, resource development, implementation assistance (e.g., personnel and funding), and advocacy outlets (chapters 3, 4, 16, and 19).

- The longevity of CSPAPs will depend on both bottom-up and top-down streams of external supports. *Bottom-up approaches* entail galvanizing school communities to become actively involved in the CSPAP. To accomplish this, each school leader, teacher, parent or guardian, or other supporting member of the school community should be able to take ownership of relevant program components and deliver PA opportunities using means and methods that feel familiar to him or her. *Top-down approaches* include establishing strong state-level policies ("big P" policies); relevant professional standards in teaching and teacher education; and other external accountability mechanisms for CSPAP implementation, effectiveness, and sustainability that reinforce work being done at the ground level (chapters 2, 3, 4, and 20).

- Central to and repeatedly emphasized throughout this book are the mutual benefits and multiplied CSPAP impacts from relationship-building approaches between university and K-12 schools (chapters 4, 16, and 19). Positive and ongoing interactions among teacher educators, researchers, and practitioners help fill knowledge gaps and overcome real-world challenges, and they are critical to changing school and community outcomes (chapters 4, 16, and 20).

What Does the Latest Evidence Say About the Effectiveness of Each CSPAP Component and Multicomponent Approaches in Promoting PA?

The bulleted response material in this section comes from mostly part III, Research on Program Effectiveness; and also part II, Conceptual Models for CSPAP Implementation; and part V, Developing, Measuring, and Promoting CSPAPs.

Effectiveness by Component

- Most CSPAP research examines the implementation of new PA opportunities by CSPAP component. Among the literature reviews available related to each CSPAP component content area, three are conceptualized within the CSPAP model (Erwin et al., 2013; Hunt & Metzler, 2017; Russ et al., 2015), and several others systematically review the evidence of school-based PA interventions generally (De Bourdeaudhuij et al., 2011; Demetriou & Höner, 2012; Dobbins et al., 2013; Kriemler et al., 2011; Metcalf et al., 2012).

- *Physical education*: Increasing opportunities for learning and PA in physical education is possible through policy, curriculum, and teacher behavior (chapter 6). Quality physical education is defined in terms of having a certified physical education teacher, manageable class sizes, adequate facilities and equipment, assessment-driven instruction, standards-based curricula, and ample opportunities for meaningful learning and PA (chapter 6). A qualified physical education teacher is at the heart of a CSPAP that not only provides increased PA for students but also links PA before, during, and after school to the knowledge, skills, and dispositions needed for healthful living across the life span (Webster et al., 2016). Despite physical education's being the foundational component of a CSPAP, physical education teachers do not always agree about CSPAP integration at their school or their place within a CSPAP (chapters 6 and 9). For some physical educators, workload and role conflict are prominent barriers for assuming expanded professional responsibilities related to promoting PA beyond teaching physical education lessons; coaching sports; or performing other assigned duties, without incentives (chapters 3, 4, and 6).

- *PA during school*: Most of the focus within the PA during-school component of a CSPAP has centered on recess and classroom movement integration within the elementary school setting. Though little is known about children's PA during typical recess periods, research demonstrates that low-cost strategies (e.g., activity zones, active supervision by recess monitors, and adding recess periods) are effective ways to increase PA. Additionally, a variety of strategies (e.g., teacher-designed lessons, specially designed equipment, and school–university partnerships) are effective at increasing children's classroom-based PA. However, classroom teachers perceived barriers to integrating movement opportunities during classroom periods, particularly lack of time (chapter 9). Because classroom teachers tend to outnumber most other CSPAP stakeholder groups and spend a considerable amount of time with children and adolescents during school, it is imperative that these professionals be provided with PA promotion options that fit neatly into their existing classroom routines (chapter 7).

- *PA before and after school*: After-school programs have received much more investigative attention than before-school programs, though it appears both types of programs can support the PA of children and adolescents. The after-school program setting provides youth with supplemental PA, but the programs typically do not meet the guidelines. Policies specific to PA in after-school programs should be combined with program-level scheduling and staff training to maximize PA opportunities. Staff should be trained to provide activities based on the interests and needs of program attendees (chapter 8).

- *Staff involvement*: Staff involvement entails offering and participating in staff wellness programs at school as well as assisting and supporting CSPAP implementation (e.g., serving on a school wellness committee and helping to promote and increase students' PA in multiple school contexts). There is a dearth of research on staff wellness programs and their impact on staff wellness, staff PA promotion, and students' PA. Wellness programs should be holistic and encompass multiple dimensions, including mental, social-emotional, physical, and spiritual wellness. Such programs should also allow for participant choice and self-direction and be aligned with organizational goals. Support from organization leaders (e.g., school principals) is important to program success, but little is known about the understandings and perceptions of school and community leaders with respect to CSPAPs (chapters 9, 12, and 14).

- Overall, research on staff PA promotion is rapidly growing and greatly eclipses research on staff wellness. To increase uptake and sustainable use of PA promotion strategies, intervention approaches that allow for staff adaptation and flexible implementation are recommended over approaches that rely on prepackaged materials or one-size-fits-all programs, which do not account for differences in context (chapter 9).

- It is clear that numerous barriers persist amid efforts to increase staff PA promotion. The application of behavioral and organizational change theories has proven helpful in better understanding what variables should be targeted in teacher education and staff professional development trainings to increase the prevalence of PA promotion in in-school and out-of-school settings (chapter 9).

- *Family and community engagement*: Relatively little research has focused on the family and community engagement component of a CSPAP. While approaches to addressing this component have varied, it is clear at this point that multiple methods of communication (including electronic and online messaging) and varied opportunities for involvement are needed to engage parents in CSPAPs. It is important to ensure that parents and other community stakeholders be included in program development from the beginning so they are invested in the program's success. Systems approaches to program implementation that bridge family and community engagement to other components of the CSPAP model are recommended to increase the influence of family and community engagement on desired PA outcomes (chapter 10).

Multicomponent Effectiveness

- Overall, few studies have investigated the implementation of a full five-component program, and even fewer studies have demonstrated the use of coordinated and synergistic efforts across components to reach program goals. It is possible to increase youth PA by increasing the number of CSPAP components used (chapter 11), although optimum uses of each component are not well understood. The processes by which CSPAP components coalesce to maximize daily PA opportunities and every student's potential to live a healthy and active life remain largely unknown. Future work must aim to uncover the most promising avenues toward creating enough opportunities for every student to reach 60 minutes of mostly moderate-to-vigorous PA each day while also meeting standards-based physical education learning outcomes.

- Multicomponent school intervention programs that have shown success, irrespective of gender, were either in increasing PA behaviors or decreasing body mass index levels of youth (chapter 18).

- Full implementation of a CSPAP as the ultimate goal may not be feasible given the many current implementation barriers, which reflect a discordance within the physical education profession. Among the barriers presented in chapter 1, several of the physical education profession barriers resonated throughout the book: *reality of current physical education teaching assignments, perceived fear of job loss, conflicting purposes of school physical education*—motor competence versus movement opportunities—and *limited knowledge and skewed messaging of CSPAPs* among physical education teachers. However, recent research suggests that some of these issues may be based on false dichotomies. For instance, Sacko and colleagues (2018) found that practicing object projection skills (e.g., kicking, throwing, and striking) and expending energy equivalent to moderate- and vigorous-intensity PA were positively related, indicating motor skill learning and PA accrual should not be viewed as antagonists. It is possible that there is undue apprehension about role fulfillment and preparedness of physical education teachers within CSPAPs because physical education teaching and PA promotion appear to overlap in significant ways.

How Does Context Factor Into Best Practices for CSPAPs?

The bulleted response material in this section comes from part IV, Contextual Considerations.

- Clearly, context matters in the design, implementation, and sustainability of a CSPAP, as demonstrated repeatedly throughout this book and particularly in chapters 12 to 15. CSPAPs are susceptible to the dynamic and transitory nature of schools. Changes in such things as a school's leadership, teachers, students and families, location, and funding can lengthen or shorten the life span of a CSPAP. Tailoring CSPAPs to fit different school contexts may increase the chances of CSPAP initiatives being sustainable (chapters 1 and 4).

- CSPAPs must be designed to support and align with the goals of the school community. Seldom has CSPAP research focused on outcomes beyond PA and other markers of physical health. For many stakeholders, the potential for a CSPAP to improve other aspects of health (e.g., social-emotional well-being, mental health, family health, and community health), school climate, or other desired outcomes may be of greater interest (chapter 12).

- Despite its rapid rate of production, CSPAP intervention research continues to be bound to a relatively narrow sphere of settings. The vast majority of CSPAP interventions have taken place in elementary school settings. The precipitous decline in a child's PA participation once he or she reaches adolescence makes CSPAP practice and research at the secondary school level a critical area of consideration (chapters 12 and 13). High school may provide many students with their last formal educational program aimed at promoting physically active lifestyles. The secondary school setting offers unique opportunities for CSPAP implementation but also poses unique challenges. An evidence base derived from interventions in elementary school settings will not provide adequate direction for CSPAP development or implementation in middle and high schools.

- There also is a need to implement CSPAPs in other settings with populations in need of increased support for PA. CSPAPs should span the educational sector, including underinvestigated settings, such as early childhood centers, alternative schools, homeschooling environments, and colleges and universities (chapter 15).

- Multicomponent PA programs that have been investigated in the United States within both urban and rural settings (chapters 12 and 13) as well as programs investigated in international settings (chapter 14) have shown positive outcomes, suggesting that there is truth to the common claim that schools are a ripe setting for PA promotion. Yet much remains to be learned about how schools effectively tap, combine, and leverage available resources to nurture long-term CSPAPs that support the needs of all students, particularly those who are less active (e.g., girls and adolescents; chapters 12, 13, and 14). A CSPAP must blend into its environment and seek sustenance in the deepest wells of available resources. Some schools may be rich in certain internal supports for a CSPAP, such as a PA champion or extensive space for PA, whereas other schools may have access to valuable external supports, such as university service learners or a strong district policy ("little p" policy) mandating whole-of-school approaches to PA promotion. Regardless of its distinct context, each school community provides a baseline infrastructure to germinate and support a CSPAP. Integrating CSPAPs into routine parts of school life may help foster program sustainability (chapters 3, 4, and 9).

- A four-part strategy for fully understanding the CSPAP experience in specific school settings includes (1) understand school context at beginning (e.g., needs assessment; chapter 16), (2) track implementation and environmental changes (e.g., establish a tracking system and implementation metrics), (3) identify and measure outcomes and impact (e.g., mode and target of evaluation), and (4) understand how changes happened (e.g., the story or process of change; chapter 18).

What Are Some Promising Strategies for Planning, Researching, Evaluating, and Promoting CSPAPs?

The bulleted response material in this section comes mostly from part V, Developing, Measuring, and Promoting CSPAPs.

Planning

- CSPAP sustainability requires planning prior to program implementation and includes decisions about how to define, enact, measure, monitor, and advocate to ensure program continuance (chapter 4).

- A central and early strategy step in the CSPAP planning process is the identification of existing policies, practices, or programs via the completion of a *needs assessment* (CDC, 2013). In addition to the many needs assessment inventories referenced in chapter 16, the CDC's School Health Index (SHI) is a prevalent assessment and planning tool adopted by several national organizations and state departments of education to examine current PA opportunities in schools. The School Physical Activity Policy Assessment (S-PAPA) is a reliable tool for elementary schools to assess existing PA policies related to physical education, recess, and other school-based PA opportunities. The CSPAP-related items from these two tools and others have been consolidated into a confirmed CSPAP-Questionnaire (CSPAP-Q) for ease of teachers' use to track CSPAP practice, policy, and program improvements in schools (Dauenhauer et al., 2018).

- Conducting a needs assessment helps organizers (ideally, a CSPAP committee) understand the greatest needs in school-based PA opportunities as well as the targeted system and subsystems at play in the school environment (chapter 16). Results are utilized to select a feasible school PA initiative to implement, which is typically charted in a stepwise action plan (or implementation or improvement plan).

- A key component of an effective needs assessment is the capacity of a team (ideally, a CSPAP committee) to carry out CSPAP development and implementation (chapter 16).

- When working with schools, CSPAP researchers and evaluators may employ the *PRECEDE-PROCEED model* (Green & Kreuter, 2005) or the *theory of community organizing* (Wallerstein et al., 2015) to inform the needs assessment and guide the decision-making process (chapters 10 and 16).

- *Asset mapping* (Allar et al., 2017) and *appreciative inquiry* (Coghlan & Brannick, 2014) provide strengths-based alternatives to the traditional needs assessment approach by flipping the focus on leveraging existing resources and support to the CSPAP planning process. Data collection examples appropriate for CSPAP asset-based assessments can be found in chapter 16.

- Practice-based evidence approaches may be the answer to the limited training school PA practitioners typically receive in program planning and evaluation and the underutilization of needs assessment data in CSPAP research or school-based PA intervention studies (chapter 16).

- Decision-making tools during the CSPAP planning and process are desired. A menu of evidence-based practices for physical education and school PA, ranked by strength of published evidence, school setting characteristics, implementation timeline, and prioritized health outcomes, is now available to aid local decision makers in selecting context-appropriate PA initiatives that address identified areas of need (Stoepker et al., 2018).

Researching and Evaluating

- The promise of CSPAP research and evaluation is to provide a robust evidence base for practitioners to use to make informed decisions about program implementation that lead to increased effectiveness and sustainability (chapter 18). The proliferation of research since 2008 has provided a sound foundation to the CSPAP knowledge base.

- Since no single measurement tool can assess all information of interest to a school, triangulation among multiple measurement tools is often needed. Measurement tools need to be easy to use, on a consistent basis, to at least assess standard outcomes to meaningfully advance CSPAP practice or knowledge. Chapter 17 provides an overview of eight measurement tools, mostly observational, that have been used to provide generalizable information about CSPAP programs.

- Emerging technologies in PA measurement, particularly among the proliferation of consumer products on the market, could shape and streamline the measurement of CSPAP outcomes (chapter 21). These technologies combined with observation protocols and established qualitative approaches could enhance CSPAP process evaluations.

- Methods of reporting CSPAP intervention research vary widely. Increased uniformity in measuring and reporting outcomes will allow comparisons to be made to other studies and to state and national policy standards (chapter 17).

- Most CSPAP interventions are designed for elementary aged students; many fewer are implemented or researched in preschool or secondary education settings (chapter 18).

- Practitioners and researchers should consider how much data (e.g., number of observation days or survey respondents) is necessary to establish accurate, representative, and convincing CSPAP findings within the scope of available resources (chapter 17).

- A substantial portion of CSPAP intervention studies lack information about the collective school environment (e.g., policies) and, longitudinally, how these cultural shifts affect youth health and academic behaviors post–CSPAP intervention. Interventions that test the effectiveness of programs designed to reach both the behavioral and educational goals of a CSPAP are needed. Understanding the effectiveness of a CSPAP on students' academic achievement in physical education and other school subjects is an immediate

- next step for the CSPAP research community (chapter 18).

- The cost associated with implementing CSPAPs in comparison to the amount of money a CSPAP saves schools and communities over the long term should be examined (chapter 18).

- A CSPAP should also be flexible in its ability to accommodate a diverse range of student interests and needs. Too often, researchers fail to consider differences in PA outcomes between groups that extend beyond comparing boys and girls. If a CSPAP is truly meant to serve all students, then future investigations also must examine the potentially differential effects of CSPAPs on more specific groups of students, such as students with and without disabilities, students who are overweight and not overweight, and students who are more and less physically active. Such research combined with studies that seek to understand the unique PA interests and needs of different groups of students will aid in the development of suitable, student-centered intervention strategies (chapters 12, 13, and 14).

- A CSPAP database, including descriptions of the kinds of initiatives being implemented and their impact and in what school settings in the United States and internationally, is needed (chapter 17). The closest database available is of data regarding CSPAP prevalence in the United States collected at the district level in the CDC's 2016 School Health Policies and Practices study and reported in the 2018 United States Report Card on Physical Activity for Children and Youth (NPAPA, 2018). Unfortunately, little research describes these programs or their origins and evolution. What brought them to life? What sustains them? What secures their future? What ensures the survival of a CSPAP in the natural selection of school policy and practice? A robust knowledge base of long-standing CSPAPs will allow future program implementation efforts to draw upon the wisdom of their forerunners and pioneers— the teachers who first pushed the boundaries of physical education and PA into uncharted territory. The construction of such a database would necessitate inquiry of school context.

Promoting

- The variety of CSPAP interventions is quickly expanding as researchers search for the most effective PA promotion strategies. Some of these approaches more closely align than others do with the multicomponent spirit of the CSPAP model.

- Promotion is one of four keys to marketing CSPAP initiatives. The other three keys are *product* (e.g., PA), *price* (e.g., cost or barriers), and *place* (e.g., location). Effective CSPAP promotion strategies, especially when resources are restricted, are media advertising (television, Internet, and print), social media outlets, print mailings, posted flyers and point-of-decision prompts, and announcements given in support programs. Promotion should occur both within the school and throughout the local community setting (chapter 19).

- When resources are limited, schools might consider employing three important messaging strategies when asking for resources: (1) *strategies* for knowing and tailoring to a specific audience; (2) the *content* of the message; and (3) a *vehicle*, or strategies for delivering the content (refer to previous bullet point for some possibilities; chapter 19).

- Advocacy strategies for CSPAPs and, more broadly, PA promotion should follow a three-step model: (1) gather and translate PA evidence into the *why* for PA; (2) create the *what*, or a central PA message or agenda; and (3) identify *how to influence support* (e.g., political forums, media outlets, and professional mobilization) and *whom to target* within the school or community. Presently, there are no known data-based publications focused on advocacy strategies specific to CSPAPs and PA outcomes (chapter 19).

- A gap in the literature and in everyday practice involves preparing in-service physical education teachers to advocate for CSPAPs (chapter 19). There are encouraging signs of progress, though. Colorado now offers a three-tiered approach to professional development for the cultivation of CSPAPs and PA leadership among in-service teachers, mostly physical educators (Dauenhauer et al., 2018).

What Are the Potential Contributions of Preservice Education and Technology Integration in CSPAP Research and Practice?

The bulleted response material in this section comes mostly from part VI, Looking to the Future.

Preservice Education

Since the 2017 special issue of the *Journal of Physical Education, Recreation & Dance* regarding CSPAPs in physical education teacher education (PETE) programs (Kulinna et al., 2017), steady progress has been made in preparing preservice physical education students in CSPAP implementation and adopting a school PA leadership role. Resultant contributions of PETE programs and potential areas for continued growth are italicized in the following bulleted items and detailed in chapter 20.

- *CSPAP knowledge, skills, and experiences* for PETE students are public health aligned; based on behavior change theory; and integrate concepts of PA promotion, PA role modeling, leadership development, cultural relevancy, and family and community engagement (Webster et al., 2015). Rather than integrating CSPAP knowledge, skills, and experiences into existing coursework, practica, and internships, PETE programs might consider offering separate or new learning experiences in CSPAPs (chapter 20).

- The depth of CSPAP integration into *graduate PETE programs* is equally important to preservice education. At the doctoral level, training students in CSPAPs and the expanded role of PA leadership is important to ensuring future PETE faculty members endorse a CSPAP-oriented approach in their teaching and research. For example, doctoral programs at the University of Utah and the University of South Carolina prepare candidates to adopt perspectives and skills inclusive of whole-of-school approaches to physical education and PA (chapter 20).

- Recruit teacher candidates who may have a *subjective warrant* for CSPAPs and the expanded role of physical education teachers in such programs (Webster et al., 2015). Seek prospective PETE students (undergraduate or graduate) who have either been predisposed to CSPAPs in their K-12 education or enacted the PA leadership role as teachers (chapter 20).

- Inconsistencies and disagreements among *current PETE faculty and mentor teachers* hinder the possibilities of CSPAPs in preservice education. PETE faculty's CSPAP knowledge and beliefs in preparing future teachers for non–physical education CSPAP components can prevent CSPAP integration in PETE programs. Very few mentor teachers implement a full CSPAP, which limits the real-world examples for teacher candidates to observe or experience (chapter 20). Moving forward, it may be critical to communicate to teacher educators how a CSPAP can serve to reinforce and strengthen physical education programs. It is imperative to dispel dichotomous or dualistic views of physical education (i.e., physical education vs. PA). All CSPAP components can be designed to support students' PA, learning, and development in ways that align with standards and grade-level outcomes in physical education (Webster et al., 2016).

- PETE curricula constraints, often driven by teacher education accreditation standards (Council for the Accreditation of Educator Preparation, 2013) and standards for initial PETE (SHAPE America, 2017), can determine the degree of CSPAP integration in preservice education. If standards for beginning physical education teachers continue to ignore CSPAP-related skills as part of the professional preparation of teacher candidates (SHAPE America, 2017), the possibilities of CSPAPs in PETE will remain spotty and confined to faculty members' subjectivities (i.e., CSPAP knowledge, values, and beliefs; chapter 20).

- Studies of PETE programs successfully integrating CSPAPs, PETE program changes related to CSPAPs and stakeholders' perceptions of these changes, and preservice student outcomes (physical education instruction, CSPAP implementation in K-12 schools, and PA levels of K-12 students) from teacher education program transformations are needed to continue to move the contributions of PETE programs forward (chapter 20).

- The promise of preservice education to CSPAPs extends to classroom teachers—both during their formal teacher education training and early career phases. Understanding ways to influence classroom teachers' PA knowledge, PA pedagogical content knowledge, and PA beliefs and perceptions—particularly when teachers lack personal wellness or student health priorities—continues to be a worthy area for study (chapters 9 and 20).

Technology Integration

The material for this section is found in chapter 21.

- Technology for CSPAPs includes active video games, online social media, mobile devices and apps, health wearables, virtual and augmented virtual reality, and global positioning systems (GPS) and geographic information systems (GIS).

- The research base on technology-facilitated CSPAP programming is still young and lacks large-scale, methodologically rigorous studies. Even so, the proliferation of technologies to support PA-related behavior already has changed the way people across society think about and engage with their own and others' PA and overall health.

- Active video games and virtual reality technologies should be promoted as alternatives to sedentary screen entertainment options but should not be viewed as a replacement for traditional forms of PA.

- The Internet and social media continue to grow as central sources of communication and education; research seeking to optimize the use of these platforms for CSPAP interventions is recommended.

- Mobile and smartphone technology is emerging as another vehicle for CSPAP interventions and merits increased attention by researchers.

- Health wearables have obtained widespread popularity among consumers and deserve increased investigation as potential devices for measurement and promotion of both personal and public PA and health.

- GPS and GIS have introduced novel possibilities for population-level research on PA behavior and the influence of the environment on such behavior.

- CSPAP interventions initiated with the aim of eventually scaling up should consider how technology can inform the design, implementation, and sustainability of the program so that the program is as effective at scale as it was when pilot tested.

Advancement Strategies

A scrutiny of the synthesized knowledge base reflected in the chapter-based responses provides many CSPAP research and practice considerations for the future. In the following text, we have summarized what are, in our estimation, the *top 10 advancement strategies*, five for research and five for practice, for stimulating the next phase of CSPAPs. These strategies may serve as the basis for putting evidence-based research into practice with CSPAPs and may be supplemented with other sources for research (Erwin et al., 2018) and practical recommendations (Active Schools, 2018).

Top Five Strategies to Advance CSPAP Research

1. Focus research on *youth outcome measures* beyond physical health indicators for the comprehensive goals of CSPAPs to be realized (e.g., Burns et al., 2016). CSPAP research might use indicators from the CDC's (2014) health and academic achievement resource to examine CSPAP linkages to students' academic performance (e.g., class grades, test scores, graduation rates, and performance related to K-12 physical education standards), education behavior (e.g., attendance, dropout rates, and on-task behavior), and cognitive skills (e.g., concentration and memory). Further, interconnections between CSPAP- and WSCC-related (ASCD, 2018) areas of development (e.g., social-emotional learning) warrant research attention (chapters 4 and 18).

2. Expand the purview of CSPAP intervention research to target and *capture the benefits of CSPAPs beyond youth*, such as staff wellness, teacher retention, and family and community health indicators. Do CSPAP efforts reach beyond students to staff, family, and the community? Research dedicated to the role and impact of the CSPAP components of staff involvement and family and community engagement is sorely needed (Chen & Gu, 2018; Hunt & Metzler, 2017; Russ et al., 2015).

3. Examine the important *process aspects* of CSPAP implementation, such as dose delivered, dose received, fidelity and quality of implementation, and cost effectiveness. Such research is critical to understanding the linkages between program implementation, uptake, and effectiveness and will provide formative data during an intervention so that CSPAP initiatives can be adjusted to better meet the needs of intended audiences in the school and community (chapters 17 and 18).

4. Apply *rigorous research designs*, such as randomized controlled groups, field-based experiments, longitudinal methods, large-scale sampling strategies, and sound and consistently used outcome measures, to fully understand the impact of CSPAPs (chapters 17 and 18).

5. Explore the influence of *simplified operationalizations of the full CSPAP model*. One possible simplification could be reducing a full CSPAP into only the components of (1) physical education, (2) PA during school, and (3) PA before and after school. In this reduced model, staff involvement and family and community engagement would serve as support mechanisms rather than be required components. Another possibility for simplification could be a three-component version of a multicomponent CSPAP model: (1) physical education, (2) student PA opportunities at school (including PA during school and PA before and after school), and (3) PA opportunities that engage adults (including staff involvement and family and community engagement). Beets and colleague's (2016) theory of expanded, extended, and enhanced

opportunities for youth PA promotion could guide research designs.

Top Five Strategies to Advance CSPAP Practice

1. Provide *professional development or in-service training opportunities* for not only physical education teachers but also for all possible PA champions in and around school communities (e.g., classroom teachers, school and district administrators, school and district wellness committees, student wellness teams, health and wellness community partners, parents, and universities). CSPAP-related professional training can raise awareness for the importance of physically active schools and, with further research evidence, possibly improve CSPAP implementation, outcomes, and sustainability (chapter 4). Sharing local needs and assets–based baseline data with multiple school stakeholders has shown early success in increasing buy-in and improving student PA outcomes (Carson et al., 2018; chapter 16).

2. Accumulate considerably more *CSPAP support from within education communities.* Within physical education, which is recognized as the cornerstone component of a CSPAP, teacher educators disagree about the role of physical education teachers in CSPAPs. Formal accountability measures for teacher education programs (e.g., PETE standards) neglect CSPAP implementation (chapter 4), and few states adopt academic standards for K-12 students that are public health–aligned or include CSPAP experiences (chapter 20).

3. Shift attention from CSPAP adoption and implementation to CSPAP sustainability and diffusion. This shift will require moving beyond proof-of-concept studies and case examples to *CSPAP initiatives designed for durability and scalability.* Utilizing the CSPAP practice- and research-based evidence shared in this book or elsewhere (Stoepker et al., 2018) is a recommended strategy for CSPAP planning and implementation longevity.

4. Certain aspects of CSPAP implementation success appear to transcend the power of building human capacity. To date, there has been an overreliance on the leader level of the CSPAP conceptual framework and the influences from a CSPAP champion and CSPAP organizers and supporters (Carson et al., 2014). In reality, schools that embrace and endorse CSPAPs may have strong cultural influences in terms of school policies ("little p" policy) and community-wide norms or physical or financial facilitators in terms of the built environment, extra work incentives, and advocacy resources. It may be time to nurture *effective CSPAP practices that stem from contextual features and environmental resources.*

5. Continue to align CSPAP practice to frameworks of multicomponent school PA promotion as well as to the overlapping *synergies and practical influences of broader healthy school models (WSCC); current national policies (ESSA); and the educational standards* (including physical education standards) schools tend to prioritize.

SUMMARY

We are hopeful for what this book can accomplish. While putting CSPAP research into practice is still in many ways a fledgling science, the growing number of diverse and exceptional scholars and practitioners is reaching a critical mass for carving a new niche in the knowledge base pertaining to the school as a vehicle for youth PA promotion. Notwithstanding the significant progress made to invigorate and energize a CSPAP field as mainstream, much work still lies ahead for CSPAPs to remain the authoritative approach for increasing PA opportunities in and around schools (CDC, 2017). It is time now to capitalize on and learn from the considerable interest, passion, and long-standing examples of CSPAPs in the United States and in international settings (chapters 1 and 14; Active Schools, 2018). Success is to be measured by the wide audience of champions adopting CSPAPs in their work, inclusive of researchers, graduate students, school and district professionals, community partners, teacher educators, teacher candidates, national and state organizations and agencies, local policy makers, parents and parent organizations, and others with a stake in educational reform and the overall health and well-being of children and adolescents. This book serves as a resource for mobilizing and supporting future progress.

REFERENCES

Preface

Centers for Disease Control and Prevention. (2015). *National framework for physical activity and physical education.* Retrieved from www.cdc.gov/healthyschools/physicalactivity/pdf/National_Framework_Physical_Activity_and_Physical_Education_Resources_Support_CSPAP_508_tagged.pdf

Centers for Disease Control and Prevention. (2017). *Increasing physical education and physical activity: A framework for schools.* Retrieved from www.cdc.gov/healthyschools/physicalactivity/pdf/17_278143-A_PE-PA-Framework_508.pdf

Chapter 1

Active Schools. (2018). *About us.* Retrieved from www.activeschoolsus.org/about

Annie E. Casey Foundation. (2017). *2017 KIDS COUNT Data Book: State Trends in Child Well-Being.* Retrieved from www.aecf.org/m/resourcedoc/aecf-2017kidscountdatabook.pdf

Barroso, C.S., Kelder, S.H., Springer, A.E., Smith, C.L., Ranjit, N., Ledingham, C., & Hoelscher, D.M. (2009). Senate Bill 42: Implementation and impact on physical activity in middle schools. *Journal of Adolescent Health, 45,* S82-S90.

Bassett, D.R., Fitzhugh, E.C., Heath, G.W., Erwin, P.C., Frederick, G.M., Wolff, D., . . . Stout, A.B. (2013). Estimated energy expenditures for school-based policies and active living. *American Journal of Preventive Medicine, 44,* 108-113.

Bauer, U.E., Briss, P.A., Goodman, R.A., & Bowman, B.A. (2014). Prevention of chronic disease in the 21st century: Elimination of the leading preventable causes of premature death and disability in the USA. *Lancet, 384,* 45-52.

Berliner, D.C., Glass, G.V., & Associates (2014). *50 Myths & Lies That Threaten America's Public Schools: The Real Crisis in Education.* New York, NY: Teachers College Press.

Biddle, S.J.H., Gorely, T., & Stensel, D.J. (2004). Health-enhancing physical activity and sedentary behavior in children. *Journal of Sports Science, 22,* 679-701.

Blankenship, B. (2013). Knowledge/skills and physical activity: Two different coins, or two sides of the same coin? *Journal of Physical Education, Recreation & Dance, 84*(6), 5-6.

Bulger, S., Jones, E.M., Taliaferro, A.R., & Wayda, V. (2015). If you build it, they will come (or not): Going the distance in teacher candidate recruitment. *Quest, 67,* 73-92.

Carson, R.L. (2018, March). *CSPAP research SIG forum.* Annual CSPAP research SIG session at the annual meeting of Society of Health and Physical Educators in America, Nashville, TN.

Carson, R.L., Castelli, D.M., Beighle, A., & Erwin, H. (2014). School-based physical activity promotion: A conceptual framework for research and practice. *Childhood Obesity, 10,* 100-106.

Carson, R.L., Castelli, D.M., Pulling Kuhn, A.C., Moore, J.B., Beets, M.W., Beighle, A., . . . Glowacki, E.M. (2014). Impact of trained champions of comprehensive school physical activity programs on school physical activity offerings, youth physical activity and sedentary behaviors. *Preventive Medicine, 69,* S12-S19.

Carson, R.L., Pulling, A.C., Castelli, D.M., & Beighle, A. (2014). Facilitators and inhibitors of the DPA program and CSPAP implementation. *Research Quarterly for Exercise and Sport, 85*(Suppl. 1), A-56.

Castelli, D.M., & Beighle, A. (2007). The physical education teacher as school activity director. *Journal of Physical Education, Recreation & Dance, 78*(5), 25-28.

Cawley, J., Meyerhoefer, C., & Newhouse, D. (2007). The correlation of youth physical activity with state policies. *Contemporary Economic Policy, 25,* 506-517.

Centers for Disease Control and Prevention (CDC). (1997). *Guidelines for school and community programs to promote lifelong physical activity among young people.* Retrieved from www.cdc.gov/mmwr/PDF/rr/rr4606.pdf

Centers for Disease Control and Prevention (CDC). (2001). *Increasing physical activity: A report on recommendations of the task force on community preventive services.* Retrieved from www.cdc.gov/mmwr/preview/mmwrhtml/rr5018a1.htm

Centers for Disease Control and Prevention (CDC). (2013). *Comprehensive school physical activity programs: A guide for schools.* Retrieved from www.cdc.gov/healthyschools/physicalactivity/pdf/13_242620-A_CSPAP_SchoolPhysActivityPrograms_Final_508_12192013.pdf

Centers for Disease Control and Prevention (CDC). (2015). *National framework for physical activity and physical education.* Retrieved from www.cdc.gov/healthyschools/physicalactivity/pdf/National_Framework_Physical_Activity_and_Physical_Education_Resources_Support_CSPAP_508_tagged.pdf

Cohen, D.A., Scribner, R.A., & Farley, T.A. (2000). A structural model of health behavior: A pragmatic approach to explain and influence health behaviors at the population level. *Preventive Medicine, 30,* 146–154.

Cordon, G., & De Bourdeaudhuij, I.M.M. (2002). Physical education and physical activity in elementary schools in Flanders. *European Journal of Physical Education, 7*(1), 5-18. doi:http://dx.doi.org/10.1080/1740898020070102

Erwin, H., Beighle, A., Carson, R.L., & Castelli, D.M. (2013). Comprehensive school-based physical activity promotion: A review. *Quest, 65*(4), 412-428.

Erwin, H., Fedewa, A., & Ahn, S. (2012). Student academic performance outcomes of a classroom physical activity intervention: Pilot study. *International Electronic Journal of Elementary Education, 4,* 473-487.

Evenson, K.R., Ballard, K., Lee, G., & Ammerman, A. (2009). Implementation of a school-based state policy to increase physical activity. *Journal of School Health, 79,* 231-238.

Goh, T.L., Hannon, J., Webster, C.A., Podlog, L.W., Brusseau, T., & Newton, M. (2014). Chapter 7: Effects of a classroom-based physical activity program on children's physical activity levels. *Journal of Teaching in Physical Education, 33*(4), 558-572.

Harvey, S., Song, Y., Baek, J., & van der Mars, H. (2016). Two sides of the same coin: Student physical activity levels during a game-centered soccer unit. *European Physical Education Review, 22,* 411–429. doi:10.1177/1356336X15614783

Heath, G.W., Parra, D.C., Sarmiento, O.L., Andersen, L.B., Owen, N., Goenka, S., . . . Brownson, R.C. (2012). Evidence-based intervention in physical activity: Lessons from around the world. *Lancet, 380,* 272–281.

Hovell, M.F., Wahlgren, D.R., & Gehrman, C.A. (2002). The behavioral ecological model: Integrating public health and behavioral science. In R.J. DeClemente, R.A. Crosby, & M. Kegler (Eds.), *Emerging theories in health promotion practice and research: Strategies for improving public health* (pp. 340-385). San Francisco, CA: Jossey-Bass.

Institute of Medicine (2013). *Educating the student body: Taking physical activity and physical education to school.* The National Academies Press. Washington, DC. Available at www.nationalacademies.org/hmd/Reports/2013/Educating-the-Student-Body-Taking-Physical-Activity-and-Physical-Education-to-School.aspx

Kahan, D., & McKenzie, T.L. (2015). The potential and reality of physical education in controlling overweight and obesity. *American Journal of Public Health, 105,* 653-659.

Katula, P. (2012). *Teachers' strikes are illegal in most states.* Retrieved from http://schoolsnapshots.org/blog/2012/09/23/teachers-strikes-are-illegal-in-most-states

Katzmarzyk, P.T., Lee, I.M., Martin, C.K., & Blair, S.N. (2017). Epidemiology of physical activity and exercise training in the United States. *Progress in Cardiovascular Diseases, 60*(1), 3-10.

Kelder, S.H., Mitchell, P.D., McKenzie, T.L., Derby, C., Strikmiller, P.K., Luepker, R.V., & Stone, E.J. (2003). Long-term implementation of the CATCH physical education program. *Health Education & Behavior, 30,* 463-475. doi:10.1177/1090198103253538

Kelder, S.H., Springer, A.E., Barroso, C.S., Smith, C.L., Sanchez, E., Ranjit, N., . . . Hoelscher, D.M. (2009). Implementation of Texas Senate Bill 19 to increase physical activity in elementary schools. *Journal of Public Health Policy, 30,* S221-S247.

Kulinna, P.H., Carson, R.L., & Castelli, D.M. (Eds.). (2017). Integrating CSPAP in PETE programs: Sharing insight and identifying strategies [Special Issue–Part 1 & 2]. *Journal of Physical Education, Recreation & Dance, 88*(1&2).

Kretchmar, R. S. (2006). Ten more reasons for quality physical education. *Journal of Physical Education, Recreation & Dance, 77*(9), 6–9. doi:10.1080/07303084.2006.10597932

Kwon, J., Kulinna, P., van der Mars, H., Beardsley, A., & Koro-Ljungberg, M. (2017, March). *CSPAP preparation in physical education teacher education programs.* Paper presented at the SHAPE America National Convention, Boston, MA.

Lohrmann, D.K. (2010). A complementary ecological model of the coordinated school health program. *Journal of School Health, 80,* 1-9.

Lorenz, K.A., van der Mars, H., Kulinna, P.H., Ainsworth, B.E., & Hovell, M.F. (2017). Environmental and behavioral influences of physical activity in junior high school students. *Journal of Physical Activity and Health, 14,* 785-792.

Lounsbery, M.A., McKenzie, T.L., Morrow, J.R., Monnat, S.M., & Holt, K.A. (2013). District and school physical education policies: Implications for physical education and recess time. *Annals of Behavioral Medicine, 45*(1), 131-141.

Lovenheim, M.F., & Willén, A. (2016). *A bad bargain.* Retrieved from www.educationnext.org/bad-bargain-teacher-collective-bargaining-employment-earnings/

Luepker, R.V., Perry, C.L., McKinlay, S.M., Nader, P.R., Parcel, G.S., Stone, E.J., . . . Kelder, S.H. (1996). Outcomes of a field trial to improve children's dietary patterns and physical activity: The Child and Adolescent Trial for Cardiovascular Health (CATCH). *Journal of the American Medical Association, 275,* 768-776.

Luntz, F. (2007). *Words that work: It's not what you say, it's what people hear.* New York, NY: Hyperion.

Mahar, M.T. (2011). Impact of short bouts of physical activity on attention-to-task in elementary school children. *Preventive Medicine, 52,* S60-S64. http://dx.doi.org/10.1016/j.ypmed.2011.01.026

Mahar, M.T., Murphy, S.K., Rowe, D.A., Golden, J., Shields, A.T., & Raedeke, T.D. (2006). Effects of a classroom-based program on physical activity and on-task behavior. *Medicine & Science in Sports & Exercise, 38,* 2086-2094. http://dx.doi.org/10.1249/01.mss.0000235359.16685.a3

Mahar, M.T., Vuchenich, M.L., Golden, J., DuBose, K.D., & Raedeke, T.D. (2011). Effects of a before-school physical activity program on physical activity and on-task behavior [Abstract]. *Medicine & Science in Sports & Exercise, 43*(5), 24. http://dx.doi.org/10.1249/01.MSS.0000402740.12322.07

Makel, M.C., & Plucker, J.A. (2014). Facts are more important than novelty: Replication in the education sciences. *Educational Researcher, 43,* 304-316.

Malin, M.H., Hodges, A.C., & Slater, E. (2012). *Public*

sector employment cases and materials (2nd ed.). Eagan, MN: West Publishing.

McKenzie, T.L., Catellier, D.J., Conway, T., Lytle, L.A., Grieser, M., Webber, L.A., . . . Elder, J.P. (2006). Girls' activity levels and lesson contexts in middle school PE: TAAG baseline. *Medicine & Science in Sports & Exercise, 38,* 1229-1235.

McKenzie, T.L., Marshall, S.J., Sallis, J.F., & Conway, T.L. (2000). Leisure-time physical activity in school environments: An observational study using SOPLAY. *Preventive Medicine, 30,* 70-77. http://10.1249/01.mss.0000227307.34149.f3

McKenzie, T.L., Nader, P.R., Strikmiller, K., Yang, M., Stone, E.J., & Perry, C.L. (1996). School physical education: Effect of the Child and Adolescent Trial for Cardiovascular Health. *Preventive Medicine, 25,* 423-431.

McMullen, J.M., Ní Chróinín, D., Tammelin, T., Pogorzelska, M., & van der Mars, H. (2015). International approaches to whole-of-school physical activity promotion. *Quest, 67,* 384-399.

Metzler, M. (2015). *Final report: Establishing a comprehensive school physical activity program.* Retrieved from https://kh.education.gsu.edu/files/2016/06/GSU-CDC-CSPAP.pdf

Metzler, M.W., McKenzie, T.L., van der Mars, H., Williams, L.H., & Ellis, S.R. (2013a). Health Optimizing Physical Education (HOPE): A new curriculum model for school programs. Part 1: Establishing the need and describing the curriculum model. *Journal of Physical Education, Recreation & Dance, 84*(4), 41-47.

Metzler, M.W., McKenzie, T.L., van der Mars, H., Williams, L.H., & Ellis, S.R. (2013b). Health Optimizing Physical Education (HOPE): A new curriculum model for school programs. Part 2: Teacher knowledge and collaboration for HOPE. *Journal of Physical Education, Recreation & Dance, 84*(5), 25-34.

Miller, A., Christensen, E., Eather, N., Gray, S., Sproule, J., Keay, J., & Lubans, D. (2016). Can physical education and physical activity outcomes be developed simultaneously using a game-centered approach? *European Physical Education Review, 22,* 113-133. http://10.1177/1356336X15594548

National Association for Sport and Physical Education (NASPE). (2008). *Comprehensive school physical activity programs* [Position statement]. Reston, VA: Author.

National Center for Education Statistics. (2016). *Elementary and secondary enrollment.* Retrieved from https://nces.ed.gov/programs/coe/indicator_cga.asp

National Physical Activity Plan Alliance (NPAPA). (2010). *U.S. national physical activity plan.* Columbia, SC: Author.

National Physical Activity Plan Alliance (NPAPA). (2014). *The 2014 United States report card on physical activity for children and youth.* Retrieved from http://physicalactivityplan.org/reportcard/NationalReportCard_longform_final%20for%20web.pdf

National Physical Activity Plan Alliance (NPAPA). (2016a). *The 2016 United States report card on physical activity for children and youth.* Retrieved from www.physicalactivityplan.org/reportcard/2016FINAL_USReportCard.pdf

National Physical Activity Plan Alliance (NPAPA). (2016b). *U.S. national physical activity plan.* Retrieved from http://physicalactivityplan.org/docs/2016NPAP_Final-forwebsite.pdf

National Physical Activity Plan Alliance (NPAPA). (2018). *The 2018 United States report card on physical activity for children and youth.* Retrieved from http://physicalactivityplan.org/projects/reportcard.html

Naylora, P.J., Macdonald, H.M., Zebedeea, J.A., Reed, K.E., & McKay, H.A. (2006). Lessons learned from Action Schools! BC—An 'active school' model to promote physical activity in elementary schools. *Journal of Science and Medicine in Sport, 9*(5), 413-423.

Ogden, C.L., Carroll, M.D., Lawman, H.G., Fryar, C.D., Kruszon-Moran, D., Kit, B.K., & Flegal, K.M. (2016). Trends in obesity prevalence among children and adolescents in the United States, 1988-1994 through 2013-2014. *Journal of the American Medical Association, 315,* 2292-2299.

Omura, J.D., Carlson, S.A., Paul, P., Sliwa, S., Onufrak, S.J., & Fulton, J.E. (2017). Shared use agreements between municipalities and public schools in the United States, 2014. *Preventive Medicine, 95,* S53-S59.

Pate, R.R., Davis, M.G., Robinson, T.N., Stone, E.J., McKenzie, T.L., & Young, J.C. (2006). Promoting physical activity in children and youth: A leadership role for schools. *Circulation, 114,* 1214-1224.

Pate, R.R., Freedson, D.S., Sallis, J.F., Taylor, W.C., Sirard, J., Trost, S.G., & Dowda, M. (2002). Compliance with physical activity guidelines: Prevalence in a population of children and youth. *Annals of Epidemiology, 12,* 303-308.

Reid, G. (2009). Delivering sustainable practice? A case study of the Scottish Active Schools programme. *Sport, Education and Society, 14,* 353-370, http://dx.doi.org/10.1080/13573320903037879

Richards, K.A.R., & Gaudreault, K.L. (Eds.). (2017). *Teacher socialization in physical education: New perspectives.* New York, NY: Routledge.

Ridgers, N.D., Stratton, G., Fairclough, S.J., & Twisk, J.W.R. (2007). Long-term effects of playground markings and physical structures on children's recess physical activity levels. *Preventive Medicine, 44,* 393-397.

Rink, J., Hall, T., & Williams, L. (2010). *Schoolwide physical activity: A comprehensive guide to designing and conducting programs.* Champaign. IL: Human Kinetics.

Russ, L.B., Webster, C.A., Beets, M.W., & Phillips, D.S. (2015). Systematic review and meta-analysis of multicomponent interventions through schools to increase physical activity. *Journal of Physical Activity and Health, 12,* 1436-1446.

Sallis, J.F. (2017). Evidence is a more fruitful approach for advancing the field than philosophy: Comment on Landi et al. (2016). *Journal of Teaching in Physical Education, 36,* 129-130. https://doi.org/10.1123/jtpe.2017-0032

Sallis, J.F., & McKenzie, T.L. (1991). Physical education's role in public health. *Research Quarterly for Exercise and Sport, 62,* 124-137. http://dx.doi.org/10.1080/02701367.1991.10608701

Sallis, J.F., McKenzie, T.L., Alcaraz, J.E., Koldy, B., Faucette, N., & Hovell, M.F. (1997). The effects of a 2-year physical education program (SPARK) on physical activity and fitness in elementary school students. *American Journal of Public Health, 87,* 1328-1334.

Sallis, J.F., McKenzie, T.L., Beets, M.W., Beighle, A., Erwin, H., & Lee, S. (2012). Physical education's role in public health: Steps forward and backward over 20 years and HOPE for the future. *Research Quarterly for Exercise and Sport, 83,* 125-135.

Sallis, J.F., Owen, N., & Fisher, E.B. (2008). Ecological models of health behavior. In K. Glanz, B.K. Rimer, & K. Viswanath (Eds.), *Health behavior and health education: Theory, research, and practice* (4th ed., pp. 465-485). San Francisco, CA: Jossey-Bass.

SHAPE America. (2013). *Comprehensive school physical activity programs: Helping students achieve 60 minutes of physical activity each day* [Position statement]. Retrieved from www.shapeamerica.org/advocacy/positionstatements/pa/upload/Comprehensive-School-Physical-Activity-programs-2013.pdf

SHAPE America. (2016). *2016 Shape of the nation: Status of physical education in the USA.* Retrieved from www.shapeamerica.org/advocacy/son/2016/upload/Shape-of-the-Nation-2016_web.pdf

SHAPE America (2017). *Initial physical education teacher education standards.* Reston, VA: Author. Retrieved from www.shapeamerica.org/accreditation/upload/National-Standards-for-Initial-Physical-Education-Teacher-Education-2017.pdf

Siedentop, D.L. (2009). National Plan for Physical Activity: Education sector. *Journal of Physical Activity and Health, 6*(Suppl. 2), S168-S180.

Siedentop, D., & van der Mars H. (2012). *Introduction to physical education, fitness, and sport* (8th ed.). St. Louis, MO: McGraw-Hill.

Slater, S.J., Nicholson, L., Chriqui, J., Turner, L., & Chaloupka, F. (2012). The impact of state laws and district policies on physical education and recess practices in a nationally representative sample of US public elementary schools. *Archives of Pediatrics & Adolescent Medicine, 166,* 311-316.

Spengler, J.O. (2012). *Promoting physical activity through the shared use of school and community recreational resources* [Research brief]. Retrieved from http://activelivingresearch.org/promoting-physical-activity-through-shared-use-school-and-community-recreational-resources

Stodden, D.F., Goodway, J.D., Langendorfer, S.J., Roberton, M.A., Rudisill, M.E., Garcia, C., & Garcia, L.E. (2008). A developmental perspective on the role of motor skill competence in physical activity: An emergent relationship. *Quest, 60,* 290-306.

Stokols, D. (1992). Establishing and maintaining healthy environments: Toward a social ecology of health promotion. *American Psychologist, 4,* 6-22.

Stratton, G., & Mullan, E. (2005). The effect of multicolor playground markings on children's physical activity level during recess. *Preventive Medicine, 41,* 828-833.

Stylianou, M., Hodges-Kulinna, P.H., van der Mars, H., Mahar, M.T., Adams, M.A., & Amazeen, E. (2016). Before-school running/walking club: Effects on student on-task behavior. *Preventive Medicine Reports, 3,* 196-202. http://10.1016/j.pmedr.2016.01.010

Stylianou, M., van der Mars, H., Hodges-Kulinna, P.H., Adams, M.A., Mahar, M.M., & Amazeen, E. (2016). Before-school running/walking club and student physical activity levels: An efficacy study. *Research Quarterly for Exercise and Sport, 87,* 342-353. http://10.1080/02701367.2016.1214665

Sutherland, R.L. Campbell, E.M., Lubans, D.R., Morgan, P.J., Nathan, N.K., Wolfenden, L., . . . Wiggers, J.H. (2016). The physical activity 4 everyone cluster randomized trial 2-year outcomes of a school physical activity intervention among adolescents. *American Journal of Preventive Medicine, 51,* 195-205.

U.S. Department of Health and Human Services (HHS). (1990). *Healthy people 2000.* Washington, DC: U.S. Government Printing Office.

U.S. Department of Health and Human Services (HHS). (2000). *Healthy people 2010.* Washington, DC: U.S. Government Printing Office.

U.S. Department of Health and Human Services (HHS). (2008). *2008 Physical activity guidelines for Americans.* Retrieved from https://health.gov/paguidelines/pdf/paguide.pdf

U.S. Department of Health and Human Services (HHS). (2018). *2018 Physical activity guidelines for Americans Advisory Committee Scientific Report.* Retrieved from https://health.gov/paguidelines/second-edition/report/pdf/PAG_Advisory_Committee_Report.pdf

U.S. Department of Health and Human Services (HHS). (2010). *Healthy people 2020.* Washington, DC: U.S. Government Printing Office.

U.S. Department of Health and Human Services (HHS). (2012). *Physical activity guidelines for Americans midcourse report: Strategies to increase physical activity among youth.* Retrieved from https://health.gov/paguidelines/midcourse/pag-mid-course-report-final.pdf

van der Mars, H. (2017). Breaking news: High schools surpass elusive goal for physical education minutes per week. *Journal of Physical Education, Recreation & Dance, 88*(4), 3-6. http://dx.doi.org/10.1080/07303084.2017.1285146

van der Mars, H. (2018). Policy development in physical education . . . our last best chance? *Quest, 70*(2), 169-191. https://doi.org/10.1080/00336297.2018.1439391

Ward, D.S. (2011). *School policies on physical education and physical activity.*Retrieved from http://activelivingresearch.org/sites/default/files/Synthesis_Ward_SchoolPolicies_Oct2011_1.pdf

Ward, P., van der Mars, H., Richards, K.A.R., Bulger, S., & Castelli, D. (2017, April). *Rethinking recruitment and retention strategies in undergraduate PETE programs.* Presented at the SHAPE America National Convention, Boston, MA.

Weaver, R.G., Webster, C.A., Erwin, H., Beighle, A., Beets, M.W., Choukroun, H., & Kaysing, N. (2016). Modifying the System for Observing Fitness Instruction Time to measure teacher practices related to physical activity promotion: SOFIT+. *Measurement in Physical Education and Exercise Science, 20,* 121-130. doi:10.10 80/1091367X.2016.1159208

Willenberg, L.J., Ashbolt, R., Holland, D., Gibbs, L., MacDougall, C., Garrard, J., . . . Waters, E. (2010). Increasing school playground physical activity: A mixed methods study combining environmental measures and children's perspectives. *Journal of Science and Medicine in Sport, 13,* 210-216.

Young, R.D., Phillips, J.A., Yu, T., & Haythornthwaite, J.A. (2006). Effects of a life skills intervention for increasing physical activity in adolescent girls. *Archives of Pediatrics & Adolescent Medicine, 160,* 1255-1261.

Chapter 2

Bartholomew, J.B., Jowers, E.M., Roberts, G., Fall, A.-M., Errisuriz, V.L., & Vaughn, S. (2018). Active learning increases children's physical activity across demographic subgroups. *Translational Journal of the American College of Sports Medicine, 3*(1), 1-9.

Belansky, E.S., Cutforth, N., Delong, E., Ross, C., Scarbro, S., Gilbert, L., . . . Marshall, J.A. (2009). Early impact of the federally mandated Local Wellness Policy on physical activity in rural, low-income elementary schools in Colorado. *Journal of Public Health Policy, 30*(Suppl. 1), S141-S160. doi:10.1057/jphp.2008.50

Boles, M., Dilley, J.A., Dent, C., Elman, M.R., Duncan, S.C., & Johnson, D.B. (2011). Changes in local school policies and practices in Washington State after an unfunded physical activity and nutrition mandate. *Preventing Chronic Disease, 8*(6), A129.

Brownson, R.C., Chriqui, J.F., & Stamatakis, K.A. (2009). Understanding evidence-based public health policy. *American Journal of Public Health, 99*(9), 1576-1583. doi:10.2105/AJPH.2008.156224

Carlson, J.A., Sallis, J.F., Chriqui, J.F., Schneider, L., McDermid, L.C., & Agron, P. (2013). State policies about physical activity minutes in physical education or during school. *Journal of School Health, 83*(3), 150-156. doi:10.1111/josh.12010

Carson, R.L., Castelli, D.M., Pulling Kuhn, A.C., Moore, J.B., Beets, M.W., Beighle, A., . . . Glowacki, E.M. (2014). Impact of trained champions of comprehensive school physical activity programs on school physical activ-

ity offerings, youth physical activity and sedentary behaviors. *Preventive Medicine, 69*(Suppl. 1), S12-S19. doi:10.1016/j.ypmed.2014.08.025

Chriqui, J.F., Eyler, A., Carnoske, C., & Slater, S. (2013). State and district policy influences on district-wide elementary and middle school physical education practices. *Journal of Public Health Management & Practice, 19*(Suppl. 1), S41-S48. doi:10.1097/PHH.0b013e31828a8bce

Cradock, A.L., Barrett, J.L., Carter, J., McHugh, A., Sproul, J., Russo, E.T., . . . Gortmaker, S.L. (2014). Impact of the Boston Active School Day policy to promote physical activity among children. *American Journal of Health Promotion, 28*(Suppl. 3), S54-S64. doi:10.4278/ajhp.130430-QUAN-204

Evenson, K.R., Ballard, K., Lee, G., & Ammerman, A. (2009). Implementation of a school-based state policy to increase physical activity. *Journal of School Health, 79*(5), 231-238. doi:10.1111/j.1746-1561.2009.00403.x

Eyler, A.A., Brownson, R.C., Aytur, S.A., Cradock, A.L., Doescher, M., Evenson, K.R., . . . Schmid, T.L. (2010). Examination of trends and evidence-based elements in state physical education legislation: A content analysis. *Journal of School Health, 80*(7), 326-332. doi:10.1111/j.1746-1561.2010.00509.x

Gamble, A., Chatfield, S.L., Cormack, M.L., & Hallam, J.S. (2017). Not enough time in the day: A qualitative assessment of in-school physical activity policy as viewed by administrators, teachers, and students. *Journal of School Health, 87*(1), 21-28.

Kelder, S.H., Springer, A.S., Barroso, C.S., Smith, C.L., Sanchez, E., Ranjit, N., & Hoelscher, D.M. (2009). Implementation of Texas Senate Bill 19 to increase physical activity in elementary schools. *Journal of Public Health Policy, 30*(Suppl. 1), S221-S247. doi:10.1057/jphp.2008.64

Kim, J. (2012). Are physical education-related state policies and schools' physical education requirement related to children's physical activity and obesity? *Journal of School Health, 82*(6), 268-276. doi:10.1111/j.1746-1561.2012.00697.x

Larson, N., Davey, C., Hoffman, P., Kubik, M.Y., & Nanney, M.S. (2016). District wellness policies and school-level practices in Minnesota, USA. *Public Health Nutrition, 19*(1), 26-35. doi:10.1017/S1368980015001500

Mahar, M.T., Murphy, S.K., Rowe, D.A., Golden, J., Shields, A.T., & Raedeke, T.D. (2006). Effects of a classroom-based program on physical activity and on-task behavior. *Medicine & Science in Sports & Exercise, 38*(12), 2086-2094. doi:10.1249/01.mss.0000235359.16685.a3

Metos, J., & Nanney, M.S. (2007). The strength of school wellness policies: One state's experience. *Journal of School Health, 77*(7), 367-372. doi:10.1111/j.1746-1561.2007.00221.x

Nanney, M.S., Nelson, T., Wall, M., Haddad, T., Kubik, M., Laska, M.N., & Story, M. (2010). State school nutrition and physical activity policy environments and youth obesity. *American Journal of Preventive Medicine, 38*(1), 9-16. doi:10.1016/j.amepre.2009.08.031

O'Brien, L.M., Polacsek, M., Macdonald, P.B., Ellis, J., Berry, S., & Martin, M. (2010). Impact of a school health coordinator intervention on health-related school policies and student behavior. *Journal of School Health, 80*(4), 176-185. doi:10.1111/j.1746-1561.2009.00484.x

Phillips, M.M., Raczynski, J.M., West, D.S., Pulley, L., Bursac, Z., Gauss, C.H., & Walker, J.F. (2010). Changes in school environments with implementation of Arkansas Act 1220 of 2003. *Obesity (Silver Spring), 18*(Suppl. 1), S54-S61. doi:10.1038/oby.2009.432

Riis, J., Grason, H., Strobino, D., Ahmed, S., & Minkovitz, C. (2012). State school policies and youth obesity. *Maternal and Child Health Journal, 16*(Suppl. 1), S111-S118. doi:10.1007/s10995-012-1000-4

Robertson-Wilson, J.E., Dargavel, M.D., Bryden, P.J., & Giles-Corti, B. (2012). Physical activity policies and legislation in schools: A systematic review. *American Journal of Preventive Medicine, 43*(6), 643-649. doi:10.1016/j.amepre.2012.08.022

Robinson, L.E., Wadsworth, D.D., Webster, E.K., & Bassett, D.R., Jr. (2014). School reform: The role of physical education policy in physical activity of elementary school children in Alabama's Black Belt Region. *American Journal of Health Promotion, 28*(Suppl. 3), S72-S76. doi:10.4278/ajhp.130430-ARB-207

Russ, L.B., Webster, C.A., Beets, M.W., & Phillips, D.S. (2015). Systematic review and meta-analysis of multicomponent interventions through schools to increase physical activity. *Journal of Physical Activity & Health, 12*(10), 1436-1446. doi:10.1123/jpah.2014-0244

SHAPE America. (2015). *The essential components of physical education.* Retrieved from www.shapeamerica.org/upload/TheEssentialComponentsOfPhysicalEducation.pdf

Taber, D.R., Chriqui, J.F., & Chaloupka, F.J. (2012). Association and diffusion of nutrition and physical activity policies on the state and district level. *Journal of School Health, 82*(5), 201-209. doi:10.1111/j.1746-1561.2012.00688.x

Webber, L.S., Catellier, D.J., Lytle, L.A., Murray, D.M., Pratt, C.A., Young, D.R., . . . Group, T.C.R. (2008). Promoting physical activity in middle school girls: Trial of Activity for Adolescent Girls. *American Journal of Preventive Medicine, 34*(3), 173-184. doi:10.1016/j.amepre.2007.11.018

Weinsier, R.L., Hunter, G.R., Heini, A.F., Goran, M.I., & Sell, S.M. (1998). The etiology of obesity: Relative contribution of metabolic factors, diet, and physical activity. *American Journal of Medicine, 105*(2), 145-150. doi:10.1016/s0002-9343(98)00190-9

Williams, A.J., Henley, W.E., Williams, C.A., Hurst, A.J., Logan, S., & Wyatt, K.M. (2013). Systematic review and meta-analysis of the association between childhood overweight and obesity and primary school diet and physical activity policies. *International Journal of Behavioral Nutrition and Physical Activity, 10*(1), 101. doi:10.1186/1479-5868-10-101

Chapter 3

Agron, P., Berends, V., Ellis, K., & Gonzalez, M. (2010). School wellness policies: Perceptions, barriers, and needs among school leaders and wellness advocates. *Journal of School Health, 80*(11), 527-535.

Allar, I., Elliott, E., Jones, E., Kristjansson, A.L., Taliaferro, A., & Bulger, S.M. (2017). Involving families and communities in CSPAP development using asset mapping. *Journal of Physical Education, Recreation & Dance, 88*(5), 7-14. doi:10.1080/07303084.2017.1280439

Association for Supervision and Curriculum Development & Centers for Disease Control and Prevention (CDC). (2014). *Whole school, whole community, whole child: A collaborative approach to learning and health.* Retrieved from www.cdc.gov/healthyschools/wscc/wsccmodel_update_508tagged.pdf

Beighle, A., Erwin, H.E., Castelli, D., & Ernst, M. (2009). Preparing physical educators for the role of physical activity director. *Journal of Physical Education, Recreation & Dance, 80*(4), 24-29.

Benjamins, M.R., & Whitman, S. (2010). A culturally appropriate school wellness initiative: Results of a 2-year pilot intervention in 2 Jewish schools. *Journal of School Health, 80*(8), 378-386. doi:10.1111/j.1746-1561.2010.00517.x

Berei, C.P. (2015). *Describing and understanding factors related to implementing comprehensive school physical activity programs by physical educators* (Doctoral dissertation). Retrieved from ProQuest Dissertations and Theses database. (UMI No. 3728945)

Buns, M.T., & Thomas, K.T. (2015). Impact of physical educators on local school wellness policies. *Physical Educator, 72*(2), 294-316.

Carson, R. (2012). Certification and duties of a director of physical activity. *Journal of Physical Education, Recreation & Dance, 83*(6), 16-19, 29.

Carson, R.L., Castelli, D.M., Beighle, A., & Erwin, H. (2014). School-based physical activity promotion: A conceptual framework for research and practice. *Childhood Obesity, 10*(2), 100-106. doi:10.1089/chi.2013.0134

Carson, R.L., Castelli, D.M., Pulling Kuhn, A.C., Moore, J.B., Beets, M.W., Beighle, A., . . . Glowacki, E.M. (2014). Impact of trained champions of comprehensive school physical activity programs on school physical activity offerings, youth physical activity, and sedentary behaviors. *Preventive Medicine, 69,* S12-S19.

Carson, R.L., Pulling, A.C., Castelli, D.M., & Beighle, A. (2014). Facilitators and inhibitors of the DPA program and CSPAP implementation. *Research Quarterly for Exercise and Sport, 85*(Suppl. 1), A-56.

Carson, R.L., Castelli, D.M., & Kulinna, P.H. (2017). CSPAP professional preparation: Takeaways from pioneering physical education teacher education programs. *Journal of Physical Education, Recreation & Dance, 88*(2), 43-51.

Castelli, D.M., & Beighle, A. (2007). The physical education teacher as school activity director. *Journal of Physical Education, Recreation & Dance, 78*(5), 25-28.

Castelli, D.M., Centeio, E.E., Beighle, A.E., Carson, R.L., & Nicksic, H.M. (2014). Physical literacy and comprehensive school physical activity programs. *Preventive Medicine, 66*, 95-100.

Castelli, D.M., Carson, R.L., & Kulinna, P.H. (2017). PETE programs creating teacher leaders to integrate comprehensive school physical activity programs. *Journal of Physical Education, Recreation & Dance, 88*(1), 8-10.

Centers for Disease Control and Prevention (CDC). (2013). *Comprehensive school physical activity programs: A guide for schools.* Retrieved from www.cdc.gov/healthyschools/professional_development/e-learning/cspap.html

Centers for Disease Control and Prevention (CDC). (2017). *Increasing physical education and physical activity: A framework for schools.* Retrieved from www.cdc.gov/healthyschools/physicalactivity/pdf/17_278143-A_PE-PA-Framework_508.pdf

Centeio, E.E., Castelli, D.M., Carson, R.L., & Beighle, A. (2014). Implementing a comprehensive school physical activity program into the school setting: Professional development outcomes. *Research Quarterly for Exercise and Sport, 85*(Suppl. 1), A56-A57.

Centeio, E.E., Erwin, H., & Castelli, D.M. (2014). Chapter 4: Comprehensive school physical activity programs: Characteristics of trained teachers. *Journal of Teaching in Physical Education, 33*(4), 492-510.

Centeio, E.E., McCaughtry, N., Gutuskey, L., Garn, A.C., Somers, C., Shen, B., . . . Kulik, N.L. (2014). Chapter 8: Physical activity change through comprehensive school physical activity programs in urban elementary schools. *Journal of Teaching in Physical Education, 33*(4), 573-591.

Chen, S., & Gu, X. (2018). Toward active living: Comprehensive school physical activity program research and implications. *Quest, 70*(2), 191-222. https://doi.org/10.1080/00336297.2017.1365002

Chriqui, J.F., & Chaloupka, F.J. (2011). Transparency and oversight in local wellness policies. *Journal of School Health, 81*(2), 114-121.

Dauenhauer, B., Carson, R.L., Krause, J., Hodgins, K., Jones, T., & Weinberger, C. (2018). Cultivating physical activity leadership in schools: A three-tiered approach to professional development. *Journal of Physical Education, Recreation, & Dance, 89*(9), 51-57.

Dauenhauer, B., Krause, J., Douglas, S., Smith, M., & Babkes Stellino, M. (2017). *Journal of Physical Education, Recreation & Dance, 88*(2), 14-19.

Deslatte, K., & Carson, R.L. (2014). Identifying the common characteristics of comprehensive school physical activity programs in Louisiana. *The Physical Educator, 71*, 610-634.

Doolittle, S.A., & Rukavina, P.B. (2014). Chapter 6: Case study of an institutionalized urban comprehensive school physical activity program. *Journal of Teaching in Physical Education, 33*(4), 528-557.

Dwyer, J.J., Allison, K.R., Barrera, M., Hansen, B., Goldenberg, E., & Boutilier, M.A. (2003). Teacher's perspective on barriers to implementing physical activity curriculum guidelines for school children in Toronto. *Canadian Journal of Public Health, 94*(6), 448-452.

Elliot, E., Erwin, H., Hall, T., & Heidorn, B. (2013). Comprehensive school physical activity programs: Helping all students achieve 60 minutes of physical activity each day. *Journal of Physical Education, Recreation & Dance, 84*(9), 9-15.

Erwin, H., Beets, M.W., Centeio, E., & Morrow, J.R., Jr. (2014). Best practices and recommendations for increasing physical activity in youth. *Journal of Physical Education, Recreation & Dance, 85*(7), 27-34.

Erwin, H., Beighle, A., Carson, R.L., & Castelli, D.M. (2013). Comprehensive school-based physical activity promotion: A review. *Quest, 65*(4), 412-428.

Goc Karp, G., Brown, H., Scruggs, P.W., & Berei, C. (2017). Cultivating leadership, pedagogy and programming for CSPAP and healthy, active lifestyles at the University of Idaho. *Journal of Physical Education, Recreation & Dance, 88*(1), 29-35.

Gollub, E.A., Kennedy, B.M., Bourgeois, B.F., Broyles, S.T., & Katzmarzyk, P.T. (2014). Engaging communities to develop and sustain comprehensive wellness policies: Louisiana's schools putting prevention to work. *Preventing Chronic Disease, 11,* E34. doi:10.5888/pcd11.130149

Heidorn, B., & Centeio, E. (2012). The director of physical activity and staff involvement. *Journal of Physical Education, Recreation & Dance, 83*(7), 13-26.

Heidorn, B.D., Hall, T.J., & Carson, R.L. (2010). Theory into practice: Comprehensive school-based physical activity program. *Strategies, 24*(2), 33-35.

Hills, A.P., Dengel, D.R., & Lubans, D.R. (2015). Supporting public health priorities: Recommendations for physical education and physical activity promotion in schools. *Progress in Cardiovascular Diseases, 57*(4), 368-374.

Hogan, L., Garcia Bengoechea, E., Salsberg, J., Jacobs, J., King, M., & Macaulay, A.C. (2014). Using a participatory approach to the development of a school-based physical activity policy in an indigenous community. *Journal of School Health, 84*(12), 786-792. doi:10.1111/josh.12214

Hughes, L.J., Savoca, L., & Grenci, A. (2015). Empowering youth to take charge of school wellness. *Journal of Extension, 53*(3), 6.

Illg, K.M. (2014). *Identification of school physical activity leader competencies using concept mapping* (Doctoral dissertation). Retrieved from ProQuest Dissertations and Theses database. (UMI No. 3637603)

Israel, B.A., Schulz, A.J., Parker, E.A., & Becker, A.B. (1998). Review of community-based research: Assessing partnership approaches to improve public health. *Annual Review of Public Health, 19*(1), 173-202. doi:10.1146/annurev.publhealth.19.1.173

Jain, A., & Langwith, C. (2013). Collaborative school-based obesity interventions: Lessons learned from 6 southern districts. *Journal of School Health, 83*(3), 213-222.

Jones, E.M., Taliaferro, A.R., Elliott, E.M., Bulger, S.M., Kristjansson, A.L., Neal, W., & Allar, I. (2014). Chapter 3: Feasibility study of comprehensive school physical activity programs in Appalachian communities: The McDowell CHOICES project. *Journal of Teaching in Physical Education, 33*(4), 467-491.

King, K.M., & Ling, J. (2015). Results of a 3-year, nutrition and physical activity intervention for children in rural, low-socioeconomic status elementary schools. *Health Education Research, 30*(4), 647-659.

Kong, A.S., Farnsworth, S., Canaca, J.A., Harris, A., Palley, G., & Sussman, A.L. (2012). An adaptive community-based participatory approach to formative assessment with high schools for obesity intervention. *Journal of School Health, 82*(3), 147-154. doi:10.1111/j.1746-1561.2011.00678.x

Kulinna, P.H., Brusseau, T., Cothran, D., & Tudor-Locke, C. (2012). Changing school physical activity: An examination of individual school designed programs. *Journal of Teaching in Physical Education, 31,* 113-130.

Kulinna, P.H., Carson, R.L., & Castelli, D.M. (Eds.). (2017). Integrating CSPAP in PETE programs: Sharing insight and identifying strategies [Special Issue–Part 1 & 2]. *Journal of Physical Education, Recreation & Dance, 88*(1&2).

Larsen, T., Samdal, O., & Tjomsland, H. (2012). Physical activity in schools: A qualitative case study of eight Norwegian schools' experiences with the implementation of a national policy. *Health Education, 113*(1), 52-63. doi:10.1108/09654281311293637

McMullen, J., Ní Chróinín, D., Tammelin, T., Pogorzelska, M., & van der Mars, H. (2015). International approaches to whole-of-school physical activity promotion. *Quest, 67*(4), 384-399.

McMullen, J., van der Mars, H., & Jahn, J.A. (2014). Chapter 2: Creating a before-school physical activity program: Pre-service physical educators' experiences and implications for PETE. *Journal of Teaching in Physical Education, 33*(4), 449-466.

Metos, J., & Nanney, M.S. (2007). The strength of school wellness policies: One state's experience. *Journal of School Health, 77*(7), 367-372.

Metzler, M.W., McKenzie, T.L., van der Mars, H., Barrett-Williams, S.L., & Ellis, R. (2013). Health Optimizing Physical Education (HOPE): A new curriculum for school programs—Part 2: Teacher knowledge and collaboration. *Journal of Physical Education, Recreation & Dance, 84*(5), 25-34.

National Association for Sport and Physical Education. (2008). *Comprehensive school physical activity programs.* Reston, VA: National Association for Sport and Physical Education.

O'Brien, L.M., Polacsek, M., MacDonald, P.B., Ellis, J., Berry, S., & Martin, M. (2010). Impact of a school health coordinator intervention on health-related school policies and student behavior. *Journal of School Health, 80*(4), 176-185.

Patton, I. (2012). Teachers' perspectives of the daily physical activity program in Ontario. *Physical and Health Education Journal, 78*(1), 14-21.

Public Law 108-265 (2004). *Child nutrition and WIC reauthorization act of 2004.* Retrieved from www.gpo.gov/fdsys/pkg/PLAW-108publ265/pdf/PLAW-108publ265.pdf

Public Law 111-296 (2010). *Healthy, hunger-free kids act of 2010.* Retrieved from www.gpo.gov/fdsys/pkg/PLAW-111publ296/pdf/PLAW-111publ296.pdf

Pulling Kuhn, A., Carson, R.L., & Beighle, A. (2015, October). *Changes in psychosocial perspectives among teachers trained as physical activity leaders: Teacher efficacy, work engagement, and affective commitment.* Research presentation at the Physical Education Teacher Education & Health Education Teacher Education triannual meeting of the Society of Health and Physical Educators (SHAPE) America, Atlanta, GA.

Rink, J.E., Hall, T.J., & Williams, L.H. (2010). *School-wide physical activity: A comprehensive guide to designing and conducting programs.* Champaign, IL: Human Kinetics.

Russ, L.B., Webster, C.A., Beets, M.W., & Phillips, D.S. (2015). Systematic review and meta-analysis of multi-component interventions through schools to increase physical activity. *Journal of Physical Activity & Health, 12*(10), 1436-1446.

SHAPE America. (2016). *Shape of the nation: Status of physical education in the USA.* Retrieved from www.shapeamerica.org/uploads/pdfs/son/Shape-of-the-Nation-2016_web.pdf

SHAPE America. (2017). *Physical activity leader (PAL) learning system.* Retrieved from https://portal.shapeamerica.org/prodev/workshops/lmas/default.aspx

Stoltz, A.D., Coburn, S., & Knickelbein, A. (2009). Building local infrastructure for coordinated school health programs: A pilot study. *Journal of School Nursing, 25,* 133-140.

Story, M., Nanney, M.S., & Schwartz, M.B. (2009). Schools and obesity prevention: Creating school environments and policies to promote healthy eating and physical activity. *Milbank Quarterly, 87*(1), 71-100. doi:10.1111/j.1468-0009.2009.00548.x

Videto, D.M., & Hodges, B.C. (2009). Use of university/school partnerships for the institutionalization of the coordinated school health program. *American Journal of Health Education, 40,* 212-219.

Ward, S.D., Saunders, R., Felton, M.G., Williams, E., Epping, N.J., & Pate, R.R. (2006). Implementation of a school environment intervention to increase physical activity in high school girls. *Health Education Research, 21*(6), 896-910.

Webster, C.A., Beets, M., Weaver, R.G., Vazou, S., & Russ, L. (2015). Rethinking recommendations for implementing comprehensive school physical activity programs: A partnership model. *Quest, 67*(2), 185-202.

Chapter 4

Beets, M.W., Weaver, R.G., Moore, J.B., Turner-McGrievy, G., Pate, R.R., Webster, C., & Beighle, A. (2014). From policy to practice: Strategies to meet physical activity standards in YMCA afterschool programs. *American Journal of Preventive Medicine, 46*(3), 281-288.

Beighle, A., Erwin, H., Castelli, D., & Ernst, M. (2009). Preparing physical educators for the role of physical activity director. *Journal of Physical Education, Recreation & Dance, 80*(4), 24-29.

Bringle, R.G., & Clayton, P.H. (2012). Civic education through service-learning: What, how, and why? In L. McIlraith, A. Lyons, & R. Munck (Eds.), *Higher education and civic engagement: Comparative perspectives* (pp. 101–124). New York, NY: Palgrave Macmillan.

Burns, R.D., Brusseau, T.A., & Hannon, J.C. (2017). Effect of comprehensive school physical activity programming on cardiometabolic health markers in children from low-income schools. *Journal of Physical Activity & Health, 14*(9), 671-676.

Cambridge, D., Kaplan, S., & Suter, V. (2005). *Community of practice design guide.* Denver, CO: EDUCAUSE. Retrieved from http://net.educause.edu/ir/library/pdf/NLI0531.pdf

Carlson, J.A., Sallis, J.F., Chriqui, J.F., Schneider, L., McDermid, L.C., & Agron, P. (2013). State policies about physical activity minutes in physical education or during school. *Journal of School Health, 83*(3), 150-156.

Carson, R. (2012). Certification and duties of a director of physical activity. *Journal of Physical Education, Recreation & Dance, 83*(6), 16-19.

Carson, R.L., Castelli, D.M., Beighle, A., & Erwin, H. (2014). School-based physical activity promotion: A conceptual framework for research and practice. *Childhood Obesity, 10*(2), 1-7.

Carson, R.L., Castelli, D.M., Pulling Kuhn, A.C., Moore, J.B., Beets, M.W., Beighle, A., ... Glowacki, E.M. (2014). Impact of trained champions of comprehensive school physical activity programs on school physical activity offerings, youth physical activity and sedentary behaviors. *Preventive Medicine, 69,* S12-S19.

Carson, R.L., & Raguse, A.L. (2014). Systematic review of service-learning in youth physical activity settings. *Quest, 66,* 57-95.

Castelli, D.M., & Beighle, A. (2007). The physical education teacher as school physical activity director. *Journal of Physical Education, Recreation & Dance, 78*(5), 25-28.

Centeio, E.E., Erwin, H., & Castelli, D.M. (2014). Chapter 4: Comprehensive school physical activity program: Characteristics of trained teachers. *Journal of Teaching in Physical Education, 33,* 492-510.

Centeio, E.E., McCaughtry, N., Gutuskey, L., Garn, A.C., Somers, C., Shen, B., ... Kulik, N. (2014). Physical activity change through comprehensive school physical activity programs in urban elementary schools. *Journal of Teaching in Physical Education, 33,* 572-591.

Centers for Disease Control and Prevention (CDC). (2013). *Comprehensive school physical activity programs: A guide for schools.* Retrieved from www.cdc.gov/healthyyouth/physicalactivity/pdf/13_242620-A_CSPAP_SchoolPhysActivityPrograms_Final_508_12192013.pdf

Cradock, A.L., Barrett, J.L., Carnoske, C., Chriqui, J.F., Evenson, K.R., Gustat, J., ... Zieff, S.G. (2013). Roles and strategies of state organizations related to school-based physical education and physical activity policies. *Journal of Public Health Management and Practice, 19*(3), S34-S40.

Crisp, B.R., Swerissen, H., & Duckett, S.J. (2000). Four approaches to capacity building in health: Consequences for measurement and accountability. *Health Promotion International, 15*(2), 99-107.

Curtner-Smith, M.D. (1999). The more things change the more they stay the same: Factors influencing teachers' interpretations and delivery of national curriculum physical education. *Sport, Education and Society, 4*(1), 75-97.

Dowda, M., Sallis, J.F., McKenzie, T.L., Rosengard, P., & Kohl, III, H.W. (2005). Evaluating the sustainability of SPARK physical education: A case study of translating research into practice. *Research Quarterly for Exercise and Sport, 76*(1), 11-19.

Egan, C.A., Webster C.A., Weaver, R.G., Russ, L., Stodden, D., Brian, A., & Stewart, G. (2018). Case study of a health-optimizing physical education-based comprehensive school physical activity program. *Evaluation and Program Planning,* Doi.org/10.1016/j.evalprogplan.2018.10.006

Evans, J., Davies, B., & Penney, D. (1996). Teachers, teaching and the social construction of gender relations. *Sport, Education, & Society, 1*(2), 165-183.

Fullan, M., & Pomfret, A. (1977). Research on curriculum and instruction implementation. *Review of Educational Research, 47*(2), 335-397.

Galvan, C., & Parker, M. (2011). Service-learning in physical education teacher education: Findings of the road less traveled. *Journal of Experiential Education, 34*(1), 55-70.

Goh, T.L., Hannon, J.C., Webster, C.A., & Podlog, L. (2017). Classroom teachers' experiences implementing a movement integration program: Barriers, facilitators, and continuance. *Teaching and Teacher Education, 66,* 88-95.

Goodman, R., Speers, M.A., McLeroy, K., Fawcett, S., Kegler, M., Parker, E., & Wallerstein, N. (1988). **Identifying and Defining the Dimensions of Community Capacity to Provide a Basis for Measurement.** *Health Education & Behavior, 25* (3), 258-278.

Heidorn, B., & Centeio, E. (2012). The director of physical activity and staff involvement. *Journal of Physical Education, Recreation & Dance, 83*(7), 13-19.

Heward, S., Hutchins, C., & Keleher, H. (2007). Organizational change: Key to capacity building and effective health promotion. *Health Promotion Journal, 22*(2), 170-178.

Hunt, K., & Metzler, M. (2017). Adoption of comprehensive school physical activity programs: A literature review. *Physical Educator, 74*(2), 315-340.

Iles, V., & Sutherland, K. (2001). *Organisational change: A review for health care managers, professionals and researchers.* London, UK: National Coordinating Centre for NHS Service Delivery and Organisation.

Israel, B.A., Schulz, A.J., Parker, E.A., & Becker, A.B. (1998). Review of community-based research: Assessing partnership approaches to improve public health. *Annual Review of Public Health, 19,* 173-202.

Johnson, K., Hays, C., Center, H., & Daley, C. (2004). Building capacity and sustainable prevention innovations: A sustainability planning model. *Evaluation and Program Planning, 27,* 135-149.

Laws, C., & Aldridge, M. (1995). Magic moments, myth or millstone: The implementation of national curriculum physical education. *British Journal of Physical Education Research Supplement, 16,* 2-12.

Lewin, K. (1951). *Field theory in social science.* New York, NY: Harper & Row.

McCullick, B.A., Baker, T.A., Tomorowski, P.D., Templin, T., Lux, K., & Isaac, T. (2012). An analysis of state physical education policies. *Journal of Teaching in Physical Education, 31*(2), 200-210.

McKenzie, T.L., Nader, P.R., Strikmiller, P.K., Yang, M., Stone, E.J., Perry, C.L, . . . Kelder, S.H. (1996). School physical education: Effect of the Child and Adolescent Trial for Cardiovascular Health. *Preventive Medicine, 25,* 423-431.

McKenzie, T.L., Sallis, J.F., Kolody, B., & Faucette, F.N. (1997). Long-term effects of a physical education curriculum and staff development program: SPARK. *Research Quarterly for Exercise and Sport, 68*(4), 280-291.

McKenzie, T.L., Sallis, J.F., & Rosengard, P. (2009). Beyond the stucco tower: Design, development, and dissemination of the SPARK physical education programs. *Quest, 61*(1), 114-127.

McLaughlin, M. (1987). Learning from experience: Lessons from policy implementation. *Educational Evaluation and Policy Analysis, 9,* 171-178.

Metzler, M.W. (2016). School-based team research to address grand challenges through P-12 physical education programs. *Research Quarterly for Exercise and Sport, 87*(4), 325-333.

Metzler, M., Barrett-Williams, S., Hunt, K., Marquis, J., & Trent, M. (2015). *Final report: Establishing a comprehensive school physical activity program.* Atlanta, GA: Centers for Disease Control and Prevention and Georgia State University Seed Award Program for Social and Behavioral Science Research.

Metzler, M.W., McKenzie, T.L., van der Mars, H., Barrett-Williams, S.L., & Ellis, R. (2013). Health Optimizing Physical Education (HOPE): A new curriculum for school programs—Part 1: Establishing the need and describing the model. *Journal of Physical Education, Recreation & Dance, 84*(4), 41-47.

Michael, R.D., Webster, C.A., Egan, C.A., Stewart, G., Nilges, L., Brian, A., . . . Vazou, S. (2018). Viability of university service learning to support movement integration in elementary classrooms: Perspectives of teachers, university students, and course instructors. *Teaching and Teacher Education, 72,* 122-132.

Nader, P.R., Stone, E.J., Lytle, L.A., Perry, C.L., Osganian, S.K., Kelder, S., . . . Wu, M. (1999). Three-year maintenance of improved diet and physical activity: The CATCH cohort. *Archives of Pediatrics & Adolescent Medicine, 153*(7), 695-704.

Owen, N., Glanz, K., Sallis, J.F., & Kelder, S.H. (2006). Evidence-based approaches to dissemination and diffusion of physical activity interventions. *American Journal of Preventive Medicine, 31*(4), 35-44.

Pettigrew, A., Ferlie, E., & McKee, L. (1992). *Shaping strategic change.* London, UK: Sage.

Rogers, E.M. (1995). *Diffusion of innovations* (4th ed.). New York, NY: Free Press.

Scheirer, M.A., & Dearing, J.W. (2011). An agenda for research on the sustainability of public health programs. *American Journal of Public Health, 101*(11), 2059-2067.

Schell, S.F., Luke, D.A., Schooley, M.W., Elliott, M.B., Herbers, S.H., Mueller, N.B., & Bunger, A.C. (2013). Public health program capacity for sustainability: A new framework. *Implementation Science, 8*(1), 15.

SHAPE America. (2017). *2017 National standards for initial physical education teacher education.* Retrieved from www.shapeamerica.org//accreditation/upload/2017-SHAPE-America-Initial-PETE-Standards-and-Components.pdf

Shediac-Rizkallah, M.C., & Bone, L.R. (1998). Planning for the sustainability of community-based health programs: Conceptual frameworks and future directions for research, practice and policy. *Health Education Research, 13,* 87-108.

Siler-Wells, G. (1987). An implementation model for health system reform. *Social Science & Medicine, 24*(10), 821-832.

Spoth, R., Greenberg, M., Bierman, K., & Redmond, C. (2004). PROSPER community–university partnership model for public education systems: Capacity-building for evidence-based, competence-building prevention. *Prevention Science, 5*(1), 31-39.

St Leger, L. (2001). Schools, health literacy and public health: Possibilities and challenges.

Health Promotion International,16, 197–205.

Vazou, S., Hutchinson, A., & Webster, C.A. (2015, March). Empowering teachers to integrate physical activity: Online communities of practice. Symposium conducted at the SHAPE America National Convention, Seattle, WA.

Weaver, R.G., Beets, M.W., Webster, C., Beighle, A., Saunders, R., & Pate, R.A. (2014). A coordinated comprehensive professional development training's effect on summer day camp staff healthy eating and physical activity promoting behaviors. *Journal of Physical Activity and Health, 11,* 1170-1177.

Weaver, R.G., Webster, C.A., Egan, C., Campos, C., Michael, R.D., & Crimarco, A. (2017). Partnerships for Active Children in Elementary Schools: Physical education outcomes after 4 months of a 2-year pilot study. *Health Education Journal, 76*(7), 763-774.

Weaver, R.G., Webster, C.A., Egan, C., Campos, C., Michael, R.D., & Vazou, S. (2017). Partnerships for Active Children in Elementary Schools: Outcomes of a 2-year pilot study to increase physical activity during the school day. *American Journal of Health Promotion, 32*(3), 621-630.

Webster, C.A., Beets, M.W., Weaver, R.G., Vazou, S., & Russ, L. (2015). Rethinking recommendations for implementing Comprehensive School Physical Activity Programs: A partnership model. *Quest, 67*(2), 185-202.

Webster, C.A., Russ, L., Vazou, S., Goh, T.L., & Erwin, H.E. (2015). Integrating movement in academic classrooms: Understanding, applying, and advancing the knowledge base. *Obesity Reviews, 16*(8), 691-701.

Webster, C.A., Nesbitt, D., Lee, H., & Egan, C. (2017). Preservice physical education teachers' service learning experiences related to comprehensive school physical activity programming. *Journal of Teaching in Physical Education, 36*, 430-444.

Webster, C.A., Russ, L., Webster, L., Molina, S., Lee, H, & Cribbs, J. (2016). PETE faculty beliefs concerning the preparation of preservice teachers for CSPAP roles: An exploratory study. *The Physical Educator, 72*(2), 315-339.

Webster, C.A., Weaver, R.G., Egan, C.A., Brian, A., & Vazou, S. (2017). Two-year process evaluation of a pilot program to increase elementary children's physical activity during school. *Evaluation and Program Planning, 61*, 134-143.

Webster, C.A., Webster, L., Russ, L., Molina, S., Lee, H., & Cribbs, J. (2015). A systematic review of public health-aligned recommendations for preparing physical education teacher candidates. *Research Quarterly for Exercise and Sport, 86*(1), 30-39.

Webster, C.A., Zarrett, N., Cook, B.S., Egan, C., Nesbitt, D., & Weaver, R.G. (2017). Movement integration in elementary classrooms: Teacher perceptions and implications for program planning. *Evaluation and Program Planning, 61,* 134-143.

Chapter 5

Ahamed, Y., Macdonald, H., Reed, K., Naylor, P.J., Liu-Ambrose, T., & McKay, H. (2007). School-based physical activity does not compromise children's academic performance. *Medicine & Science in Sports & Exercise, 39*(2), 371-376.

Ajzen, I. (1985). From intentions to actions: A theory of planned behavior. In J. Kubland & J. Beckman (Eds.), *Action-control: From cognitions to behavior* (pp. 11-39). Heidelberg: Springer.

Ames, C. (1992a). Achievement goals and the classroom motivational climate. In D.H. Schunk & J.L. Meece (Eds.), *Student perceptions in the classroom* (pp. 327-348). Hillsdale, NJ: Lawrence Erlbaum Associates, Inc.

Ames, C.A. (1992b). Achievement goals, motivational climate, and motivational processes. In G.C. Roberts (Ed.), *Motivation in sport and exercise* (pp. 161-172). Champaign IL: Human Kinetics.

Amorose, A.J. (2007). Coaching effectiveness: Exploring the relationship between coaching behavior and motivation from a self-determination theory perspective. In N. Chatzisarantis & M.S. Hagger (Eds.), *Self-determination theory in sport and exercise* (pp. 209-227). Champaign, IL: Human Kinetics.

Annesi, J.J. (2004). Relationship between self-efficacy and changes in rated tension and depression for 9- to 12-yr.-old children enrolled in a 12-wk. after-school physical activity program. *Perceptual and Motor Skills, 99*(1), 191-194.

Annesi, J.J. (2006). Relations of physical self-concept and self-efficacy with frequency of voluntary physical activity in preadolescents: Implications for after-school care programming. *Journal of Psychosomatic Research, 61*(4), 515-520.

Annesi, J.J., Faigenbaum, A.D., Westcott, W.L., Smith, A.E., Unruh, J.L., & Hamilton, F.G. (2007). Effects of the Youth Fit for Life protocol on physiological, mood, self-appraisal, and voluntary physical activity changes in African American preadolescents: Contrasting after-school care and physical education formats. *International Journal of Clinical Health Psychology, 7*(3), 641-659.

Annesi, J.J., Westcott, W.L., Faigenbaum, A.D., & Unruh, J.L. (2005). Effects of a 12-week physical activity protocol delivered by YMCA after-school counselors (Youth Fit for Life) on fitness and self-efficacy changes in 5-12-year-old boys and girls. *Research Quarterly for Exercise and Sport, 76*(4), 468-476.

Babkes Stellino, M., & Sinclair, C.D. (2013). Psychological predictors of children's recess physical activity motivation and behavior. *Research Quarterly for Exercise and Sport, 84*(2), 167-176.

Babkes Stellino, M., Thornton, M., & Erwin, H. (2015). Elementary teacher autonomy support for children's recess physical activity motivation. [Abstract]. *Research Quarterly for Exercise and Sport, XX*(S1), A.

Bandura, A. (1977). Self-efficacy: Toward a unifying theory of behavioral change. *Psychological Review, 84*(2), 191-215.

Bandura, A. (1986). *Social foundations of thought and action: A social cognitive theory.* Englewood Cliffs, NJ: Prentice Hall.

Bartholomew, J.B., & Jowers, E.M. (2011). Physically active academic lessons in elementary children. *Preventive Medicine, 52,* S51-S54.

Baumeister, R., & Leary, M.R. (1995). The need to belong: Desire for interpersonal attachments as fundamental human motive. *Psychological Bulletin, 117,* 497-529.

Boyle-Holmes, T., Grost, L., Russell, L., Laris, B.A., Robin, L., Haller, E., . . . Lee, S. (2010). Promoting elementary physical education: Results of a school-based evaluation study. *Health Education & Behavior, 37*(3), 377-389.

Bronfenbrenner, U. (1977). Toward an experimental ecology of human development. *American Psychologist, 32,* 513-531.

Bronfenbrenner, U., & Morris, P.A. (1998). The ecology of developmental processes. In W. Damon & R.M. Lerner (Eds.), *Handbook of child psychology: Theoretical models of human development* (pp. 993-1028). Hoboken, NJ: John Wiley.

Carson, R.L., Castelli, D.M., Beighle, A., & Erwin, H. (2014). School-based physical activity promotion: A conceptual framework for research and practice. *Childhood Obesity, 10*(2), 100-106. doi:10.1089/chi.2013.0134

Cliff, D.P., Wilson, A., Okely, A.D., Mickle, K.J., & Steele, J.R. (2007). Feasibility of SHARK: A physical activity skill-development program for overweight and obese children. *Journal of Science and Medicine in Sport, 10*(4), 263-267.

Cohen, K.E., Morgan, P.J., Plotnikoff, R.C., Callister, R., & Lubans, D.R. (2015). Physical activity and skills intervention: SCORES cluster randomized controlled trial. *Medicine & Science in Sports & Exercise, 47*(4), 765-774.

Deci, E.L. (1975). *Intrinsic motivation.* New York, NY: Plenum.

Deci, E.L., & Ryan, R.M. (1985). *Intrinsic motivation and self-determination in human behavior.* New York, NY: Springer.

Deci, E.L., & Ryan, R.M. (2000). The "what" and "why" of goal pursuits: Human needs and the self-determination of behavior. *Psychological Inquiry, 11*(4), 227-268.

Dishman, R.K., Motl, R.W., Saunders, R., Felton, G., Ward, D.S., Dowda, M., & Pate, R.R. (2004). Self-efficacy partially mediates the effect of a school-based physical-activity intervention among adolescent girls. *Preventive Medicine, 38*(5), 628-636.

Donnelly, J.E., Greene, J.L., Gibson, C.A., Smith, B.K., Washburn, R.A., Sullivan, D.K., . . . Williams, S.L. (2009). Physical Activity Across the Curriculum (PAAC): A randomized controlled trial to promote physical activity and diminish overweight and obesity in elementary school children. *Preventive Medicine, 49*(4), 336-341.

Donnelly, J.E., & Lambourne, K. (2011). Classroom-based physical activity, cognition, and academic achievement. *Preventive Medicine, 52,* S36-S42.

DuBose, K.D., Mayo, M.S., Gibson, C.A., Green, J.L., Hill, J.O., Jacobsen, D.J., . . . Donnelly, J.E. (2008). Physical Activity Across the Curriculum (PAAC): Rationale and design. *Contemporary Clinical Trials, 29*(1), 83-93.

Duda, J.L. (2001). Goal perspective research in sport: Pushing some boundaries and clarifying some misunderstandings. In G.C. Roberts (Ed.), *Advances in motivation in sport and exercise* (pp. 129-182). Champaign, IL: Human Kinetics.

Eather, N., Morgan, P.J., & Lubans, D.R. (2013). Social support from teachers mediates physical activity behavior change in children participating in the Fit-4-Fun intervention. *International Journal of Behavioral Nutrition and Physical Activity, 10*(1), 68. doi.org/10.1186/1479-5868-10-68

Emmons, K. (2000). Health behaviours in a social context. In L. Berkman & I. Kawachi (Eds.), *Social epidemiology* (pp. 242-266). New York, NY: Oxford University Press.

Epstein, J.L. (1989). Family structures and student motivation: A developmental perspective. In C. Ames & R. Ames (Eds.), *Research on motivation in education* (Vol. 3, pp. 259-295). Orlando, FL: Academic Press.

Fishbein, M., & Ajzen, I. (1975). *Belief, attitude, intention and behavior: An introduction to theory and research.* Reading, MA: Addison-Wesley.

Fitzgerald, A., Fitzgerald, N., & Aherne, C. (2012). Do peers matter? A review of peer and/or friends' influence on physical activity among American adolescents. *Journal of Adolescence, 35,* 941-958.

Gibson, C.A., Smith, B.K., DuBose, K.D., Greene, J.L., Bailey, B.W., Williams, S.L., . . . Mayo, M.S. (2008). Physical activity across the curriculum: Year one process evaluation results. *International Journal of Behavioral Nutrition and Physical Activity, 5*(1), 36.

Harter, S. (1978). Effectance motivation reconsidered: Toward a developmental model. *Human Development, 21*(1), 34-64.

Harter, S. (1981). A model of intrinsic mastery motivation in children: Individual differences and developmental change. In W.A. Collins (Ed.), *Minnesota symposium on child psychology* (Vol. 14, pp. 215-255). Hillsdale, NJ: Erlbaum.

Harwood, C.G., Keegan, R.J., Smith, J.M., & Raine, A.S. (2015). A systematic review of the intrapersonal correlates of motivational climate perceptions in sport and physical activity. *Psychology of Sport and Exercise, 18,* 9-25.

Hyndman, B.P., Benson, A.C., Ullah, S., & Telford, A. (2014). Evaluating the effects of the Lunchtime Enjoyment Activity and Play (LEAP) school playground intervention on children's quality of life, enjoyment and participation in physical activity. *BMC Public Health, 14*(1), 164.

Jamner, M.S., Spruijt-Metz, D., Bassin, S., & Cooper, D.M. (2004). A controlled evaluation of a school-based intervention to promote physical activity among sedentary adolescent females: Project FAB. *Journal of Adolescent Health, 34*(4), 279-289.

Jones, L., Karageorghis, C.I., & Ekkekakis, P. (2014). Can high-intensity exercise be more pleasant? Attentional dissociation using music and video. *Journal of Sport & Exercise Psychology, 36*(5), 528-541.

Langille, J.D., & Rodgers, W.M. (2010). Exploring the influence of a social ecological model on school-based physical activity. *Health Education & Behavior, 37*(6), 879-894. doi:10.1177/1090198110367877

Lonsdale, C., Rosenkranz, R.R., Sanders, T., Peralta, L.R., Bennie, A., Jackson, B., . . . Lubans, D.R. (2013). A cluster randomized controlled trial of strategies to increase adolescents' physical activity and motivation in physical education: Results of the Motivating Active Learning in Physical Education (MALP) trial. *Preventive Medicine, 57*(5), 696-702.

Lubans, D.R., Morgan, P.J., Weaver, K., Callister, R., Dewar, D.L., Costigan, S.A., . . . Plotnikoff, R.C. (2012). Rationale and study protocol for the Supporting Children's Outcomes Using Rewards, Exercise and Skills (SCORES) group randomized controlled trial: A physical activity and fundamental movement skills intervention for primary schools in low-income communities. *BMC Public Health, 12*(1), 427.

Mageau, G.A., & Vallerand, R.J. (2003). The coach-athlete relationship: A motivational model. *Journal of Sports Sciences, 21,* 883-904.

Mantis, K., Vazou, S., Saint-Maurice, P.F., & Welk, G.J. (2014). Integrated physical activity with academics: Objectively-measured activity levels in the classroom. *Medicine & Science in Sports & Exercise, 46*(5S), 232.

National Institute on Out-of-School Time (NIOST). (n.d.). *BOKS longitudinal evaluation.* Retrieved from https://niost.org/Active-Projects/boks-longitudinal-evaluation

Naylor, P.J., Macdonald, H.M., Warburton, D.E., Reed, K.E., & McKay, II.A. (2008). An active school model to promote physical activity in elementary schools: Action Schools! BC. *British Journal of Sports Medicine, 42*(5), 338-343.

Naylor, P.J., Macdonald, H.M., Zebedee, J.A., Reed, K.E., & McKay, H.A. (2006). Lessons learned from Action Schools! BC—an 'active school' model to promote physical activity in elementary schools. *Journal of Science and Medicine in Sport, 9*(5), 413-423.

Neumark-Sztainer, D.R., Friend, S.E., Flattum, C.F., Hannan, P.J., Story, M.T., Bauer, K.W, . . . Petrich, C.A. (2010). New moves—preventing weight-related problems in adolescent girls: A group-randomized study. *American Journal of Preventive Medicine, 39*(5), 421-432.

Neumark-Sztainer, D.R., Story, M., Hannan, P.J., & Rex, J. (2003a). New Moves: A school-based obesity prevention program for adolescent girls. *Preventive Medicine, 37*(1), 41-51.

Neumark-Sztainer, D.R., Story, M., Hannan, P.J., Tharp, T., & Rex, J. (2003b). Factors associated with changes in physical activity: A cohort study of inactive adolescent girls. *Archives of Pediatrics & Adolescent Medicine, 157*(8), 803-810.

Nicholls, J.G. (1984). Achievement motivation: Conceptions of ability, subjective experience, task choice, and performance. *Psychological Review, 91,* 328-346.

Norris, E., Dunsmuir, S., Duke-Williams, O., Stamatakis, E., & Shelton, N. (2016a). Protocol for the 'Virtual Traveller' cluster-randomised controlled trial: A behaviour change intervention to increase physical activity in primary-school math and English lessons. *BMJ Open, 6*(6), e011982.

Norris, E., Shelton, N., Dunsmuir, S., Duke-Williams, O., & Stamatakis, E. (2015). Teacher and pupil perspectives on the use of virtual field trips as physically active lessons. *BMC Research Notes, 8*(1), 719.

Norris, E., Shelton, N., Dunsmuir, S., Duke-Williams, O., & Stamatakis, E. (2016b). Virtual traveller: A behaviour change intervention to increase physical activity during primary school lessons. *European Health Psychologist, 18*(S), 556.

Pangrazi, R.P., Beighle, A., Vehige, T., & Vack, C. (2003). Impact of Promoting Lifestyle Activity for Youth (PLAY) on children's physical activity. *Journal of School Health, 73*(8), 317-321.

Pate, R.R., Saunders, R., Dishman, R.K., Addy, C., Dowda, M., & Ward, D.S. (2007). Long-term effects of a physical activity intervention in high school girls. *American Journal of Preventive Medicine, 33*(4), 276-280.

Pate, R.R., Ward, D.S., Saunders, R.P., Felton, G., Dishman, R.K., & Dowda, M. (2005). Promotion of physical activity among high-school girls: A randomized controlled trial. *American Journal of Public Health, 95*(9), 1582-1587.

Priebe, C.S., & Spink, K. (2011). When in Rome: Descriptive norms and physical activity. *Psychology of Sport and Exercise, 12,* 93-98.

Prochaska, J.O., & Velicer, W.F. (1997). The transtheoretical model of health behavior change. *American Journal of Health Promotion, 12*(1), 38-48.

Rosenkranz, R.R., Lubans, D.R., Peralta, L.R., Bennie, A., Sanders, T., & Lonsdale, C. (2012). A cluster-randomized controlled trial of strategies to increase adolescents' physical activity and motivation during physical education lessons: The Motivating Active Learning in Physical Education (MALP) trial. *BMC Public Health, 12*(1), 834.

Ryan, R.M., & Connell, J.P. (1989). Perceived locus of causality and internalization: Examining reasons for activating in two domains. *Journal of Personality and Social Psychology, 57,* 749-761.

Ryan, R.M., & Deci, E.L. (2000a). Intrinsic and extrinsic motivations: Classic definitions and new directions. *Contemporary Educational Psychology, 25*(1), 54-67.

Ryan, R.M., & Deci, E.L. (2000b). Self-determination theory and the facilitation of intrinsic motivation, social development, and well-being. *American Psychologist, 55,* 68-78.

Ryan, R.M., & Deci, E.L. (2002). An overview of self-determination theory: An organismic-dialectical perspective. In E.L. Deci & R.M. Ryan (Eds.), *Handbook of self-determination research* (pp. 3-33). Rochester, NY: University of Rochester Press.

Saunders, R.P., Ward, D., Felton, G.M., Dowda, M., & Pate, R.R. (2006). Examining the link between program implementation and behavior outcomes in the Lifestyle Education for Activity Program (LEAP). *Evaluation and Program Planning, 29*(4), 352-364.

Schneider, M., & Cooper, D.M. (2011). Enjoyment of exercise moderates the impact of a school-based physical activity intervention. *International Journal of Behavioral Nutrition and Physical Activity, 8*(1), 64.

Schneider, M., Dunton, G.F., Bassin, S., Graham, D.J., Eliakim, A., & Cooper, D.M. (2007). Impact of a school-based physical activity intervention on fitness and bone in adolescent females. *Journal of Physical Activity and Health, 4*(1), 17-29.

Shilts, M.K., Horowitz, M., & Townsend, M.S. (2009). Guided goal setting: Effectiveness in a dietary and physical activity intervention with low-income adolescents. *International Journal of Adolescent Medicine and Health, 20*(1), 111-122.

Silva, P., Lott, R., Mota, J., & Welk, G. (2014). Direct and indirect effects of social support on youth physical activity behavior. *Pediatric Exercise Science, 26*(1), 86-94.

Silverman, S., Keating, X.D., & Phillips, S.R. (2008). A lasting impression: A pedagogical perspective on youth fitness testing. *Measurement in Physical Education and Exercise Science, 12*(3), 146-166.

Simon, C., Kellou, N., Dugas, J., Platat, C., Copin, N., Schweitzer, B., . . . Blanc, S. (2014). A socio-ecological approach promoting physical activity and limiting sedentary behavior in adolescence showed weight benefits maintained 2.5 years after intervention cessation. *International Journal of Obesity, 38*(7), 936-943. doi:10.1038/ijo.2014.23

Spence, J.C., & Lee, R.E. (2003). Toward a comprehensive model of physical activity. *Psychology of Sport and Exercise, 4*(1), 7-24. doi:10.1016/S1469-0292(02)00014-6

Springer, A.E., Kelder, S.H., Ranjit, N., Hochberg-Garrett, H., Crow, S., & Delk, J. (2012). Promoting physical activity and fruit and vegetable consumption through a community-school partnership: The effects of Marathon Kids® on low-income elementary school children in Texas. *Journal of Physical Activity and Health, 9*(5), 739-753.

Standage, M., Duda, J.L., & Ntoumanis, N. (2005). A test of self-determination theory in school physical education. *British Journal of Educational Psychology, 75*, 411-433.

Sterdt, E., Liersch, S., & Walter, U. (2014). Correlates of physical activity of children and adolescents: A systematic review of reviews. *Health Education Journal, 73*(1), 72-89.

Stock, S., Miranda, C., Evans, S., Plessis, S., Ridley, J., Yeh, S., & Chanoine, J.P. (2007). Healthy Buddies: A novel, peer-led health promotion program for the prevention of obesity and eating disorders in children in elementary school. *Pediatrics, 120*(4), e1059-e1068.

Story, M., Sherwood, N.E., Himes, J.H., Davis, M., Jacobs, D.R., Cartwright, Y., . . . Rochon, J. (2003). An after-school obesity prevention program for African-American girls: The Minnesota GEMS pilot study. *Ethnicity and Disease, 13*(Suppl. 1), S1-54.

Stych, K., & Parfitt, G. (2011). Exploring affective responses to different exercise intensities in low-active young adolescents. *Journal of Sport & Exercise Psychology, 33*(4), 548-568.

Sylvester, B.D., Standage, M., Ark, T.K., Sweet, S.N., Crocker, P.R., Zumbo, B.D., & Beauchamp, M.R. (2014). Is variety a spice of (an active) life?: Perceived variety, exercise behavior, and the mediating role of autonomous motivation. *Journal of Sport & Exercise Psychology, 36*(5), 516-527.

van Beurden, E., Barnett, L.M., Zask, A., Dietrich, U.C., Brooks, L.O., & Beard, J. (2003). Can we skill and activate children through primary school physical education lessons? "Move It Groove It"—a collaborative health promotion intervention. *Preventive Medicine, 36*(4), 493-501.

Vazou, S., Mischo, A., & Ekkekakis, P. (2015). Reimagining fitness testing in schools: Enjoyment, need satisfaction, and intention. *Journal of Sport & Exercise Psychology, 37*, S149.

Vazou, S., Ntoumanis, N., & Duda, J.L. (2006). Predicting young athlete's motivational indices from perceived coach and peer climate. *Psychology of Sport and Exercise, 7*, 215-233.

Vazou, S., & Skrade, M.A. (2016). Intervention integrating physical activity with math: Math performance, perceived competence, and need satisfaction. *International Journal of Sport and Exercise Psychology, 15*(5), 508-522.

Weaver, R.G., Webster, C.A., Egan, C., Campos, C.M., Michael, R.D., & Vazou, S. (2017). Partnerships for active children in elementary schools: Outcomes of a 2-year pilot study to increase physical activity during the school day. *American Journal of Health Promotion, 76*(7), 763-744.

Webber, L.S., Catellier, D.J., Lytle, L.A., Murray, D.M., Pratt, C.A., Young, D.R., . . . Pate, R.R. (2008). Promoting physical activity in middle school girls: Trial of Activity for Adolescent Girls. *American Journal of Preventive Medicine, 34*(3), 173-184.

Wiersma, L.D., & Sherman, C.P. (2008). The responsible use of youth fitness testing to enhance student motivation, enjoyment, and performance. *Measurement in Physical Education and Exercise Science, 12*, 167-183.

Welk, G.J. (2008). The role of physical activity assessments for school-based physical activity promotion. *Measurement in Physical Education and Exercise Science, 12*(3), 184-206. doi: 10.1080/10913670802216130

Wilson, D.K., Evans, A.E., Williams, J., Mixon, G., Sirard, J.R., & Pate, R. (2005). A preliminary test of a student-centered intervention on increasing physical activity in underserved adolescents. *Annals of Behavioral Medicine, 30*(2), 119.

Chapter 6

Agron, P., Berends, V., Ellis, K., & Gonzalez, M. (2010). School wellness policies: Perceptions, barriers, and needs among school leaders and wellness advocates. *Journal of School Health, 80*, 527-535.

Alderman, B.L., Benham-Deal, T., Beighle, A., Erwin, H.E., & Olson, R.L. (2012). Physical education's contribution to daily physical activity among middle school youth. *Pediatric Exercise Science, 24,* 634-648.

Angela, T., & Hannon, J.C. (2012). Health-related fitness knowledge and physical activity of high school students. *The Physical Educator, 69,* 71-88.

Beighle, A., Erwin, H., Castelli, D., & Ernst, M. (2009). Preparing physical educators for the role of physical activity director. *Journal of Physical Education, Recreation & Dance, 80*(4), 24-29.

Bulger, S. M., & Housner, L.D. (2009). Relocating from easy street: Strategies for moving physical education forward. *Quest, 61,* 442-469.

Centers for Disease Control and Prevention (CDC). (2013). *Comprehensive school physical activity programs: A guide for schools.* Retrieved from www.cdc.gov/healthyyouth/physicalactivity/pdf/13_242620-A_CSPAP_SchoolPhysActivityPrograms_Final_508_12192013.pdf

Chen, S., Yang, L., & Schaben, J. (2017). To move more and sit less: Does physical activity/fitness knowledge matter in youth? *International Journal of Sports Nutrition and Exercise Metabolism, 32,* 1-44. http://doi.org/10.1123/ijspp.2015-0012

Dale, D., & Corbin, C.B. (2000). Physical activity participation of high school graduates following exposure to conceptual or traditional physical education. *Research Quarterly for Exercise and Sport, 71,* 61-68.

Ennis, C.D. (2011). Physical education curriculum priorities: Evidence for education and skillfulness. *Quest, 63,* 5-18.

Erwin, H., Beighle, A., Carson, R.L., & Castelli, D.M. (2013). Comprehensive school-based physical activity promotion: A review. *Quest, 65,* 412-428.

Gallahue, D.L., & Ozmun, J.C. (1998). *Understanding motor development: Infants, children, adolescents, adults.* McGraw-Hill.

Graber, K.C., Woods, A.M., & O'Connor, J.A. (2012). Impact of wellness legislation on comprehensive school health programs. *Journal of Teaching in Physical Education, 31,* 163-181.

Institute of Medicine. (2013). *Educating the student body: Taking physical activity and physical education to school.* Retrieved from https://www.nap.edu/read/18314/chapter/1

Kniffin, K.M., & Baert, H. (2015). Maximizing learning through assessment in middle and high school physical education. *Journal of Physical Education, Recreation & Dance, 86,* 7-16.

Lee, S.M., Burgeson, C.R., Fulton, J.E., & Spain, C.G. (2007). Physical education and physical activity: Results from the School Health Policies and Programs Study 2006. *Journal of School Health, 77,* 435-463.

Levin, S., McKenzie, T.L., Hussey, J.R., Kelder, S.H., & Lytle, L.A. (2001). Variability of physical activity during physical education lessons across elementary school grades. *Measurement in Physical Education and Exercise Science, 5,* 207-218.

McCullick, B.A., Baker, T., Tomporowski, P.D., Templin, T.J., Lux, K., & Isaac, T. (2012). An analysis of state physical education policies. *Journal of Teaching in Physical Education, 31,* 200-210.

McKenzie, T.L., & Lounsbery, M.A. (2013). Physical education teacher effectiveness in a public health context. *Research Quarterly for Exercise and Sport, 84,* 419-430.

McKenzie, T.L., Marshall, S.J., Sallis, J.F., & Conway, T.L. (2000). Student activity levels, lesson context, and teacher behavior during middle school physical education. *Research Quarterly for Exercise and Sport, 71,* 249-259.

McKenzie, T.L., Nader, P.R., Strikmiller, P.K., Yang, M., Stone, E.J., Perry, C.L., . . . Kelder, S.H. (1996). School physical education: Effect of the Child and Adolescent Trial for Cardiovascular Health (CATCH). *Preventive Medicine, 25,* 423-431.

McKenzie, T.L., Sallis, J.F., & Nader, P.R. (1991). SOFIT: System for Observing Fitness Instruction Time. *Journal of Teaching in Physical Education, 11,* 195-205.

McKenzie, T.L., Sallis, J.F., Prochaska, J.J., Conway, T.L., Marshall, S.J., & Rosengard, P. (2004). Evaluation of a 2-year middle-school physical education intervention: M-SPAN. *Medicine & Science in Sports & Exercise, 36,* 1382-1388.

McKenzie, T.L., Sallis, J.F., & Rosengard, P. (2009). Beyond the stucco tower: Design, development, and dissemination of the SPARK physical education programs. *Quest, 61*(1), 114-127.

Metzler, M.W., McKenzie, T.L., van der Mars, H., Barrett-Williams, S.L., & Ellis, R. (2013a). Health Optimizing Physical Education (HOPE): A new curriculum for school programs—Part 1: Establishing the need and describing the model. *Journal of Physical Education, Recreation & Dance, 84*(4), 41-47.

Metzler, M.W., McKenzie, T.L., van der Mars, H., Barrett-Williams, S.L., & Ellis, R. (2013b). Health Optimizing Physical Education (HOPE): A new curriculum for school programs—Part 2: Teacher knowledge and collaboration. *Journal of Physical Education, Recreation & Dance, 84*(5), 25-34.

Napper-Owen, G.E., Marston, R., Volkinburg, P.V., Afeman, H., & Brewer, J. (2008). What constitutes a highly qualified physical education teacher? *Journal of Physical Education, Recreation & Dance, 79,* 26-51.

National Association for Sport and Physical Education (NASPE). (2006). *Opposing substitution and waiver/exemptions for required physical education* [Position statement]. Reston, VA: Author.

National Association for Sport and Physical Education (NASPE). (2007). *What constitutes a highly qualified physical education teacher* [Position statement]. Reston, VA: Author.

Rink, J. (2014). *Teaching physical education for learning* (7th ed.). New York, NY: McGraw-Hill.

Robinson, L.H., Stodden, D.F., Barnett, L.M., Lopes, V., Logan, S.W., Rodrigues, L.P., & D'Hondt, E. (2015). Motor competence and its effect on positive developmental trajectories of health. *Sports Medicine, 45,* 1273-1284.

Rowe, P.J., Schuldheisz, J.M., & van der Mars, H. (1997). Validation of SOFIT for measuring physical activity of first- to eighth-grade students. *Pediatric Exercise Science, 9,* 136-149.

Rowe, P., van der Mars, H., Schuldheisz, J., & Fox, S. (2004). Measuring students' physical activity levels: Validating SOFIT for use with high-school students. *Journal of Teaching in Physical Education, 23,* 235-251.

Sallis, J.F., McKenzie, T.L., Alcaraz, J.E., Kolody, B., Faucette, N., & Hovell, M.F. (1997). The effects of a 2-year physical education program (SPARK) on physical activity and fitness in elementary school students. Sports, Play and Active Recreation for Kids. *American Journal of Public Health, 87,* 1328-1334.

Sallis, J.F., McKenzie, T.L., Beets, M.W., Beighle, A., Erwin, H., & Lee, S. (2012). Physical education's role in public health: Steps forward and backward over 20 years and HOPE for the future. *Research Quarterly for Exercise and Sport, 83,* 125-135.

SHAPE America. (2009). *Appropriate instructional practice guidelines, K-12: A side-by-side comparison.* Retrieved from www.shapeamerica.org/standards/guidelines/upload/Appropriate-Instructional-Practices-Grid.pdf

SHAPE America. (2010). *Opportunity to learn: Guidelines for elementary, middle & high school physical education: A side-by-side comparison.* Retrieved from www.shapeamerica.org/standards/guidelines/upload/Opportunity-to-Learn-Grid.pdf

SHAPE America. (2013). *Grade-level outcomes for K-12 physical education.* Retrieved from www.shapeamerica.org/standards/pe/upload/Grade-Level-Outcomes-for-K-12-Physical-Education.pdf

SHAPE America. (2015a). *The essential components of physical education.* Retrieved from www.shapeamerica.org/upload/TheEssentialComponentsofPhysicalEducation.pdf

SHAPE America. (2015b). *Guide for physical education policy.* Retrieved from www.shapeamerica.org/advocacy/upload/Guide-for-Physical-Education-Policy-9-23-14.pdf

SHAPE America. (2016). *2016 SHAPE of the nation: Status of physical education in the USA.* Retrieved from www.shapeamerica.org/uploads/pdfs/son/Shape-of-the-Nation-2016_web.pdf

Shephard, R.J., & Trudeau, F. (2000). The legacy of physical education: Influences on adult lifestyle. *Pediatric Exercise Science, 12*(1), 34-50.

Stodden, D.F., Goodway, J.D., Langendorfer, S.J., Roberton, M.A., Rudisill, M.E., Garcia, C., & Garcia, L.E. (2008). A developmental perspective on the role of motor skill competence in physical activity: An emergent relationship. *Quest, 60,* 290-306.

Stodden, D., Langendorfer, S., & Roberton, M.A. (2009). The association between motor skill competence and physical fitness in young adults. *Research Quarterly for Exercise and Sport, 80,* 223-229.

Trudeau, F., & Shephard, R.J. (2008). Physical education, school physical activity, school sports and academic performance. *International Journal of Behavioral Nutrition and Physical Activity, 5.* http://doi.org/10.1186/1479-5868-5-10

Webster, C.A., Beets, M., Weaver, R.G., Vazou, S., & Russ, L. (2015). Rethinking recommendations for implementing comprehensive school physical activity programs: A partnership model. *Quest, 67,* 185-202.

Webster, C.A., Stodden, D.F., Carson, R.L., Egan, C., & Nesbitt, D. (2016). Integrative public health-aligned physical education and implications for the professional preparation of future teachers and teacher educators/researchers in the field. *Quest, 68,* 457-474. doi:10.1080/00336297.2016.1229628

Williams, S.M., Phelps, D., Laurson, K.R., Thomas, D.Q., & Brown, D.D. (2013). Fitness knowledge, cardiorespiratory endurance and body composition of high school students. *Biomedical Human Kinetics, 5*(1), 17-21. http://doi.org/10.2478/bhk-2013-0004

Chapter 7

Babkes Stellino, M., Sinclair, C.D., Partridge, J.A., & King, K.M. (2010). Differences in children's recess physical activity: Recess Activity of the Week intervention. *Journal of School Health, 80*(9), 436-444.

Beets, M.W., Okely, A., Weaver, R.G., Webster, C., Lubans, D., Brusseau, T., . . . Cliff, D.P. (2016). The theory of expanded, extended, and enhanced opportunities for youth physical activity promotion. *International Journal of Behavioral Nutrition and Physical Activity, 13*(1), 120.

Beighle, A. (2012). *Increasing physical activity through recess.* Retrieved from https://activelivingresearch.org/sites/default/files/ALR_Brief_Recess.pdf

Beighle, A., Morgan, C.F., Le Masurier, G., & Pangrazi, R.P. (2006). Children's physical activity during recess and outside of school. *Journal of School Health, 76*(10), 516-520.

Brusseau, T.A., Kulinna, P.H., Tudor-Locke, C., Ferry, M., van der Mars, H., & Darst, P.W. (2011). Pedometer-determined segmented physical activity patterns of fourth and fifth grade children. *Journal of Physical Activity and Health, 8*(2), 279-286.

Centers for Disease Control and Prevention. (2018). *Physical activity and health.* Retrieved from www.cdc.gov/physicalactivity/basics/pa-health/index.htm

Donnelly, J.E., Greene, J.L., Gibson, C.A., Smith, B.K., Washburn, R.A., Sullivan, D.K., . . . Williams, S.L. (2009). Physical Activity Across the Curriculum (PAAC): A randomized controlled trial to promote physical activity and diminish overweight and obesity in elementary school children. *Preventive Medicine, 49*(4), 336-341.

Dunn, L.L., Venturanza, J.A., Walsh, R.J., & Nonas, C.A. (2012). An observational evaluation of Move-To-Improve, a classroom-based physical activity program, New York City schools, 2010. *Preventing Chronic Disease, 9,* E146. http://dx.doi.org/10.5888/pcd9.120072

Erwin, H.E., Abel, M.G., Beighle, A., & Beets, M.W. (2011). Promoting children's health through physically active math classes. *Health Promotion Practice, 12*(2), 244-251.

Erwin, H.E., Abel, M.G., Beighle, A., Noland, M.P., Worley, B., & Riggs, R. (2012). The contribution of recess to children's school-day physical activity. *Journal of Physical Activity and Health, 9,* 442-448.

Erwin, H.E., Beets, M.W., Centeio, E., & Morrow, J.R. (2014). Best practices and recommendations for increasing physical activity in youth. *Journal of Physical Education, Recreation & Dance, 87*(7), 27-34.

Erwin, H.E., Beighle, A., Routen, A.C., & Montemayor, B. (2017). Perceptions of using sit-to-stand desks in a middle school classroom. *Health Promotion Practice, 19*(1), 68-74. doi:1524839917730046

Erwin, H.E., Fedewa, A.L., Ahn, S., & Thornton, M. (2016). Elementary students' physical activity levels and behavior when using stability balls. *American Journal of Occupational Therapy, 70*(2), 700220010.

Erwin, H.E., Fedewa, A., Beighle, A., & Soyeon, A. (2012). A quantitative review of physical activity, health, and learning outcomes associated with classroom-based physical activity interventions. *Journal of Applied School Psychology, 28*(1), 14-36.

Erwin, H.E., Ickes, M., Ahn, S., & Fedewa, A. (2014). Impact of recess interventions on children's physical activity: A meta-analysis. *American Journal of Health Promotion, 28*(3), 159-167.

Fedewa, A.L., Abel, M., & Erwin, H.E. (2017). The effects of using stationary bicycle desks in classrooms on adolescents' physical activity. *Journal of Occupational Therapy, Schools, & Early Intervention, 10*(1), 78-89. https://doi.org/10.1080/19411243.2016.126645

Fedewa, A.L., & Erwin, H.E. (2011). Stability balls and students with attention and hyperactivity concerns: Implications for on-task and in-seat behavior. *American Journal of Occupational Therapy, 63,* 393-399.

Gopher Sport. (2017). *Active & Healthy Schools*™. Retrieved from www.gophersport.com/resources/active-healthy-schools

Hood, N.E., Colabianchi, N., Terry-McElrath, Y.M., O'Malley, P.M., & Johnston, L.D. (2014). Physical activity breaks and facilities in US secondary schools. *Journal of School Health, 84*(11), 697-705.

Huberty, J.L., Siahpush, M., Beighle, A., Fuhrmeister, E., Silva, P., & Welk, G. (2011). Ready for Recess: A pilot study to increase physical activity in elementary school children. *Journal of School Health, 81*(5), 251-257.

Ickes, M.J., Erwin, H., & Beighle, A. (2013). Systematic review of recess interventions to increase physical activity. *Journal of Physical Activity and Health, 10*(6), 910-926.

Israel, B.A., Schulz, A.J., Parker, E.A., Becker, A.B., Allen, A.J., & Guzman, R. (2003). Critical issues in developing and following community based participatory research principles. In M.

Minkler & N. Wallerstein (Eds.), *Community-based participatory research for health* (pp. 47–66). San Francisco, CA: Jossey-Bass.

Jarrett, O.S., Maxwell, D.M., Dickerson, C., Hoge, P., Davies, G., & Yetley, A. (1998). Impact of recess on classroom behavior: Group effects and individual differences. *The Journal of Educational Research, 92*(2), 121-126.

Katz, D.L. Cushman, D., Reynolds, J., Nijke, V., Treu, J.A., Walker, J., . . . Katz, C. (2010). Putting physical activity where it fits in the school day: Preliminary results of the ABC (Activity Bursts in the Classroom) for fitness program. *Preventing Chronic Disease, 7*(4), A82.

Kibbe, D.L., Hackett, J., Hurley, M., McFarland, A., Schubert, K.G., Schultz, A., & Harris, S. (2011). Ten years of Take 10!: Integrating physical activity with academic concepts in elementary school classrooms. *Preventive Medicine, 52*(Suppl.1), S43-S50.

Loucaides, C.A., Jago, R., & Charalambous, I. (2009). Promoting physical activity during school break times: Piloting a simple, low cost intervention. *Preventive Medicine, 48*(4), 332-334.

Lorenz, K.A., van der Mars, H., Kulinna, P.H., & Ainstworth, B.E. (2017). Environmental and behavioral influences of physical activity in Junior High students. *Journal of Physical Activity and Health, 14*(1), 785-792.

Mahar, M.T., Murphy, S.K., Rowe, D.A., Golden, J., Shields, A.T., & Raedeke, T.D. (2006). Effects of a classroom-based program on physical activity and on-task behavior. *Medicine & Science in Sports & Exercise, 38*(12), 2086-2094.

McKenzie, T.L., Sallis, J.F., Elder, J.P., Berry, C.C., Hoy, P.L., Nader, P.R., . . . Broyles, S.L. (1997). Physical activity levels and prompts in young children at recess: A two-year study of a bi-ethnic sample. *Research Quarterly for Exercise and Sport, 68*(3), 195-202.

Norlander, T., Moas, L., & Archer, T. (2005). Noise and stress in primary and secondary school children: Noise reduction and increased concentration ability through a short but regular exercise and relaxation program. *School Effectiveness and School Improvement, 16*(1), 91-99.

Pellegrini, A.D., & Bohn, C.M. (2005). The role of recess in children's cognitive performance and school adjustment. *Educational Researcher, 34*(1), 13-19.

Ridgers, N.D., Stratton, G., & Fairclough, S.J. (2005). Assessing physical activity during recess using accelerometry. *Preventive Medicine, 41*(1), 102-107.

Ridgers, N.D., Stratton, G., Fairclough, S.J., & Twisk, J.W.R. (2007). Long-term effects of playground markings and physical structures on children's recess physical activity levels. *Preventive Medicine, 44,* 393-397.

Russ, L.B., Webster, C.A., Beets, M.W., Weaver, R.G., Egan, C.A., Harvey, R., & Phillips, D. (2017). Development of the System for Observing Student Movement in Academic Routines and Transitions (SOSMART). *Health Education & Behavior, 44*(2), 304-315.

Stratton, G., & Mullan, E. (2005). The effect of multicolor playground markings on children's physical activity level during recess. *Preventive Medicine, 41*(5), 828-833.

Strong, W.B., Malina, R.M., Blimkie, C.J., Daniels, S.R., Dishman, R.K., Gutin, B., . . . Rowland, T. (2005). Evidence based physical activity for school-age youth. *Journal of Pediatrics, 146*(6), 732-737.

Szabo-Reed, A.N., Willis, E.A., Lee, J., Hillman, C.H., Washburn, R.A., & Donnelly, J.E. (2017). Impact of 3 years of classroom physical activity bouts on time-on-task behavior. *Medicine & Science in Sports & Exercise, 49*(11), 2343-2350. doi:10.1249/MSS.0000000000001346

Tudor-Locke, C., Lee, S.M., Morgan, C.F., Beighle, A., & Pangrazi, R.P. (2006). Children's pedometer-determined physical activity during the segmented school day. *Medicine & Science in Sports & Exercise, 38*(10), 1732-1738.

Turner, L., & Chaloupka, F.J. (2016). Reach and implementation of physical activity breaks and active lessons in elementary school classrooms. *Health Education & Behavior, 44*(3), 370-375.

Verstraete, S.J., Cardon, G.M., De Clercq, D.L., & De Bourdeaudhuij, I.M. (2006). Increasing children's physical activity levels during recess periods in elementary schools: The effects of providing game equipment. *European Journal of Public Health, 16*(4), 415-419.

Waite-Stupiansky, S., & Findlay, M. (2001). The fourth R: Recess and its link to learning. *Educational Forum, 66*(1), 16-25.

Watson, A., Timperio, A., Brown, H., Best, K., & Hesketh, K.D. (2017). Effect of classroom-based physical activity interventions on academic and physical activity outcomes: A systematic review and meta-analysis. *International Journal of Behavioral Nutrition and Physical Activity, 14*, 114. doi.org/10.1186/s12966-017-0569-9

Weaver, R.G., Webster, C.A., Egan, C., Campos, C.M.C., Michael, R.D., & Vazou, S. (2017). Partnerships for active children in elementary schools: Outcomes of a 2-year pilot study to increase physical activity during the school day. *American Journal of Health Promotion, 32*(3), 621-630. doi:10.1177/0890117117707289

Webster, C.A., Beets, M.W., Weaver, R.G., Vazou, S., & Russ, L. (2015). Rethinking recommendations for implementing Comprehensive School Physical Activity Programs: A partnership model. *Quest, 67*(2), 185-202.

Chapter 8

Afterschool Alliance. (2014). *America after 3pm: Afterschool programs in demand.* Retrieved from http://afterschoolalliance.org/documents/AA3PM-2014/AA3PM_National_Report.pdf

Ajja, R., Beets, M.W., Huberty, J., Kaczynski, A.T., & Ward, D.S. (2012). The Healthy Afterschool Activity and Nutrition Documentation Instrument. *American Journal of Preventive Medicine, 43*(3), 263-271. https://doi.org/10.1016/j.amepre.2012.05.020

Ajja, R., Clennin, M.N., Weaver, R.G., Moore, J.B., Huberty, J.L., Ward, D.S., . . . Beets, M. W. (2014). Association of environment and policy characteristics on children's moderate-to-vigorous physical activity and time spent sedentary in afterschool programs. *Preventive Medicine, 69*(Suppl.), S49-S54. https://doi.org/10.1016/j.ypmed.2014.09.010

Annesi, J.J., Tennant, G., Westcott, W.L., Faigenbaum, A.D., & Smith, A.E. (2009). Effects of the Youth Fit for Life protocol on physiological, psychological, and behavioral factors at YMCA Calgary after-school care sites. *Psychological Reports, 104*(3), 879-895. https://doi.org/10.2466/PR0.104.3.879-895

Annesi, J.J., Unruh, J.L., & Smith, A.E. (2007). Relations of sex differences in initial body mass index and physical activity with observed changes over 12 weeks among children in the Youth Fit for Life after-school care intervention. *Perceptual and Motor Skills, 105*(3), 1196-1202. https://doi.org/10.2466/PMS.105.7.1196-1202

Annesi, J.J., Walsh, S.M., Greenwood, B.L., Mareno, N., & Unruh-Rewkowski, J.L. (2017). Effects of the Youth Fit 4 Life physical activity/nutrition protocol on body mass index, fitness and targeted social cognitive theory variables in 9- to 12-year-olds during after-school care. *Journal of Paediatrics and Child Health, 53*(4), 365-373. https://doi.org/10.1111/jpc.13447

Annesi, J.J., Westcott, W.L., & Faigenbaum, A.D. (2005). Effects of a 12-week physical activity protocol delivered by YMCA after-school counselors (Youth Fit For Life) on fitness and self-efficacy changes in 5-12-year-old boys and girls. *Research Quarterly for Exercise and Sport, 76*(4), 468-476.

Atkin, A.J., Gorely, T., Biddle, S.J.H., Cavill, N., & Foster, C. (2011). Interventions to promote physical activity in young people conducted in the hours immediately after school: A systematic review. *International Journal of Behavioral Medicine, 18*(3), 176-187. https://doi.org/10.1007/s12529-010-9111-z

Babkes Stellino, M., & Dauenhauer, B. (2015). Before school physical activity programming: Evidence for policy inclusion. Research presented at Active Living Research, San Diego, CA.

Babkes Stellino, M., Dauenhauer, B., Stoepker, P., & Kuhn, A.C. (2017). Structured before-school physical activity: Impact on student behaviors and experiences [Abstract]. *Research Quarterly for Exercise and Sport, 88*(S1), A107-A108.

Bassett, D.R., Fitzhugh, E.C., Heath, G.W., Erwin, P.C., Frederick, G.M., Wolff, D.L., . . . Stout, A.B. (2013). Estimated energy expenditures for school-based policies and active living. *American Journal of Preventive Medicine, 44*(2), 108-113. https://doi.org/10.1016/j.amepre.2012.10.017

Beets, M.W. (2012a). Enhancing the translation of physical activity interventions in afterschool programs. *American Journal of Lifestyle Medicine, 6*(4), 328-341. https://doi.org/10.1177/1559827611433547

Beets, M.W. (2012b). *Policies and standards for promoting physical activity in after-school programs: A research brief.* Retrieved from https://activelivingresearch.org/sites/default/files/ALR_Brief_Afterschool_May2012_0.pdf

Beets, M.W., Beighle, A., Erwin, H.E., & Huberty, J.L. (2009). After-school program impact on physical activity and fitness: A meta-analysis. *American Journal of Preventive Medicine, 36*(6), 527-537. https://doi.org/10.1016/j.amepre.2009.01.033

Beets, M.W., Huberty, J., & Beighle, A. (2012). Physical activity of children attending afterschool programs. *American Journal of Preventive Medicine, 42*(2), 180-184. https://doi.org/10.1016/j.amepre.2011.10.007

Beets, M.W., Huberty, J., & Beighle, A. (2013). Systematic observation of physical activity in afterschool programs: Preliminary findings from Movin' Afterschool intervention. *Journal of Physical Activity & Health, 10*(7), 974-981.

Beets, M.W., Huberty, J., Beighle, A., Moore, J.B., Webster, C., Ajja, R., & Weaver, G. (2013). Impact of policy environment characteristics on physical activity and sedentary behaviors of children attending afterschool programs. *Health Education & Behavior, 40*(3), 296-304.

Beets, M.W., Shah, R., Weaver, R.G., Huberty, J., Beighle, A., & Moore, J.B. (2015). Physical activity in afterschool programs: Comparison with physical activity policies. *Journal of Physical Activity & Health, 12*(1), 1-7.

Beets, M.W., Wallner, M., & Beighle, A. (2010). Defining standards and policies for promoting physical activity in afterschool programs. *Journal of School Health, 80*(8), 411-417. https://doi.org/10.1111/j.1746-1561.2010.00521.x

Beets, M.W., Weaver, R.G., Moore, J.B., Turner-McGrievy, G., Pate, R.R., Webster, C., & Beighle, A. (2014). From policy to practice: Strategies to meet physical activity standards in YMCA afterschool programs. *American Journal of Preventive Medicine, 46*(3), 281-288. https://doi.org/10.1016/j.amepre.2013.10.012

Beets, M.W., Weaver, R.G., Turner-McGrievy, G., Huberty, J., Ward, D.S., Freedman, D.A., . . . Moore, J.B. (2014). Making healthy eating and physical activity policy practice: The design and overview of a group randomized controlled trial in afterschool programs. *Contemporary Clinical Trials, 38*(2), 291-303. https://doi.org/10.1016/j.cct.2014.05.013

Beets, M.W., Weaver, R.G., Turner-McGrievy, G., Huberty, J., Ward, D.S., Pate, R.R., . . . Beighle, A. (2015). Making policy practice in afterschool programs: A randomized controlled trial on physical activity changes. *American Journal of Preventive Medicine, 48*(6), 694-706. https://doi.org/10.1016/j.amepre.2015.01.012

Beets, M.W., Weaver, R.G., Turner-McGrievy, G., Huberty, J., Ward, D.S., Pate, R.R., . . . Beighle, A. (2016). Physical activity outcomes in afterschool programs: A group randomized controlled trial. *Preventive Medicine, 90,* 207-215. https://doi.org/10.1016/j.ypmed.2016.07.002

Beets, M.W., Weaver, R.G., Turner-McGrievy, G., Moore, J.B., Webster, C., Brazendale, K., . . . Beighle, A. (2016). Are we there yet? Compliance with physical activity standards in YMCA afterschool programs. *Childhood Obesity, 12*(4), 237-246. https://doi.org/10.1089/chi.2015.0223

Beets, M.W., Webster, C., Saunders, R., & Huberty, J.L. (2013). Translating policies into practice: A framework to prevent childhood obesity in afterschool programs. *Health Promotion Practice, 14*(2), 228-237. https://doi.org/10.1177/1524839912446320

Beighle, A., Beets, M.W., Erwin, H.E., Huberty, J.L., Moore, J.B., & Stellino, M.B. (2010). Promoting physical activity in afterschool programs. *Afterschool Matters, 11,* 24-32.

Bocarro, J., Kanters, M.A., Casper, J., & Forrester, S. (2008). School physical education, extracurricular sports, and lifelong active living. *Journal of Teaching in Physical Education, 27*(2), 155-166.

Bocarro, J.N., Kanters, M.A., Cerin, E., Floyd, M.F., Casper, J.M., Suau, L.J., & McKenzie, T.L. (2012). School sport policy and school-based physical activity environments and their association with observed physical activity in middle school children. *Health & Place, 18*(1), 31-38. https://doi.org/10.1016/j.healthplace.2011.08.007

Bocarro, J.N., Kanters, M.A., Edwards, M.B., Casper, J.M., & McKenzie, T.L. (2014). Prioritizing school intramural and interscholastic programs based on observed physical activity. *American Journal of Health Promotion, 28,* S65-S71.

Brazendale, K., Beets, M.W., Weaver, R.G., Huberty, J., Beighle, A.E., & Pate, R.R. (2015). Wasting our time? Allocated versus accumulated physical activity in afterschool programs. *Journal of Physical Activity & Health, 12*(8), 1061-1065.

Brazendale, K., Chandler, J.L., Beets, M.W., Weaver, R.G., Beighle, A., Huberty, J.L., & Moore, J.B. (2015). Maximizing children's physical activity using the LET US Play principles. *Preventive Medicine, 76,* 14-19. https://doi.org/10.1016/j.ypmed.2015.03.012

Centers for Disease Control and Prevention (CDC). (2015). *Results from the School Health Policies and Practices Study 2014.* Retrieved from www.cdc.gov/healthyyouth/data/shpps/pdf/SHPPS-508-final_101315.pdf

Chaufan, C., Yeh, J., & Fox, P. (2012). The Safe Routes to School program in California: An update. *American Journal of Public Health, 102*(6), e8-e11. https://doi.org/10.2105/AJPH.2012.300703

Chillón, P., Evenson, K.R., Vaughn, A., & Ward, D.S. (2011). A systematic review of interventions for promoting active transportation to school. *International Journal of Behavioral Nutrition and Physical Activity, 8,* 10. https://doi.org/10.1186/1479-5868-8-10

Cradock, A.L., Barrett, J.L., Giles, C.M., Lee, R.M., Kenney, E.L., deBlois, M.E., . . . Gortmaker, S.L. (2016). Promoting physical activity with the Out of School Nutrition and Physical Activity (OSNAP) Initiative: A cluster-randomized controlled trial. *JAMA Pediatrics, 170*(2), 155-162. https://doi.org/10.1001/jamapediatrics.2015.3406

Davison, K.K., Werder, J.L., & Lawson, C.T. (2008). Children's active commuting to school: Current knowledge and future directions. *Preventing Chronic Disease, 5*(3), A100. Retrieved from www.ncbi.nlm.nih.gov/pmc/articles/PMC2483568/

DeBate, R.D., Pettee Gabriel, K., Zwald, M., Huberty, J., & Zhang, Y. (2009). Changes in psychosocial factors and physical activity frequency among third- to eighth-grade girls who participated in a developmentally focused youth sport program: A preliminary study. *The Journal of School Health, 79*(10), 474-484. https://doi.org/10.1111/j.1746-1561.2009.00437.x

Demetriou, Y., Gillison, F., & McKenzie, T. (2017). After-school physical activity interventions on child and adolescent physical activity and health: A review of reviews. *Advances in Physical Education, 7*(2), 191-215.

D'Haese, S., Vanwolleghem, G., Hinckson, E., De Bourdeaudhuij, I., Deforche, B., Van Dyck, D., & Cardon, G. (2015). Cross-continental comparison of the association between the physical environment and active transportation in children: A systematic review. *International Journal of Behavioral Nutrition and Physical Activity, 12*, 1-14. https://doi.org/10.1186/s12966-015-0308-z

DiMaggio, C., & Li, G. (2013). Effectiveness of a Safe Routes to School program in preventing school-aged pedestrian injury. *Pediatrics, 131*(2), 2012-2182. https://doi.org/10.1542/peds.2012-2182

Dohle, S., & Wansink, B. (2013). Fit in 50 years: Participation in high school sports best predicts one's physical activity after age 70. *BMC Public Health, 13*, 1100. https://doi.org/10.1186/1471-2458-13-1100

Dzewaltowski, D.A., Rosenkranz, R.R., Geller, K.S., Coleman, K.J., Welk, G.J., Hastmann, T.J., & Milliken, G.A. (2010). HOP'N after-school project: An obesity prevention randomized controlled trial. *International Journal of Behavioral Nutrition and Physical Activity, 7*, 90. https://doi.org/10.1186/1479-5868-7-90

Edwards, M.B., Bocarro, J.N., Kanters, M., & Casper, J. (2011). Participation in interscholastic and intramural sport programs in middle schools: An exploratory investigation of race and gender. *Recreational Sports Journal, 35*(2), 157-173.

Edwards, M.B., Kanters, M.A., & Bocarro, J.N. (2014). Policy changes to implement intramural sports in North Carolina middle schools: Simulated effects on sports participation rates and physical activity intensity, 2008-2009. *Preventing Chronic Disease, 11*. https://doi.org/10.5888/pcd11.130195

Edwards, M.J., May, T., Kesten, J.M., Banfield, K., Bird, E.L., Powell, J.E., . . . Jago, R. (2016). Lessons learnt from the Bristol Girls Dance Project cluster RCT: Implications for designing and implementing after-school physical activity interventions. *BMJ Open, 6*(1), e010036. https://doi.org/10.1136/bmjopen-2015-010036

Eime, R.M., Young, J.A., Harvey, J.T., Charity, M.J., & Payne, W.R. (2013). A systematic review of the psychological and social benefits of participation in sport for children and adolescents: Informing development of a conceptual model of health through sport. *The International Journal of Behavioral Nutrition and Physical Activity, 10*, 98. https://doi.org/10.1186/1479-5868-10-98

Faulkner, G.E.J., Buliung, R.N., Flora, P.K., & Fusco, C. (2009). Active school transport, physical activity levels and body weight of children and youth: A systematic review. *Preventive Medicine, 48*(1), 3-8. https://doi.org/10.1016/j.ypmed.2008.10.017

Galeotti, S. (2015). Empowering pre-adolescent girls: Girls on the Run experiential learning program exploratory study. *Journal of Experiential Education, 38*(4), 407-423. https://doi.org/10.1177/1053825915603578

Garn, A.C., McCaughtry, N., Kulik, N.L., Kaseta, M., Maljak, K., Whalen, L., . . . Fahlman, M. (2014). Successful after-school physical activity clubs in urban high schools: Perspectives of adult leaders and student participants. *Journal of Teaching in Physical Education, 33*(1), 112-133. https://doi.org/10.1123/jtpe:2013-0006

Gortmaker, S.L., Lee, R.M., Mozaffarian, R.S., Sobol, A.M., Nelson, T.F., Roth, B.A., & Wiecha, J.L. (2012). Effect of an after-school intervention on increases in children's physical activity. *Medicine & Science in Sports & Exercise, 44*(3), 450-457. https://doi.org/10.1249/MSS.0b013e3182300128

Goudeau, S., Baker, B., & Garn, A.C. (2014). Teacher perceptions of barriers to implementing a school-based physical activity club: A qualitative investigation. *The Global Journal of Health and Physical Education Pedagogy, 3*(3), 256-269.

Hamer, M., & Chida, Y. (2008). Active commuting and cardiovascular risk: A meta-analytic review. *Preventive Medicine, 46*(1), 9-13. https://doi.org/10.1016/j.ypmed.2007.03.006

Heelan, K.A., Abbey, B.M., Donnelly, J.E., Mayo, M.S., & Welk, G.J. (2009). Evaluation of a Walking School Bus for promoting physical activity in youth. *Journal of Physical Activity & Health, 6*(5), 560-567. https://doi.org/10.1123/jpah.6.5.560

Herrick, H., Thompson, H., Kinder, J., & Madsen, K.A. (2012). Use of SPARK to promote after-school physical activity. *Journal of School Health, 82*(10), 457-461. https://doi.org/10.1111/j.1746-1561.2012.00722.x

Huberty, J.L., Beets, M.W., Beighle, A., & McKenzie, T.L. (2013). Association of staff behaviors and afterschool program features to physical activity: Findings from Movin' After School. *Journal of Physical Activity & Health, 10*(3), 423-429. https://doi.org/10.1123/jpah.10.3.423

Huberty, J.L., Dinkel, D.M., & Beets, M.W. (2014). Evaluation of GoGirlGo!: A practitioner based program to improve physical activity. *BMC Public Health, 14,* 118. https://doi.org/10.1186/1471-2458-14-118

Hughey, S.M., Weaver, R.G., Saunders, R., Webster, C., & Beets, M.W. (2014). Process evaluation of an intervention to increase child activity levels in afterschool programs. *Evaluation and Program Planning, 45,* 164-170. https://doi.org/10.1016/j.evalprogplan.2014.04.004

Institute of Medicine. (2013). *Educating the student body: Taking physical activity and physical education to school.* Retrieved from www.nap.edu/read/18314/chapter/1

Iversen, C.S.S., Nigg, C., & Titchenal, C.A. (2011). The impact of an elementary after-school nutrition and physical activity program on children's fruit and vegetable intake, physical activity, and body mass index: Fun 5. *Hawaii Medical Journal, 70*(7 Suppl. 1), 37-41.

Jago, R., Edwards, M.J., Sebire, S.J., Cooper, A.R., Powell, J.E., Bird, E.L., . . . Blair, P.S. (2013). Bristol Girls Dance Project (BGDP): Protocol for a cluster randomised controlled trial of an after-school dance programme to increase physical activity among 11-12 year old girls. *BMC Public Health, 13,* 1003. https://doi.org/10.1186/1471-2458-13-1003

Jago, R., Edwards, M.J., Sebire, S.J., Tomkinson, K., Bird, E.L., Banfield, K., . . . Blair, P.S. (2015). Effect and cost of an after-school dance programme on the physical activity of 11-12 year old girls: The Bristol Girls Dance Project, a school-based cluster randomised controlled trial. *International Journal of Behavioral Nutrition and Physical Activity, 12,* 128. https://doi.org/10.1186/s12966-015-0289-y

Jago, R., Sebire, S.J., Cooper, A.R., Haase, A.M., Powell, J., Davis, L., . . . Montgomery, A.A. (2012). Bristol Girls Dance Project feasibility trial: Outcome and process evaluation results. *International Journal of Behavioral Nutrition and Physical Activity, 9,* 83. https://doi.org/10.1186/1479-5868-9-83

Johnston, L.D., Delva, J., & O'Malley, P.M. (2007). Sports participation and physical education in American secondary schools: Current levels and racial/ethnic and socioeconomic disparities. *American Journal of Preventive Medicine, 33*(4 Suppl.), S195-S208. https://doi.org/10.1016/j.amepre.2007.07.015

Jones, S.E., & Sliwa, S. (2016). School factors associated with the percentage of students who walk or bike to school, School Health Policies and Practices Study, 2014. *Preventing Chronic Disease, 13.* https://doi.org/10.5888/pcd13.150573

Kanters, M., Bocarro, J., Casper, J., & Forrester, S. (2008). Determinants of sport participation in middle school children and the impact of intramural sports. *Recreational Sports Journal, 32*(2), 134-151.

Kanters, M., Bocarro, J., Edwards, M., Casper, J., & Floyd, M. (2013). School sport participation under two school sport policies: Comparisons by race/ethnicity, gender, and socioeconomic status. *Annals of Behavioral Medicine, 45,* 113-121. https://doi.org/10.1007/s12160-012-9413-2

Kanters, M.A., Bocarro, J.N., Greenwood, P.B., Casper, J.M., Suau, L., & McKenzie, T.L. (2012). Determinants of middle school sport participation: A comparison of different models for school sport delivery. *International Journal of Sport Management and Marketing, 12*(3/4), 159-179.

Kelder, S., Hoelscher, D.M., Barroso, C.S., Walker, J.L., Cribb, P., & Hu, S. (2005). The CATCH Kids Club: A pilot after-school study for improving elementary students' nutrition and physical activity. *Public Health Nutrition, 8*(2), 133-140. https://doi.org/10.1079/PHN2004678

Kenney, E.L., Giles, C.M., deBlois, M.E., Gortmaker, S.L., Chinfatt, S., & Cradock, A.L. (2014). Improving nutrition and physical activity policies in afterschool programs: Results from a group-randomized controlled trial. *Preventive Medicine, 66,* 159-166. https://doi.org/10.1016/j.ypmed.2014.06.011

Larouche, R., Saunders, T.J., John Faulkner, G.E., Colley, R., & Tremblay, M. (2014). Associations between active school transport and physical activity, body composition, and cardiovascular fitness: A systematic review of 68 studies. *Journal of Physical Activity & Health, 11*(1), 206-227. https://doi.org/10.1123/jpah.2011-0345

Lee, M.C., Orenstein, M.R., & Richardson, M.J. (2008). Systematic review of active commuting to school and children's physical activity and weight. *Journal of Physical Activity & Health, 5*(6), 930-949.

Maljak, K., Garn, A., McCaughtry, N., Kulik, N., Martin, J., Shen, B., . . . Fahlman, M. (2014). Challenges in offering inner-city after-school physical activity clubs. *American Journal of Health Education, 45*(5), 297-307. https://doi.org/10.1080/19325037.2014.934414

McDonald, N.C. (2007). Active transportation to school: Trends among U.S. schoolchildren, 1969-2001. *American Journal of Preventive Medicine, 32*(6), 509-516. https://doi.org/10.1016/j.amepre.2007.02.022

McDonald, N.C. (2015). *Impact of Safe Routes to School programs on walking and biking.* Retrieved from http://activelivingresearch.org/sites/default/files/ALR_Review_SRTS_May2015_0.pdf

McDonald, N.C., Steiner, R.L., Lee, C., Smith, T.R., Zhu, X., & Yang, Y. (2014). Impact of the Safe Routes to School program on walking and bicycling. *Journal of the American Planning Association, 80*(2), 153-167. https://doi.org/10.1080/01944363.2014.956654

McDonald, N.C., Yang, Y., Abbott, S.M., & Bullock, A.N. (2013). Impact of the Safe Routes to School program on walking and biking: Eugene, Oregon study. *Transport Policy, 29,* 243-248. https://doi.org/10.1016/j.tranpol.2013.06.007

Mears, R., & Jago, R. (2016). Effectiveness of after-school interventions at increasing moderate-to-vigorous physical activity levels in 5- to 18-year olds: A systematic review and meta-analysis. *British Journal of Sports Medicine, 50*(21). https://doi.org/10.1136/bjsports-2015-094976

Mendoza, J.A., Levinger, D.D., & Johnston, B.D. (2009). Pilot evaluation of a walking school bus program in a low-income, urban community. *BMC Public Health, 9*, 122. https://doi.org/10.1186/1471-2458-9-122

Mendoza, J.A., Watson, K., Baranowski, T., Nicklas, T.A., Uscanga, D.K., & Hanfling, M.J. (2011). The Walking School Bus and children's physical activity: A pilot cluster randomized controlled trial. *Pediatrics, 128*(3), e537-e544. https://doi.org/10.1542/peds.2010-3486

National AfterSchool Association. (2011). *National AfterSchool Association HEPA standards.* Retrieved from https://naaweb.org/images/NAA_HEPA_Standards_new_look_2015.pdf

National Center for Safe Routes to School. (2015). *Creating healthier generations: A look at the 10 years of federal Safe Routes to School program.* Retrieved from www.pedbikeinfo.org/pdf/Community_SRTSfederal_CreatingHealthierGenerations.pdf

National Federation of State High School Associations (NFSHSA). (2016). *2015-16 High school athletics participation survey.* Retrieved from www.nfhs.org/ParticipationStatistics/PDF/2015-16_Sports_Participation_Survey.pdf

National Institute on Out-of-School Time (NIOST). (n.d.). *BOKS longitudinal evaluation.* Retrieved from www.niost.org/Active-Projects/boks-longitudinal-evaluation

Nichol, M.E., Pickett, W., & Janssen, I. (2009). Associations between school recreational environments and physical activity. *Journal of School Health, 79*(6), 247-254. https://doi.org/10.1111/j.1746-1561.2009.00406.x

Pate, R.R., & O'Neill, J.R. (2009). After-school interventions to increase physical activity among youth. *British Journal of Sports Medicine, 43*(1), 14-18.

Pate, R.R., Trost, S.G., Levin, S., & Dowda, M. (2000). Sports participation and health-related behaviors among US youth. *Archives of Pediatrics & Adolescent Medicine, 154*(9), 904-911. https://doi.org/10.1001/archpedi.154.9.904

Perkins, D.F., Jacobs, J.E., Barber, B.L., & Eccles, J.S. (2004). Childhood and adolescent sports participation as predictors of participation in sports and physical fitness activities during young adulthood. *Youth & Society, 35*(4), 495-520. https://doi.org/10.1177/0044118X03261619

Pojednic, R., Peabody, S., Carson, S., Kennedy, M., Bevans, K., & Phillips, E.M. (2016). The effect of before school physical activity on child development: A study protocol to evaluate the Build Our Kids Success (BOKS) program. *Contemporary Clinical Trials, 49,* 103-108. https://doi.org/10.1016/j.cct.2016.06.009

Pont, K., Ziviani, J., Wadley, D., Bennett, S., & Abbott, R. (2009). Environmental correlates of children's active transportation: A systematic literature review. *Health & Place, 15*(3), 849-862. https://doi.org/10.1016/j.healthplace.2009.02.002

Ratey, J. (2008). *SPARK: The revolutionary new science of exercise and the brain.* New York, NY: Little, Brown and Company.

Robbins, L.B., Ling, J., Toruner, E.K., Bourne, K.A., & Pfeiffer, K.A. (2016). Examining reach, dose, and fidelity of the "Girls on the Move" after-school physical activity club: A process evaluation. *BMC Public Health, 16.* https://doi.org/10.1186/s12889-016-3329-x

Robbins, L., Pfeiffer, K.A., Maier, K., Lo, Y.-J., & Wesolek (LaDrig), S. (2012). Pilot intervention to increase physical activity among sedentary urban middle school girls: A two-group pretest-posttest quasi-experimental design. *Journal of School Nursing, 28*(4), 302-315. https://doi.org/10.1177/1059840512438777

Robbins, L.B., Pfeiffer, K.A., Vermeesch, A., Resnicow, K., You, Z., An, L., & Wesolek, S.M. (2013). "Girls on the Move" intervention protocol for increasing physical activity among low-active underserved urban girls: A group randomized trial. *BMC Public Health, 13,* 474. https://doi.org/10.1186/1471-2458-13-474

Safe Routes to School (SRTS) National Partnership. (n.d.a). *The 6 Es of safe routes to school.* Retrieved from www.saferoutespartnership.org/safe-routes-school/101/6-Es

Safe Routes to School (SRTS) National Partnership. (n.d.b). *Safe routes to school.* Retrieved www.saferoutespartnership.org/safe-routes-school

Sebire, S.J., Kesten, J.M., Edwards, M.J., May, T., Banfield, K., Tomkinson, K., . . . Jago, R. (2016). Using self-determination theory to promote adolescent girls' physical activity: Exploring the theoretical fidelity of the Bristol Girls Dance Project. *Psychology of Sport and Exercise, 24,* 100-110. https://doi.org/10.1016/j.psychsport.2016.01.009

SHAPE America. (2013). Schools should provide before- and after-school physical activity and intramural sports programs. Retrieved from www.shapeamerica.org/advocacy/positionstatements/pe/upload/Before-and-After-School-Physical-Activity-in-new-SA-template.pdf

Sharpe, E.K., Forrester, S., & Mandigo, J. (2011). Engaging community providers to create more active after-school environments: Results from the Ontario CATCH Kids Club implementation project. *Journal of Physical Activity & Health, 8,* S26-S31.

Slusser, W.M., Sharif, M.Z., Erausquin, J.T., Kinsler, J.J., Collin, D., & Prelip, M.L. (2013). Improving overweight among at-risk minority youth: Results of a pilot intervention in after-school programs. *Journal of Health Care for the Poor and Underserved, 24*(Suppl. 2), 12-24.

Stewart, O., Moudon, A.V., & Claybrooke, C. (2014). Multistate evaluation of safe routes to school programs. *American Journal of Health Promotion, 28*(3 Suppl.), S89-S96. https://doi.org/10.4278/ajhp.130430-QUAN-210

Stylianou, M., Hodges-Kulinna, P., & Kloeppel, T. (2014). Healthy living initiative: Running/walking club. *Physical Educator, 71*(2), 157-184.

Stylianou, M., Kulinna, P.H., van der Mars, H., Mahar, M.T., Adams, M.A., & Amazeen, E. (2016). Before-school running/walking club: Effects on student on-task behavior.

Preventive Medicine Reports, 3, 196-202. https://doi.org/10.1016/j.pmedr.2016.01.010

Stylianou, M., van der Mars, H., Kulinna, P.H., Adams, M.A., Mahar, M., & Amazeen, E. (2016). Before-school running/walking club and student physical activity levels: An efficacy study. *Research Quarterly for Exercise and Sport, 87*(4), 342-353. https://doi.org/10.1080/02701367.2016.1214665

Timperio, A., Ball, K., Salmon, J., Roberts, R., Giles-Corti, B., Simmons, D., . . . Crawford, D. (2006). Personal, family, social, and environmental correlates of active commuting to school. *American Journal of Preventive Medicine, 30*(1), 45-51. https://doi.org/10.1016/j.amepre.2005.08.047

Trost, S.G., Rosenkranz, R.R., & Dzewaltowski, D. (2008). Physical activity levels among children attending after-school programs. *Medicine & Science in Sports & Exercise, 40*(4), 622-629. https://doi.org/10.1249/MSS.0b013e318161eaa5

Trudeau, F., & Shephard, R.J. (2008). Physical education, school physical activity, school sports and academic performance. *International Journal of Behavioral Nutrition and Physical Activity, 5,* 10. https://doi.org/10.1186/1479-5868-5-10

U.S. Department of Health and Human Services. (2008) *2008 physical activity guidelines for Americans.* Retrieved from www.health.gov/paguidelines/pdf/paguide.pdf

Weaver, R.G., Beets, M.W., Beighle, A., Webster, C., Huberty, J., & Moore, J.B. (2016). Strategies to increase afterschool program staff skills to promote healthy eating and physical activity. *Health Promotion Practice, 17*(1), 88-97. https://doi.org/10.1177/1524839915589732

Weaver, R.G., Beets, M.W., Huberty, J., Freedman, D., Turner-McGrievy, G., & Ward, D. (2015). Physical activity opportunities in afterschool programs. *Health Promotion Practice, 16*(3), 371-382. https://doi.org/10.1177/1524839914567740

Weaver, R.G., Beets, M.W., Hutto, B., Saunders, R.P., Moore, J.B., Turner-McGrievy, G., . . . Freedman, D. (2015). Making healthy eating and physical activity policy practice: Process evaluation of a group randomized controlled intervention in afterschool programs. *Health Education Research, 30*(6), 849-865. https://doi.org/10.1093/her/cyv052

Weaver, R.G., Beets, M.W., Saunders, R.P., Beighle, A., & Webster, C. (2014). A comprehensive professional development training's effect on afterschool program staff behaviors to promote healthy eating and physical activity. *Journal of Public Health Management and Practice, 20*(4), E6-E14. https://doi.org/10.1097/PHH.0b013e3182a1fb5d

Weaver, R.G, Beets, M.W., Webster, C., Beighle, A., & Huberty, J. (2012). A conceptual model for training after-school program staffers to promote physical activity and nutrition. *Journal of School Health, 82*(4), 186-195. https://doi.org/10.1111/j.1746-1561.2011.00685.x

Weaver, R.G., Moore, J.B., Huberty, J., Freedman, D., Turner-McGrievy, B., Beighle, A., . . . Beets, M.W. (2016). Process evaluation of making HEPA policy practice.

Health Promotion Practice, 17(5), 631-647. https://doi.org/10.1177/1524839916647331

Weaver, R.G., Moore, J.B., Turner-McGrievy, B., Saunders, R., Beighle, A., Khan, M.M., . . . Beets, M.W. (2016). Identifying strategies programs adopt to meet healthy eating and physical activity standards in afterschool programs. *Health Education & Behavior, 44*(4), 536-547. https://doi.org/10.1177/1090198116676252

Weaver, R.G., Webster, C., & Beets, M.W. (2013). LET US Play: Maximizing physical activity in physical education. *Strategies, 26*(6), 33-37. https://doi.org/10.1080/08924562.2013.839518

Westcott, W.L., Puhala, K., Colligan, A., Loud, R.L., & Cobbett, R. (2015). Physiological effects of the BOKS before-school physical activity program for preadolescent youth. *Journal of Exercise, Sports & Orthopedics, 2*(2), 1-7.

Whalen, L., McCaughtry, N., Garn, A., Kulik, N., Centeio, E. E., Maljak, K., . . . Martin, J. (2016). Why inner-city high-school students attend after-school physical activity clubs. *Health Education Journal, 75*(6), 639-651.

Wiecha, J.L., Hall, G., & Barnes, M. (2014). Uptake of National Afterschool Association physical activity standards among US after-school sites. *Preventive Medicine, 69*(Suppl.), S61-S65. https://doi.org/10.1016/j.ypmed.2014.07.010

Wong, B.Y.-M., Faulkner, G., & Buliung, R. (2011). GIS measured environmental correlates of active school transport: A systematic review of 14 studies. *International Journal of Behavioral Nutrition and Physical Activity, 8,* 39. https://doi.org/10.1186/1479-5868-8-39

Young, D.R., Felton, G.M., & Grieser, M. (2007). Policies and opportunities for physical activity in middle school environments. *Journal of School Health, 77*(1), 41-47. https://doi.org/10.1111/j.1746-1561.2007.00161.x

Yu, C.Y., & Zhu, X. (2016). From attitude to action: What shapes attitude toward walking to/from school and how does it influence actual behaviors? *Preventive Medicine, 90,* 72-78. https://doi.org/10.1016/j.ypmed.2016.06.036

Chapter 9

Allegrante, J.P., & Michela, J.L. (1990). Impact of a school-based workplace health promotion program on morale of inner-city teachers. *Journal of School Health, 60*(1), 25-29.

Allison, K.R., Vu-Nguyen, K., Ng, B., Schoueri-Mychasiw, N., Dwyer, J.J., Manson, H., . . . Robertson, J. (2016). Evaluation of Daily Physical Activity (DPA) policy implementation in Ontario: Surveys of elementary school administrators and teachers. *BMC Public Health, 16*(1), 746.

Anderson, D.R., & Staufacker, M.J. (1996). The impact of worksite-based health risk appraisal on health-related outcomes: A review of the literature. *American Journal of Health Promotion, 10*(6), 499-508.

Anderson, L.M., Quinn, T.A., Glanz, K., Ramirez, G., Kahwati, L.C., Johnson, D.B., . . . Katz, D.L. (2009). The effectiveness of worksite nutri tion and physical activity interventions for controlling employee overweight and obesity: A systematic review. *American Journal of Preventive Medicine, 37*(4), 340-357.

Annesi, J.J., Marti, C.N., & Stice, E. (2010). A meta-analytic review of the Youth Fit For Life intervention for effects on body mass index in 5- to 12-year-old children. *Health Psychology Review, 4*(1), 6-21.

Ayala, A.M.C., Salmon, J., Timperio, A., Sudholz, B., Ridgers, N.D., Sethi, P., & Dunstan, D.W. (2016). Impact of an 8-month trial using height-adjustable desks on children's classroom sitting patterns and markers of cardio-metabolic and musculoskeletal health. *International Journal of Environmental Research and Public Health, 13*(12), 1227.

Barnett, T.A., O'Loughlin, J.L., Gauvin, L., Paradis, G., Hanley, J., McGrath, J.J., & Lambert, M. (2009). School opportunities and physical activity frequency in nine year old children. *International Journal of Public Health, 54*(3), 150-157.

Beets, M.W., Beighle, A., Erwin, H.E., & Huberty, J.L. (2009). Impact of after-school programs to increase physical activity: A meta-analysis. *American Journal of Preventive Medicine, 36*(6), 527-537.

Beets, M.W., Weaver, R.G., Moore, J.B., Turner-McGrievy, G., Pate, R.R., Webster, C., & Beighle, A. (2014). From policy to practice: Strategies to meet physical activity standards in YMCA afterschool programs. *American Journal of Preventive Medicine, 46*(3), 281-288.

Beets, M.W., Weaver, R.G., Turner-McGrievy, G., Huberty, J., Ward, D.S., Pate, R.R., . . . Beighle, A. (2015). Making physical activity policy practice: A group randomized controlled trial on changes in moderate-to-vigorous physical activity in afterschool programs. *American Journal of Preventive Medicine, 48,* 694-706.

Beets, M.W., Weaver, R.G., Turner-McGrievy, G., Huberty, J., Ward, D.S., Pate, R.R., . . . Beighle, A. (2016). Physical activity outcomes in afterschool programs: A group randomized controlled trial. *Preventive Medicine, 90,* 207-215.

Beighle, A., Erwin, H., Castelli, D., & Ernst, M. (2009). Preparing physical educators for the role of physical activity director. *Journal of Physical Education, Recreation & Dance, 80*(4), 24-29.

Benden, M.E., Zhao, H., Jeffrey, C E., Wendel, M.L., & Blake, J.J. (2014). The evaluation of the impact of a stand-biased desk on energy expenditure and physical activity for elementary school students. *International Journal of Environmental Research and Public Health, 11*(9), 9361-9375.

Berei, C.P. (2015). *Describing and understanding factors related to implementing comprehensive school physical activity programs by physical educators.* (Unpublished doctoral dissertation). University of Northern Colorado, Greeley, CO.

Blair, S.N., Collingwood, T.R., Reynolds, R., Smith, M., Hagan, R.D., & Sterling, C.L. (1984). Health promotion for educators: Impact on health behaviors, satisfaction, and general well-being. *American Journal of Public Health, 74*(2), 147-149.

Blair, S.N., Smith, M., Collingwood, T.R., Reynolds, R., Prentice, M.C., & Sterling, C.L. (1986). Health promotion for educators: Impact on absenteeism. *Preventive Medicine, 15*(2), 166-175.

Brazendale, K., Chandler, J.L., Beets, M.W., Weaver, R.G., Beighle, A., Huberty, J.L., & Moore, J.B. (2015). Maximizing children's physical activity using the LET US Play principles. *Preventive Medicine, 76,* 14-19.

Brown, K.M., & Elliott, S.J. (2015). "It's not as easy as just saying 20 minutes a day": Exploring teacher and principal experiences implementing a provincial physical activity policy. *Universal Journal of Public Health, 3*(2), 71-83.

Carson, R. (2012). Certification and duties of a director of physical activity. *Journal of Physical Education, Recreation & Dance, 83,* 16-29.

Castelli, D.M., & Beighle, A. (2007). The physical education teacher as school activity director. *Journal of Physical Education, Recreation & Dance, 78*(5), 25-28.

Cavanagh, B.D., & Meinen, A. (2015). Utilizing Wisconsin afterschool programs to increase physical activity in youth. *Journal of School Health, 85*(10), 697-703.

Centeio, E.E., Erwin, H., & Castelli, D.M. (2014). Comprehensive school physical activity programs: Characteristics of trained teachers. *Journal of Teaching in Physical Education, 33*(4), 492-510.

Cheval, B., Courvoisier, D.S., & Chanal, J. (2016). Developmental trajectories of physical activity during elementary school physical education. *Preventive Medicine, 87,* 170-174.

Conn, V.S., Hafdahi, A.R., Cooper, P.S., Brown, L.M., & Lusk, S.L. (2009). Meta-analysis of workplace physical activity interventions. *American Journal of Preventive Medicine, 37*(4), 330-339.

Corbin, C.B., Welk, G.J., Corbin, W.R., & Welk, K.A. (2016). *Concepts of fitness and wellness: A comprehensive lifestyle approach* (12th ed.). New York, NY: McGraw-Hill.

Cothran, D.J., Kulinna, P.H., & Garn, A.C. (2010). Classroom teachers and physical activity integration. *Teaching and Teacher Education, 26*(7), 1381-1388.

Cullen, K.W., Baranowski, T., Baranowski, J., Hebert, D., DeMoor, C., Hearn, M.D., & Resnicow, K. (1999). Influence of school organizational characteristics on the outcomes of a school health promotion program. *Journal of School Health, 69*(9), 376-380.

Curry, J.R., & O'Brien, E.R. (2012). Shifting to a wellness paradigm in teacher education: A promising practice for fostering teacher stress reduction, burnout resilience, and promoting retention. *Ethical Human Psychology and Psychiatry, 14*(3), 178-191.

DeFrank, R.S., & Stroup, C.A. (1989). Teacher stress and health: Examination of a model. *Journal of Psychosomatic Research, 33*(1), 99-109.

Delk, J., Springer, A.E., Kelder, S.H., & Grayless, M. (2014). Promoting teacher adoption of physical activity breaks in the classroom: Findings of the Central Texas CATCH Middle School Project. *Journal of School Health, 84*(11), 722-730.

Demissie, Z., Brener, N.D., & Goekler, S.F. (2013). Chapter 10: Faculty and staff health promotion. In *Results from the school health policies and practices study* (pp. 123-128). Retrieved from www.cdc.gov/healthyyouth/shpps/2012/pdf/shpps-results_2012.pdf

Dinkel, D.M., Lee, J., & Schaffer, C. (2016). Examining the knowledge and capacity of elementary teachers to implement classroom physical activity breaks. *International Electronic Journal of Elementary Education*. Retrieved from http://works.bepress.com/danae-dinkel/10/

Dzewaltowski, D.A., Rosenkranz, R.R., Geller, K.S., Coleman, K.J., Welk, G.J., Hastmann, T.J., & Milliken, G.A. (2010). HOP'N after-school project: An obesity prevention randomized controlled trial. *International Journal of Behavioral Nutrition and Physical Activity, 7*(1), 1.

Eaton, D.K., Marx, E., & Bowie, S.E. (2007). Faculty and staff health promotion: Results from the School Health Policies and Programs Study 2006. *Journal of School Health, 77*(8), 557-566.

Erickson, J.A., & Gillespie, C.W. (2000). Reasons women discontinued participation in an exercise and wellness program. *Physical Educator, 57*(1), 2.

Erwin, H., Beighle, A., Carson, R.L., & Castelli, D.M. (2013). Comprehensive school-based physical activity promotion: A review. *Quest, 65*(4), 412-428.

Fröberg, A., Raustorp, A., Pagels, P., Larsson, C., & Boldemann, C. (2017). Levels of physical activity during physical education lessons in Sweden. *Acta Paediatrica, 106*(1), 135-141.

Gately, P., Curtis, C., & Hardaker, R. (2013). An evaluation in UK schools of a classroom-based physical activity programme—TAKE 10!®: A qualitative analysis of the teachers' perspective. *Education and Health, 31*(4), 72-78.

Goetzel, R.Z., & Ozminkowski, R.J. (2008). The health and cost benefits of work site health-promotion programs. *Annual Review of Public Health, 29*, 303-323.

Goetzel, R.Z., Ozminkowski, R.J., Asciutto, A.J., Chouinard, P., & Barrett, M. (2001). Survey of Koop Award winners: Life-cycle insights. *The Art of Health Promotion, 5*(2), 1-8.

Gortmaker, S.L., Lee, R.M., Mozaffarian, R.S., Sobol, A.M., Nelson, T.F., Roth, B.A., & Wiecha, J.L. (2012). Effect of an after-school intervention on increases in children's physical activity. *Medicine & Science in Sports & Exercise, 44*(3), 450-457.

Griva, K., & Joekes, K. (2003). UK teachers under stress: Can we predict wellness on the basis of characteristics of the teaching job? *Psychology and Health, 18*(4), 457-471.

Hagger, M.S., Chatzisarantis, N., Culverhouse, T., & Biddle, S.J.H. (2003). The processes by which perceived autonomy support in physical education promotes leisure-time physical activity intentions and behaviour: A trans-contextual model. *Journal of Educational Psychology, 95*, 784-795.

Hastmann, T.J., Bopp, M., Fallon, E.A., Rosenkranz, R.R., & Dzewaltowski, D.A. (2013). Factors influencing the implementation of organized physical activity and fruit and vegetable snacks in the HOP'N after-school obesity prevention program. *Journal of Nutrition Education and Behavior, 45*(1), 60-68.

Hattie, J.A., Myers, J.E., & Sweeney, T.J. (2004). A factor structure of wellness: Theory, assessment, analysis, and practice. *Journal of Counseling & Development, 82*(3), 354-364.

Heaney, C.A., & Goetzel, R.Z. (1997). A review of health-related outcomes of multi-component worksite health promotion programs. *American Journal of Health Promotion, 11*(4), 290-307.

Heidorn, B., & Centeio, E. (2012). The director of physical activity and staff involvement. *Journal of Physical Education, Recreation & Dance, 83*(7), 13-26.

Herrick, H., Thompson, H., Kinder, J., & Madsen, K.A. (2012). Use of SPARK to promote after-school physical activity. *Journal of School Health, 82*(10), 457-461.

Holt, E., Bartee, T., & Heelan, K. (2013). Evaluation of a policy to integrate physical activity into the school day. *Journal of Physical Activity & Health, 10*(4), 480-487.

Huberty, J., Dinkel, D., Coleman, J., Beighle, A., & Apenteng, B. (2012). The role of schools in children's physical activity participation: Staff perceptions. *Health Education Research, 27*(6), 986-995.

Iversen, C.S., Nigg, C., & Titchenal, C.A. (2011). The impact of an elementary after-school nutrition and physical activity program on children's fruit and vegetable intake, physical activity, and body mass index: Fun 5. *Hawaii Medical Journal, 70*(7 Suppl. 1), 37-41.

Johnson, C.C., Lai, Y.L., Rice, J., Rose, D., & Webber, L.S. (2010). ACTION live: Using process evaluation to describe implementation of a worksite wellness program. *Journal of Occupational and Environmental Medicine, 52*(Suppl. 1), S14.

Kaldy, J. (1985). Schools shape up with employee wellness. *School Administrator, 42*(4), 12-15.

Kelder, S., Hoelscher, D.M., Barroso, C.S., Walker, J.L., Cribb, P., & Hu, S. (2005). The CATCH Kids Club: A pilot after-school study for improving elementary students' nutrition and physical activity. *Public Health Nutrition, 8*(02), 133-140.

Kittel, F., & Leynen, F. (2003). A study of work stressors and wellness/health outcomes among Belgian school teachers. *Psychology and Health, 18*(4), 501-510.

Lai, S.K., Costigan, S.A., Morgan, P.J., Lubans, D.R., Stodden, D.F., Salmon, J., & Barnett, L.M. (2014). Do school-based interventions focusing on physical activity, fitness, or fundamental movement skill competency produce a sustained impact in these outcomes in children and adolescents? A systematic review of follow-up studies. *Sports Medicine, 44*(1), 67-79.

Lander, N., Eather, N., Morgan, P.J., Salmon, J., & Barnett, L.M. (2017). Characteristics of teacher training in school-based physical education interventions to improve fundamental movement skills and/or physical activity: A systematic review. *Sports Medicine, 47*(1), 135-161.

Langille, J.L., & Rodgers, W.M. (2010). Exploring the influence of a social ecological model on school-based physical activity. *Health Education & Behavior, 37*(6), 879-894.

Lau, P.S., Chan, R.M.C., Yuen, M., Myers, J.E., & Lee, Q.A. (2008). Wellness of teachers: A neglected issue in teacher development. In J.C.-K. Lee & L.-P. Shiu (Eds.), *Developing teachers and developing schools in changing contexts* (pp. 101-116). Hong Kong, China: The Chinese University Press.

Lauzon, L. (1992). *Teacher wellness: An interpretive inquiry.* (Unpublished doctoral dissertation). University of Victoria, Victoria, Canada.

Lerner, D., Rodday, A.M., Cohen, J.T., & Rogers, W.H. (2013). A systematic review of the evidence concerning the economic impact of employee-focused health promotion and wellness programs. *Journal of Occupational and Environmental Medicine, 55*(2), 209-222.

Lloyd, M., Saunders, T.J., Bremer, E., & Tremblay, M.S. (2014). Long-term importance of fundamental motor skills: A 20-year follow-up study. *Adapted Physical Activity Quarterly, 31*(1), 67-78.

Lonsdale, C., Rosenkranz, R.R., Sanders, T., Peralta, L.R., Bennie, A., Jackson, B., . . . Lubans, D.R. (2013). A cluster randomized controlled trial of strategies to increase adolescents' physical activity and motivation in physical education: Results of the Motivating Active Learning in Physical Education (MALP) trial. *Preventive Medicine, 57*(5), 696-702.

Martin, J.J., & Kulinna, P.H. (2004). Self-efficacy theory and the theory of planned behavior: Teaching physically active physical education classes. *Research Quarterly for Exercise and Sport, 75*(3), 288-297.

Martin, J.J., & Kulinna, P.H. (2005). A social cognitive perspective of physical-activity-related behavior in physical education. *Journal of Teaching in Physical Education, 24*(3), 265-281.

Martin, J.J., Kulinna, P.H., Eklund, R.C., & Reed, B. (2001). Determinants of teachers' intentions to teach physically active physical education classes. *Journal of Teaching in Physical Education, 20*(2), 129-143.

Maslach, C., & Jackson, S.E. (1986). *Maslach Burnout Inventory manual* (2nd ed.). Palo Alto, CA: Consulting Psychologists Press.

Mâsse, L.C., McKay, H., Valente, M., Brant, R., & Naylor, P.J. (2012). Physical activity implementation in schools: A 4-year follow-up. *American Journal of Preventive Medicine, 43*(4), 369-377.

Mâsse, L.C., Naiman, D., & Naylor, P.J. (2013). From policy to practice: Implementation of physical activity and food policies in schools. *International Journal of Behavioral Nutrition and Physical Activity, 10*(1), 1.

McCrady-Spitzer, S.K., Manohar, C.U., Koepp, G.A., & Levine, J.A. (2015). Low-cost and scalable classroom equipment to promote physical activity and improve education. *Journal of Physical Activity & Health, 12*(9), 1259-1263.

McKenzie, T.L., LaMaster, K.J., Sallis, J.F., & Marshall, S.J. (1999). Classroom teachers' leisure physical activity and their conduct of physical education. *Journal of Teaching in Physical Education, 19*(1), 126-132.

McMullen, J.M., Martin, R., Jones, J., & Murtagh, E.M. (2016). Moving to learn Ireland: Classroom teachers' experiences of movement integration. *Teaching and Teacher Education, 60*, 321-330.

Parks, M., Solmon, M., & Lee, A. (2007). Understanding classroom teachers' perceptions of integrating physical activity: A collective efficacy perspective. *Journal of Research in Childhood Education, 21*(3), 316-328.

Patton, I.T. (2012). *School-based physical activity in children: An evaluation of the Daily Physical Activity program in Ontario elementary schools.* (Unpublished doctoral dissertation). University of Western Ontario, Ontario, Canada.

Pelletier, K.R. (1996). A review and analysis of the health and cost-effective outcome studies of comprehensive health promotion and disease prevention programs at the worksite: 1993-1995 update. *American Journal of Health Promotion, 10*(5), 380-388.

Pelletier, K.R. (2001). A review and analysis of the clinical- and cost-effectiveness studies of comprehensive health promotion and disease management programs at the worksite: 1998-2000 update. *American Journal of Health Promotion, 16*(2), 107-116.

Pelletier, K.R. (2011). A review and analysis of the clinical- and cost-effectiveness studies of comprehensive health promotion and disease management programs at the worksite: Update VIII 2008 to 2010. *Journal of Occupational and Environmental Medicine, 53*(11), 1310-1331.

Racette, S.B., Dill, T.C., White, L. Castillo, J.C., Uhrich, M.L., Inman, C.L., . . . Clark, R. (2015). Influence of physical education on moderate-to-vigorous physical activity of urban public school children in St. Louis, Missouri, 2011-2014. *Preventing Chronic Disease, 12*, 140458. doi: http://dx.doi.org/10.5888/pcd12.140458

Rasku, A., & Kinnunen, U. (2003). Job conditions and wellness among Finnish upper secondary school teachers. *Psychology & Health, 18*(4), 441-456.

Resnicow, K., Davis, M., Smith, M., Baranowski, T., Lin, L.S., Baranowski, J., Doyle, C., & Wang, D.T. (1998). Results of the TeachWell worksite wellness program. *American Journal of Public Health, 88*(2), 250-257.

Richardson, K.M., & Rothstein, H.R. (2008). Effects of occupational stress management intervention programs: A meta-analysis. *Journal of Occupational Health Psychology, 13*(1), 69.

Russ, L.B., Webster, C.A., Beets, M.W., Egan, C., Weaver, R.G., Harvey, R., & Phillips, D.S. (2016). Development of the System for Observing Student Movement in Academic Routines and Transitions (SOSMART). *Health Education & Behavior, 44*(2), 304-315.

Russ, L.B., Webster, C.A., Beets, M.W., & Phillips, D.S. (2015). Systematic review and meta-analysis of multicomponent interventions through schools to increase physical Activity. *Journal of Physical Activity & Health, 12*(10), 1436-1446 doi:10.1123/jpah.2014-0244

Sallis, J.F., McKenzie, T.L., Beets, M.W., Beighle, A., Erwin, H., & Lee, S. (2012). Physical education's role in public health: Steps forward and backward over 20 years and HOPE for the future. *Research Quarterly for Exercise and Sport, 83*(2), 125-135.

Saunders, R.P., Ward, D., Felton, G.M., Dowda, M., & Pate, R.R. (2006). Examining the link between program implementation and behavior outcomes in the lifestyle education for activity program (LEAP). *Evaluation and Program Planning, 29*(4), 352-364.

Sharpe, E.K., Forrester, S., & Mandigo, J. (2011). Engaging community providers to create more active after-school environments: Results from the Ontario CATCH Kids Club implementation project. *Journal of Physical Activity & Health, 8*(1), S26.

Slusser, W.M., Sharif, M.Z., Erausquin, J.T., Kinsler, J.J., Collin, D., & Prelip, M.L. (2013). Improving overweight among at-risk minority youth: Results of a pilot intervention in after-school programs. *Journal of Health Care for the Poor and Underserved, 24*(2), 12-24.

Stylianou, M., Kulinna, P.H., & Naiman, T. (2016). ". . . Because there's nobody who can just sit that long": Teacher perceptions of classroom-based physical activity and related management issues." *European Physical Education Review, 22*(3), 390-408.

Sudholz, B., Timperio, A., Ridgers, N.D., Dunstan, D.W., Baldock, R., Holland, B., & Salmon, J. (2016). The impact and feasibility of introducing height-adjustable desks on adolescents' sitting in a secondary school classroom. *AIMS Public Health, 3*(2), 274-287.

Task Force on Community Preventive Services. (2009). A recommendation to improve employee weight status through worksite health promotion programs targeting nutrition, physical activity, or both. *American Journal of Preventive Medicine, 37*(4), 358-359.

Thomas, H.M., Fellner, L., Tucker, P., & Irwin, J.D. (2011). Healthy eating and physical activity challenges and opportunities in after-school programs: Providers' perspectives. *Child Health and Education, 3*(2), 106-121.

Troiano, R., Berrigan, D., Dodd, K., Masse, L., Tilert, T., & McDowell, M. (2008). Physical activity in the U.S. measured by accelerometer. *Medicine & Science in Sports & Exercise, 40,* 181-188.

Turner, L., & Chaloupka, F.J. (2017). Reach and implementation of physical activity breaks and active lessons in elementary school classrooms. *Health Education & Behavior, 44*(3), 370-375. https://doi.org/10.1177/1090198116667714

Vazou, S., & Vlachopoulos, S.P. (2014). Motivation and intention to integrate physical activity into daily school life: The JAM World Record event. *Health Promotion Practice, 15*(6), 819-827. https://doi.org/10.1177/1524839914541278

Vercambre, M.N., Brosselin, P., Gilbert, F., Nerrière, E., & Kovess-Masféty, V. (2009). Individual and contextual covariates of burnout: A cross-sectional nationwide study of French teachers. *BMC Public Health, 9*(1), 1.

Weaver, R.G., Beets, M.W., Hutto, B., Saunders, R., Moore, J.B., Turner-McGrievy, G., . . . Freedman, D. (2015). Making healthy eating and physical activity policy practice: Process evaluation of a group randomized controlled intervention in afterschool programs. *Health Education Research, 30*(6), 849-865.

Weaver, R.G., Beets, M.W., Saunders, R., Beighle, A., & Webster, C. (2014). A comprehensive professional development training's effect on afterschool program staff behaviors to promote healthy eating and physical activity. *Journal of Public Health Management and Practice, 20*(4), E6-E14.

Weaver, R.G., Beets, M.W., Turner-McGrievy, G., Webster, C.A., & Moore, J. (2014). Effects of a competency-based professional development training on children's physical activity and staff physical activity promotion in summer day camps. *New Directions for Youth Development, 143,* 57-78.

Weaver, R.G., Moore, J.B., Huberty, J., Freedman, D., Turner-McGrievy, B., Beighle, A., . . . Brazendale, K. (2016). Process evaluation of making HEPA policy practice: A group randomized trial. *Health Promotion Practice, 17*(5), 631-647.

Weaver, R.G., Webster, C., & Beets, M.W. (2013). LET US Play: Maximizing physical activity in physical education. *Strategies, 26*(6), 33-37.

Webster, C.A., Buchan, H., Perreault, M., Doan, R., Doutis, P., & Weaver, R.G. (2015). An exploratory study of elementary classroom teachers' physical activity promotion from a social learning perspective. *Journal of Teaching in Physical Education, 34*(3), 474-495.

Webster, C.A., Caputi, P., Perreault, M., Doan, R., Weaver, G., & Doutis, P. (2013). Elementary classroom teachers' adoption of physical activity promotion in the context of a statewide policy: An innovation diffusion and socio-ecologic perspective. *Journal of Teaching in Physical Education, 32*(4), 419-440.

Webster, C.A., Russ, L., Vazou, S., Goh, T.L., & Erwin, H.E. (2015). Integrating movement in academic classrooms: Understanding, applying, and advancing the knowledge base. *Obesity Reviews, 16*(8), 691-701.

Webster, C.A., Zarrett, N., Cook, B.S., Egan, C., Nesbitt, D., & Weaver, R.G. (2017). Movement integration in elementary classrooms: Teacher perceptions and implications for program planning. *Evaluation and Program Planning, 61,* 134-143.

Woynarowska-Solden, M. (2016). Outcomes evaluation of the school staff health promotion project. *Medycyna Pracy, 67*(2), 187-200.

Zarrett, N., Skiles, B., Wilson, D.K., & McClintock, L. (2012). A qualitative study of staff's perspectives on implementing an after school program promoting youth physical activity. *Evaluation and Program Planning, 35*(3), 417-426.

Chapter 10

Baker, P.R., Francis, D.P., Soares, J., Weightman, A.L., & Foster, C. (2015). Community wide interventions for increasing physical activity. *Cochrane Database of Systematic Reviews.* https://doi.org/10.1002/14651858. CD008366.pub3

Brown, H.E., Atkin, A.J., Panter, J., Wong, G., Chinapaw, M.J.M., & Van Sluijs, E.M.F. (2016). Family-based interventions to increase physical activity in children: A systematic review, meta-analysis and realist synthesis. *Obesity Reviews, 17*(4), 345-360. https://doi.org/10.1111/obr.12362

Brownson, R.C., Colditz, G.A., & Proctor, E.K. (Eds). (2012). *Dissemination and implementation research in health: Translating science to practice.* Oxford, UK: Oxford University Press.

Caballero, B., Clay, T., Davis, S.M., Ethelbah, B., Rock, B.H., Lohman, T., . . . Stevens, J. (2003). Pathways: A school-based, randomized controlled trial for the prevention of obesity in American Indian schoolchildren. *The American Journal of Clinical Nutrition, 78*(5), 1030-1038.

Carson, R.L., Castelli, D.M., Beighle, A., & Erwin, H. (2014). School-based physical activity promotion: A conceptual framework for research and practice. *Childhood Obesity, 10*(2), 100-106. https://doi.org/10.1089/chi.2013.0134

Carson, R.L., Castelli, D.M., Pulling Kuhn, A.C., Moore, J.B., Beets, M.W., Beighle, A., . . . Glowacki, E.M. (2014). Impact of trained champions of comprehensive school physical activity programs on school physical activity offerings, youth physical activity and sedentary behaviors. *Preventive Medicine, 69*(Suppl.), S12-S19. https://doi.org/10.1016/j.ypmed.2014.08.025

Centers for Disease Control and Prevention (CDC). (2011). *School health guidelines to promote healthy eating and physical activity.* Retrieved from www.cdc.gov/mmwr/pdf/rr/rr6005.pdf

Centers for Disease Control and Prevention (CDC). (2012). *Parent engagement: Strategies for involving parents in school health.* Retrieved from www.cdc.gov/healthyyouth/protective/pdf/parent_engagement_strategies.pdf

Centers for Disease Control and Prevention (CDC). (2013). *Comprehensive school physical activity programs: A guide for schools.* Retrieved from www.cdc.gov/healthyschools/physicalactivity/pdf/13_242620-A_CSPAP_SchoolPhysActivityPrograms_Final_508_12192013.pdf

Cipriani, K., Richardson, C., & Roberts, G. (2012). Family and community involvement in the Comprehensive School Physical Activity Program. *Journal of Physical Education, Recreation & Dance, 83*(7), 20-26. https://doi.org/10.1080/07303084.2012.10598807

Deslatte, K., & Carson, R.L. (2014). Identifying the common characteristics of comprehensive school physical activity programs in Louisiana. *Physical Educator, 71*(4), 610-634.

Dobbins, M., Husson, H., DeCorby, K., & LaRocca, R.L. (2013). School-based physical activity programs for promoting physical activity and fitness in children and adolescents aged 6 to 18. *Cochrane Database of Systematic Reviews.* https://doi.org/10.1002/14651858. CD007651.pub2

Dzewaltowski, D.A., Estabrooks, P.A., Welk, G.J., Hill, J., Milliken, G., Karteroliotis, K., & Johnston, J.A. (2009). Healthy Youth Places: A randomized controlled trial to determine the effectiveness of facilitating adult and youth leaders to promote physical activity and fruit and vegetable consumption in middle schools. *Health Education & Behavior, 36*(3), 583-600. https://doi.org/10.1177/1090198108314619

Dzewaltowski, D.A., Rosenkranz, R.R., Geller, K.S., Coleman, K.J., Welk, G.J., Hastmann, T.J., & Milliken, G.A. (2010). HOP'N after-school project: An obesity prevention randomized controlled trial. *International Journal of Behavioral Nutrition and Physical Activity, 7,* 90. https://doi.org/10.1186/1479-5868-7-90

Eisenmann, J.C., Gentile, D.A., Welk, G.J., Callahan, R., Strickland, S., Walsh, M., & Walsh, D.A. (2008). SWITCH: Rationale, design, and implementation of a community, school, and family-based intervention to modify behaviors related to childhood obesity. *BMC Public Health, 8,* 223. https://doi.org/10.1186/1471-2458-8-223

Elder, J.P., Lytle, L., Sallis, J.F., Young, D.R., Steckler, A., Simons-Morton, D., . . . Ribisl, K. (2007). A description of the social-ecological framework used in the Trial of Activity for Adolescent Girls (TAAG). *Health Education Research, 22*(2), 155-165. https://doi.org/10.1093/her/cyl059

Epstein, J.L. (1987). *Toward a theory of family-school connections: Teacher practices and parent involvement.* In K. Hurrelmann, F. Kaufmann, & F. Losel (Eds.), *Social intervention: Potential and constraints.* New York, NY: De Gru.

Epstein, J.L. (1995). School/family/community partnerships: Caring for the children we share. *Phi Delta Kappan, 76*(9), 701-712.

Epstein, J.L. (2010). *School, family, and community partnerships: Preparing educators and improving schools.* Boulder, CO: Westview Press.

Epstein, J.L., & Sanders, M.G. (2006). Prospects for change: Preparing educators for school, family, and community partnerships. *Peabody Journal of Education, 81*(2), 81-120. https://doi.org/10.1207/S15327930pje8102_5

Garriguet, D., Colley, R., & Bushnik, T. (2017). Parent-child association in physical activity and sedentary behaviour. *Health Reports, 28*(6), 3-11.

Gentile, D.A., Welk, G.J., Eisenmann, J.C., Reimer, R.A., Walsh, D.A., Russell, D.W., . . . Fritz, K. (2009). Evaluation of a multiple ecological level child obesity prevention program: Switch® what you Do, View, and Chew. *BMC Medicine, 7,* 49. https://doi.org/10.1186/1741-7015-7-49

Gunawardena, N., Kurotani, K., Indrawansa, S., Nonaka, D., Mizoue, T., & Samarasinghe, D. (2016). School-based intervention to enable school children to act as change agents on weight, physical activity and diet of their mothers: A cluster randomized controlled trial. *International Journal of Behavioral Nutrition and Physical Activity, 13,* 45. https://doi.org/10.1186/s12966-016-0369-7

Hawe, P., Shiell, A., & Riley, T. (2009). Theorising interventions as events in systems. *American Journal of Community Psychology, 43*(3-4), 267-276. https://doi.org/10.1007/s10464-009-9229-9

Hills, A.P., Dengel, D.R., & Lubans, D.R. (2015). Supporting public health priorities: Recommendations for physical education and physical activity promotion in schools. *Progress in Cardiovascular Diseases, 57*(4), 368-374.

IOM (Institute of Medicine). 2013. *Educating the student body: Taking physical activity and physical education to school.* Washington, DC: The National Academies Press.

https://doi.org/10.1016/j.pcad.2014.09.010

Kitzman-Ulrich, H., Wilson, D.K., St. George, S.M., Lawman, H., Segal, M., & Fairchild, A. (2010). The integration of a family systems approach for understanding youth obesity, physical activity, and dietary programs. *Clinical Child and Family Psychology Review, 13*(3), 231-253. https://doi.org/10.1007/s10567-010-0073-0

Krishnaswami, J., Martinson, M., Wakimoto, P., & Anglemeyer, A. (2012). Community-engaged interventions on diet, activity, and weight outcomes in U.S. schools: A systematic review. *American Journal of Preventive Medicine, 43*(1), 81-91. https://doi.org/10.1016/j.amepre.2012.02.031

Langer, S.L., Crain, A.L., Senso, M.M., Levy, R.L., & Sherwood, N.E. (2014). Predicting child physical activity and screen time: Parental support for physical activity and general parenting styles. *Journal of Pediatric Psychology, 39*(6), 633-642. https://doi.org/10.1093/jpepsy/jsu021

Lee, S.M., Nihiser, A., Strouse, D., Das, B., Michael, S., & Huhman, M. (2010). Correlates of children and parents being physically active together. *Journal of Physical Activity & Health, 7*(6), 776-783.

Leeman, J., Aycock, N., Paxton-Aiken, A., Lowe-Wilson, A., Sommers, J., Farris, R., . . . Ammerman, A. (2015). Policy, systems, and environmental approaches to obesity prevention: Translating and disseminating evidence from practice. *Public Health Reports, 130*(6), 616-622.

Luepker, R.V., Perry, C.L., McKinlay, S.M., Nader, P.R., Parcel, G.S., Stone, E.J., . . . Johnson, C.C. (1996). Outcomes of a field trial to improve children's dietary patterns and physical activity: The Child and Adolescent Trial for Cardiovascular Health. CATCH collaborative group. *JAMA, 275*(10), 768-776.

Neumark-Sztainer, D.R., Friend, S.E., Flattum, C.F., Hannan, P.J., Story, M.T., Bauer, K.W., . . . Petrich, C.A. (2010). New Moves—Preventing weight-related problems in adolescent girls. *American Journal of Preventive Medicine, 39*(5), 421-432. https://doi.org/10.1016/j.amepre.2010.07.017

Patino-Fernandez, A.M., Hernandez, J., Villa, M., & Delamater, A. (2013). School-based health promotion intervention: Parent and school staff perspectives. *Journal of School Health, 83*(11), 763-770. https://doi.org/10.1111/josh.12092

Rebholz, C.E., Chinapaw, M.J.M., van Stralen, M.M., Bere, E., Bringolf, B., De Bourdeaudhuij, I., . . . te Velde, S.J. (2014). Agreement between parent and child report on parental practices regarding dietary, physical activity and sedentary behaviours: The ENERGY cross-sectional survey. *BMC Public Health, 14,* 918. https://doi.org/10.1186/1471-2458-14-918

Remington, P.L., & Brownson, R.C. (2011). *Fifty years of progress in chronic disease epidemiology and control.* Retrieved from www.cdc.gov/mmwr/preview/mmwrhtml/su6004a12.htm

Rowe, D.A., Raedeke, T.D., Wiersma, L.D., & Mahar, M.T. (2007). Investigating the youth physical activity promotion model: Internal structure and external validity evidence for a potential measurement model. *Pediatric Exercise Science, 19*(4), 420-435.

Russ, L.B., Webster, C.A., Beets, M.W., & Phillips, D.S. (2015). Systematic review and meta-analysis of multi-component interventions through schools to increase physical activity. *Journal of Physical Activity & Health, 12*(10), 1436-1446. https://doi.org/10.1123/jpah.2014-0244

Sallis, J.F., & Owen, N. (2015). Ecological models of health behavior. In K. Glanz, B.K. Rimer, & K. Viswanath (Eds.), *Health behavior: Theory, research, and practice* (pp. 43-64, 5th ed.). San Francisco: Jossey-Bass.

Sanders, M.G. (2001). The role of "community" in comprehensive school, family, and community partnership programs. *The Elementary School Journal, 102*(1), 19-34. https://doi.org/10.2307/1002167

Schaben, J.A., Welk, G.J., Joens-Matre, R., & Hensley, L. (2006). The predictive utility of the Children's Physical Activity Correlates (CPAC) Scale across multiple grade levels. *Journal of Physical Activity & Health, 3*(1), 59-69. https://doi.org/10.1123/jpah.3.1.59

Silva, P., Lott, R., Mota, J., & Welk, G.J. (2014). Direct and indirect effects of social support on youth physical activity behavior. *Pediatric Exercise Science, 26*(1), 86-94. https://doi.org/10.1123/pes.2012-0207

Straker, L.M., Smith, K.L., Fenner, A.A., Kerr, D.A., McManus, A., Davis, M.C., . . . Abbott, R.A. (2012). Rationale, design and methods for a staggered-entry, waitlist controlled clinical trial of the impact of a community-based, family-centered, multidisciplinary program focused on activity, food and attitude habits (Curtin University's Activity, Food and Attitudes Program—CAFAP) among overweight adolescents. *BMC Public Health, 12,* 471. https://doi.org/10.1186/1471-2458-12-471

Van Sluijs, E.M.F., McMinn, A.M., & Griffin, S.J. (2007). Effectiveness of interventions to promote physical activity in children and adolescents: Systematic review of controlled trials. *British Medical Journal, 335*(7622), 703. https://doi.org/10.1136/bmj.39320.843947.BE

Webster, C.A., Beets, M., Weaver, R.G., Vazou, S., & Russ, L. (2015). Rethinking recommendations for implementing Comprehensive School Physical Activity Programs: A partnership model. *Quest, 67*(2), 185-202. https://doi.org/10.1080/00336297.2015.1017588

Welk, G.J. (1999). The youth physical activity promotion model: A conceptual bridge between theory and practice. *Quest, 51*(1), 5.

Welk, G.J., Chen, S., Nam, Y.H., & Weber, T.E. (2015). A formative evaluation of the SWITCH® obesity prevention program: Print versus online programming. *BMC Obesity, 2*, 20. https://doi.org/10.1186/s40608-015-0049-1

Welk, G.J., Wood, K., & Morss, G. (2003). Parental influences on physical activity in children: An exploration of potential mechanisms. *Pediatric Exercise Science, 15*(1), 19-33. https://doi.org/10.1123/pes.15.1.19

Williamson, D.A., Copeland, A.L., Anton, S.D., Champagne, C., Han, H., Lewis, L., . . . Ryan, D. (2007). Wise Mind project: A school-based environmental approach for preventing weight gain in children. *Obesity, 15*(4), 906-917. https://doi.org/10.1038/oby.2007.597

Young, D.R., Phillips, J.A., Yu, T., & Haythornthwaite, J.A. (2006). Effects of a life skills intervention for increasing physical activity in adolescent girls. *Archives of Pediatrics & Adolescent Medicine, 160*(12), 1255-1261. https://doi.org/10.1001/archpedi.160.12.1255

Chapter 11

Active Schools. (2014). *Let's Move!* Active Schools assessment guide. Retrieved from https://schools.healthiergeneration.org/_asset/dhgkpk/13-5959_PE01_20Toolkit.pdf

Baker, T.B., Collins, L.M., Mermelstein, R., Piper, M.E., Schlam, T.R., Cook, J.W., . . . Fiore, M.C. (2016). Enhancing the effectiveness of smoking treatment research: Conceptual bases and progress. *Addiction, 111*(1), 107-116.

Bassett, D.R., Fitzhugh, E.C., Heath, G.W., Erwin, P.C., Fredrick, G.M., Wolff, D.L., Welch, W.A., & Stout, A.B. (2013). Estimated energy expenditure for school-based policies and active living. *American Journal of Preventive Medicine, 44*(2), 108-113.

Beets, M.W., Beighle, A., Erwin, H.E., & White, J. (2009). Review of after-school programs to increase physical activity: A meta-analysis. *American Journal of Preventive Medicine, 36*, 527-537.

Beighle, A., Erwin, H., Castelli, D., & Ernst, M. (2009). Preparing physical educators for the role of physical activity director. *Journal of Physical Education, Recreation & Dance, 80*(4), 24-29.

Brusseau, T.A., Hannon, J., & Burns, R.D. (2016). The effect of a comprehensive school physical activity program on physical activity and health-related fitness in children from low-income families. *Journal of Physical Activity & Health, 13*, 888-894.

Burns, R.D., Brusseau, T.A., & Fu, Y. (2017). Influence of goal setting on physical activity and cardiorespiratory endurance in low-income children enrolled in CSPAP schools. *American Journal of Health Education, 48*(1), 32-40.

Burns, R.D., Brusseau, T.A., & Hannon, J.C. (2017). Effect of comprehensive school physical activity programming on cardio-metabolic health markers in children from low-income schools. *Journal of Physical Activity & Health, 14*(9), 671-676.

Castelli, D.M., & Beighle, A. (2007). The physical education teacher as school physical activity director. *Journal of Physical Education, Recreation & Dance, 78*(5), 25-28.

Castelli, D.M., Centeio, E.E., Boehrnsen, H., Barclay, D., & Bundy, C. (2012). School-university partnership: The Wwizard, the warrior, and the wagoner. *Journal of Physical Education, Recreation & Dance, 83*(9), 15-18.

Castelli, D.M., Centeio, E.E., & Nicksic, H.M. (2013). Preparing educators to promote and provide physical activity in schools. *American Journal of Lifestyle Medicine, 7*(5), 324-332.

Centeio, E.E., Erwin, H., & Castelli, D.M. (2014). Comprehensive school physical activity programs: Characteristics of trained teachers. *Journal of Teaching in Physical Education, 33*(4), 492-510.

Centeio, E.E., McCaughtry, N., Gutuskey, L., Garn, A.C., Somers, C., Shen, B., . . . Kulik, N.L. (2014). Physical activity change through comprehensive school physical activity programs in urban elementary schools. *Journal of Teaching in Physical Education, 33*(4), 573-591.

Centers for Disease Control and Prevention (CDC). (2013). *Comprehensive school physical activity programs: A guide for schools.* Retrieved from www.cdc.gov/healthyyouth/physicalactivity/pdf/13_242620-A_CSPAP_SchoolPhysActivityPrograms_Final_508_12192013.pdf

Chen, W., Mason, S.A., Hypnar, A.J., Zalmout, S., & Hammond-Benett, A. (2014). Students' daily physical activity behaviors: The role of quality physical education in a comprehensive school physical activity program. *Journal of Teaching in Physical Education, 33*, 592-610.

Colabianchi, N., Griffin, J.L., Slater, S.J., O'Malley, P.M., & Johnston, L.D. (2015). The Whole-of-School approach to physical activity: Findings from a national sample of US secondary students. *American Journal of Preventive Medicine, 49*(3), 387-394.

Collins, L.M., Baker, T.B., Mermelstein, R.J., Piper, M.E., Jorenby, D.E., Smith, S.S., . . . Fiore, M.C. (2011). The multiphase optimization strategy for engineering effective tobacco use interventions. *Annals of Behavioral Medicine, 41*(2), 208-226.

Collins, L.M., Murphy, S.A., Nair, V.N., & Strecher, V.J. (2005). A strategy for optimizing and evaluating behavioral interventions. *Annals of Behavioral Medicine, 30*(1), 65-73.

Collins, L.M., Murphy, S.A., & Strecher, V.J. (2007). The Multiphase Optimization Strategy (MOST) and the

Sequential Multiple Assignment Randomized Trial (SMART). *American Journal of Preventive Medicine, 32*(5), S112-S118.

Collins, L.M., Nahum-Shani, I., & Almirall, D. (2014). Optimization of behavioral dynamic treatment regimens based on the Sequential, Multiple Assignment, Randomized Trial (SMART). *Clinical Trials, 11*(4), 426-434.

Danielson, L.M. (2009). Fostering reflection. *Educational Leadership, 66*(5), 1-5.

Doolittle, S., & Rukavina, P. (2014). Case study of an institutionalized Comprehensive School Physical Activity Program. *Journal of Teaching in Physical Education, 33,* 528-557.

Fu, Y., Brusseau, T.A., Hannon, J.C., & Burns, R.D. (2017). Effect of a 12-week summer break on school day physical activity and health-related fitness in low-income children from CSPAP schools. *Journal of Environmental and Public Health,* 1-7. doi:10.1155/2017/9760817

Glowacki, E.M., Centeio, E.E., Van Dongen, D.J., Carson, R.L., & Castelli, D.M. (2016). Health promotion efforts as predictors of opportunities for physical activity: An application of the Diffusion of Innovations model. *Journal of School Health, 86*(6), 399-406.

Goc Karp, G., Scruggs, P.W., Brown, H., & Kelder, S.H. (2014). Implications for Comprehensive School Physical Activity Program implementation. *Journal of Teaching in Physical Education, 33,* 611-623.

Institute of Medicine. (2005). *Preventing childhood obesity: Health in the balance.* Washington, DC: National Academies Press.

Institute of Medicine. (2013). *Educating the student body: Taking physical activity and physical education to school.* Washington, DC: National Academies Press.

Lewallen, T.C., Hunt, H., Potts-Datema, W., Zaza, S., & Giles, W. (2015). The Whole School, Whole Community, Whole Child model: A new approach for improving educational attainment and healthy development for students. *Journal of School Health, 85,* 729-739. doi:10.1111/josh.12310

McMullen, J., van der Mars, H., & Jahn, J.A. (2014). Creating a before-school physical activity program: Pre-service physical educators' experiences and implications for PETE. *Journal of Teaching in Physical Education, 33*(4), 449-466.

National Association for Sport and Physical Education (NASPE). (2008). *Comprehensive school physical activity programs* [Position statement]. Retrieved https://files.eric.ed.gov/fulltext/ED541610.pdf

Pellegrini, C.A., Hoffman, S.A., Collins, L.M., & Spring, B. (2014). Optimization of remotely delivered intensive lifestyle treatment for obesity using the multiphase optimization strategy: Opt-IN study protocol. *Contemporary Clinical Trials, 38*(2), 251-259.

Strecher, V.J., McClure, J.B., Alexander, G.L., Chakraborty, B., Nair, V.N., Konkel, J.M., . . . Pomerleau, O.F. (2008). Web-based smoking-cessation programs: Results of a randomized trial. *American Journal of Preventive Medicine, 34*(5), 373-381.

Chapter 12

Adams, J.M. (2015). Lawsuit agreement to force schools to provide physical education. Retrieved from https://edsource.org/2015/lawsuit-agreement-to-force-schools-to-provide-physical-education/73544

Allar, I., Elliott, E., Jones, E., Krisjansson, A.L., Taliaferro, A., & Bulger, S. (2017). Involving families and communities in CSPAP development using asset mapping. *Journal of Physical Education, Recreation & Dance, 88*(5), 7-14.

Aspen Institute. (2017). State of play: Trends and developments. Retrieved from https://assets.aspeninstitute.org/content/uploads/2017/12/FINAL-SOP2017-report.pdf

Bai, Y., Saint-Maurice, P., Welk, G., Russell, D., Allums-Featherston, K., & Candelaria, N. (2017). The longitudinal impact of NFL PLAY 60 programming on youth aerobic capacity and BMI. *American Journal of Preventive Medicine, 52*(3), 311-323.

Basch, C.E. (2011). Physical activity and the achievement gap among urban minority youth. *Journal of School Health, 81*(10), 626-634.

Bauman, A.E., Reis, R.S., Sallis, J.F., Wells, J.C., Loos, R.J., & Martin, B.W. (2012). Correlates of physical activity: Why are some people physically active and others not? *Lancet, 380*(9838), 258-271.

Bleeker, M., Beyler, N., James-Burdumy, S., & Fortson, J. (2015). The impact of Playworks on boys' and girls' physical activity during recess. *Journal of School Health, 85*(3), 171-178.

Carlson, J.A., Schipperijn, J., Kerr, J., Saelens, B.E., Natarajan, L., Frank, L.D., . . . Sallis, J.F. (2016). Locations of physical activity as assessed by GPS in young adolescents. *Pediatrics, 137*(1). doi:10.1542/peds.2015-2430

Castelli, D.M., Glowacki, E., Barcelona, J.M., Calvert, H.G., & Hwang, J. (2015). Active education: Growing evidence on physical activity and academic performance. Active Living Research, 1-5.

Centeio, E.E., McCaughtry, N., Gutuskey, L., Garn, A.C., Somers, C., Shen, B., & Kulik, N.L. (2014). Physical activity change through Comprehensive School Physical Activity Programs in urban elementary schools. *Journal of Teaching in Physical Education, 33*(4), 573-591.

Centeio, E.E., McCaughtry, N., Moore, E.W.G., Kulik, N., Garn, A., Martin, J., . . . Fahlman, M. (2018). Building healthy cmmunities: A comprehensive school health program to prevent obesity in elementary schools. *Preventive Medicine, 111,* 210-215. doi:10.1177/1559827613490488

Centers for Disease Control and Prevention (CDC). (2012). *Comprehensive school physical activity program (CSPAP) policy continuum.* Retrieved from https://c.ymcdn.com/sites/www.chronicdisease.org/resource/resmgr/school_health/cspap_policy_continuum_final.pdf

Centers for Disease Control and Prevention (CDC). (2013). *Comprehensive school physical activity programs: A guide for schools.* Retrieved from www.cdc.gov/healthyyouth/physicalactivity/pdf/13_242620-A_CSPAP_SchoolPhysActivityPrograms_Final_508_12192013.pdf

Centers for Disease Control and Prevention (CDC). (2014). *Physical education profiles: Physical education and physical activity practices and policies among secondary schools at select US sites.* Retrieved from www.cdc.gov/healthyyouth/physicalactivity/pdf/PE_Profile_Book_2014.pdf

Chin, J.J., & Ludwig, D. (2013). Increasing children's physical activity during school recess periods. *American Journal of Public Health, 103*(7), 1229-1234.

Coppola, A., Hancock, D., Allan, V., Vierimaa, M., & Côté, J. (2018) Enhancing university practicum students' roles in implementing the Ontario Daily Physical Activity (DPA) policy. *Qualitative Research in Sport, Exercise and Health.* https://doi.org/10.1080/2159676X.2018.1445660

Cothran, D.J., & Ennis, C.D. (2010). Alone in a crowd: Meeting students' needs for relevance and connection in urban high school physical education. *Journal of Teaching in Physical Education, 18*(2), 234-247.

Culp, B. (2017). "Illegitimate" Bodies in Legitimate Times: Life, Liberty, and the Pursuit of Movement: National Association for Kinesiology in Higher Education 26th Delphine Hanna Commemorative Lecture 2017. *Quest, 69*(2), 143-156.

Dauenhauer, B.D., & Keating, X.D. (2011). The influence of physical education on physical activity levels of urban elementary students. *Research Quarterly for Exercise and Sport, 82*(3), 512-520.

Davison, K.K., & Lawson, C.T. (2006). Do attributes in the physical environment influence children's physical activity? A review of the literature. *International Journal of Behavioral Nutrition and Physical Activity, 3*(1), 19.

DeBate, R., Koby, E., Looney, T., Trainor, J., Zwald, M., Bryant, C., & McDermott, R. (2011). Utility of the Physical Activity Resource Assessment for child-centric physical activity intervention planning in two urban neighborhoods. *Journal of Community Health, 36,* 132-140.

Diamond, C., & Freudenberg, N. (2016). Community schools: A public health opportunity to reverse urban cycles of disadvantage. *Journal of Urban Health, 93*(6), 923-939.

Donnelly, J.E., Hillman, C.H., Castelli, D., Etnier, J. ., Lee, S., Tomporowski, P., ... & Szabo-Reed, A. N. (2016). Physical activity, fitness, cognitive function, and academic achievement in children: a systematic review. *Medicine and science in sports and exercise, 48*(6), 1197.

Doolittle, S.A., & Rukavina, P.B. (2014). Case study of an institutionalized urban Comprehensive School Physical Activity Program. *Journal of Teaching in Physical Education, 33*(4), 528-557.

Eime, R.M., & Payne, W.R. (2009). Linking participants in school-based sport programs to community clubs. *Journal of Science and Medicine in Sport, 12*(2), 293-299.

Ennis, C.D. (1999). Communicating the value of active, healthy lifestyles to urban students. *Quest, 51*(2), 164-169.

Evaluation of Mayor de Blasio's unprecedented investment in middle school afterschool shows 98 percent of surveyed parents say children like the program (2016, April 11). Retrieved from www1.nyc.gov/office-of-the-mayor/news/343-16/evaluation-mayor-de-blasio-s-unprecedented-investment-middle-school-afterschool-shows-98

Fernandez, M., & Sturm, R. (2010). Facility provision in elementary schools: Correlates with physical education, recess and obesity. *Preventive Medicine, 50,* 530-535.

Flory, S.B., & McCaughtry, N. (2011). Culturally relevant physical education in urban schools: Reflecting cultural knowledge. *Research Quarterly for Exercise and Sport, 82*(1), 49-60.

Garn, A.C., Martin, J.J., Boyd, B., & McCaughtry, N. (2017). Underserved urban minority children: Overcoming the challenges and enhancing the benefits of engaging in physical activity. In A.J.S. Morin, C. Maïano, D. Tracey, & R.G. Craven (Eds.), *International advances in education: Global initiatives for equity and social justice.* Charlotte, NC: Information Age Publishing.

Garn, A.C., McCaughtry, N., Kulik, N.L., Kaseta, M., Maljak, K., Whalen, L., & Fahlman, M. (2014). Successful afterschool physical activity clubs in urban high schools: Perspectives of adult leaders and student participants. *Journal of Teaching in Physical Education, 33*(1), 112-133.

Gordon-Larsen, P., Nelson, M., Page, P., & Popkin, B. (2006). Inequality in the built environment underlies key health disparities in physical activity and obesity. *Pediatrics, 117*(2), 417-424.

Griffin, P.S. (1985). Teaching in an urban, multiracial physical education program: The power of context. *Quest, 37*(2), 154-165.

Gutuskey, L., Centeio, E., Shen, B., McCaughtry, N., & Murphy, A. (2014). An examination of student leadership impacts on youth participants. *Research Quarterly for Exercise and Sport, 85,* A67.

Hogan, A., & Stylianou, M. (2018). School-based sports development and the role of NSOs as 'boundary spanners': Benefits, disbenefits and unintended consequences of the *Sporting Schools* policy initiative. *Sport, Education and Society, 23*(4), 367-380.

Institute of Medicine (2013). *Educating the student body: Taking physical activity and physical activity to school.* Retrieved from www.nap.edu/read/18314/chapter/1

James-Burdumy, S., Beyler, N., Borradaile, K., Bleeker, M., Maccarone, A., & Fortson, J. (2016). The impact of Playworks on students' physical activity by race/ethnicity: Findings from a randomized controlled trial. *Journal of Physical Activity & Health, 13,* 275-280.

Joens-Matre, R.R., Welk, G.J., Calabro, M.A., Russell, D.W., Nicklay, E., & Hensley, L.D. (2008). Rural-urban differences in physical activity, physical fitness, and overweight prevalence of children. *The Journal of Rural Health, 24*(1), 49-54.

Johnston, L.D., Delva, J., & O'Malley, P.M. (2007). Sports participation and physical education in American secondary schools: Current levels and racial/ethnic and socioeconomic disparities. *American Journal of Preventive Medicine, 33*(4), S195-S208.

Jones, S.E., & Wendel, A.M. (2015). Peer reviewed: Characteristics of joint use agreements in school districts in the United States: Findings from the School Health Policies and Practices Study, 2012. *Preventing Chronic Disease, 12.* doi:10.5888/pcd12.140560

Kahan, D. & McKenzie, T. (2018). Physical activity and psychological correlates during an afterschool running club. *American Journal of Health Education, 49*(2). https://doi.org/10.1080/19325037.2017.1414646.

Kimbro, R.T., Brooks-Gunn, J., & McLanahan, S. (2011). Young children in urban areas: Links among neighborhood characteristics, weight status, outdoor play, and television watching. *Social Science & Medicine, 72*(5), 668-676.

Kulinna, P.H., McCaughtry, N., Cothran, D., & Martin, J. (2006). What do urban/inner-city physical education teachers teach? A contextual analysis of one elementary/primary school district. *Physical Education & Sport Pedagogy, 11*(1), 45-68.

Lawson, H.A. (2005). Empowering people, facilitating community development, and contributing to sustainable development: The social work of sport, exercise, and physical education programs. *Sport, Education and Society, 10*(1), 135-160.

Lee, B.Y., Adam, A., Zenkov, E., Hertenstein, D., Ferguson, M.C., Wang, P.I., & Brown, S.T. (2017). Modeling the economic and health impact of increasing children's physical activity in the United States. *Health Affairs, 36*(5), 902-908.

MacDonald, S., Clennin, M., & Pate, R. (2018). Specific strategies for promotion of physical activity in kids—which ones work? A Systematic Review of the Literature. *American Journal of Lifestyle Medicine, 12*(1), 51-82. https://doi.org/10.1177/1559827615616381

Maljak, K., Garn, A.C., McCaughtry, N., Kulik, N., Martin, J., Shen, B., & Fahlman, M. (2014). Challenges in offering inner-city after-school physical activity clubs. *American Journal of Health Education, 45*, 297-307.

Massey, W.V., Babkes Stellino, M., Wilkison, M., & Whitley, M. (2018). The impact of a recess-based leadership program on urban elementary school students. *Journal of Applied Sport Psychology, 30*(1), 45-63.

Mayor de Blasio, Speaker Mark-Viverito, Chancellor Fariña announce universal physical education initiative. (2017, June 5). Retrieved from www1.nyc.gov/office-of-the-mayor/news/390-17/mayor-de-blasio-speaker-mark-viverito-chancellor-fari-a-universal-physical-education#/0

McCaughtry, N., Barnard, S., Martin, J., Shen, B., & Kulinna, P.H. (2006). Teachers' perspectives on the challenges of teaching physical education in urban schools: The student emotional filter. *Research Quarterly for Exercise and Sport, 77*(4), 486-497.

McKenzie, T.L., Marshall, S.J., Sallis, J.F., & Conwat, T.L. (2000). Leisure time physical activity in school environments: An observational study using SOPLAY. *Preventive Medicine, 30*, 70-77.

McMullen, J., van der Mars, H., & Jahn, J.A. (2014). Creating a before-school physical activity program: pre-service physical educators' experiences and implications for PETE. *Journal of Teaching in Physical Education, 33*(4), 449-466.

Moore, J.B., Jilcott, S.B., Shores, K.A., Evenson, K.R., Brownson, R.C., & Novick, L.F. (2010). A qualitative examination of perceived barriers and facilitators of physical activity for urban and rural youth. *Health Education Research, 25*(2), 355-367.

Office of the New York City Comptroller. (2014). *Dropping the Ball: Disparities in Physical Education in New York City Schools*. Retrieved from https://comptroller.nyc.gov/wp-content/uploads/documents/Phys_Ed.pdf

Phillips, J.A., & Young, D.R. (2009). Past-year sports participation, current physical activity and fitness in urban adolescent girls. *Journal of Physical Activity & Health, 6*(1), 105-111.

Sagas, M., & Cunningham, G.B. (2014). *Sport participation rates among underserved American youth* [Research brief]. Retrieved from https://assets.aspeninstitute.org/content/uploads/files/content/docs/pubs/Project_Play_Underserved_Populations_Roundtable_Research_Brief.pdf

Sallis, J.F., & McKenzie, T.L. (1991). Physical education's role in public health. *Research Quarterly for Exercise and Sport, 62*, 124-137.

Sallis, J.F., Owen, N., & Fisher, E.B. (2008). Ecological models of health behavior. In K. Glanz, B.K. Rimer, & K. Viswanath (Eds.), *Health behavior and health education: Theory, research, and practice* (4th ed., pp. 465-486). San Francisco, CA: Jossey-Bass.

Staurowsky, E., DeSousa, M., Miller, K., Sabo, D., Shakib, S., Thebarge, N., Veliz, P., Weaver, A., & Williams, N. (2015). *Her life depends on it III: Sport, physical activity, and the health and well-being of American girls and women*. East Meadow, NY: Women's Sports Foundation.

Sterdt, E., Liersch, S., & Walter, U. (2014). Correlates of physical activity of children and adolescents: A systematic review of reviews. *Health Education Journal, 73*(1), 72-89.

Tisch Center for Food, Education, & Policy. (2018). *Wellness in the Schools (WITS) evaluation final report*. Retrieved from www.tc.columbia.edu/media/media-library-2014/centers/tisch-center/WITS-Evaluation-TFC-Final-Report-March-12-2018-(1).pdf

Turner, L., Johnson, T., Calvert, H., & Chaloupka, F. (2017). Stretched too thin? The relationship between insufficient resource allocation and physical education instructional time and assessment practices. *Teaching and Teacher Education, 68,* 210-219.

Turner, L., Johnson, T.G., Slater, S.J., & Chaloupka, F.J. (2015). *Physical education professionals play a key role in promoting important physical activity practices in elementary schools* [Research brief]. Retrieved from www.bridgingthegapresearch.org/_asset/x3ygtj/BTG_PE_brief_FINAL_25June2015.pdf

U.S. Department of Education. (2017). *Revised state template for the consolidated state plan: The Elementary and Secondary Education Act of 1965, as amended by the Every Student Succeeds Act.* Retrieved from www.alsde.edu/sites/boe/Attachments/Draft%20ESSA%20Plan.pdf

U. S. Department of Health and Human Services (HHS) (2013) Educating the student body: Taking physical activity and physical education to school [Report brief] Retrieved from www.nap.edu/read/18314/chapter 1

Webster, C.A., Beets, M., Weaver, R.G., Vazou, S., & Russ, L. (2015). Rethinking recommendations for implementing comprehensive school physical activity programs: A partnership model. *Quest, 67,* 185-202.

Whooten, R., Perkins, M., Gerber, M., & Taveras, E. (2018). Effects of before-school physical activity on obesity prevention and wellness. *American Journal of Preventive Medicine, 54*(4), 510-518.

Wilkinson, S.D., & Penney, D. (2016). The involvement of external agencies in extra-curricular physical education: Reinforcing or challenging gender and ability inequities? *Sport, Education and Society, 21*(5), 741-758.

Yancey, A.K., Fielding, J.E., Flores, G.R., Sallis, J.F., McCarthy, W.J., & Breslow, L. (2007).

Creating a robust public health infrastructure for physical activity promotion. *American Journal of Preventive Medicine, 32*(1), 68-78.

Yancey, A.K., & Kumanyika, S.K. (2007). Bridging the gap: Understanding the structure of social inequities in childhood obesity. *American Journal of Preventive Medicine, 33,* S172-S174.

Chapter 13

Babey, S.H., Hastert, T.A., Huang, W., & Brown, R.E. (2009). Sociodemographic, family, and environmental factors associated with active commuting to school among US adolescents. *Journal of Public Health Policy, 30*(Suppl. 1), S203-S220.

Baker, E.A., Elliott, M., Barnidge, E., Estlund, A., Brownson, R.C., Milne, A., . . . Hashimoto, D. (2017). Implementing and evaluating environmental and policy interventions for promoting physical activity in rural schools. *Journal of School Health, 87*(7), 538-545.

Barnidge, E.K., Baker, E.A., Estlund, A., Motton, F., Hipp, P.R., & Brownson R.C. (2015). A participatory regional partnership approach to promote nutrition and physi-cal activity through environmental and policy change in rural Missouri. *Preventing Chronic Disease, 12,* 140593. doi:http://dx.doi.org/10.5888/pcd12.140593

Bershwinger, T., & Brusseau, T.A. (2013). The impact of classroom activity breaks on the school-day physical activity of rural children. *International Journal of Exercise Science, 6*(2), 134-143.

Brusseau, T.A., Kulinna, P.H., Tudor-Locke, C., Ferry, M., van der Mars, H., & Darst, P.W. (2011). Pedometer-determined segmented physical activity patterns of fourth- and fifth-grade children. *Journal of Physical Activity and Health, 8*(2), 279-286.

Byun, S.Y., Meece, J.L., Irvin, M.J., & Hutchins, B.C. (2012). The role of social capital in educational aspirations of rural youth. *Rural Sociology, 77*(3), 355-379.

Centeio, E.E., Glowacki, E., & Castelli, D.M. (2014). Predictors of physical activity opportunities: Educational policy and administrative support. *Research Quarterly for Exercise and Sport, 85,* 57-57.

Centers for Disease Control and Prevention. (2013). *Comprehensive school physical activity programs: A guide for schools.* Retrieved from www.cdc.gov/healthyyouth/physicalactivity/pdf/13_242620-A_CSPAP_SchoolPhysActivityPrograms_Final_508_12192013.pdf

Corbin, C.B., Le Masurier, G.C., & Lambdin, D.D. (2007). *Fitness for life: Middle school.* Champaign, IL: Human Kinetics Publishers.

Corbin, C.B., LeMasurier, G.C., Lambdin, D.D., & Greiner, M. (2010). *Fitness for life for elementary school: Guide for wellness coordinators.* Champaign, IL: Human Kinetics Publishers.

Cox, M., Schofield, G., Greasley, N., & Kolt, G.S. (2006). Pedometer steps in primary school-aged children: A comparison of school-based and out-of-school activity. *Journal of Science and Medicine in Sport, 9*(1), 91-97.

Fan J.X., Wen, M., & Kowaleski-Jones, L. (2014). Rural-urban differences in objective and subjective measures of physical activity: Findings from the National Health and Nutrition Examination Survey (NHANES) 2003-2006. *Preventing Chronic Disease, 11,* E141.

Guskey, T.R. (2002). Professional development and teacher change. *Teachers and teaching: Theory and practice, 8,* 381-391.

Heelan, K.A., Bartee, R.T., Nihiser, A., & Sherry, B. (2015). Healthier school environment leads to decreases in childhood obesity: The Kearney Nebraska story. *Childhood Obesity, 11*(5), 600-607.

Ismailov, R.M., & Leatherdale, S.T. (2010). Rural-urban differences in overweight and obesity among a large sample of adolescents in Ontario. *International Journal of Pediatric Obesity, 5*(4), 351-360.

Johnson, J.A., & Johnson, A.M. (2015). Urban-rural differences in childhood and adolescent obesity in the United States: A systematic review and meta-analysis. *Childhood Obesity, 11*(3), 233-241. doi:10.1089/chi.2014.0085

Jones, E.M., Taliaferro, A.R., Elliott, E.M., Bulger, S.M., Kirstjansson, A.L., Neal, W., . . . Allar, I. (2014). Feasibility study of comprehensive school PA programs in Appalachian Communities: the McDowell CHOICES Project. *Journal of Teaching in Physical Education, 33,* 467-491.

Jordan, M., Lorenz, K.A., Stylianou, M., & Kulinna, P.H. (2016). Examining student social capital in a comprehensive school-based health intervention. *Journal of Classroom Interaction, 51*(2), 36-49.

Kulinna, P.H. (2004). Physical activity and fitness knowledge: How much 1-6 grade students know. *International Journal of Physical Education, 41,* 111-121.

Langley, K., & Kulinna, P.H. (2018). Developing a staff physical activity program at your school: Implementing the lesser used component of the CSPAP model. *Journal of Physical Education, Recreation & Dance, 89*(2), 49-55.

Liu, J., Bennett, K.J., Harun, N., & Probst, J.C. (2008). Urban-rural differences in overweight status and physical inactivity among US children aged 10-17 years. *Journal of Rural Health, 24,* 407-415.

Liu, J., Bennett, K.J., Harun, N., Zheng, X., Probst, J.C., & Pate, R.R. (2007). *Overweight and physical inactivity among rural children aged 10-17: A national and state portrait.* Retrieved from https://sc.edu/study/colleges_schools/public_health/research/research_centers/sc_rural_health_research_center/documents/71obesitychartbook2007.pdf

Molefe, A., Burke, M.R., Collins, N., Sparks, D., & Hoyer, K. (2017). *Postsecondary education expectations and attainment of rural and nonrural students.* Retrieved from https://ies.ed.gov/ncee/edlabs/regions/midwest/pdf/REL_2017257.pdf

Moore J., Jilcott S., Shores K., Evenson K., Brownson R., & Novick L. (2010). A qualitative examination of perceived barriers and facilitators of physical activity for urban and rural youth. *Health Education Research, 24*(2), 355-367.

Moreno, L.A., Sarria, A., Fleta, J., Rodriguez, G., Gonzalez, J.M., & Bueno, M. (2001). Sociodemographic factors and trends on overweight prevalence in children and adolescents in Aragon (Spain) from 1985 to 1995. *Journal of Clinical Epidemiology, 54*(9), 921-927.

Murimi, M., & Harpel T. (2010). Practicing preventive health: The underlying culture among low-income rural populations. *Journal of Rural Health, 26*(3), 273-282.

National Association for Sport and Physical Education. (2008). *Comprehensive school physical activity programs* [Position statement]. Retrieved from https://files.eric.ed.gov/fulltext/ED541610.pdf

Stylianou, M., Kulinna, P.H., van der Mars, H., Mahar, M.T., Adams, M.A., & Amazeen, E. (2016). Before-school running/walking club: Effects on student on-task behavior. *Preventive Medicine Reports, 3,* 196-202.

Stylianou, M., Lorenz, K.A., & Kulinna, P.H. (2015). Teacher training and implementation of CSPAP components. *Research Quarterly for Exercise and Sport, 86,* A6.

Stylianou, M., van der Mars, H., Kulinna, P.H., Adams, M.A., Mahar, M., & Amazeen, E. (2016). Before-school running/walking club and student physical activity levels: An efficacy study. *Research Quarterly for Exercise and Sport, 87*(4), 342-353.

Teatro, C., Kulinna, P.H., Zhu, W., Boiarskaia, E., & Wilde, B. (2013). *Validating middle school fitness knowledge assessments: The Fitness for Life Test Bank Validation Project.* Paper presented at the American Alliance for Health, Physical Education, Recreation & Dance meeting, Charlotte, NC.

Tremblay, M.S., Barnes, J.D., González, S.A., Katzmarzyk, P.T., Onywera, V.O., Reilly, J.J., . . . Global Matrix 2.0 Research Team. (2016). Global Matrix 2.0: Report card grades on the physical activity of children and youth comparing 38 countries. *Journal of Physical Activity and Health, 13*(11), S343-S366.

U.S. Department of Health and Human Services (HHS). (2008). *Physical activity guidelines for americans.* Retrieved from https://health.gov/paguidelines/pdf/paguide.pdf

Chapter 14

Active Healthy Kids Global Alliance. (2016). *Global Matrix 2.0.* Retrieved from www.activehealthykids.org/the-global-matrix-2-0-on-physical-activity-for-children-and-youth/

Ahamed, Y., Macdonald, H., Reed, K., Naylor, P.-J., Liu-Ambrose, T., & McKay, H. (2007). School-based physical activity does not compromise children's academic performance. *Medicine & Science in Sports & Exercise, 39*(2), 371.

Audit Office of New South Wales. (2012). *New South Wales auditor-general's report, performance audit: Physical activity in government primary schools.* Sydney, NSW: Department of Education and Communities.

Bowles, R., Ní Chróinín, D., & Murtagh, E. (2017). Attaining the Active School Flag: How physical activity provision can be enhanced in Irish primary schools. *European Physical Education Review.* http://dx.doi.org/10.1177%2F1356336X17706091

Cale, L. (2000a). Physical activity promotion in schools: PE teachers' views. *European Journal of Physical Education, 5,* 158-168.

Cale, L. (2000b). Physical activity promotion in secondary schools. *European Physical Education Review, 6*(1), 71-90.

Cale, L., & Harris, J. (2006). School-based physical activity interventions: Effectiveness, trends, issues, implications and recommendations for practice. *Sport, Education and Society, 11,* 401-420.

Centers for Disease Control and Prevention (CDC). (2013). *Comprehensive school physical activity programs: A guide for schools.* Retrieved from www.cdc.gov/healthyyouth/physicalactivity/pdf/13_242620-A_CSPAP_SchoolPhysActivityPrograms_Final_508_12192013.pdf

Coppinger, T., Lacey, S., O'Neill, C., & Burns, C. (2016). 'Project Spraoi': A randomized control trial to improve nutrition and physical activity in school children. *Contemporary Clinical Trials Communication, 3*(15), 94-101.

Day, M.E., Strange, K.S., McKay, H.A., & Naylor, P-J. (2008). Action schools! BC-Healthy Eating: Effects of a whole-school model to modifying eating behaviours of elementary school children. *Canadian Journal of Public Health/Revue Canadienne de Sante'e Publique,* 328-331.

Department of Education and Training. (2012). *Smart Moves: Physical activity programs in Queensland state schools evaluation summary.* Retrieved from http://education.qld.gov.au/schools/healthy/docs/smart-moves-summary-report.pdf

Dobbins, M., Husson, H., DeCorby, K., & LaRocca, R.L. (2013). School-based physical activity programs for promoting physical activity and fitness in children and adolescents aged 6 to 18 [Review]. *Cochrane Database of Systematic Reviews, 2,* CD007651.

Dyson, B. (2006). Students' perspectives of physical education. In D. Kirk, D. MacDonald, & M. O'Sullivan (Eds.), *Handbook of physical education* (pp. 326-346). London, UK: Sage.

European Commission. (2014). *EU action plan on childhood obesity 2014-2020.* Retrieved from https://ec.europa.eu/health/sites/health/files/nutrition_physical_activity/docs/childhoodobesity_action-plan_2014_2020_en.pdf

Haapala, H.L., Hirvensalo, M.H., Kulmala, J., Hakonen, H., Kankaanpää, A. Laine, K., . . . Tammelin, T.H. (2016). Changes in physical activity and sedentary time in the Finnish Schools on the Move program: A quasi-experimental study. *Scandinavian Journal of Medicine & Science in Sports.* Advance online publication. doi:10.1111/sms.12790

Haapala H.L., Hirvensalo, M.H., Laine, K., Hakonen, H., Lintunen, T., & Tammelin, T.H. (2014). Adolescents' physical activity at recess and actions to promote a physically active school day in four Finnish schools. *Health Education Research, 5,* 840-852.

Institute of Medicine. (2013). *Educating the student body: Taking physical activity and physical education to school.* Retrieved from www.nap.edu/read/18314/chapter/1

Kämppi, K., Asanti, R., Hirvensalo, M., Laine, K., Pönkkö, A., Romar, J-A., & Tammelin, T. (2013). A more pleasant and peaceful learning environment—School staff's experiences and views on promoting a physical activity based operating culture in school. *LIKES Research Reports on Sport and Health,* 269. Jyväskylä, Finland: LIKES—Foundation for Sport and Health Sciences. [Report in Finnish, abstract in English]. Retrieved from www.likes.fi/filebank/887-viihtyvyytta_ja_tyorauhaa_summary.pdf

Kriemler, S., Meyer, U., Martin, E., van Sluijs, E. M., Andersen, L.B., & Martin, B.W. (2011). Effect of school-based interventions on physical activity and fitness in children and adolescents: a review of reviews and systematic update. *British journal of sports medicine, 45*(11), 923-30.

McBride, N., & Midford, R. (1999). Encouraging schools to promote health: Impact of the Western Australia School Health Project (1992-1995). *Journal of School Health, 69,* 220-226.

McMullen, J., Ní Chróinín, D., Tammelin, T., Pogorzelska, M., & van der Mars, H. (2015). International approaches to whole-of-school physical activity promotion. *Quest, 67,* 384-399.

Naylor, P-J. Macdonald, H.M., Reed, K.E., & McKay, H.A. (2006b). Action Schools! BC: A socioecological approach to modifying chronic disease risk factors in elementary school children. *Preventing Chronic Disease, 3*(2), A60.

Naylor, P-J. Macdonald, H.M., Warburton, D.E., Reed, K.E., & McKay, H.A. (2008). An active school model to promote physical activity in elementary schools: Action Schools! BC. *British Journal of Sports Medicine, 42*(5), 338-343.

Naylor, P.-J., Macdonald, H.M., Zebedee, J.A., Reed, K.E., & McKay, H.A. (2006a). Lessons learned from Action Schools! BC—An 'active school' model to promote physical activity in elementary schools. *Journal of Science and Medicine in Sport, 9*(5), 413-423.

Naylor, P-J., & McKay, H.A. (2009). Prevention in the first place: Schools a setting for action on physical inactivity. *British Journal of Sports Medicine, 43*(1), 10-13.

Naylor, P.-J., Scott, J., Drummond, J., Bridgewater, L., McKay, H., & Panagiotopoulos, C. (2010). Implementing a whole school physical activity and healthy eating model in rural and remote First Nations schools: A process evaluation of Action Schools! BC. *Rural Remote Health, 10*(2), 1296.

Ní Chróinín, D., Murtagh, E., & Bowles, R. (2012). Flying the 'Active School Flag': Physical activity promotion through self-evaluation in primary schools in Ireland. *Irish Educational Studies, 31*(3), 281-296.

Nutbeam, D. (1992). The health promoting school: Closing the gap between theory and practice. *Health Promotion International, 7*(3), 151-153.

Prime Minister's Office, Finland. (2015). *Finland, a land of solutions.* Strategic Programme of Prime Minister Juha Sipilä's Government. 29 May 2015. Retrieved from http://vnk.fi/en/publication?pubid=6407

Pühse, U. (1995). Bewegte Schule-eine bewegungspädagogische Perspektive. *Sportunterricht, 44*(10), 416-425.

Queensland School Sport. (2015). *CQ sporty schools.* Retrieved from https://queenslandschoolsport.eq.edu.au/Sportsinformation/cqsportyschools/Pages/cqsportyschools.aspx

Reed, K.E., Warburton, D.E., Macdonald, H.M., Naylor, P., & McKay, H.A. (2008). Action Schools! BC: A school-based physical activity intervention designed to decrease cardiovascular disease risk factors in children. *Preventive Medicine, 46*(6), 525-531.

Reid, G. (2009). Delivering sustainable practice? A case study of the Scottish Active Schools programme. *Sport, Education and Society, 14*, 353-370.

Rush, E., Cairncross, C., Williams, M.H., Tseng, M., Coppinger, T., McLennan, S., & Latimer, K. (2016). Project Energize: Intervention development and 10 years of progress in preventing childhood obesity. *BMC Research Notes, 9.* doi:10.1186/s13104-016-1849-1

Rush, E., McLennan, S., Obolonkin, V., Vandal, A.C., Hamlin, M., Simmons, D., & Graham, D. (2014a). Project Energize: Whole-region primary school nutrition and physical activity programme; evaluation of body size and fitness 5 years after the randomised control trial. *British Journal of Nutrition, 111*, 363-371.

Rush, E., Obolonkin, V., McLennan, S., Graham, D., Harris, J.D., Mernagh, P., & Weston, A.R. (2014b). Lifetime cost effectiveness of a through-school nutrition and physical programme: Project Energize. *Obesity Research and Clinical Practice, 8,* e115-e122.

Rush, E., Reed, P., McLennan, S., Coppinger, T., Simmons, D., & Graham, D. (2011). A school-based obesity control programme: Project energize. Two-year outcomes. *British Journal of Nutrition, 107*, 581-587.

Schranz, N.K., Olds, T., Boyd, R., Evans, J., Gomersall, S.R., Hardy, L., . . . Vella, S. (2016). Results from Australia's 2016 Report Card on Physical Activity for Children and Youth. *Journal of Physical Activity & Health, 13*(Suppl. 2), S87-S94.

Sutherland, R.L., Campbell, E.M., Lubans, D.R., Morgan, P.J., Nathan, N.K., Wolfenden, L., . . . Wiggers, J.H. (2016). The Physical Activity 4 Everyone cluster randomized trial, 2-year outcomes of a school physical activity intervention among adolescents. *American Journal of Preventive Medicine, 51,* 195-205.

Sutherland, R.L., Campbell, E.M., Lubans, D.R., Morgan, P.J., Okely, A.D., Nathan, N., . . . Wiggers, J. (2015). 'Physical Activity 4 Everyone' school-based intervention to prevent decline in adolescent physical activity levels: 12 month (mid-intervention) report on a cluster randomised trial. *British Journal of Sports Medicine, 50,* 488-495.

Tammelin, T., Laine, K., & Turpeinen, S. (2012). Final report on the Finnish Schools on the Move programme's pilot phase 2010-2012. *LIKES Research Reports on Sport and Health, 261.* Jyväskylä, Finland: LIKES—Foundation for Sport and Health Sciences. [Report in Finnish, abstract in English]. Retrieved from https://www.likes.fi/filebank/884-Liikkuvakoulu_loppuraportti_web_enkku.pdf

Tomlin, D., Naylor, P., McKay, H., Zorzi, A., Mitchell, M., & Panagiotopoulos, C. (2012). The impact of Action Schools! BC on the health of Aboriginal children and youth living in rural and remote communities in British Columbia. *International Journal of Circumpolar Health, 71,* 17999. doi:10.3402/ijch.v71i0.17999

Tremblay, M.S., Gray, C.E., Akinroye, K., Harrington, D.M., Katzmarzyk, P.T., Lambert, E.V., . . . Tomkinson, G. (2014). Physical activity of children: A global matrix of grades comparing 15 countries. *Journal of Physical Activity & Health, 11,* S113-S125.

World Health Organization (WHO). (2015). *Factsheets on health-enhancing physical activity in the 28 European Union member states of the WHO European region.* Retrieved from www.euro.who.int/__data/assets/pdf_file/0007/288106/Factsheets-on-health-enhancing-physical-activity-in-the-28-European-Union-Member-States-of-the-WHO-European-Region.pdf?ua=1

Chapter 15

Andre, E.K., Williams, N., Schwartz, F., & Bullard, C. (2017). Benefits of campus outdoor recreation programs: A review of the literature. *Journal of Outdoor Recreation, Education, and Leadership, 9*(1), 15-25.

Baicker, K., Cutler, D., & Song, Z. (2010). Workplace wellness programs can generate savings. *Health Affairs, 29*(2), 304-311.

Biddle, S., & Goudas, M. (1996). Analysis of children's physical activity and its association with adult encouragement and social cognitive variables. *Journal of School Health, 66*(2), 75-78.

Bornstein, D.B., Beets, M.W., Byun, W., & McIver, K. (2011). Accelerometer-derived physical activity levels of preschoolers: A meta-analysis. *Journal of Science and Medicine in Sport, 14*(6), 504 511.

Brock, S.J., Wadsworth, D., Hollett, N., & Rudisill, M.E. (2016). Using Movband technology to support online learning: An effective approach to maximizing resources in kinesiology. *Kinesiology Review, 5,* 289-294.

Brusseau, T.A., Burns, R.D., & Hannon, J.C. (2016). Physical activity and health-related fitness of adolescents within the juvenile justice system. *BioMed Research International,6.*

Brusseau, T.A., Burns, R.D., & Hannon, J.C. (submitted for publication). Effectiveness of SPARK program on the physical activity of youth in custody.

Butler, C.E., Clark, B.R., Burlis, T.L., Castillo, J.C., & Racette, S.B. (2015). Physical activity for campus employees: A university worksite wellness program. *Journal of Physical Activity & Health, 12,* 470-476.

Cardinal, B.J., Sorensen, S.D., & Cardinal, M.K. (2012). Historical perspective and current status of the physical education graduation requirement at American 4-year colleges and universities. *Research Quarterly for Exercise and Sport, 83*(4), 503-512.

Chuang, R., Sharma, S.V., Perry, C., & Diamond, P. (2017). Does the CATCH early childhood program increase physical activity among low-income preschoolers? Results from a pilot study. *American Journal of Health Promotion, 32*(2), 344-348.

Collier, D. (2011). Instructional strategies for adapted physical education. In J.P. Winnick (Ed.), *Adapted physical education and sport* (p. 121). Champaign, IL: Human Kinetics.

Curry, J., Jenkins, J.M., & Weatherford, J. (2015). Focus on freshmen: Basic instruction programs enhancing physical activity. *The Physical Educator, 72,* 621-639.

Dinger, M.K., Brittain, D.R., & Hutchinson, S.R. (2014). Associations between physical activity and health-related factors in a national sample of college students. *Journal of American College Health, 62*(1), 67-72.

Ferrer, M.E., & Laughlin, D.D. (2017). Increasing college students' engagement and physical activity with classroom brain breaks. *Journal of Physical Education, Recreation & Dance, 88*(3), 53-57.

Gagne, C., & Harnois, I. (2014). How to motivate childcare workers to engage preschoolers in physical activity. *Journal of Physical Activity & Health, 11,* 364-374.

Gordon, E.S., Tucker, P., Burke, S.M., & Carron, A.V. (2013). Effectiveness of physical activity interventions for preschoolers: A meta-analysis. *Research Quarterly for Exercise and Sport, 84,* 287-294.

Gordon-Larsen, P., Nelson, M.C., & Popkin, B.M. (2004). Longitudinal physical activity and sedentary behavior trends: adolescence to adulthood. *American Journal of Preventive Medicine, 27,* 277-283.

Grunbaum, J.A., Lowry, R., & Kann, L. (2001). Prevalence of health-related behaviors among alternative high school students as compared with students attending regular high schools. *Journal of Adolescent Health, 29*(5), 337-343.

Haines, D.J., Davis, L., Rancour, P., Robinson, M., Neel-Wilson, T., & Wagner, S. (2007). A pilot intervention to promote walking and wellness and to improve the health of college faculty and staff. *Journal of American College Health, 55,* 219-225.

Hannon, J.C., & Brown, B.B. (2008). Increasing preschoolers' physical activity intensities: An activity-friendly preschool playground intervention. *Preventive Medicine, 46*(6), 532-536.

Hellison, D.R. (2011). *Teaching personal and social responsibility through physical activity.* Champaign, IL: Human Kinetics Publishers.

Houston, J., & Kulinna, P.H. (2014). Health-related fitness models in physical education. *Strategies, 27*(2), 20-26.

Institute of Medicine. (2011). *Early childhood obesity prevention policies.* Retrieved from www.nap.edu/read/13124/chapter/1

Kirk, S.M., & Kirk, E.P. (2016). Sixty minutes of physical activity per day included within preschool academic lessons improves early literacy. *Journal of School Health, 86,* 155-163.

Kubik, M.Y., Lytle, L., & Fulkerson, J.A. (2004). Physical activity, dietary practices, and other health behaviors of at-risk youth attending alternative high schools. *Journal of School Health, 74*(4), 119.

Law, M., King, G., King, S., Kertoy, M., Hurley, P., Rosenbaum, P., ... & Hanna, S. (2006). Patterns of participation in recreational and leisure activities among children with complex physical disabilities. *Developmental Medicine and Child Neurology, 48*(5), 337-342.

Lieberman, L.J., Dunn, J.M., van der Mars, H., & McCubbin, J. (2000). Peer tutors' effects on activity levels of deaf students in inclusive elementary physical education. *Adapted Physical Activity Quarterly, 17*(1), 20-39.

Lieberman, L., & Houston-Wilson, C. (2009). *Strategies for inclusion: A handbook for physical educators* (2nd ed.). Champaign, IL: Human Kinetics Publishers.

Ling, J., Robbins, L.B., Wen, F., & Peng, W. (2015). Interventions to increase physical activity in children aged 2-5 years: A systematic review. *Pediatric Exercise Science, 27,* 314-333.

Lubans, D.R., Plotnikoff, R.C., & Lubans, N.J. (2012). Review: A systematic review of the impact of physical activity programmes on social and emotional wel;\l-being in at-risk youth. *Child and Adolescent Mental Health, 17*(1), 2-13.

Martinek, T., & Hellison, D. (2016). Teaching personal and social responsibility: Past, present and future. *Journal of Physical Education, Recreation & Dance, 87*(5), 9-13.

McElveen, M., & Rossow, A. (2014). Relationship of intramural participation to GPA and retention in first-time-in-college students. *Recreational Sports Journal, 38,* 50-54.

Melton, B., Bland, H., Harris, B., Kelly, D., & Chandler, K. (2015). Evaluating a physical activity app in the classroom: A mixed methodological approach among university students. *The Physical Educator, 72,* 601-620.

Miramontez, S.K., & Schwartz, I.S. (2016). The effects of physical activity on the on-task behavior of young children with autism spectrum disorders. *International Electronic Journal of Elementary Education, 9*(2), 405-418.

Neter, J.E., Schokker, D.F., de Jong, E., Renders, C.M., Seidell, J.C., & Visscher, T.L.S. (2011). The prevalence of overweight and obesity and its determinants in children with and without disabilities. *Journal of Pediatrics, 158*(5), 735-739.

Nicaise, V., Kahan, D., Reuben, K., & Sallis, J.F. (2012). Evaluation of a redesigned outdoor space on preschool children's physical activity during recess. *Pediatric Exercise Science, 24,* 507-518.

Ogden, C.L., Carroll, M.D., Kit, B.K., & Flegal, K.M. (2014). Prevalence of childhood and adult obesity in the United States, 2011-2012. *JAMA, 311*(8), 806-814.

Palmer, K.K., Miller, M.W., & Robinson, L.E. (2013). Acute exercise enhances preschoolers' ability to sustain attention. *Journal of Sport & Exercise Psychology, 35,* 433-437.

Pate, R.R., & O'Neill, J.R. (2012). Physical Activity Guidelines for Young

Children: An Emerging Consensus. *Archives of Pediatric and Adolescent Medicine, 166,* 1095-1096.

Pate, R.R., O'Neill, J.R., Brown, W.H., McIver, K.L., Howie, E.K., & Dowda, M. (2013). Top 10 research questions related to physical activity in preschool children. *Research Quarterly for Exercise and Sport, 84,* 448-455.

Prewitt, S.L., Hannon, J.C., Colquitt, G., Brusseau, T.A., Newton, M., & Shaw, J. (2015). Effect of personalized system of instruction on health-related fitness knowledge and class time physical activity. *The Physical Educator, 72,* 23-39.

Pugliese, J., & Tinsley, B. (2007). Parental socialization of child and adolescent physical activity: A meta-analysis. *Journal of Family Psychology, 21,* 331-343.

Raywid, M. (1994). Alternative schools: The state of the art. *Educational Leadership, 52*(1), 26-31.

Redford, J., Battle, D., & Bielick, S. (2016). *Homeschooling in the United States: 2012.* Retrieved from https://nces.ed.gov/pubs2016/2016096rev.pdf

Reilly, J.J. (2010). Low levels of objectively measured physical activity in preschoolers in child care. *Medicine & Science in Sports & Exercise, 42*(3), 502-507.

Reimer, M.S., & Cash, T. (2003). *Alternative schools: Best practices for development and evaluation.* Retrieved from https://files.eric.ed.gov/fulltext/ED481475.pdf

Rimmer, J.H. (2006). Use of the ICF in identifying factors that impact participation in physical activity/rehabilitation among people with disabilities. *Disability and Rehabilitation, 28*(17), 1087-1095.

Rimmer, J.H., & Marques, A.C. (2012). Physical activity for people with disabilities. *Lancet, 380*(9838), 193-195.

Sharma, S., Chuang, R.J., & Hedberg, A.M. (2011). Pilot testing CATCH early childhood: A preschool-based healthy nutrition and physical activity program. *American Journal of Health Education, 42*(1), 12-23.

Sherrill, C. (1997). Disability, identity, and involvement in sport and exercise. In K.R. Fox (Ed.), *The physical self: From motivation to well-being* (pp. 257-286). Champaign, IL: Human Kinetics Publishers.

Siedentop, D., Hastie, P.A., & van der Mars, H. (2011). *Complete guide to sport education.* Champaign, IL: Human Kinetics Publishers.

Sirard, J.R., Kubik, M.Y., Fulkerson, J.A., & Arcan, C. (2008). Objectively measured physical activity in urban alternative high school students. *Medicine & Science in Sports & Exercise, 40*(12), 2088.

Sit, C.H., McKenzie, T.L., Cerin, E., Chow, B.C., Huang, W.Y., & Yu, J. (2017). Physical activity and sedentary time among children with disabilities at school. *Medicine & Science in Sports & Exercise, 49*(2), 292-297.

Sit, C.H., McKenzie, T.L., Lian, J.M., & McManus, A. (2008). Activity levels during physical education and recess in two special schools for children with mild intellectual disabilities. *Adapted Physical Activity Quarterly, 25*(3), 247-259.

Sit, C.H., McManus, A., McKenzie, T. L., & Lian, J. (2007). Physical activity levels of children in special schools. *Preventive Medicine, 45*(6), 424-431.

Swenson, S., Pope, Z., & Zeng, N. (2016). Objectively-measured physical activity levels in physical education among homeschool children. *Journal of Teaching, Research, and Media in Kinesiology, 2,* 1-9.

Trost, S.G., Fees, B., & Dzewaltowski, D. (2008). Feasibility and efficacy of a "Move and Learn" physical activity curriculum in preschool children. *Journal of Physical Activity & Health, 5,* 88-103.

U.S. Department of Education. (2016). *Digest of education statistics: 2015.* Retrieved from https://nces.ed.gov/programs/digest/d15/

Van Stan, S., Lessard, L., & Dupont, P.K. (2013). The impact of statewide training to increase child care providers' knowledge of nutrition and physical activity rules in Delaware. *Childhood Obesity, 9,* 43-50.

Wachob, D.A., & Alman, R.E. (2014). Influence of the parent-teacher on the cardiovascular health and body composition of homeschooling children. *Medicine & Science in Sports & Exercise, 46*(5), 471-472.

Webb, E., & Forrester, S. (2015). Affective outcomes of intramural sport participation. *Recreational Sports Journal, 39,* 69-81.

Welk, G., & Meredith, M.D. (Eds.). (2010). *FitnessGram & ActivityGram test administration manual: Updated 4th edition.* Champaign, IL: Human Kinetics Publishers.

Welk, G.J., Schaben, J.A., & Shelley, M. (2004). Physical activity and physical fitness in children schooled at home and in public schools. *Pediatric Exercise Science, 16*(4), 310-323.

Chapter 16

Allar, I., Elliott, E., Jones, E., Kristjansson, A.L., Taliaferro, A., & Bulger, S.M. (2017). Involving families and communities in CSPAP development using asset mapping. *Journal of Physical Education, Recreation & Dance, 88*(5), 7-14.

Allegrante, J.P., Hyden, C., & Kristjansson, A.L. (in press). Research approaches of education, applied psychology, and behavioral science and their application to behavioral medicine. In E. Fisher, L.D. Cameron, A. Christensen, U. Ehlert, Y. Guo, B. Oldenburg, & F. Snoek (Eds.), *Principles and concepts of behavioral medicine: A global handbook.* New York, NY: Springer.

Anderson, R.E., Carter, I., & Lowe, G.R. (1999). *Human behavior in the social environment* (5th ed.). New York, NY: Aldine de Gruyter.

Baker, I.R., Dennison, B.A., Boyer, P.S., Sellers, K.F., Russo, T.J., & Sherwood, N.A. (2007). An asset-based community initiative to reduce television viewing in New York state. *Preventive Medicine, 44,* 437–441.

Bartholomew, L.K., Markham, C., Mullen, P., & Fernandez, M.E. (2015). Planning models for theory-based health promotion interventions. In K. Glanz, K. Rimer, & K. Viswanath (Eds.), *Health behavior: Theory, research, and practice* (pp. 359-388, 5th ed.). San Francisco, CA: Jossey-Bass.

Beaulieu, L.J. (2002). *Mapping the assets of your community: A key component for building local capacity.* Retrieved from http://srdc.msstate.edu/trainings/educurricula/asset_mapping/asset_mapping.pdf

Beighle, A., Erwin, H., Castelli, D., & Ernst, M. (2009). Preparing physical educators for the role of physical activity director. *Journal of Physical Education, Recreation & Dance, 80*(4), 24-29.

Blank, M.J., Melaville, A., & Shah, B.P. (2003). *Making the difference: Research and practice in community schools.* Retrieved from https://files.eric.ed.gov/fulltext/ED499103.pdf

Brusseau, T.A., Bulger, S.M., Elliott, E., Hannon, J.C., & Jones, E. (2015). University and community partnerships to implement comprehensive school physical activity programs: Insights and impacts for kinesiology departments. *Kinesiology Review, 4*(4), 370-377.

Bulger, S.M., & Housner, L. (2009). Relocating from easy street: Strategies for moving physical education forward. *Quest, 61,* 442-469.

Burke, W.W. (2002). *Organizational change: Theory and practice.* Thousand Oaks, CA: Sage.

Carson, R.L., Castelli, D.M., Beighle, A., & Erwin, H. (2014). School-based physical activity promotion: A conceptual framework for research and practice. *Childhood Obesity, 10*(2), 100-106.

Castelli, D.M., Centeio, E.E., & Nicksic, H.M. (2013). Preparing educators to promote and provide physical activity in schools. *American Journal of Lifestyle Medicine, 7,* 324-332.

Centers for Disease Control and Prevention. (2013). *Comprehensive school physical activity programs: A guide for schools.* Retrieved from www.cdc. gov/healthyyouth/physicalactivity/pdf/13_242620-A_CSPAP_SchoolPhysActivityPrograms_Final_508_12192013.pdf

Coghlan, D., & Brannick, T. (2014). *Doing action research in your own organization* (4th ed.). Thousand Oaks, CA: Sage.

Dillman, D.A., Smyth, J.D., & Christian, L.M. (2008). *Internet, mail, and mixed-mode surveys: The tailored design method* (3rd ed.). Hoboken, NJ: John Wiley & Sons, Inc.

Dorfman, D. (1998). *Mapping community assets workbook. Strengthening community education: The basis for sustainable renewal.* Retrieved from https://resources.depaul.edu/abcd-institute/resources/Documents/DorfmanMappingCommunityAssetsWorkBook.pdf

Fowler, F.J., Jr. (2014). *Survey research methods* (5th ed.). Thousand Oaks, CA: Sage.

Gates, M., Hanning, R., Gates, A., Stephen, J., Fehst, A., & Tsuji, L. (2016). Physical activity and fitness of First Nations youth in a remote and isolated northern Ontario community: A needs assessment. *Journal of Community Health, 41,* 46-56.

Glanz, K., Rimer, K., & Viswanath K. (Eds.). (2015). *Health behavior: Theory, research, and practice* (5th ed.). San Francisco, CA: Jossey-Bass.

Goldman, K.D., & Schmalz, K.J. (2005). "Accentuate the positive!": Using an asset-mapping tool as part of a community-health needs assessment. *Health Promotion Practice, 6*(2), 125-128.

Green, L. (2006). Public health asks of systems science: To advance of evidence-based practice, can you help us get more practice-based evidence? *American Journal of Public Health, 96*(3), 406-409.

Green, L.W., & Kreuter, M. (2005). *Health program planning: An educational and ecological approach* (4th ed.). New York, NY: McGraw-Hill.

Hanson, E. (1996). *Educational administration and organizational behavior* (4th ed.). Boston, MA: Allyn and Bacon.

Hays, R.T. (2006). *The science of learning: A systems theory perspective.* Boca Raton, FL: BrownWalker Press.

Hunt, K., & Metzler, M. (2017). Adoption of comprehensive school PA programs: A literature review. *Physical Educator, 74*(2), 315-340.

Hursen, C., & Birinci, C.M. (2013). Educational needs assessment of art teachers during teaching process. *Procedia - Social and Behavioral Sciences, 83,* 1068-1072.

Institute of Medicine (IOM). (2013). *Educating the student body: Taking physical activity and physical education to school.* Retrieved from www.nap.edu/read/18314/chapter/1

Jones, E.M., Taliaferro, A.R., Elliott, E.M., Bulger, S.M., Kristjansson, A.L., Neal, W., & Allar, I. (2014). Feasibility study of comprehensive school physical activity programs in Appalachian communities: The McDowell CHOICES project. *Journal of Teaching in Physical Education, 33,* 467-491.

Kaufman, R., & English, F.W. (1979). *Needs assessment: Concept and application.* Englewood Cliffs, NJ: Educational Technology Publications, Inc.

Kretzmann, J.P., McKnight, J.L., Dobrowolski, S., & Puntenney, D. (2005). *Discovering community power: A guide to mobilizing local assets and your organization's capacity.* Retrieved from https://resources.depaul.edu/abcd-institute/publications/publications-by-topic/Documents/kelloggabcd.pdf

Kristjansson, A.L., Elliott, E., Bulger, S., Jones, E., Taliaferro, A.R., & Neal, W. (2015). Needs assessment of child and adolescent physical activity opportunities in rural West Virginia: The McDowell CHOICES planning effort. *BMC Public Health, 15,* 327.

Laszlo, S., & Krippner, S. (1998). Systems theories: Their origins, foundations, and development. In J.S. Jordan (Ed.), *Systems theories and a priori aspects of perception* (pp. 47-74). Amsterdam, The Netherlands: Elsevier Science.

Livingood, W.C., Allegrante, J.P., Airhihenbuwa, C.O., Clark, N.M., Windsor, R.C., Zimmerman, M.A., & Green, L.W. (2011). Applied social and behavioral science to address complex health problems. *American Journal of Preventative Medicine, 41*(5), 525-531.

Lohrmann, D.K. (2010). A complementary ecological model of the coordinated school health program. *Journal of School Health, 80*(1), 1-9.

Misra, S.M., Nepal, V.P., Banerjee, D., & Giardino, A.P. (2016). Chronic health conditions, physical activity and dietary behaviors of Bhutanese refugees: A Houston-based needs assessment. *Journal of Immigrant and Minority Health, 18,* 1423-1431.

Moore, K.J., Garbacz, A., Gau, J.M., Dishion, T.J., Brown, K.L., Stormshak, E.A., & Seeley, J.R. (2016). Proactive parent engagement in public schools: Using a brief strengths and needs assessment in a multiple-gating risk management strategy. *Journal of Positive Behavior Interventions, 18*(4), 230-240.

Page, T.F., Beck-Sague, C.M., Pinzon-Iregui, M.C., Cuddihy, A., Tyler, T., Forno, E., . . . Gasana, J. (2013). Asthma in underserved schoolchildren in Miami, Florida: Results of a school- and community-based needs assessment. *Journal of Asthma, 50*(5), 480-487.

Pavri, S. (2004). General and special education teachers' preparation needs in providing social support: A needs assessment. *Teacher Education and Special Education, 27*(4), 433-443.

Robinson, J.P. (2003). Asset mapping: A tool for building capacity in communities. *Journal of Family & Consumer Sciences, 95*(3), 52-53.

Shaked, H., & Schechter, C. (2013). Seeing wholes: The concept of systems thinking and its implementation in school leadership. *International Review of Education, 59*(6), 771-791.

Sharpe, P.A., Greaney, M.L., Lee, P.R., & Royce, S.W. (2000). Assets-oriented community assessment. *Public Health Reports, 115*, 205-211.

Soriano, F. (2012). *Conducting needs assessments: A multidisciplinary approach.* Thousand Oaks, CA: Sage.

Wallerstein, N.B., & Duran, B. (2006). Using community-based participatory research to address health disparities. *Health Promotion Practice, 7*(3), 312-323.

Wallerstein, N., Minkler, M., Carter-Edwards, L., Avila, M., & Sanchez, V. (2015). Improving health through community engagement, community organization, and community building. In K. Glanz, K. Rimer, & K. Viswanath (Eds.), *Health behavior: Theory, research, and practice* (5th ed.). San Francisco, CA: Jossey-Bass.

Warren, M., & Mapp, K. (2011). *A Match on Dry Grass: Community Organizing as a Catalyst for School Reform.* Oxford: Oxford University Press.

Webster, C.A., Beets, M., Weaver, R.G., Vazou, S., & Russ, L. (2015). Rethinking recommendations for implementing comprehensive school physical activity programs: A partnership model. *Quest, 67*, 185-202.

Witkin, B.R., & Atlschuld, J.W. (1995). *Planning and conducting needs assessments: A practical guide.* Thousand Oaks, CA: Sage.

World Health Organization. (2009). *Systems thinking for health systems strengthening.* Retrieved from http://apps.who.int/iris/bitstream/handle/10665/44204/9789241563895_eng.pdf;jsessionid=11A3F08F3A73A62C1A79B372578B3696?sequence=1

Chapter 17

Bingham, D.D., Boddy, L.M., Ridgers, N.D., & Stratton, G. (2015). The physical activity levels and play behaviours of children with special needs: An exploratory cross-sectional study. *Archives of Exercise in Health and Disease, 5*(1-2), 359-365. doi:10.5628/aehd.v5i1-2.172

Bocarro, J.N., Kanters, M.A., Cernin, E., Floyd, M.F., Casper, J.M., Suau, L.J., & McKenzie, T.L. (2012). School sport policy and school-based physical activity environments and their association with observed physical activity in middle school children. *Health & Place, 18*(1), 31-38. *doi:101016/j.healthplace.2011.08.007*

Bocarro, J.N., Kanters, M., Edwards, M., Casper, J., & McKenzie, T.L. (2014). Prioritizing school intramural and interscholastic programs based on observed physical activity. *American Journal of Health Promotion, 28*(Suppl. 3), S65-S71. doi:10.4278/ajhp.130430-QUAN-205

Carlton, T.A., Kanters, M.A., Bocarro J.N., Floyd, M.F., Edwards, M.B., & Suau, L.J. (2017). Shared use agreements and leisure time physical activity in North Carolina public schools. *Preventive Medicine, 95*, S10-S16. http://dx.doi.org/10.1016/j.ypmed.2016.08.037

Centers for Disease Control and Prevention. (2013). *Comprehensive school physical activity programs: A guide for schools.* Retrieved from www.cdc.gov/healthyyouth/physicalactivity/pdf/13_242620-A_CSPAP_SchoolPhysActivityPrograms_Final_508_12192013.pdf

Curtner-Smith, M.D., Sofo, S., Chouinard, J., & Wallace, S. (2007). Health-promoting physical activity and extra-curricular sport. *European Physical Education Review, 13*(2), 131-144.

Demissie, Z., Brener, N.D., McManus, T., Shanklin, S.L., Hawkins, J., & Kann, L. (2015). *School health profiles 2014: Characteristics of health programs among secondary schools.* Retrieved from www.cdc.gov/healthyyouth/data/profiles/pdf/2014/2014_profiles_report.pdf

Evenson K., Jones, S., Holliday, K., Cohen, D., & McKenzie, T.L. (2016). Park characteristics, use, and physical activity: A review of studies using SOPARC (System for Observing Play and Recreation in Communities). *Preventive Medicine, 86*, 153-166. http://dx.doi.org/10.1016/j.ypmed.2016.02.029

Huberty, J.L., Beets, M.W., Beighle, A., Saint-Maurice, P.F., & Welk, G. (2014). Effects of Ready for Recess, an environmental intervention, on physical activity in third- through sixth-grade children. *Journal of Physical Activity & Health, 11*(2), 384-395.

Institute of Medicine. (2013). *Educating the student body: Taking physical activity and physical education to school.* Retrieved from https://www.nap.edu/read/18314/chapter/1

Kahan, D., & McKenzie, T.L. (2017). Physical education policies and practices in California private secondary schools. *Journal of Physical Activity & Health, 14*, 130-137. https://doi.org/10.1123/jpah.2016-0171

Kanters, M.A., Bocarro, J.N., Filardo, M., Edwards, M., McKenzie, T.L., & Floyd, M. (2014). Shared use of school facilities with community organizations and afterschool physical activity program participation: A cost-benefit assessment. *Journal of School Health, 84*, 302-309.

Kanters, M.A., McKenzie, T.L., Edwards, M., Bocarro, J.N., Mahar, M., Martel, K., & Hodge, C. (2015). Youth sport practice model gets kids more active with more time practicing skills. *Retos, 28*, 173-177.

Katzmarzyk, P.T., Denstel, K.D., Beals, K., Bolling, C., Braxton, C., Crouter, S.E., . . . Sisson, S.B. (2016). Results from the United States of America's report card on physical activity for children and youth. *Journal of Physical Activity & Health, 13*(11, Suppl. 2), S307-S313. doi:10.1123/jpah.2016-0321

Lounsbery, M.A.F., McKenzie, T.L., Morrow, J.R., Holt, K.A., & Budnar, R.G. (2013). School physical activity policy assessment. *Journal of Physical Activity & Health, 10*(4), 496-503. doi:10.1123/jpah.10.4.496

Lounsbery, M.A., McKenzie, T.L., Morrow, J.R., Monnat, S., & Holt, K. (2013). District and school physical education policies: Implications for physical education and recess time. *Annals of Behavioral Medicine, 45*(Suppl. 1), S131-S141. doi:10.1007/s12160-012-9427-9

Lounsbery, M.A.F., Holt, K.A., Monnat, S.A., Funk, B., & McKenzie, T.L. (2014). JROTC as a substitute for PE: Really? *Research Quarterly for Exercise and Sport, 85,* 413-419. doi:10.1080/02701367.2014.930408

Mayfield, C.A., Child, S., Weaver, R.G., Zarret, N., Beets, M., & Moore, J.B. (2017). Effectiveness of a playground intervention for antisocial, prosocial, and physical activity behaviors. *Journal of School Health, 87,* 338-345.

McKenzie, T.L. (2016). Context matters: Systematic observation of place-based physical activity. *Research Quarterly for Exercise and Sport, 87*(4), 334-341. doi:10.1080/02701367.2016.1234302

McKenzie, T.L., Alcaraz, J.E., Sallis, J.F., & Faucette, F.N. (1998). Effects of a physical education program on children's manipulative skills. *Journal of Teaching in Physical Education, 17*(3), 327-341. doi.org/10.1123/jtpe.17.3.327

McKenzie, T.L., Cohen, D.A., Sehgal, A., Williamson, S., & Golinelli, D. (2006). System for Observing Play and Recreation in Communities (SOPARC): Reliability and feasibility measures. *Journal of Physical Activity & Health, 3*(Suppl. 1), S208-222. doi:10.1123/jpah.3.s1.s208

McKenzie, T.L., Li, D., Derby, C., Webber, L., Luepker, R.V., & Cribb, P. (2003). Maintenance of effects of the CATCH physical education program: Results from the CATCH-ON study. *Health Education & Behavior, 30*(4), 447-462.

McKenzie, T.L., & Lounsbery, M.A.F. (2014). *PASS: Physical activity school score: Background and technical manual.* Retrieved from http://activelivingresearch.org/sites/default/files/PASS_Manual_April2014_0.pdf

McKenzie, T.L., Marshall, S.J., Sallis, J.F., & Conway, T.L. (2000). Leisure-time physical activity in school environments: An observational study using SOPLAY. *Preventive Medicine, 30,* 70-77.

McKenzie, T.L., Sallis, J.F., Kolody, B., & Faucette, N. (1997). Long term effects of a physical education curriculum and staff development program: SPARK. *Research Quarterly for Exercise and Sport, 68,* 280-291.

McKenzie, T.L., Sallis, J.F., & Nader, P.R. (1991). SOFIT: System for Observing Fitness Instruction Time. *Journal of Teaching in Physical Education, 11,* 195-205.

McKenzie, T.L., Sallis, J.F., Rosengard, P.R., & Ballard, K. (2016). The SPARK programs: A public health model of physical education research and dissemination. *Journal of Teaching in Physical Education, 35*(4), 381-389. doi.10.1123/jtpe.2016-0100

McKenzie, T.L., & Smith, N.J. (2017). Studies of physical education in the United States using SOFIT: A review. *Research Quarterly for Exercise and Sport, 88*(4), 492-502. doi:10.1080/02701367.2017.1376028

McKenzie, T.L., Strikmiller, P.K., Stone, E.J., Woods, S.E., Ehlinger, S., Romero, K.A., & Budman, S.T. (1994). CATCH: Physical activity process evaluation in a multicenter trial. *Health Education Quarterly, Suppl. 2,* S73-S89.

McKenzie, T.L., & van der Mars, H. (2015). Top 10 research questions related to assessing physical activity and its contexts using systematic observation. *Research Quarterly for Exercise and Sport, 86*(1), 13-29. doi:10.1080/02701367.2015.991264

Monnat, S.M., Lounsbery, M.A.F., McKenzie, T.L., & Chandler, R.F. (2017). Associations between demographic characteristics and physical activity practices in Nevada schools. *Preventive Medicine, 95,* S4-S9. doi:10.1016/j.ypmed.2016.08.029

National Physical Activity Plan Alliance (NPAPA). (2018). *The 2018 United States report card on physical activity for children and youth.* Retrieved from http://physicalactivityplan.org/projects/reportcard.html

Powers, H.S., Conway, T.L., McKenzie, T.L., Sallis, J.F., & Marshall, S.J. (2002). Participation in extracurricular physical activity programs in middle schools. *Research Quarterly for Exercise and Sport, 73,* 187-192.

Ridgers, N.D., Carter, L.M., Stratton, G., & McKenzie, T.L. (2011). Examining children's physical activity and play behaviors during school playtime over time. *Health Education Research, 26,* 586-595.

Ridgers, N.D., Stratton, G., & McKenzie, T.L. (2010). Reliability and validity of the System for Observing Children's Activity and Relationships during Play (SOCARP). *Journal of Physical Activity & Health, 7,* 17-25.

Sallis, J.F., Conway, T.L., Prochaska, J.J., McKenzie, T.L., Marshall, S., & Brown, M. (2001). The association of school environments with youth physical activity. *American Journal of Public Health, 91*(4), 618-620.

Sallis, J.F., McKenzie, T.L., Alcaraz, J.E., Kolody, B., Faucette, N., & Hovell, M.F. (1997). The effects of a 2-year physical education program (SPARK) on physical activity and fitness in elementary school students. *American Journal of Public Health, 87,* 1328-1334.

Sallis, J.F., McKenzie, T.L., Alcaraz, J.E., Kolody, B., Hovell, M.F., & Nader, P.R. (1993). Project SPARK: Effects of physical education on adiposity in children. *Annals of the New York Academy of Sciences, 699,* 127-136.

Sallis, J.F., McKenzie, T.L., Conway, T.L., Elder, J.P., Prochaska, J.J., Brown, M., . . . Alcaraz, J.E. (2003). Environmental interventions for eating and physical activity: A randomized controlled trial in middle schools. *American Journal of Preventive Medicine, 24*, 209-217.

Sallis, J.F., McKenzie, T.L., Kolody, B., Lewis, M., Marshall, S., & Rosengard, P. (1999). Effects of health-related physical education on academic achievement: Project SPARK. *Research Quarterly for Exercise and Sport, 70*, 127-134.

Strelow, J.S., Larson, J.J., Sallis, J.F., Conway, T.L., Powers, H.S., & McKenzie, T.L. (2002). Factors influencing the performance of volunteers who provide physical activity in middle schools. *Journal of School Health, 72*, 147-151.

U.S. Department of Health and Human Services & Centers for Disease Control and Prevention. (2015). *Results from the School Health Policies and Practices Study 2014.* Retrieved from www.cdc.gov/healthyyouth/data/shpps/pdf/shpps-508-final_101315.pdf

Woods, A., Graber, K., & Daum, D. (2012). Children's recess physical activity: Movement patterns and preferences. *Journal of Teaching in Physical Education, 31*, 146-162.

Chapter 18

Brusseau, T.A., Hannon, J.C., & Burns, R.D. (2016). The effect of a comprehensive school physical activity program on physical activity and health-related fitness in children from low-income families. *Journal of Physical Activity & Health, 13*, 888-894.

Burns, R.D., Brusseau, T.A., Fu, Y., Myrer, R., & Hannon, J.C. (2016). Impact of CSPAP on children on-task behavior at school. *American Journal of Health Behavior, 40*(1), 100-107. http://dx.doi.org/10.5993/AJHB.40.1.11

Burns, R.D., Brusseau, T.A., & Hannon, J.C. (2015). Effect of a comprehensive school physical activity program on school day step counts in children. *Journal of Physical Activity & Health, 12*, 1536-1542. doi:10.1123/jpah.2014-0578

Burns, R.D., Brusseau, T.A., & Hannon, J.C. (2017). Effect of comprehensive school physical activity programming on cardiometabolic health markers in children from low-income schools. *Journal of Physical Activity & Health, 14*(9), 671-676. https://doi.org/10.1123/jpah.2016-0691

Caballero, B., Clay, T., Davis, S.M., Ethelbah, B., Rock, B.H., Lohman, T., . . . Stevens, J. (2003). Pathways: A school-based, randomized controlled trial for the prevention of obesity in American Indian schoolchildren. *American Journal of Clinical Nutrition, 78*(5), 1030-1038.

Carson, R.L., Castelli, D.M., Pulling Kuhn, A.C., Moore, J.B., Beets, M.W., Beighle, A., . . . Glowacki, E.M. (2014). Impact of trained champions of comprehensive school physical activity programs on school physical activity offerings, youth physical and sedentary behaviors. *Preventive Medicine, 69*, S12-S19. doi:10.1016/j.ypmed.2014.08.025

Carson, R.L., Pulling, A.C., Castelli, D.M., & Beighle, A. (2014). Facilitators and inhibitors of the DPA program and CSPAP implementation. *Research Quarterly for Exercise and Sport, 85*(Suppl. 1), A-56.

Centeio, E.E., Kulik, N.L., McCaughtry, N., Garn, A.C., Somers, C., Martin, J., . . . Fahlman, M. (2016). *The role of principals in increasing physical activity through comprehensive school physical activity programs.* Presented at the annual meeting for SHAPE America, Minneapolis, MN.

Centeio, E.E., McCaughtry, N., Gutuskey, L., Garn, A.C., Somers, C., Shen, B., . . . Kulik, N. (2014). Physical activity change through comprehensive school physical activity programs in urban elementary schools. *Journal of Teaching in Physical Education, 33*, 572-591. doi:10.1123/jtpe.2014-0067

Centeio, E.E., McCaughtry, N., Moore, E.W.G., Kulik, N., Garn, A., Martin, J., . . . Fahlman, M. (2018). Building healthy communities: A comprehensive school health program to prevent obesity in elementary schools. *Preventive Medicine, 111*, 210-215. https://doi.org/10.1016/j.ypmed.2018.03.005

Centeio, E.E., Somers, C., Moore, E.W., Kulik, N., Garn, A., Martin, J., & McCaughtry, N. (2018). Relationship between academic achievement and healthy school transformations in urban elementary schools in the United States. *Physical Education and Sport Pedagogy, 23*(4), 402-417. https://doi.org/10.1080/17408989.2018.1441395

Centers for Disease Control and Prevention. (2010). *The association between school-based physical activity, including physical education, and academic performance.* Retrieved from www.cdc.gov/healthyyouth/health_and_academics/pdf/pa-pe_paper.pdf

Demetriou, Y., Gillison, F., & McKenzie, T.L. (2017). After-school physical activity interventions on child and adolescent physical activity and health: A review of reviews. *Advances in Physical Education, 7*, 191-215.

Institute of Medicine. (2013). *Educating the student body: Taking physical activity and physical education to school.* Retrieved from https://www.nap.edu/read/18314/chapter/1

Kulik, N., Moore, E.W.G., Centeio, E.E., Garn, A., Martin, J., Shen, B., . . . McCaughtry, N*Knowledge, attitudes, self-efficacy and healthy eating behavior among children: Results from the Building Healthy Communities Trial.* Manuscript submitted for publication.

Lubans, D.R., Morgan, P.J., Aguiar, E.J., & Callister, R. (2011). Randomized controlled trial of the physical activity leaders (PALs) program for adolescent boys from disadvantaged secondary schools. *Preventive Medicine, 52*, 239-246.

Luepker, R.V., Perry, C.L., McKinlay, S.M., Nader, P.R., Parcel, G.S., Stone, E.J., . . . Kelder, S.H. (1996). Outcomes of a field trial to improve children's dietary patterns and physical activity: The Child and Adolescent Trial for Cardiovascular Health (CATCH). *JAMA, 275*(10), 768-776.

Murray, R., Ramstetter, C., Devore, C., Allison, M., Ancona, R., Barnett, S., . . . Okamoto, J. (2013). The crucial role of recess in school. *Pediatrics, 131*(1), 183-188.

Nader, P.R., Stone, E.J., Lytle, L.A., Perry, C.L., Osganian, S.K., Kelder, S., . . . Wu, M. (1999). Three-year maintenance of improved diet and physical activity: The CATCH cohort. *Archives of Pediatrics & Adolescent Medicine, 153*(7), 695-704.

Pate, R.R., Ward, D.S., Saunders, R.P., Felton, G., Dishman, R.K., & Dowda, M. (2005). Promotion of physical activity among high-school girls: A randomized controlled trial. *American Journal of Public Health, 95*(9), 1582-1587.

Puder, J.J., Marques-Vidal, P., Schindler, C., Zahner, L., Niederer, I., Bürgi, F., . . . Kriemler, S. (2011). Effect of multidimensional lifestyle intervention on fitness and adiposity in predominantly migrant preschool children (Ballabeina): Cluster randomised controlled trial. *British Medical Journal, 343,* d6195. doi:10.1136/bmj.d6195

Pulling Kuhn, A., Carson, R.L., & Beighle, A. (2015). *Changes in psychosocial perspectives among teachers trained as physical activity leaders: Teacher efficacy, work engagement, and affective commitment.* Research presentation at the Physical Education Teacher Education and Health Education Teacher Education triannual meeting of SHAPE America, Atlanta, GA.

Sallis, J.F., & McKenzie, T.L. (1991). Physical education's role in public health. *Research Quarterly for Exercise and Sport, 62*(2), 124-137.

Sallis, J.F., McKenzie, T.L., Alcaraz, J.E., Kolody, B., Faucette, N., & Hovell, M.F. (1997). The effects of a 2-year physical education program (SPARK) on physical activity and fitness in elementary school students. Sports, Play and Active Recreation for Kids. *American Journal of Public Health, 87*(8), 1328-1334.

Seo, D.C., King, M.H., Kim, N., Sovinski, D., Meade, R., & Lederer, A.M. (2013). Predictors for moderate- and vigorous-intensity physical activity during an 18-month coordinated school health intervention. *Preventive Medicine, 57*(5), 466-470.

Wallerstein, N., & Berstein, E. (1988). Empowerment education: Freire's ideas adapted to health education. *Health Education & Behavior, 15*(4), 379-394.

Chapter 19

Advocacy. (n.d.). *Merriam-Webster's online dictionary.* Retrieved from www.merriam-webster.com/dictionary/advocacy

Bauman, A.E., Bellew, B., Owen, N., & Vita, P. (2001). Impact of an Australian mass media campaign targeting physical activity in 1998. *American Journal of Preventive Medicine, 21*(1), 41-47.

Bryan, C., & Sims, S. (2011). K-12 and university partnerships: Bridging the advocacy gap. *Strategies, 25*(1), 36-37.

Carson, R.L., Castelli, D.M., Beighle, A., & Erwin, H. (2014). School-based physical activity promotion: A conceptual framework for research and practice. *Childhood Obesity, 10*(2), 100-106. doi: 10.1089/chi.2013.0134

Carson, R.L., Castelli, D.M., & Kulinna, P.H. (2017). CSPAP professional preparation: Takeaways from pioneering physical education teacher education programs. *Journal of Physical Education, Recreation & Dance, 88*(2), 43-51.

Centers for Disease Control and Prevention (CDC). (2010). *The association between school-based physical activity, including physical education, and academic performance.* Retrieved from www.cdc.gov/healthyyouth/health_and_academics/pdf/pa-pe_paper.pdf

Centers for Disease Control and Prevention (CDC). (2011). *Strategies to prevent obesity and other chronic diseases: The CDC guide to strategies to increase physical activity in the community.* Retrieved from www.cdc.gov/obesity/downloads/PA_2011_WEB.pdf

Centers for Disease Control and Prevention (CDC). (2013a). *Comprehensive school physical activity programs: A guide for schools.* Retrieved from www.cdc.gov/healthyschools/physicalactivity/pdf/13_242620-A_CSPAP_SchoolPhysActivityPrograms_Final_508_12192013.pdf

Centers for Disease Control and Prevention (CDC). (2013b). *Make a difference at your school.* Retrieved from https://digitalcommons.hsc.unt.edu/cgi/viewcontent.cgi?article=1030&context=disease

Darst, P.W., Pangrazi, R.P., Brusseau, T.A., & Erwin, H. (2014). *Dynamic physical education for secondary school students* (8th ed.). San Francisco, CA: Pearson.

Designed to Move. (2015). *Designed to move* [web page]. Retrieved November 16, 2018, from www.designedtomove.org

Huhman, M., Potter, L.D., Wong, F.L., Banspach, S.W., Duke, J.C., & Heitzler, C.D. (2005). Effects of a mass media campaign to increase physical activity among children: Year 1 results of the VERB campaign. *Pediatrics, 116,* e277-e284.

Kahn, E.B., Ramsey, L.T., Brownson, R.C., Heath, G.W., Howze, E.H., Powell, K.E., . . . Corso, P. (2002). The effectiveness of interventions to increase physical activity: A systematic review. *American Journal of Preventive Medicine, 22*(4), 73-107.

Loland, S. (2006). Morality, medicine, and meaning: Toward an integrated justification of physical education. *Quest, 58,* 60-70.

National Board for Professional Teaching Standards. (2014). *Physical education standards* (2nd ed.). Washington, DC: U.S. Department of Education.

Physical Activity Guidelines Advisory Committee. (2008). *Physical activity guidelines advisory committee report, 2008.* Retrieved from https://health.gov/paguidelines/report/pdf/CommitteeReport.pdf

Shilton, T. (2006). Advocacy for physical activity: From evidence to influence. *Promotion and Education, 13*(2), 118-126.

Shilton, T. (2008). Creating and making the case: Global advocacy for physical activity. *Journal of Physical Activity and Health, 5,* 765-776.

Soler, R.E., Leeks, K.D., Buchanan, L.R., Brownson, R.C., Heath, G.W., & Hopkins, D.H. (2010). Point-of-decision prompts to increase stair use. *American Journal of Preventive Medicine, 38*(2), S292-S300.

Tannehill, D., van der Mars, H., & MacPhail, A. (2015). Comprehensive school physical activity programs. In D. Tannehill, H. van der Mars, & A. MacPhail (Eds.), *Building effective physical education programs.* Burlington, MA: Jones & Bartlett Learning.

World Health Organization. (1995). *Report of the interagency meeting on advocacy strategies for health and development: Development communication in action.* Geneva, Switzerland: World Health Organization.

Chapter 20

American Heart Association. (n.d.). *Kids heart challenge* [Web page]. Retrieved from http://american.heart.org/kidsheartchallenge/

Beighle, A., Erwin, H., Castelli, D.M., & Ernst, M. (2009). Preparing physical educators for the role of PA director. *Journal of Physical Education, Recreation & Dance, 80*(4), 24-29.

Berei, C.P., Goc Karp, G., & Kauffman, K. (2018). Physical activity opportunities in Idaho schools. *The Physical Educator, 75*(2), 282-301.

Berei, C.P., Goc Karp, G., Olsen, S., Fennell, M., & Drake, E. (2017). *Perceptions of PEP grant influences on CSPAP implementation.* Paper presented at the annual meeting of the Society of Health and Physical Educators, Boston, MA.

Brazendale, K., Chandler, J.L., Beets, M.W., Weaver, R.G., Beighle, A., Huberty, J.L., & Moore, J.B. (2015). Maximizing children's physical activity using the LET US Play principles. *Preventive Medicine, 76,* 14-19. https://doi.org/10.1016/j.ypmed.2015.03.012

Brusseau, T.A. (2017). Infusing CSPAP knowledge, training and research into doctoral PETE. *Journal of Physical Education, Recreation & Dance, 88*(2), 20-24. http://dx.doi.org/10.1080/07303084.2017.1260974

Carson, R.L. (2012). Certification and duties of a director of physical activity. *Journal of Physical Education, Recreation & Dance, 83*(6), 16-29. https://doi.org/10.1080/07303084.2012.10598790

Carson, R.L., Castelli, D.M., Beighle, A., & Erwin, H. (2014). School-based physical activity promotion: A conceptual framework for research and practice. *Childhood Obesity, 10*(2), 100-106.

Carson, R., Castelli, D.M., & Kulinna, P.H. (2017). CSPAP professional preparation: Takeaways from pioneering physical education teacher education programs. *Journal of Physical Education, Recreation & Dance, 88*(2), 43-51. http://dx.doi.org/10.1080/07303084.2017.1260986

Carson, R.L., Erwin, H., Goc Karp, G., Heidorn, B., Webster, C.A., van der Mars, H., . . . Brusseau, T.A. (2015). *Integrating CSPAP in PETE programs: Sharing insights and identifying strategies.* Symposium conducted at the annual meeting of the Society of Health and Physical Educators America, Seattle, WA.

Carson, R.L., & Raguse, A.L. (2014). Systematic review of service-learning in youth physical activity settings. *Quest, 66*(1), 57-95.

Castelli, D.M., & Beighle, A. (2007). The physical education teacher as school activity director. *Journal of Physical Education, Recreation & Dance, 78*(5), 25-28.

Centeio, E.E., Castelli, D.M., Carson, R.L., Beighle, A., & Glowacki, E. (2014). *Comprehensive school physical activity programs: Current practice and promise.* Paper presented at the American Alliance for Health, Physical Education, Recreation and Dance, National Convention, St. Louis, MO.

Centeio, E.E., Erwin, H., & Castelli, D.M. (2014). Comprehensive school physical activity programs: Characteristics of trained teachers. *Journal of Teaching in Physical Education, 33*(4), 492-510. https://doi.org/10.1123/jtpe.2014-0066

Centeio, E.E., & McCaughtry, N. (2017). Implementing comprehensive school physical activity programs: A Wayne State University case study. *Journal of Physical Education, Recreation & Dance, 88*(1), 47-49. http://dx.doi.org/10.1080/07303084.2017.1250536

Centers for Disease Control and Prevention (CDC). (2006). *Physical Education Curriculum Analysis Tool.* Atlanta, GA. Retrieved from www.cdc.gov/healthyschools/pecat/index.htm

Centers for Disease Control and Prevention (CDC). (2013). *Comprehensive school physical activity programs: A guide for schools.* Retrieved from www.cdc.gov/healthyschools/physicalactivity/pdf/13_242620-A_CSPAP_SchoolPhysActivityPrograms_Final_508_12192013.pdf

Centers for Disease Control and Prevention (CDC). (2014). *Physical education and activity questionnaire.* Retrieved from www.cdc.gov/healthyyouth/shpps/2014/questionnaires/pdf/physed12014questionnaire.pdf

Centers for Disease Control and Prevention (CDC). (2015). *School Health Index.* Retrieved from www.cdc.gov/healthyschools/shi/index.htm#

Centers for Disease Control and Prevention (CDC) (2017). *Increasing physical education and physical activity: A framework for schools.* Atlanta, GA: U.S. Department of Health and Human Sciences. Retrieved from www.cdc.gov/healthyschools/physicalactivity/index.htm

Center for Strengthening the Teaching Profession. (2009). *Teacher leadership skills framework.* Retrieved from http://cstp-wa.org/cstp2013/wp-content/uploads/2018/07/2018-Teacher-Leadership-Framework.pdf

Ciotto, C.M., & Fede, M.H. (2017). Integrating CSPAP into the PETE programs at Southern Connecticut State University and Central Connecticut State University. *Journal of Physical Education, Recreation & Dance, 88*(1), 20-28. http://dx.doi.org/10.1080/0730 3084.2017.1250520

Cothran, D.J., Kulinna, P.H., & Garn, A.C. (2010). Classroom teachers and physical activity integration. *Teaching and Teacher Education, 26*(7), 1381-1388.

Dauenhauer, B., Stellino, M.B., & Smith, M.A. (2015). *Service learning lessons from a before school physical activity program.* Paper presented at the annual meeting of the Society of Health and Physical Educators America, Seattle, WA.

DePauw, K.P., & Goc Karp, G. (1994). Integrating knowledge of disability throughout the physical education curriculum: An infusion approach. *Adapted Physical Activity Quarterly, 11*, 3-13.

Doolittle, S.A., & Virgilio, S.J. (2017). Moving toward integration of CSPAP in a highly regulated PETE context. *Journal of Physical Education, Recreation & Dance, 88*(2), 8-13. http://dx.doi.org/10.1080/07303 084.2017.1260957

Dweck, C.S. (2006). *Mindset: The new psychology of success.* New York, NY: Random House.

Erwin, H.E. (n.d.). *Implementing classroom-based physical activity.* Retrieved from www.pelinks4u.org/articles/erwin0610.htm

Erwin, H.E., Beighle, A., Carson, R.L., & Castelli, D.M. (2013). Comprehensive school-based physical activity programs: A review. *Quest, 65*, 412.

Erwin, H.E., Beighle, A., & Eckler, S. (2017). PETE preparation for CSPAP at the University of Kentucky. *Journal of Physical Education, Recreation & Dance, 88*(1), 36-41. http://dx.doi.org/10.1080/07303 084.2017.1250532

Erwin, H., Goc Karp, G., & Carson, R. (2015). *Professional preparation programs for CSPAP leaders.* Symposium conducted at the annual meeting of the Society of Health and Physical Educators, Physical Education Teacher Education & Health Education Teacher Education Conference, Atlanta, GA.

Goc Karp, G., Brown, H., Scruggs, P.W., & Berei, C. (2017). Cultivating leadership, pedagogy and programming for CSPAP and healthy, active lifestyles at the University of Idaho. *Journal of Physical Education, Recreation & Dance, 88*(1), 29-35. http://dx.doi.org/10.1080/0730 3084.2017.1250523

Goc Karp, G., & Scruggs, P. (2012). *Integrating comprehensive school PA leadership into PETE and beyond.* NASPE Conference on Physical Education Teacher Education, Las Vegas, NV.

Goh, T.L., Hannon, J.C., Newton, M., Webster, C., Podlog, L., & Pillow, W. (2013). "I'll squeeze it in": Transforming preservice classroom teachers' perceptions toward movement integration in schools. *Action in Teacher Education, 35*(4), 286-300.

Hargreaves, A., & Fullan, M. (2012). *Professional capital: Transforming teaching in every school.* New York, NY: Teachers College Press.

Heidorn, B., & Centeio, E. (2012). The director of physical activity and staff involvement. *Journal of Physical Education, Recreation & Dance, 83*(7), 13-19, 25-26.

Heidorn, B., & Mosier, B. (2017). Sharing insights and strategies from the University of West Georgia. *Journal of Physical Education, Recreation & Dance, 88*(1), 50-56. http://dx.doi.org/10.1080/07303084.201 7.1250538

HOPSports. (n.d.). [Web page]. Retrieved from http://hopsports.com/

Institute of Medicine (IOM). (1988). *The future of public health.* Washington, DC: The National Academies Press.

Institute of Medicine (IOM). (2003). *The future of public health in the 21st century.* Washington, DC: The National Academies Press.

Jackson, T., Burrus, J., Bassett, K., & Roberts, R.D. (2010). *Teacher leadership: An assessment framework for and emerging area of professional practice.* Princeton, NJ: Center for New Constructs.

Jones, E.M., Taliaferro, A.R., Elliott, E.M., Bulger, S.M., Kristjansson, A.L., Neal, W., . . . Allar, I. (2014). Feasibility study of comprehensive school physical activity programs in Appalachian communities: The McDowell CHOICES project. *Journal of Teaching in Physical Education, 33*(4), 467-491.

Kibbe, D.L., Hackett, J., Hurley, M., McFarland, A., Schubert, K.G., Schultz, A., & Harris, S. (2011). Ten years of Take 10!: Integrating physical activity with academic concepts in elementary school classrooms. *Preventive Medicine, 52*(Suppl.1), S43-S50.

Kwon, J.Y. (2016). *How current physical education teacher education programs prepare pre-service teachers for comprehensive school physical activity programs (CSPAP)* (Unpublished doctoral dissertation). Arizona State University, Tempe.

Kwon, J.Y., Kulinna, P.H., van der Mars, H., Koro-Ljungberg, M., Amrein-Beardsley, A., & Norris, J. (in press). Physical education preservice teachers' perceptions about preparation for comprehensive school physical activity programs. *Research Quarterly for Exercise and Sport.*

Lounsbery, M.A.F., McKenzie, T.L., Morrow, J.R., Holt, K.A., & Budnar, R.G. (2013). School physical activity policy assessment. *Journal of Physical Activity & Health, 10*(4), 496-503. doi:10.1123/jpah.10.4.496

MacPhail, A., Patton, K., Parker, M., & Tannehill, D. (2014). Leading by example: Teacher educators' professional learning through communities of practice. *Quest, 66*(1), 39-56.

Mahar, M.T., Murphy, S.K., Rowe, D.A., Golden, J., Shields, A.T., & Raedeke, T.D. (2006). Effects of a classroom-based program on physical activity and on-task behavior. *Medicine & Science in Sports & Exercise, 38*(12), 2086-2094. Doi: 10.1249/01.mss.0000235359.16685.a3

McKenzie, T.L. (2007). The preparation of physical educators: A public health perspective. *Quest, 59*(4), 345-357. doi:10.1080/00336297.2007.10483557

McKenzie, T., & Kahan, D. (2004). Impact of Surgeon General's Report: Through the eyes of physical education teacher educators. *Journal of Teaching in Physical Education, 23*(4), 300-317.

McLeroy, K.R., Bibeau, D., Steckler, A., & Glanz, K. (1988). An ecological perspective on health promotion programs. *Health Education Quarterly, 15*(4), 351-377.

McMullen, J., Kulinna, P.H., & Cothran, D. (2014). Physical activity opportunities during the school day: Classroom teachers' perceptions of using activity breaks in the classroom. *Journal of Teaching in Physical Education, 33*(4), 511-527. doi:10.1123/jtpe.2014-0062

McMullen, J., van der Mars, H., & Jahn, J. (2014). Promoting student ownership in a non-traditional physical education teacher education internship course. *Physical Education and Sport Pedagogy, 19*(3), 337-348. doi:10.1080/17408989.2012.761684

McTighe, J., & Wiggins, G. (2012). *Understanding by design framework.* Alexandria, VA: ASCD.

Mosier, B., & Heidorn, B. (2013). Theory into practice: Training others to lead comprehensive school physical activity programs. *Strategies, 26*(5), 43-45.

National Association for Sport and Physical Education. (2004). *Physical activity for children: A statement of guidelines for children ages 5-12.* Reston, VA: Author.

National Center for Safe Routes to School. (n.d.). [Web page]. Retrieved from http://www.saferoutesinfo.org/

Office of Disease Prevention and Health Promotion. (n.d.). *Healthy People tools and resources.* Retrieved from www.healthypeople.gov/2020/tools-resources

Pate, R. (2014). An inside view of the U.S. national physical activity plan. *Journal of Physical Activity and Health, 11*(3), 461-462.

Rowitz, L. (2013). *Public health leadership: Putting principles into practice.* Sudbury, MA: Jones and Bartlett Publishers.

Russ, L., Webster, C.A., Beets, M.W., & Phillips, D. (2015). Systematic review and meta-analysis of multi-component interventions through schools to increase physical activity. *Journal of Physical Activity & Health, 12*(10), 1436-1446.

Sallis, J.F., & McKenzie, T.L. (1991). Physical education's role in public health. *Research Quarterly for Exercise and Sport, 62*(2), 124-137.

Scruggs, P.W., Goc Karp, G., & Johnson, T. (2010). *The changing role of physical educators as PA specialists in Idaho.* Paper presented at the annual meeting of the Idaho Association for Health, Physical Education, Recreation & Dance, Boise, ID.

SHAPE America. (2013). *Comprehensive school physical activity programs: Helping all students log 60 minutes of physical activity each day.* Retrieved from www.shapeamerica.org/uploads/pdfs/2018/advocacy/position-statements/CSPAP-final.pdf

SHAPE America. (2017). *National standards for initial physical education teacher education.* Retrieved from www.shapeamerica.org/accreditation/peteacherprep.cfm

Talbert, J.E., & McLaughlin, M. (1994). Teacher professionalism in local school contexts. *American Journal of Education, 102*(2), 123-153.

Tannehill, D., Parker, M., Tindall, D., Moody, B., & MacPhail, A. (2015). Looking across and within: Studying ourselves as teacher educators. *Asia-Pacific Journal of Health, Sport and Physical Education, 6*(3), 299-311. http://dx.doi.org/10.1080/18377122.2015.1092726

van der Mars, H., Lorenz, K.A., & Kwon, J.Y. (2017). Building CSPAP development into Arizona State University's PETE program: A work in progress. *Journal of Physical Education, Recreation & Dance, 88*(1), 11-19. http://dx.doi.org/10.1080/07303084.2017.1250518

Weaver, R.G., Webster, C., & Beets, M.W. (2013). LET US Play: Maximizing physical activity in physical education. *Strategies, 26*(6), 33-37. https://doi.org/10.1080/08924562.2013.839518

Webster, C. (2017). CSPAP professional preparation and research initiatives at the University of South Carolina. *Journal of Physical Education, Recreation & Dance, 88*(2), 25-36. doi:10.1080/07303084.2017.1260979

Webster, C.A., Beets, M., Weaver, R.G., Vazou, S., & Russ, L. (2015). Rethinking recommendations for implementing comprehensive school physical activity programs: A partnership model. *Quest, 67*(2), 185-202.

Webster, C.A., Erwin, H., & Parks, M. (2013). Relationships between and changes in preservice classroom teachers' efficacy beliefs, willingness to integrate movement and perceived barriers to movement integration. *Physical Educator, 70*(3), 314-335.

Webster, C.A., Monsma, E., & Erwin, H.E. (2010). The role of biographical characteristics of classroom teachers' school physical activity promotion attitudes. *Journal of Teaching in Physical Education, 29*, 358-377.

Webster, C.A., & Nesbitt, D. (2017). Expanded roles of physical education teachers within a CSPAP and implications for PETE. *Journal of Physical Education, Recreation & Dance, 88*(3), 22-28.

Webster, C.A., Nesbitt, D., Lee, H., & Egan, C. (2017). Preservice physical education teachers' service learning experiences related to comprehensive school physical activity programs. *Journal of Teaching in Physical Education, 36*(4), 430-444.

Webster, C.A., Russ, L., Webster, L., Molina, S., Lee, H., & Cribbs, J. (2014). *Preparing preservice teachers for comprehensive school physical activity programs: A view from PETE.* Manuscript submitted for publication.

Webster, C.A., Russ, L., Webster, L., Molina, S., Lee, H., & Cribbs, J. (2016). PETE faculty beliefs concerning the preparation of preservice teachers for CSPAP roles: An exploratory study. *The Physical Educator, 73*(2), 315-339.

Webster, C.A., Stodden, D.F., Carson, R.L., Nesbitt, D., & Egan, C. (2016). Integrative public health-aligned physical education and implications for the professional preparation of future teachers and teacher educators/researchers in the field. *Quest, 68*(4), 457-474. doi:10.1080/00336297.2016.1229628

York-Barr, J., & Duke, K. (2004). What do we know about teacher leadership: Findings from two decades of scholarship. *Review of Educational Research, 74*(3), 255-316.

Chapter 21

Almalki, M., Gray, K., & Sanchez, F.M. (2015). The use of self-quantification systems for personal health information: Big data management activities and prospects. *Health Information Science and Systems, 3*(1), 1-11.

Baranowski, T. (2016). Pokémon Go, go, go, gone? *Games for Health Journal, 5*(5), 293-294. http://doi.org/10.1089/g4h.2016.01055.tbp

Cadmus-Bertram, L.A., Marcus, B.H., Patterson, R.E., Parker, B.A., & Morey, B.L. (2015). Randomized trial of a Fitbit-based physical activity intervention for women. *American Journal of Preventive Medicine, 49*(3), 414-418.

Castelli, D., & Fiorentino, L.H. (2008). *Physical education technology playbook.* Champaign, IL: Human Kinetics Publishers.

Charara, S. (2016). *Fashion tech: 20 wearables that are more chic than geek.* Retrieved from www.wareable.com/fashion/wearable-tech-fashion-style

Christison, A., & Khan, H.A. (2012). Exergaming for health: A community-based pediatric weight management program using active video gaming. *Clinical Pediatrics, 51*(4), 382-388.

Dominic, D., Hounkponou, F., Doh, R., Ansong, E., & Brighter, A. (2013). Promoting physical activity through persuasive technology. *International Journal of Inventive Engineering and Sciences, 2*(1), 16-22.

Duncan, M., & Staples, V. (2010). The impact of a school-based active video game play intervention on children's physical activity during recess. *Human Movement, 11*(1), 95-99. http://doi.org/10.2478/v10038-009-0023-1

Flett, M., Moore, R., Pfeiffer, K., Belonga, J., & Navarre, J. (2010). Connecting children and family with nature-based physical activity. *American Journal of Health Education, 41*(5), 292-300.

Fogel, V.A., Miltenberger, R.G., Graves, R., & Koehler, S. (2010). The effects of exergaming on physical activity among inactive children in a physical education classroom. *Journal of Applied Behavior Analysis, 43*(4), 591-600. http://doi.org/10.1901/jaba.2010.43-591

Fogg, B.J. (2003). *Persuasive technology: Using computers to change what we think and do.* New York, NY: Morgan Kaufmann Publishers.

Gao, Z. (2012). Motivated but not active: The dilemmas of incorporating interactive dance into gym class. *Journal of Physical Activity & Health, 9*(6), 794-800.

Gao, Z. (2017a). Fight fire with fire: Promoting physical activity and health through active video games. *Journal of Sport and Health Science, 6,* 1-3.

Gao, Z. (2017b). *Technology in physical activity and health promotion.* London, UK: Routledge.

Gao, Z., & Chen, S. (2014). Are field-based exergames useful in preventing childhood obesity? A systematic review. *Obesity Reviews, 5,* 1-16. http://doi.org/10.1111/obr.12164

Gao, Z., Chen, S., Pasco, D., & Pope, Z. (2015). A meta-analysis of active video games on health outcomes among children and adolescents. *Obesity Reviews, 16*(9), 783-794. http://doi.org/10.1111/obr.12287

Gao, Z., Hannan, P., Xiang, P., Stodden, D.F., & Valdez, V.E. (2013). Video game–based exercise, Latino children's physical health, and academic achievement. *American Journal of Preventive Medicine, 44*(3), S240-S246. http://doi.org/10.1016/j.amepre.2012.11.023

Gao, Z., Hannon, J.C., Newton, M., & Huang, C. (2011). Effects of curricular activity on students' situational motivation and physical activity levels. *Research Quarterly for Exercise and Sport, 82*(3), 536-544.

Gao, Z., Huang, C., Liu, T., & Xiong, W. (2012). Impact of interactive dance games on urban children's physical activity correlates and behavior. *Journal of Exercise Science & Fitness, 10*(2), 107-112. http://doi.org/10.1016/j.jesf.2012.10.009

Gao, Z., & Podlog, L. (2012). Urban Latino children's physical activity levels and performance in interactive dance video games: Effects of goal difficulty and goal specificity. *Archives of Pediatrics & Adolescent Medicine, 166*(10), 933-937. http://doi.org/10.1001/archpediatrics.2012.649

Gao, Z., Pope, Z., Lee, J., Stodden, D., Roncesvalles, N., Pasco, D., Huang, C., & Feng, D. (2017). Impact of exergaming on young children's school day energy expenditure and moderate-to-vigorous physical activity levels. *Journal of Sport and Health Science, 6,* 11-16.

Gao, Z., & Xiang, P. (2014). Effects of exergaming based exercise on urban children's physical activity participation and body composition. *Journal of Physical Activity & Health, 11*(5), 992-998. http://doi.org/10.1123/jpah.2012-0228

Gao, Z., Zhang, T., & Stodden, D. (2013). Children's physical activity levels and psychological correlates in interactive dance versus aerobic dance. *Journal of Sport and Health Science, 2*(3), 146-151. http://doi.org/10.1016/j.jshs.2013.01.005

Graham, D.J., & Hipp, J.A. (2014). Emerging technologies to promote and evaluate physical activity: Cutting-edge research and future directions. *Frontiers in Public Health, 2,* 66.

Graham, M., Zook, M., & Boulton, A. (2013). Augmented reality in urban places: Contested content and the duplicity of code. *Transactions of the Institute of British Geographers, 38*(3), 464-479.

Groundspeak. (2016). *Geocaching 101.* Retrieved from www.geocaching.com/guide/

Hansen, L., & Sanders, S.W. (2012). Active gaming: Is "virtual" reality right for your physical education program? *Strategies, 25*(6), 24-27.

Isaac, J. (2016). *Step into a new world: Virtual reality (VR)*. Retrieved from www.completegate.com/2016070154/blog/virtual-reality-explained

Kervin, L., Verenikina, I., Jones, P., & Beath, O. (2013). Investigating synergies between literacy, technology and classroom practice. *Australian Journal of Language and Literacy, 36*(3), 135-147.

King, A., Glanz, K., & Patrick, K. (2015). Technologies to measure and modify physical activity and eating environments. *American Journal of Preventive Medicine, 48*(5), 630-638.

Kohl, H., & Murray, T. (2012). School-based approaches to promoting physical activity. In H.W. Kohl III & T.D. Murray (Eds.), *Foundations of physical activity and public health* (pp. 195-211). Champaign, IL: Human Kinetics Publishers.

Leight, J.M. (2014). *Technology for physical education teacher education: Student handbook of technology skills instruction and assessment* (2nd ed). Lavergne, TN: CreateSpace.

Liao, T. (2015). Application of virtual reality technology to sports. *Proceedings of the 2015 AASRI International Conference on Circuits and Systems*. Atlantis Press.

Lobelo, F., Kelli, H., Tejedor, S., Pratt, M., McConnell, M., Martin, S., & Welk, G. (2016). The wild wild west: A framework to integrate mHealth software applications and wearables to support physical activity assessment, counseling, and interventions for cardiovascular disease risk reduction. *Progress in Cardiovascular Diseases, 58*(6), 584-594.

Lubans, D., Smith, J., Skinner, G., & Morgan, P. (2014). Development and implementation of a smartphone application to promote physical activity and reduce screen-time in adolescent boys. *Frontiers in Public Health, 2*. doi:10.3389/fpubh.2014.00042

Lubans, D., Smith, J., Peralta, L., Plotnikoff, R., Okely, A., Salmon, J., . . . Morgan, P. (2016). A school-based intervention incorporating smartphone technology to improve health-related fitness among adolescents: Rationale and study protocol for the NEAT and ATLAS 2.0 cluster randomised controlled trial and dissemination study. *BMJ Open, 6*, 6. doi:10.1136/bmjopen-2015-010448

Lyons, E.J., Lewis, Z.H., Mayrsohn, B.G., & Rowland, J.L. (2014). Behavior change techniques implemented in electronic lifestyle activity monitors: A systematic content analysis. *Journal of Medical Internet Research, 16*(8), e192.

Mahar, M. (2011). Impact of short bouts of physical activity on attention-to-task in elementary school children. *Preventive Medicine, 52*, S60-S64.

Martin, N., Ameluxen-Coleman, E., & Heinrichs, D. (2015). Innovative ways to use modern technology to enhance, rather than hinder, physical activity among youth. *Journal of Physical Education, Recreation & Dance, 86*(4), 46-53.

Mears, D., & Hansen, L. (2009). Active gaming: Definitions, options and implementation. *Strategies, 23*(2), 26-29.

Michie, S., Ashford, S., Sniehotta, F.F., Dombrowski, S.U., Bishop, A., & French, D.P. (2011). A refined taxonomy of behaviour change techniques to help people change their physical activity and healthy eating behaviours: The CALO-RE taxonomy. *Psychology & Health, 26*(11), 1479-1498.

Miller, T.A., Vaux-Bjerke, A., McDonnell, K.A., & DiPietro, L. (2013). Can e-gaming be useful for achieving recommended levels of moderate- to vigorous-intensity physical activity in inner-city children? *Games for Health Journal, 2*(2), 96-102. http://doi.org/10.1089/g4h.2012.0058

Mossberg, W.S. (2012). "Google Stores, Syncs, Edits in the Cloud." Retrieved from www.wsj.com/articles/SB10001424052702303459004577362111867730108

Pasco, D. (2013). The potential of using virtual reality technology in physical activity settings. *Quest, 65*(4), 429-441.

Patel, M.S., Asch, D.A., & Volpp, K.G. (2015). Wearable devices as facilitators, not drivers, of health behavior change. *JAMA, 313*(5), 459-460.

Powell, A.C., Landman, A.B., & Bates, D.W. (2014). In search of a few good apps. *JAMA, 311*(18), 1851-1852.

Richardson, J., & Ancker, J. (2015). *Public health perspectives of mobile phones' effects on healthcare quality and medical data security and privacy: A 2-year nationwide survey*. Paper presented at the AMIA Annual Symposium.

Rodriguez, D., Brown, A., & Troped, P. (2005). Portable global positioning units to complement accelerometry-based physical activity monitors. *Medicine & Science in Sports & Exercise, 37*(11), S572-S581.

Ruotsalainen, H., Kyngas, H., Tammelin, T., Heikkinen, H., & Kaariainen, M. (2015). Effectiveness of Facebook-delivered lifestyle counselling and physical activity self-monitoring on physical activity and body mass index in overweight and obese adolescents: A randomized controlled trial. *Nursing Research and Practice, 159205*. http://doi.org/10.1155/2015/159205

Serino, M., Cordrey, K., McLaughlin, L., & Milanaik, R. (2016). Pokemon Go and augmented virtual reality games: A cautionary commentary for parents and pediatricians. *Current Opinions in Pediatrics, 28*(5), 673-677.

Sheehan, D.P., & Katz, L. (2013). The effects of a daily, 6-week exergaming curriculum on balance in fourth grade children. *Journal of Sport and Health Science, 2*(3), 131-137. http://doi.org/10.1016/j.jshs.2013.02.002

Smith, A. (2015). U.S. smartphone use in 2015. Retrieved from www.pewinternet.org/2015/04/01/us-smartphone-use-in-2015/

Smith, J., Morgan, P., Plotnikoff, R., Dally, K., Salmon, J., Okely, A., . . . Lubans, D. (2014). Smart-phone obesity prevention trial for adolescent boys in low-income communities: The ATLAS RCT. *Pediatrics, 134*(3), e723-e731.

Statista. (2016). *Worldwide tablet shipments from 2nd quarter 2010 to 2nd quarter 2016 (in million units).* Retrieved from www.statista.com/statistics/272070/global-tablet-shipments-by-quarter/

Sun, H. (2012). Exergaming impact on physical activity and interest in elementary school children. *Research Quarterly for Exercise and Sport, 83,* 212-220.

Sun, H. (2013). Impact of exergames on physical activity and motivation in elementary school students: A follow-up study. *Journal of Sport and Health Science, 2*(3), 138-145. http://doi.org/10.1016/j.jshs.2013.02.003

Terrel, K. (2015). *The history of social media: Social networking evolution.* Retrieved from http://history-cooperative.org/the-history-of-social-media

Troped, P., Oliveira, M., Matthews, C., Cromley, E., Melly, S., & Craig, B. (2008). Prediction of activity mode with global positioning system and accelerometer data. *Medicine & Science in Sports & Exercise, 40*(5), 972-978.

Troped, P., Saunders, R., Pate, R., Reininger, B., Ureda, J., & Thompson, S. (2001). Associations between self-reported and objective physical environmental factors and use of a community rail-trail. *Preventive Medicine, 32*(2), 191-200.

Valle, C.G., Tate, D.F., Mayer, D.K., Allicock, M., & Cai, J. (2013). A randomized trial of a Facebook-based physical activity intervention for young adult cancer survivors. *Journal of Cancer Survivors, 7,* 355-368.

Van Kessel, G., Kavanagh, M., & Maher, C. (2016). A qualitative study to examine feasibility and design of an online social networking intervention to increase physical activity in teenage girls. *PloS One, 11*(3), e0150817.

Wang, J.B., Cadmus-Bertram, L.A., Natarajan, L., White, M.M., Madanat, H., Nichols, J.F., . . . Pierce, J. P. (2015). Wearable sensor/device (Fitbit One) and SMS text-messaging prompts to increase physical activity in overweight and obese adults: A randomized controlled trial. *Telemedicine and e-Health, 21*(10), 782-792.

Watterson, T. (2012). *Changes in attitudes and behaviors toward physical activity, nutrition, and social support for middle school students using the AFIT app as a supplement to instruction in a physical education class.* (Doctoral dissertation). Retrieved from https://scholarcommons.usf.edu/cgi/viewcontent.cgi?referer=https://duckduckgo.com/&httpsredir=1&article=5614&context=etd

West, D. (2012). How mobile devices are transforming healthcare. *Issues in Technology Innovation, 18*(1), 1-11.

Whittman, G. (2010). Video gaming increases physical activity. *Journal of Extension, 48*(2), 1-4.

Zeng, N., Pope, Z., & Gao, Z. (2017). Acute effect of virtual reality exercise bike games on college students' physiological and psychological outcomes. *Cyberpsychology, Behavior, and Social Networking, 20*(7), 453-457.

Chapter 22

Active Schools. (2018). *Active schools: The movement.* Retrieved from https://www.activeschoolsus.org/about

Allar, I., Elliott, E., Jones, E., Kristjansson, A.L., Taliaferro, A., & Bulger, S.M. (2017). Involving families and communities in CSPAP development using asset mapping. *Journal of Physical Education, Recreation & Dance, 88*(5), 7-14.

Allensworth, D.D., & Kolbe, L.J. (1987). The comprehensive school health program: Exploring an expanded concept. *Journal of School Health, 57*(10), 409-412.

Association for Supervision and Curriculum Development (ASCD). (2018). *Whole school, whole community, whole child.* Retrieved from http://www.ascd.org/programs/learning-and-health/wscc-model.aspx

Bandura, A. (1986). *Social foundations of thought and action: A social cognitive theory.* Englewood Cliffs, NJ: Prentice Hall.

Beets, M., Okely, A., Weaver, R.G., Webster, C., Lubans, D., Brusseau, T., . . . Cliff, D.P. (2016). The theory of expanded, extended, and enhanced opportunities for youth physical activity promotion. *International Journal of Behavioral Nutrition and Physical Activity, 13,* 120. doi:10.1186/s12966-016-0442-2

Burns, R., Brusseau, T., Fu, Y., Myrer, R., & Hannon, J. (2016). Comprehenisve school physical activity programming and classroom behavior. *American Journal of Health Behavior, 40*(1), 100-107. doi:10.5993/AJHB.40.1.11

Carson, R. L., Castelli, D. M., Beighle, A., & Erwin, H. (2014). School-based physical activity promotion: A conceptual framework for research and practice. *Childhood Obesity, 10*(2), 100-106. doi: 10.1089/chi.2013.0134

Carson, R.L., Dauenhauer, B., Stoepker, P., Pulling Kuhn, A.C., von Klinggraeff, L.E., Capps, M.J., . . . McMullen, J.M. (2018, February). *Data-sharing with classroom teachers and elementary children's physical activity at school.* Oral research presentation at the annual meeting of Active Living Research, Banff, Alberta, Canada.

Centers for Disease Control and Prevention (CDC). (2013). *Comprehensive school physical activity programs: A guide for schools.* Retrieved from https://www.cdc.gov/healthyschools/professional_development/e-learning/cspap.html

Centers for Disease Control and Prevention (CDC). (2014). *Health and academic achievement.* Retrieved from https://www.cdc.gov/healthyyouth/health_and_academics/pdf/health-academic-achievement.pdf

Centers for Disease Control and Prevention (CDC). (2017). *Increasing physical education and physical activity: A framework for schools.* Retrieved from https://www.cdc.gov/healthyschools/physicalactivity/pdf/17_278143-A_PE-PA-Framework_508.pdf

Centers for Disease Control and Prevention (CDC). (2018). *Comprehensive school physical activity programs: A guide for schools.* Retrieved from https://www.cdc.gov/healthyschools/physicalactivity/pdf/13_242620-A_CSPAP_SchoolPhysActivityPrograms_Final_508_12192013.pdf

Chen, S., & Gu, X. (2018). Toward active living: Comprehensive school physical activity program research and implications. *Quest, 70*(2), 191–212. doi:10.1080/00336297.2017.1365002

Coghlan, D., & Brannick, T. (2014). *Doing action research in your own organization* (4th ed.). Thousand Oaks, CA: Sage Publications.

Council for the Accreditation of Educator Preparation. (2013). *The CAEP standards.* Received from http://caepnet.org/standards/introduction

Dauenhauer, B., Carson, R.L., Krause, J., Hodgins, K., Jones, T., & Weinberger, C. (2018). Cultivating physical activity leadership in schools: A three-tiered approach to professional development. *Journal of Physical Education, Recreation & Dance, 89*(9), 51-57.

De Bourdeaudhuij, I., Van Cauwenberghe, E., Spittaels, H., Oppert, J.M., Rostami, C., Brug, J., . . . Maes, L. (2011). School-based interventions promoting both physical activity and healthy eating in Europe: A systematic review within the HOPE project. *Obesity Reviews, 12*(3), 205-216. doi:10.1111/j.1467-789X.2009.00711.x

Deci, E.L., & Ryan, R.M. (1985). *Intrinsic motivation and self-determination in human behavior.* New York, NY: Plenum Press.

Demetriou, Y., & Höner, O. (2012). Physical activity interventions in the school setting: A systematic review. *Psychology of Sport and Exercise, 13*(2), 196. doi:10.1016/j.psychsport.2011.11.006

Dobbins, M., Husson, H., DeCorby, K., & LaRocca, R.L. (2013). School-based physical activity programs for promoting physical activity and fitness in children and adolescents aged 6 to 18. *Cochrane Database of Systematic Reviews, 2,* CD007651. doi:10.1002/14651858.CD007651.pub2

Erwin, H., Beighle, A., Carson, R.L., & Castelli, D.M. (2013). Comprehensive school-based physical activity promotion: A review. *Quest, 65*(4), 412-428. doi:10.1080/00336297.2013.791872

Erwin, H., Brusseau, T.A., Carson, R.L., Hodge, S., & Kang, M. (2018). SHAPE America's 50 Million Strong™: Critical research questions related to youth physical activity. *Research Quarterly for Exercise and Sport, 89*(3), 286-297. doi:10.1080/02701367.2018.1490607

Green, L.W., & Kreuter, M. (2005). *Health program planning: An educational and ecological approach* (4th ed.). New York, NY: McGraw-Hill.

Greenberg, J.D., & LoBianco, J.L. (in press). *Organization and administration of physical education: Theory and practice.* Champaign, IL: Human Kinetics.

Hunt, K., & Metzler, M. (2017). Adoption of comprehensive school physical activity programs: A literature review. *Physical Educator, 74*(2), 315-340. http://dx.doi.org/10.18666/TPE-2017-V74-I2-7167

Kriemler, S., Meyer, U., Martin, E., van Sluijs, E.M.F., Andersen, L.B., & Martin, B.W. (2011). Effect of school-based interventions on physical activity and fitness in children and adolescents: A review of reviews and systematic update. *British Journal of Sports Medicine, 45*(11), 923-930. doi:10.1136/bjsports-2011-090186

Kulinna, P.H., Carson, R.L., & Castelli, D.M. (Eds.). (2017). Integrating CSPAP in PETE programs: Sharing insight and identifying strategies [Special Issue–Part 1 & 2]. *Journal of Physical Education, Recreation & Dance, 88*(1&2).

Metcalf, B., Henley, W., & Wilkin, T. (2012). Effectiveness of intervention on physical activity of children: Systematic review and meta-analysis of controlled trials with objectively measured outcomes (EarlyBird 54). *BMJ, 345,* e5888. doi:10.1136/bmj.e5888

National Physical Activity Plan Alliance (NPAPA). (2016). *The plan—NPAP sectors: Education.* Retrieved from http://www.physicalactivityplan.org/theplan/education.html

National Physical Activity Plan Alliance (NPAPA). (2018). *The 2018 United States report card on physical activity for children and youth.* Retrieved from http://physicalactivityplan.org/projects/PA/2018/2018%20US%20Report%20Card%20Full%20Version_WEB.PDF?pdf=header-image

Rogers, E.M. (1995). *Diffusion of innovations* (4th ed.). New York, NY: Free Press.

Russ, L., Webster, C.A., Beets, M.W., & Phillips, D. (2015). Systematic review and meta-analysis of multi-component interventions through schools to increase physical activity. *Journal of Physical Activity & Health, 12*(10), 1436-1446. doi:10.1123/jpah.2014-0244

Sacko, R.S., McIver, K., Brian, A., & Stodden, D.F. (2018). New insight for activity intensity relativity, metabolic expenditure during object projection skill performance. *Journal of Sports Sciences, 21*(36), 2412-2418. https://doi.org/10.1080/02640414.2018.1459152

SHAPE America. (2017). *National standards for initial physical education teacher education.* Retrieved from https://www.shapeamerica.org/accreditation/upload/National-Standards-for-Initial-Physical-Education-Teacher-Education-2017.pdf

Stoepker, P., Carson, R.L., Pulling Kuhn, A., Lorenz, K., George, M.W., Graham, D., . . . the Advancing IDEAS for School Health Collaborative. (2018). *Menu of evidence-based practices for school health: Physical education and physical activity.* Retrieved from https://s3.amazonaws.com/org-healthyschoolshub/wp-content/uploads/2018/08/30064305/PhysicalEducationPhysicalActivity.pdf

Wallerstein, N., Minkler, M., Carter-Edwards, L., Avila, M., & Sanchez, V. (2015). Improving health through community engagement, community organization, and community building. In K. Glanz, B.K. Rimer, & K. Viswanath (Eds), *Health behavior: Theory, research, and practice* (5th ed, pp. 277-300). San Francisco, CA: Jossey-Bass.

Webster, C.A., Stodden, D.F., Carson, R.L., Egan, C., & Nesbitt, D. (2016). Integrative public health-aligned physical education and implications for the professional preparation of future teachers and teacher educators/researchers in the field. *Quest, 68*(4), 457-474. https://doi.org/10.1080/00336297.2016.1229628

Webster, C.A., Webster, L., Russ, L., Molina, S., Lee, H., & Cribbs, J. (2015). A systematic review of public health-aligned recommendations for preparing physical education teacher candidates. *Research Quarterly for Exercise and Sport, 86*(1), 30-39. https://doi.org/10.1080/02701367.2014.980939

INDEX

Note: The italicized *f* and *t* following page numbers refer to figures and tables, respectively.

ABOUT THE EDITORS

Russ Carson, PhD, has 20 years of academic experience, as a secondary physical education and health teacher, teacher educator, accomplished scholar, professor, and founding director of the University of Northern Colorado Active Schools Institute. He is a long-standing leader of the comprehensive school physical activity program (CSPAP)

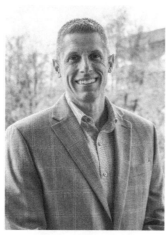

Courtesy of Lauren Smart, and edited by Miao-Ju Olsen.

model and its corresponding training programs. He earned his doctorate in health and kinesiology from Purdue University.

Collin Webster, PhD, earned his doctorate in physical education and sport studies from the University of Georgia in 2006 and has held academic appointments at the University of South Carolina and the University of Wollongong in Australia. He is a nationally and internationally recognized scholar in the area of youth physical activity promotion, particularly compre-

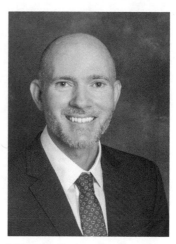

Office of Communications and Public Affairs at the University of South Carolina.

hensive school physical activity programs.

CONTRIBUTORS

Catherine P. Abel-Berei, PhD
Southern Connecticut State University

Megan Babkes Stellino, EdD
University of Northern Colorado

Aaron Beighle, PhD
University of Kentucky

Kevin Brabham
Jesse Boyd Elementary School

Helen Brown, MPH, RDN
University of Idaho

Timothy A. Brusseau, PhD
University of Utah

Sean Bulger, EdD
West Virginia University

Martha Carman
Ashburn Elementary School

Darla M. Castelli, PhD
The University of Texas at Austin

Erin E. Centeio, PhD
Wayne State University

Déirdre Ní Chróinín, PhD
Mary Immaculate College

Brian Dauenhauer, PhD
University of Northern Colorado

Sarah Doolittle, EdD
Adelphi University

Cate A. Egan, PhD
University of Idaho

Eloise Elliott, PhD
West Virginia University

Heather Erwin, PhD
University of Kentucky

Jung Eun Lee, PhD
University of Minnesota–Duluth

Alan Everett, MBA
HealthWorks Foundation of Arizona

Abigail Gamble, PhD
University of Mississippi Medical Center

David Gardner, DA
North Carolina Division of Public Health

Zan Gao, PhD
University of Minnesota–Twin Cities

Grace Goc Karp, PhD
University of Idaho

Kim C. Graber, EdD
University of Illinois at Urbana-Champaign

James C. Hannon, PhD
Kent State University

Pamela Hodges Kulinna, PhD
Arizona State University

Katie Hodgin, PhD
University of Northern Colorado

Emily Jones, PhD
Illinois State University

Yeonhak Jung, MS
The University of Texas at Austin

Chad M. Killian, MA
University of Illinois at Urbana-Champaign

Lyndsie M. Koon, PhD
University of Illinois at Urbana-Champaign

Alfgeir Kristjansson, PhD
West Virginia University

Joey A. Lee
University of Colorado at Colorado Springs

Tan Leng Goh, PhD
Central Connecticut State University

Kent A. Lorenz, PhD
San Francisco State University

Athanasios (Tom) Loulousis
Edison Park School

Lee Marcheschi
Ashburn Elementary School

Amelia Mays Woods, PhD
University of Illinois at Urbana-Champaign

Nate McCaughtry, PhD
Wayne State University

Daniel McDonough
University of Minnesota–Twin Cities

Thomas L. McKenzie, PhD
Professor Emeritus, San Diego State University

Jaimie M. McMullen, PhD
University of Northern Colorado

Kevin Mercier, EdD
Adelphi University

Justin B. Moore, PhD, MS, FACSM
Wake Forest School of Medicine

Shannon C. Mulhearn, MS
Arizona State University

Shawn Orme, MA, MS
HealthWorks Foundation of Arizona

Tanya Peal
Soaring Heights PK-8

Alexandra Peluso, BS
University of Texas at Austin

Danny Perry, MAEd, MSA
Bertie County Schools

Ashley Phelps, MPE
The University of Texas at Austin

Zachary Pope, PhD
University of Minnesota–Twin Cities

Paul Rukavina, PhD
Adelphi University

Laura Russ, PhD
Augusta University

Jessica Shawley
Moscow Middle School

Chuck Steinfurth
South Carolina Alliance of YMCAs

Michalis Stylianou, PhD
The University of Queensland

Tuija Tammelin, PhD
LIKES Research Centre for Physical Activity and Health, Finland

Tom Taylor, BS
HealthWorks Foundation of Arizona

Hans van der Mars, PhD
Arizona State University

Spyridoula Vazou, PhD
Iowa State University

Ja Youn Kwon, PhD
Arizona State University

R. Glenn Weaver, PhD
University of South Carolina

Michelle A. Webster
Rosewood Elementary School

Cyrus Weinberger
Soaring Heights PK-8

Gregory J. Welk, PhD
Iowa State University

Nan Zeng
Colorado State University

About SHAPE America

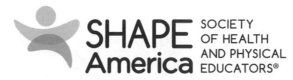

SHAPE America – Society of Health and Physical Educators is the nation's largest membership organization of health and physical education professionals. Since its founding in 1885, the organization has defined excellence in physical education, and our National Standards for K-12 Physical Education serve as the foundation for well-designed physical education programs across the country. We provide programs, resources and advocacy to support health and physical educators at every level, from preschool to university graduate programs. For more information, visit www.shapeamerica.org.

The organization has most recently created the National Standards & Grade-Level Outcomes for K-12 Physical Education (2014), National Standards for Initial Physical Education Teacher Education (2016), National Standards for Health Education Teacher Education (2017) and National Standards for Sport Coaches (2006). Also, SHAPE America participated as a member of the Joint Committee on National Health Education Standards, which published National Health Education Standards, Second Edition: Achieving Excellence (2007).

The SHAPE America website, www.shapeamerica.org, holds a treasure trove of free resources for health and physical educators, adapted physical education teachers, teacher trainers and coaches, including activity calendars, curriculum resources, tools and templates, assessments and more. Visit www.shapeamerica.org and search for Teacher's Toolbox.

Every spring, SHAPE America hosts its National Convention & Expo, the premier national professional-development event for health and physical educators.

Advocacy is an essential element in the fulfillment of our mission. By speaking out for the school health and physical education professions, SHAPE America strives to make an impact on the national policy landscape.

Our Vision: A nation where all children are prepared to lead healthy, physically active lives.

Our Mission: To advance professional practice and promote research related to health and physical education, physical activity, dance and sport.

Our Commitment: 50 Million Strong by 2029

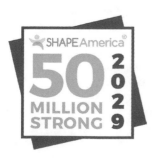

50 Million Strong by 2029 is SHAPE America's commitment to put all children on the path to health and physical literacy through effective health and physical education programs. We believe that through effective teaching, health and physical educators can help students develop the ability and confidence to be physically active and make healthy choices. As educators, our guidance can also help foster their desire to maintain an active and healthy lifestyle in the years to come. To learn more visit www.shapeamerica.org/50Million.

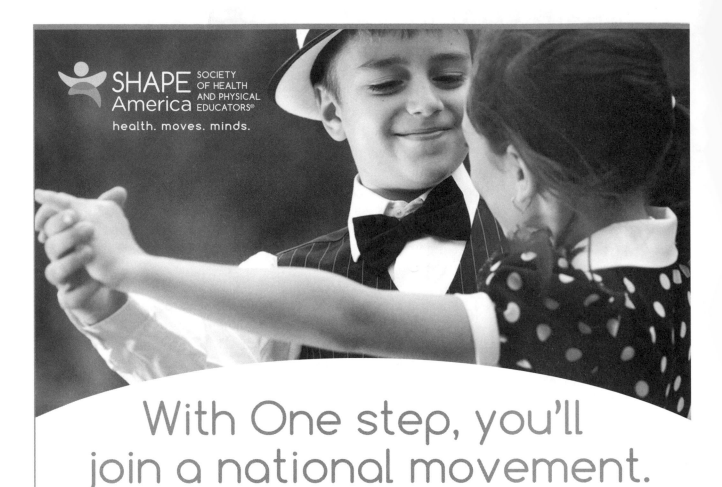   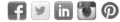